W9-AMT-634

Hearing in Children

THIRD EDITION

Hearing in Children

THIRD EDITION

Jerry L. Northern, Ph.D.

Professor
Department of Otolaryngology/Pediatrics
University of Colorado
School of Medicine
Denver, Colorado

Head
Audiology Services
University Hospital
Denver, Colorado

Marion P. Downs, Dr.H.S.

Professor Emerita
Department of Otolaryngology
University of Colorado
School of Medicine
Denver, Colorado

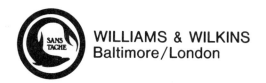

WILLIAMS & WILKINS
Baltimore/London

Editor: William R. Hensyl
Copy Editor: William Vinck
Design: Bert Smith
Illustration Planning: Reginald R. Stanley
Production: Raymond E. Reter

First Edition 1974
Second Edition 1978
  Reprinted 1979

Accurate indications, adverse reactions, and dosage schedules for drugs are provided
in this book, but it is possible that they may change. The reader is urged to review
the package information data of the manufacturers of the medications mentioned.

Made in the United States of America

Library of Congress Cataloging in Publication Data

Northern, Jerry L.
  Hearing in children.

  Bibliography: p.
  Includes indexes.
  1. Hearing disorders in children. I. Downs, Marion P. II. Title. [DNLM:
1. Hearing disorders—In infancy and childhood. 2. Hearing tests—In infancy and
childhood. WV 271 N874h]
RF291.5.C45N67   1984   618.92′0978   83-10378
ISBN 0-683-06573-4

Composed and printed at the
Waverly Press, Inc.
Mt. Royal and Guilford Aves.
Baltimore, MD 21202, U.S.A.

Preface
for Third Edition

Times change and progress continues. A decade ago, we wrote the initial edition of *Hearing in Children* because we felt a need existed for a thorough textbook about the audiological problems encountered by children with ear and hearing problems. We wanted to present information from a medically-oriented point of view, primarily for students of hearing, speech, and language studies, but also hoped to draw the interest and concern of various medical specialists to the problems of hearing-impaired youngsters.

Since the mid-1970s we have seen a veritable flood of textbooks dealing with the many aspects of problems encountered by children who have hearing problems. Complete textbooks have now been devoted to materials we initially presented in individual chapters. College graduate-level courses have been developed in many areas of concern to train clinicians and educators to evaluate and manage the auditory impairments of children of all ages. We cannot hope to provide complete coverage of all specialty topics, in the necessary depth, for all the technical aspects of children and their hearing problems. We do provide, however, in this Third Edition, an updated and current overview of the problems of hearing in children to help students and professionals understand the complexities involved with each child who suffers from hearing impairment or deafness.

Many textbooks are written with an implicit assumption that contained within are the eternal verities of scientific knowledge. Time has proven that even the most accepted scientific theories are not written in stone by an infallible hand, without which the truth would never be known. Individuals contribute in various ways to the development of knowledge. Einstein is attributed with the statement that, " ... even if Newton and Leibniz had not lived the world would still have had the calculus, although if Beethoven had not lived we would never have had the C-Minor Symphony."

We feel that there is room in any profession for personal statements—for an individual point of view in observing the contemporary scene. We have traveled many miles around the country, meeting countless members of our profession. What has filled us with awe and respect is that even the most wide-eyed recent graduate potentially has an individual statement to make—a personal viewpoint that will ultimately make a fresh contribution to the profession. To attain the freedom to make that statement, the individual must learn to read critically to keep his mind open, and to select those professional ways that let him be true to himself.

As you read this book, we hope you will recognize that it contains our own personal statements of our reactions to the scientific knowledge in the field. Nowhere do we imply, "Believe as we do. Do as we say." What we hope you will infer is, "Here is a body of knowledge to which we have reacted in our way. Please react to it in your way."

Acknowledgments
for First Edition

A book of this magnitude cannot be assembled and written without the help of many other people. We would like to pay special tribute and thanks to five of our colleagues and good friends who gave graciously of their valuable time and personal material for our benefit—LaVonne Bergstrom, M.D.; Isamu Sando, M.D.; Janet M. Stewart, M.D.; Marlin Weaver, M.D.; and Winfield McChord, Jr., M.S.

Many others responded to our needs, willingly and unselfishly, to provide requested information at a moment's notice: Carol Amon, M.A.; Owen Black, M.D.; Carol Cox, M.A.; Kathleen O. Foust, M.A.; William K. Frankenberg, M.D.; W. G. Hemenway, M.D.; Brian Hersch, M.D.; Aram Glorig, M.D.; Mrs. Page T. Jenkins; Darrel Teter, Ph.D.; Pat Tesauro, M.A.; and Harold Weber, M.A. Connie H. Knight, M.A., Audiologist at the Georgia Retardation Center, Atlanta, was our Research Associate and gathered much of the material presented in the "Index of Selected Birth Defect Syndromes," Sharon Mraz was our Editorial Assistant. Patricia Jenkins Thompson, M.A., diligently proofread and critiqued our efforts.

Y. Oishi, M.D., served as our primary photographer, Miriam Eliachar illustrated the chapter pictures and embryology figures; and Anita McGuire typed the entire manuscript. We would also like to acknowledge the cooperation of the publishing staff at Williams & Wilkins, especially William R. Hensyl who encouraged us to write this textbook.

And finally, we would like to extend our appreciation and thanks to our spouses, families, children, and friends, who will long remember (as will we!) this period of time during which we were too busy, too preoccupied, or too tired—our Year of the Book, 1973.

JLN and MPD (1973)

for Second Edition

Once again numerous colleagues came to our aid to provide advice, share materials, and labor in the libraries to help prepare this Second Edition of *Hearing in Children*. We would like to express our warmest thanks to Jeff Adams, Marlin Cohrs, Roni Halpern, Donna Lutz, Winfield McChord, Deborah Smith, Steven Staller, Darrel Teter, Harold Weber, and Janet Zarnoch. We are particularly grateful for the contributions of Mrs. Kathleen Bryant, Speech Pathologist at the University of Colorado Medical Center. Patsy Tormey, our helpful secretary, typed the manuscript and quietly tolerated our many revisions. Ruby Richardson at Williams & Wilkins nudged us gently, but firmly, throughout this revision. And finally, we appreciate the helpful comments and critique provided by our professional friends who took time to respond to a lengthy questionnaire regarding the first edition. Their guidance and suggestions have greatly influenced this second edition of *Hearing in Children*.

JLN and MPD (1978)

for Third Edition

We are again grateful to a new cadre of friends, students, and associates who have responded to our requests for help with this third edition. We would like to thank David Asher, James R. Curran, Sandra Abbott Gabbard, Marianne Geisler, Christine Gerhardt, Kathryn Grose, Katherine Pike Gerkin, Deanie Johnson, Deborah Kinder, Sharon A. Mitchell, Patrick Sullivan, M.D., and Ann Wilson. Patsy Tormey-Meredith typed the new manuscripts again, but this time during maternity leave. We were delighted to work again with William R. Hensyl, of Williams & Wilkins, who was the original perpetrator of *Hearing in Children*.

JLN and MPD (1983)

Contents

Chapter 9 **Education for Hearing-Impaired Children**

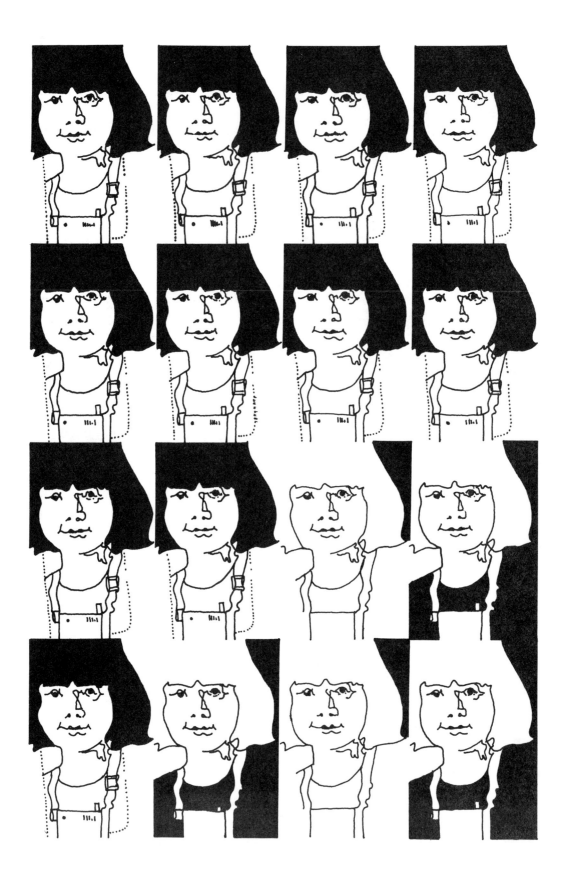

CHAPTER 1

What Is a Hearing Loss?

Long ago the function of hearing became the building stone upon which our intricate human communication system was constructed. If predawn man had not inherited an ear, he might have resorted instead to signing with his fingers or scratching marks upon the sand to share his thoughts with others. The result would have been an awkward method of communication that could have slowed, for millennia, our so-called progress. For good or bad, we have developed the ear and the vocal mechanism as the media through which language is customarily learned and communicated. An illustration of the interdependence of the ear and speech is found in the direct relationship between the frequencies which make speech intelligible and the differential sensitivity of the human ear—most sensitive at those same speech frequencies. The question of which of these factors came first is an ontogenic mystery no one has yet solved.

The structure of language is unique to *Homo sapiens*, although recent experimenters have demonstrated that signed symbols and other visual language forms can be taught to chimpanzees and believe that the beginnings of true language are evidenced in these primates (Gardner and Gardner, 1969; Premack and Premack, 1972; Savage-Rumbaugh et al., 1980). Other investigators insist that the conceptual system learned by these primates is not linguistic, i.e., they do not "think in words," they use instead a signalization system that is far removed from the higher symbolization and syntax of human language (Terrace et al., 1979). But neither group would question that between the laboriously learned signal response of the chimpanzee and the first voluntary sentence of the 18-month-old baby lies, as Langer (1957) stated, a whole day of creation.

The human baby appears to be born with "preexistent knowledge" of language—specialized neural structures in the brain that await auditory experience with language to trigger them into functioning (Hunt, 1982). These structures are dependent on auditory stimulation for their emergence, providing of course that other developmental factors are normal.

The auditory-linked acquisition of language is further unique to human beings because it is a time-locked function, related to early maturational periods in the infant's life. The longer auditory language stimulation is delayed, the less efficient will be the language facility. The reason is that critical periods exist for the development of biological functions, and language is one of the biological functions of humans (Lenneberg, 1967; Chomsky, 1966). A baby who is deprived of appropriate language stimulation during this first 2 or 3 years of life will never fully attain his best potential language function, whether the deprivation is from lack of hearing or from lack of high quality language experience.

It is for these reasons that it is urgent to attack the hearing problems of children with all the skill, knowledge and insights of which we are capable. The prevention of hearing loss in children protects the right of children to their essential humanity, which lies in optimal language function.

WHAT IS A HANDICAPPING HEARING LOSS?

It is first necessary to ask if there is a definition for hearing loss in children. At what point does hearing in children cease to be normal and become abnormal? This question has never been satisfactorily resolved. The problem is that no one has adequately defined the parameters of a hearing handicap nor described the best method of securing the necessary data for such definition. Thus it has been extremely difficult to estimate the prevalence of hearing handicaps, for unless there are agreed upon criteria there is no way to determine the rate of occurrence. A review of governmental attempts to resolve this dilemma reveals what is involved.

The Health Examination Survey of the Department of Health, Education and Welfare undertook, in 1963–1970 (Leske, 1981) to collect hearing data on a representative sample of children 6–11 years of age. Ear, nose, and throat examinations, audiologic tests, and a parental health questionnaire were given to a sample of the United States child population. The estimate of the prevalence of "hearing handicaps" was obtained from the parents' questionnaire, which inquired if the child had "trouble hearing?" An equivalent of one million children, 6–11 years old (4%), was judged to be hearing handicapped on the basis of this question. Yet the audiometric tests collected by the survey revealed fewer than 1% to be handicapped, using a criterion of average loss (500—2000 Hz) of 26 dB (ANSI) as a beginning hearing loss. A National Speech and Hearing Survey in 1968–1969 used the same criterion on a sample of children tested in grades 1–12 (Hull et al., 1971) and found a prevalence of 0.73%.

On the ear examinations of the Health Examination Survey, the children found to have abnormalities of the eardrum were significantly more likely to have had trouble hearing as reported by their parents. Yet the audiometric findings showed small differences between those with normal and those with abnormal eardrum findings.

Thus, even when chronic otitis media existed, as evidenced by perforated eardrums, less than 15 dB difference was found between those ears and the normal ears. Can it be that there has been a gross misevaluation as to what constitutes a significant hearing loss?

Evidently a credibility gap existed in the survey between what parents thought and what the government team decreed as hearing handicap. Either the parents misjudged their children's ability to hear, or the scientific criterion of adequacy was in error. Which? Resolving this question is critical to the activities of schools, government agencies, and health facilities whose task it is to identify hearing loss in children.

A classic survey reported by Jordan and Eagles (1961) obtained otoscopic examinations and auditory thresholds on 4067 5–10-year-old school children. They found that 6% of the children who could be examined otoscopically had bilateral, abnormal findings, and 12% had unilateral abnormalities. Some 13% of the children could not be given otoscopic examination because of cerumen in the ear canal. When the individual pathologies were compared with the threshold audiometry it was found that 50% of the children with serous otitis media had hearing better than 15 dB hearing level (HL) (ANSI). In other words, even a 15-dB HL screening criterion would have missed more than half of the children with serous otitis media. Another comparison revealed that of 30 children with dry perforations of the drum, 40% would have been missed by a 15-dB HL screening criterion.

These authors pointed out that audiometric screening—and even threshold audiometry—may not identify the majority of children with significant ear pathology. Does this mean that there is no relationship between ear disease and hearing loss? Most certainly not. It merely means that one of them has been incorrectly defined. Inasmuch as ear disease is an observable fact, while "hearing loss" is only a concept, the concept is the one to be changed to fit the fact.

Kessner et al. (1974) for the National

Academy of Science examined a sample numbering 1639 of the children in health agencies in the Washington, D.C., area, conducting audiometric studies on the 4–11-year-old group. They chose as their criterion for a significant hearing loss the level of 15 dB or greater (500–2000 Hz). Their results are summarized in Table 1.1. This chart shows that 2.2% of the children had bilateral losses in the speech range (500–2000 Hz) of 15 dB or greater; 4.5% had unilateral losses in the speech range of over 15 dB, or a total of 6.7% with significant hearing losses in one ear or both. Most interesting is the fact that in the 4–5-year-old group, 4.1% had significant hearing losses in both ears—a figure almost identical with that of the Health Examination Survey derived from the parents' questionnaire.

In the Kessner study the mean threshold difference between the normal ears and those diagnosed as having serous otitis media was only 7.4 dB in the speech range. Mean threshold for the normals was 7.8 dB while children with definite serous otitis had mean thresholds of 15.2 dB. The survey found that it was serous otitis media (or middle ear effusion, MEE) that was present in the majority of children with middle ear infection. Serous otitis is an asymptomatic disease, which makes it an insidious threat to the welfare of children. It must be searched out and found by vigorous innovative screening programs. Crisis health care does not identify all the cases of MEE.

The occurrence of both ear pathology and hearing loss is age-related in all studies of prevalence. Kessner's report demonstrated the relationship of both factors to age in Figure 1.1. The rate of ear pathology peaks at age 2 with 30% abnormal ears, and declines to 15% abnormal ears by age 11. It can be seen that the age trend for hearing loss parallels that for ear pathology. Although no hearing data were obtained for children under 4, the strong correlation between hearing loss and ear pathology in the 4–11-year-olds led the authors to assume the same trend in the under-4-year group. If one extrapolates from the data for the 4–11-year-olds, it appears that 15% of the 2-year-olds will have losses in the speech range greater than 15 dB in at least one ear. Further extrapolation from the Table 1.1 shows that one third of the total speech-range losses (4–11 years) are bilateral. Applying this rate to the children 2 years and under leaves 5% of the 2-year-olds with significant bilateral hearing loss. This is not to say that unilateral hearing losses are innocuous. On the contrary, most clinical observers feel that unilateral losses are a great deal more handicapping than any available measure can show. A study by Boyd (1974) did demonstrate that 30% of a group of children with unilateral deafness but normal hearing in the other ear had a mean academic achievement lag of 1.12 years. Bess (1982) also found a sig-

Table 1.1.
Distribution of Hearing Test Results in Children Age 4–11 Years by Age: Community Sample, Selected Areas in Washington, D.C., 1971[a]

Hearing Test Result	Age of Child (Percent Distribution)				Total All Ages
	4–5 yr	6–7 yr	8–9 yr	10–11 yr	
Bilateral normal	76.2	78.8	84.8	84.8	81.1
Bilateral speech loss	4.1	1.7	1.1	1.9	2.2
Unilateral speech loss	5.1	4.6	3.7	4.5	4.5
Bilateral nonspeech loss	4.8	4.5	4.1	5.2	4.6
Unilateral nonspeech loss	9.7	10.4	6.2	3.7	7.6
Total:	99.9	100.0	99.9	100.1	100.0
Total number	402	443	406	388	1639[b]

[a] From D. M. Kessner, C. K. Snow, and J. Singer: *Assessment of Medical Care in Children*, National Academy of Sciences, Washington, D.C., 1974.
[b] Excludes 31 who could not be tested.

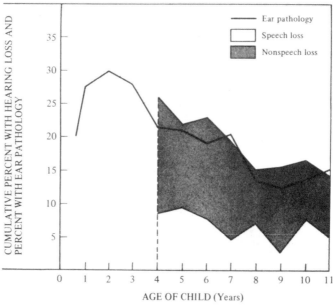

Figure 1.1. Prevalence of ear pathology in children 6 months through 11 years of age and prevalence of hearing loss by type of loss in children 4–11 years of age. (Reprinted with premission from D. M. Kessner, C. K. Snow, and F. Singer: *Assessment of Medical Care for Children.* Washington, D.C., National Academy of Sciences, 1974.)

nificant effect of unilateral hearing loss on the educational, linguistic, and auditory perceptual development of children.

Other variables, besides ear disease and unilaterality and bilaterality, should be mentioned when looking at prevalence rates. One of the most interesting demographic findings in these large sample studies was that there were not the expected hearing loss differences between the various races. In fact, the Kessner study found the prevalence rates of both ear pathology and hearing loss to be almost twice as high in white children as in black children—a condition which may be unique to the Washington, D.C., area. The most consistent demographic association was the education level of parents: the higher the educational attainment, the lower the prevalence of hearing loss (Fig. 1.2). There is a lesser but significant association with family income: the higher the income, the lower the rate of hearing loss (Fig. 1.3).

Another demographic association was found in the National Health Survey between regions of the United States and hearing loss. Children living in the South had less sensitive hearing in the middle frequencies (for frequencies below 6000 Hz), with children in the West having the most sensitive hearing in those frequencies (frequencies lower than 4000 Hz). To add to the confusion on prevalence rates there is the report (Human Communication and Its Disorders, 1969) that showed 10% of children at 12 months of age failed an auditory stimuli response test. This figure corresponds a little more closely with the estimate from Kessner and Kalk (1973) of a prevalence of 15% in the under-2-years of age group that may have hearing loss.

MINIMAL CRITERIA FOR HEARING LOSS

Can we afford to be complacent if a 15-dB hearing level is accepted as the criterion for a handicapping hearing loss? An examination of different proposals is relevant here.

In 1979 the American Academy of Otolaryngology's Committee on Hearing and Equilibrium and the American Council of

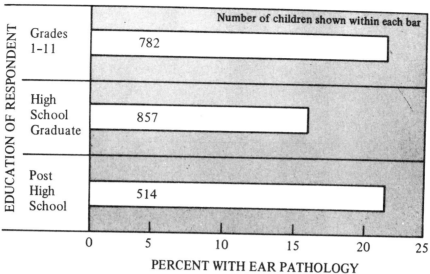

Figure 1.2. Education level of parents and prevalence of hearing loss in children. (Reprinted with permission from D. M. Kessner, C. K. Snow, and F. Singer: *Assessment of Medical Care for Children.* Washington, D.C., National Academy of Sciences, 1974.)

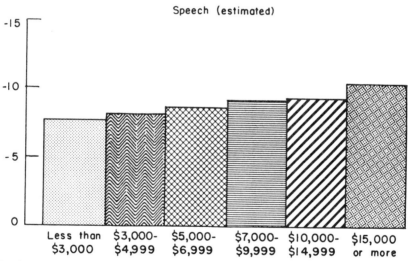

Figure 1.3. Income level of parents and hearing levels of children. (Reprinted with permission from *Hearing Levels of Children by Demographic and Socioeconomic Characteristics.* Washington, D.C., U.S. Department of HEW, 1972.)

Otolaryngology Committee on the Medical Aspects of Noise (1979) revised their *Guide for the Evaluation of Hearing Handicap.* This *Guide* gives directions to compensation agencies for rating the percentage of hearing loss in industrial compensation, and concerns adults only. Handicap was rated in terms of the ability to hear every-

day speech in quiet and noise, but was interpreted in terms of pure tone threshold. The average of the thresholds at 500, 1000, 2000, and 3000 Hz was felt to reflect a realistic degree of the understanding of speech in both quiet and noise. Although 3000 Hz was a new addition to the previous criteria, it was selected because of its importance to hearing speech in noise or when speech is distorted.

In the Committee's Guide, every dB over 25 dB average (500–3000 Hz) was given 1.5% weight in a compensation rating. The poorer ear was given a weight of 5 out of 6, the better ear a weight of 1. Such a 25-dB "low fence" for hearing handicapped adults has been accepted for many years. But how realistic is it to apply this low fence to children's hearing needs? If hearing for speech is the basis of the criterion for adult hearing loss, should it be the same for children? The answer depends on what are the speech needs of various ages (Fig. 1.4).

For the adult all the contextual strategies of interpreting speech have been firmly implanted—indeed, an adult does not have to hear all of the speech sounds in order to put together the concept of what is said. Speech can be badly distorted or interrupted and still be intelligible to an adult (Berlin and Lowe, 1972; Bocca and Calearo, 1963). But a child who is just learning to interpret speech and language needs to hear

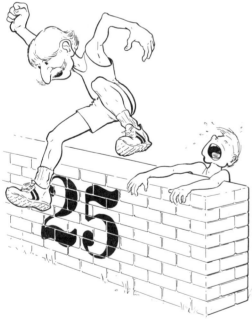

Figure 1.4. The 25-dB "low fence," established to define the beginning of hearing loss in adults, may be too severe to serve as the "low fence" figure for children's hearing loss.

acutely in order to develop the strategies necessary to his adult skills. Even year-old infants must hear well if they are to lay the groundwork for later language skills.

Many people may question why a 15-dB loss or mere early recurrent otitis media results in such language delays. The reasons lie in the nature of speech sounds, with the major amount of speech energy residing in the voiced vowels and consonants. The unvoiced consonants (s, p, t, k, th, f, sh) contain so little speech energy that they often fall below even normal hearing thresholds in average rapid conversation (Fig. 1.5). Those of us who have learned speech and language know so well all the strategies for understanding speech-in-context that our brains can fill in automatically for the missing sounds. But the child or infant just learning speech relationships has a need to hear all sounds clearly in order to implant the perceptions solidly.

Skinner (1978) listed a number of liabilities to a child's language learning when a mild hearing loss exists:

Lack of Constancy of Auditory Clues when Acoustic Information Fluctuates. When a child does not hear speech sounds in the same way from one time to another there is a confusion in abstracting the meanings of words due to inconsistent categorization of speech sounds.

Confusion of Acoustic Parameters in Rapid Speech. Even the normal hearing child suffers from variations of speech occurring between speakers and even in the same speaker. Frequency, duration and intensity vary as a result of differences between speakers of age, sex, and personality. The child with mild hearing loss will be confused in language learning as a result.

Confusion in Segmentation and Prosody. The child with a mild loss may miss linguistic boundaries such as plurals, tenses, intonation and stress patterns. These factors are requisite to meaningful interpretation of speech.

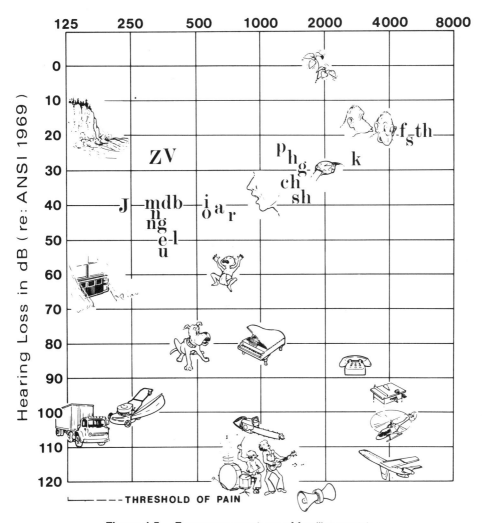

Figure 1.5. Frequency spectrum of familiar sounds.

Masking of Ambient Noise. According to French and Steinberg (1947) the normal child required a signal-to-noise ratio of +30 dB at 200–6000 Hz in order for speech learning to take place. It is rare in our modern culture for such a ratio to be present. Public school classes have no better signal-to-noise ratio than +12. A child with even mild loss is handicapped in such situations.

Breakdown of Early Ability to Perceive Speech Sounds. Almost at birth the infant begins to learn to discriminate speech sounds. Studies have shown that at 1–4 months the infant makes discrimination between most of the English speech sound pairs. By 6 months he recognizes many of the speech sounds of his language, and is making ongoing cataloging of speech sounds as discussed in Chapter 4. If these sounds are not perceived clearly due to a hearing loss, learning can be impeded.

Breakdown in Early Perceptions of Meanings. Often, during ordinary speech the normal listener misses some unstressed or elided words or sounds that he is able to fill in by context. But when an infant's hearing loss causes him to miss many of these soft or inaudible sounds, there is confusion in word naming, difficulty in developing classes of objects, and misunderstanding of multiple meanings.

Faulty Abstraction of Grammatical Rules. When short words are soft or elided as they often are it becomes more difficult for a slightly hearing impaired child to identify the relationships between words and to understand word orders.

Subtle Stress Patterns Missing. The mild hearing loss of a conductive loss has worse hearing in the low frequencies than in the high frequencies. The emotional content of speech, its rhythm and intonation are communicated through the low frequencies. When these are lost the emotional content of speech is confused—a condition which would impair learning of the speech milieu.

Contrary to conventional wisdom, mild conductive losses may even be more handicapping than mild sensorineural losses. A conductive loss muffles the sound that is heard, whereas in a sensorineural loss, the full loudness sensation of the sound is heard (Fig. 1.6). In a conductive loss of 30 dB, speech of 50 dB will be heard at 20-dB loudness sensation, whereas in a sensorineural loss of 30 dB, 50-dB speech will be heard at almost 50-dB loudness sensation.

Others have questioned the use of a 25-dB low fence even for adults. Kryter (1973) felt that it was too high because it failed to account for hearing in the presence of background noise. He proposed a low fence of 15 dB (ANSI) for 500, 1000, and 2000 Hz average. Suter (1978) looked at speech performance of normal and hearing-impaired adult listeners and also found the 25 dB criterion unrealistic. She showed that a low fence that would differentiate handicap from nonhandicap would be appropriate if set at 10 dB for 1000, 2000, and 3000 Hz and at 22 dB for 1000, 2000, and 4000 Hz. Again, these low-fence figures are for adults who have learned their language strategies well.

An ingenious scheme to show what happens with a mild 20-dB conductive loss was devised by Dobie and Berlin (1979). Knowing that a child with a 20-dB HL loss would pass a screening test that used 20-dB HL as the criterion intensity level, Dobie and Berlin undertook to find out what kind of speech perception problems such a child would have in language learning situations. They treated recorded speech sample utterances, first by recording them through correcting filters which shaped the signal as if it were processed through an ear at about the 40 phon level. They then displayed these utterances oscillographically and attenuated them by 20 dB, to simulate how a 20-dB conductive hearing loss would receive the material. These oscillographic samples were then displayed underneath the unattenuated samples, and spectral analyses of each 600 msec of the speech samples were prepared. A number of readers then examined the oscillographs to segment and mark the onsets of the various phonetic utterances.

The readings of these treated utterances revealed the following two observations: (1) there was a potential loss of transitional information, especially plural endings and related final-position fricatives; and (2) very brief utterances or high-frequency information could conceivably either be distorted or degraded if signal-to-noise conditions were less than satisfactory.

Dobie and Berlin reasoned that on the basis of their findings, a child with a 20-dB hearing loss from otitis media might be handicapped acoustically in the following ways:

1. Morphological markers might be lost or sporadically misunderstood; for example, "Where are Jack's gloves to be placed?" might be perceived as "Where Jack glove be place?"
2. Very short words that are often elided in connected speech (see "are" and "to" above) will lose considerable loudness because of the critical relationship between intensity, duration, and loudness.

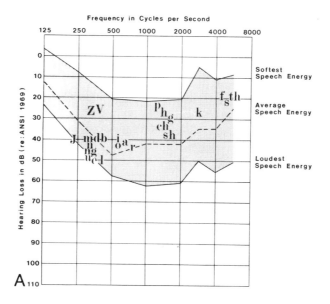

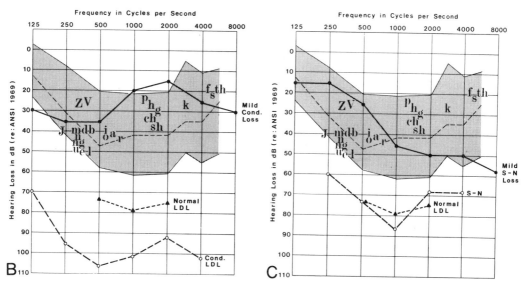

Figure 1.6. Average range of speech energy in dB HL is shown in audiogram (*A*); loudness discomfort level (LDL) of mild conductive hearing loss compared to that of normal ear is shown in audiogram (*B*); loudness discomfort level for mild sensorineural hearing loss is shown in audiogram (*C*). (Audiograms adapted from Skinner (1978) and Dudich et al. (1975).)

3. Inflections, or markers, carrying subtle nuances such as questioning and related intonation contouring can at the very best be expected to come through inconsistently.

What, then, is the beginning of a handicapping loss for a child? Is it 10 dB, 15 dB, 20 dB? Certainly it is lower than 25 dB. But it may be that a specific measure can-

not be applied for children. The American Academy of Otolaryngology committee (1979) defined a permanent handicap as "The disadvantage imposed by an impairment sufficient to affect a person's efficiency in the activities of daily living." Handicap implies a material impairment. Evidently the committee felt it could place a number on what would affect efficiency in daily living—the 25-dB low fence. But at the same time the commitee recognized the difficulty of measuring efficiency in understanding speech, and it deplored the fact that methods for assessing the ability to understand speech have not been well standardized because the "understanding of speech is affected by such variables as vocabulary, education, intelligence and nature of speech test material, in addition to hearing ability per se."

The foregoing concepts, then, can be used in proposing a realistic definition of hearing loss in children, namely: "A handicapping hearing loss in a child is any degree of hearing that reduces the intelligibility of a speech message to a degree inadequate for accurate interpretation or learning." Such a definition recognizes that it may not be possible to place a specific measure on what handicaps a child's ability to learn. Too may variables are present in the learning process of children: amount of parental stimulation, quality of parental stimulation, innate intelligence, age of onset of hearing loss, personality factors, health conditions, and, socioeconomic status. These variables may so affect the learning abilities of children that a 10-dB loss will be a handicap to one child, whereas a 25-dB loss will not handicap another (Fig. 1.7).

This definition places the onus on the audiologist or the managing physician to discover in any given case whether the degree of hearing loss is in fact affecting the child's ability to learn language and speech. A great deal of effort has been devoted in recent years to show restrospectively that certain types of mild hearing losses resulting from middle ear effusion do impair children's learning skills and ultimately their language abilities.

MINIMAL AUDITORY DEFICIENCY

Many infants and young children go for months with mild hearing losses due to middle ear effusion (MEE). Bluestone (1981) has suggested that the increase in MEE in the past 20 years may be because

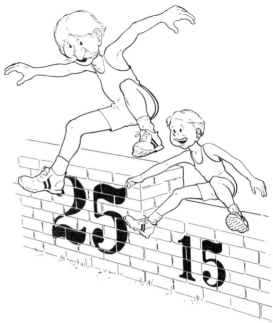

Figure 1.7. Normal hearing "low fence" for children may be more appropriate at 15 dB HL because of their more critical need for hearing *all* the intricacies of speech.

doctors are prescribing antibiotics too freely.

Some clinicians believe that MEE follows the vigorous application of antibiotics for acute otitis media attacks. The antimicrobial clears the bacterial infection, but some fluid remains in the ear and can result in a chronic secretion, or effusion. There is no evidence that MEE exists in similar incidence in populations where no antimicrobials are used. In this country and in Western Europe the condition has almost become endemic in nature.

For these reasons it is important to devote an entire section to review some of the studies concerning the disease of MEE. If auditory language learning is affected by MEE, the audiologist's and language pathologist's responsibility becomes manifestly important in identifying and remediating the language effects. The reader should evaluate these studies carefully, for most are retrospective in nature, and based on fairly small populations.

One of the first reports on the effect of early ear disease was made by a psychologist working with language learning problems (Eisen, 1962). He identified a child with auditory learning difficulties who had had a history of otitis media in early childhood, starting in infancy. Although this child now had normal hearing Eisen blamed the early otitis media for causing irreversible auditory language learning problems. He felt that a new syndrome had been identified, and called it the "quondam hard-of-hearing" syndrome ("at one-time" hard-of-hearing).

In a classic study by Holm and Kunze (1969) an experimental group of children 5½–9 years old was identified who had had no other medical problems but middle ear disease that had had its onset before the age of 2. Hearing levels had fluctuated from normal to greater than 25 dB. A well-matched control group of children with no history of ear disease was used for comparison. Each group was given a battery of tests, including the Illinois Test of Psycholinguistic Abilities (ITPA), the Peabody Picture Vocabulary test, the Templin-Darley Picture Articulation Screening test, and the Mecham Verbal Language Development Scale. As shown in Figure 1.8 the otitis media group showed significant lowered scores in all tests requiring the receiving or processing of auditory stimuli or the production of a verbal response. But essentially no differences were found in tests requiring visual skills. All language skills were lower in the experimental groups.

The exact type of otitis media that was present in the children in this study is not known. It was described as "recurrent and chronic" otitis media. However, the concomitant hearing loss fluctuated from normal to over 25 dB from time to time. This fact would indicate that the disease was either acute otitis media that recurred often, or recurrent serous otitis media. If it had been genuine chronic otitis, which is characterized by perforated eardrum and drainage the hearing would not have returned to normal. Holm and Kunze expressed concern that the signficance of fluctuating hearing loss from otitis media occurring during early critical periods may be overlooked by physicians who are not aware of the educational implications of such losses.

Eskimo children have been found to have an unusually high prevalence of otitis media (Beal, 1972) and thus provide natural material for studying the disease. Kaplan et al. (1973), in a cohort study of 489 Eskimo children, followed their development from birth to 7 through 10 years of age. Hearing tests showed 16% with hearing levels (500–2000 Hz) worse than 26 dB in at least one ear, more than 8% worse in both ears; 25% had hearing better than 25 dB ("normal") in at least one ear but had measurable air-bone gaps of 15 dB or more. Eight percent had bilateral air-bone gaps of 15 dB or more, but were considered to have "normal" hearing. The hearing loss group (>26 dB) averaged 5–7 attacks of otitis media, the air-bone gap group (>15 dB) averaged 5 attacks, and a group with normal hearing and no air-bone gap averaged 2.4 attacks. Of the 76% with history of otitis media, 78% had had their first attack before their second birthday, 22% after age 2. All the children were given Wechsler Intelligence Scale for Children (WISC) intelligence tests, Bender-Gestalt tests for perceptual problems, the Draw-a-Person test, and most were given the Metropolitan Achievement Test.

As expected, those children with a history of otitis media before age 2 and hearing levels of 26 dB or greater had statistically significant loss of verbal ability and were retarded in total reading, total math, and language. Even those with hearing better than 26 dB, but measurable air-bone gaps of 15 dB, had lower verbal and achievement scores than the completely normal group.

In terms of school placement it seemed that neither hearing levels nor numbers of attacks of otitis were as important as time of initial occurrence: 34% of all the children

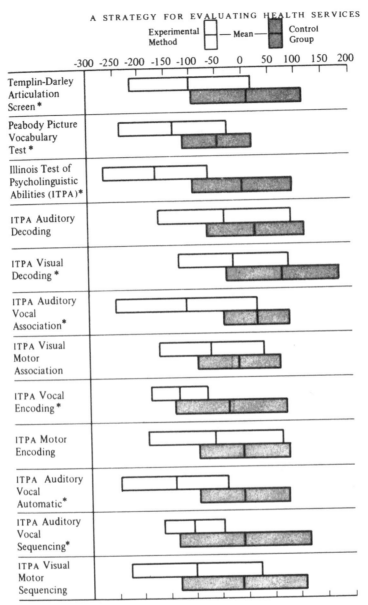

Figure 1.8.   Holme and Kunze study of matched groups (see text). (Reprinted with permission from D. M. Kessner and C. E. Kalk: *A Strategy for Evaluating Health Services*. Washington, D.C., National Academy of Sciences, 1973.)

were behind in their school placement. Of these, 63% had had their first otitis episode before age 2, 17% after age 2, and 20% had no history of otitis media.

Kaplan's team noted that since the 15-dB air-bone gap is "now in what is considered normal range, it can only be their past history of otitis media and transient hearing loss that has continued to have deleterious effects on them."

What is perhaps most significant in Kaplan's findings is that the school achievement gap between the early otitis media group and the nonaffected children showed a tendency to widen with increasing grade level, so the differences could become even greater at an older age. Here is evidence that not only may the effect of otitis media on language be a permanent one, but an increasingly greater one. These concerned

Table 1.2.
Relationship of the Incidence of Otitis Media to Age at the First Acute Episode[a]

Total Episodes of Otitis	Number of Patients	
	First episode at 0–18 months	First episode at 19–72 months
1	98	22
2	62	14
3	34	2
4	24	2
5	26	1
6	18	0
7	9	
8	8	
9	2	
10	2	
11	1	
12	3	
13	1	
14	2	
15	1	
16	0	
17	1	

[a] From V. M. Howie: Natural history of otitis media. *Annals of Otology, Rhinology, and Laryngology, Suppl. 19,* 67–72, 1975.

physicians in Alaska also predicted what is now becoming more and more evident: "A history of early and recurrent otitis media can identify those who will need special assistance in a regular classroom." They also suggest that special skills may need to be developed to habilitate these children.

Pediatricians seem to have been more acutely conscious of the effects of otitis media than any other specialists. Joining Holm, Kaplan and cohorts, and others that will be mentioned, was another concerned pediatrician, Virgil Howie. In Howie's study of some 488 children, he reported the prevalence and effects of otitis media prospectively. He identified a group of children in his practice whom he titled "otitis-prone" (Howie et al., 1975). These were children who had had 6 or more recurrent bouts of otitis media before age 6, as against a "non-otitis-prone" group who had had fewer than 6 episodes of otitis media. Howie (1975) identified 149 of these patients who were otitis prone. All of these patients had had their first episode of otitis media in the first 18 months. Only 5 of the 41 patients

whose first bout occurred after 18 months had more than 1 additional episode (Table 1.2). In addition it was found that those patients whose ears were aspirated and found to contain pneumococcus were 2½ times as likely to go on to become otitis-prone. Therefore there appeared to be two conditions predisposing children to become otitis-prone: occurrence of the first attack before 18 months, and presence of pneumococcus in the aspirate at the first episode.

Howie (1979) was also interested in the effects of otitis media. From his practice he identified two matched groups of paired children: one group having had no otitis media in the first year of life, the other group having had at least three recorded episodes of otitis media in the first year. Figure 1.9 shows the results of WISC IQ tests on the children at 7 years. The mean scores of the otitis group were significantly lower than those of the nonotitis group. Here Howie has pinpointed an age that

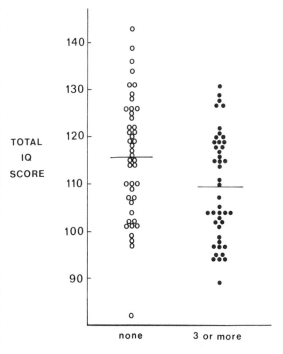

Figure 1.9. IQ comparison with "otitis prone" children and nonotologic history children. (Courtesy of V. M. Howie, Huntsville, Alabama, 1976.)

appears to be critical to mental development when there is recurrent otitis media.

Paradise (1976b) looked at a group of 32 cleft plate children who had had aggressive otologic management early in life. By this he meant myringotomy and tube placement as young as 2 or 3 months of age. Two thirds of his children maintained good or fair levels of follow-up care and otologic status, one third had poor levels of follow-up. All children at age 4 or 5 years were given both the Stanford-Binet IQ tests and the ITPA. The mean IQ of the children in the good-care group was 110, as compared with 98 in the poor-care group. On the ITPA, in all but one of the subtests, the mean scores of the children with good care were higher than those with poor care.

A study by Lewis (1976) identified a group of 14 aboriginal children between 6 and 9 years of age who had suffered documented ear infections over a 4-year period. The otitis media was presumed to have appeared initially before age 2. Another group of 18 aboriginal children aged 7–9 years were found who had been disease-free over a period of 4 years. A similar control group of European children 6–7 years old was also identified who had had no evidence of ear disease. The audiometric differences between the three groups are shown in Figure 1.10. If one averages the thresholds in the speech range it appears that there is no more than a 10-dB difference between the two aboriginal groups and around 12-dB difference between the aboriginal otitis group and the normal European group. All the children were given a variety of auditory skills tests including speech hearing in quiet (phonetically balanced (PB) lists), speech hearing in noise (S/N ratio of 0), Wepman Auditory Discrimination test, a phonemic synthesis test similar to the sound-blending subtest of the ITPA, a dichotic digits test, Enticknap Picture Vocabulary test, and the Goodenough Draw-a-man test (Table 1.3).

Significant differences between the two aboriginal groups were shown on the Wepman Auditory Discrimination test, on the phonemic synthesis task, and on the Enticknapp Picture Vocabulary test. There was a general tendency in all the other tests for the control group to perform better than experimental group, even where there was no statistical significance. Lewis reported that the magnitude of the pure-tone sensitivity differences are not necessarily responsible for the effects demonstrated in the study. The important consideration seems to be the existence of a middle ear disorder of early origin which apparently tends "to encourage inefficient listening strategies that can persist well beyond the

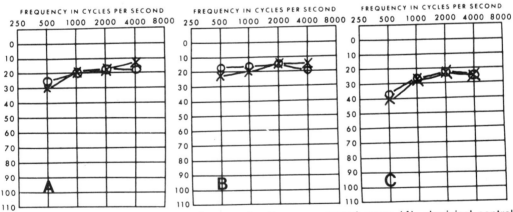

Figure 1.10. Average pure-tone audiograms for European control group (A), aboriginal control group (B) and aboriginal experimental group (C). (Reprinted with permission from N. Lewis: *Archives of Otolaryngology, 102*:387–390, © 1976, American Medical Association.)

episodes of active ear disease. In other words, it can be said that the mere presence of otitis media may be considered as presumptive evidence that a hearing disability exists.

Teele et al. (1981) studied 218 3-year-old white children with normal developmental history. They were stratified according to duration of persistent MEE, sex, type of health care, and socioeconomic status (SES). Table 1.4 shows the results of speech and language examination results for children with more than 130 days of purulent MEE and those with purulent MEE less than 30 days in a private practice (I) and an urban clinic (II).

These data suggest that purulent MEE (PMEE) early in life is associated with significant impairment of speech and language, but that children from higher SES appear at greater risk. It is difficult to understand why the effects here would appear in a group with presumably the best parental background rather than in a lower level functioning group. Perhaps the answer lies in the fact that the entire lower SES group II already had an auditory deprivation factor due to the lower levels of language input that were present in the environment of group II. Such a generalized depression in language learning could wipe out differences in the effects of PMEE. Note that the PMEE children in group I had higher levels of functioning in all tests than did the normal subjects from group II.

Teele et al. also reported that their data show that it is the history of otitis media in the first 6 months of life that accounts for the significant differences as found—that if only later history of otitis media

Table 1.3.
Mean Listening Scores for Performance on Various Tests by European Control Group, Aboriginal Control Group and Aboriginal Experimental Group[a]

Tests	Mean Score		
	European control	Aboriginal control	Aboriginal experimental
Speech-in-quiet (% correct)	93.6	94.8	91.6
Speech-in-noise (% correct)	74.4	69.2	58.4
Wepman (% correct)	78.0	77.7	58.7
Phonemic synthesis (% correct)	47.9	37.8	25.9
Dichotic listening (IAD score)[b]	21.8	13.6	23.9
DAM-IQ[c]	92.2	82.5	78.3
EPV-IQ	92.2	80.9	74.7

[a] From N. Lewis: *Archives of Otolargyngology*, 102: 387–390, 1976.
[b] Dichotic listening performance is expressed as an interaural difference score (IAD) reflecting the magnitude but not the direction of hemispherical asymmetry.
[c] DAM, Draw-a-man test; IQ, intelligence quotient; EPV, Enticknap Picture Vocabulary.

Table 1.4.
Effects of Persistent Middle Ear Effusion on Development of Speech and Language[a]

Test[b]	Group I			Group II		
	>130 days	<30 days	p[c]	>130 days	<30 days	p[c]
PPVT	103	113	0.003	92	94	NS
PSLS-AC	121	135	0.004	116	115	NS
PSLS-VA	113	130	0.006	115	112	NS

[a] From D. W. Teele, J. O. Klein, and B. Rosner: *Research in Pediatrics*, April 1981.
[b] PPVT, Peabody Picture Vocabulary Test; PSLS-AC, Pre-School Language Scale-Auditory Comprehension; and PSLA-VA, Pre-School Language Scale-Verbal Ability.
[c] Degree of significance.

were figured in, all significance would be wiped out. A previous study by Klein (1979), however, tends to suggest that the low level of auditory input from the environment of low SES children would tend to wipe out the marked differences that were found in higher income groups.

Brandes and Ehinger (1981) studied 15 children aged 7–9 years, with histories of early MEE, in a middle class suburban school. They were contrasted with a matched group of non-otitis media children by means of 12 auditory perceptual tests, academic achievement tests, nonverbal IQ and visual perception tests. The overall performance on all tests was significantly lower in the MEE group. Most significant difference in performance of this group was on the Goldman-Fristoe-Woodcock Selective Attention Total Test measuring the ability to attend to a listening in noise most particularly. There were no significant differences between the two groups in their academic achievement, a fact which the authors related to the fact that this group had had more special support services than had the other group. However, it should be noted that, in the Sak and Ruben (1982) study (described below), the middle class children in their MEE group also showed no functional differences in classroom performance. However, in most of the studies that follow there are clearly demonstrated major deficiencies in the academic performance of children who have had early serous otitis. It is apparent that the effects of the disease are extremely variable and that, when samples are taken from various populations, this variability results in some disparate effects.

Kessler and Randolph (1979) studied two groups of children who had been culled from the third grades in a school district, one group with histories of early otitis media and the other group with no history of otitis. The SES was matched, and a wide variety was represented. Nine measures of auditory abilities were tested on these groups, and in most of the measures of auditory ability the early otitis group scored statistically significantly lower than did the control group. On measures of academic achievement of the children as assessed by the Word Study Skills and Reading Comprehension Subtest of the Stanford Achievement Tests, the otitis media group scored significantly lower than the total third grade population on both subtests. These authors concluded that early middle ear disease can result in difficulty in acquiring adequate language and academic skills.

Needleman (1977) identified 20 children age 3–8 years with recurrent serous otitis media that had begun between birth and 18 months and continued for at least 2 years. She compared this group with a matched group of otitis-free children, studying the comprehension and production of aspects of the phonological system as measured by various tests. She found the otitis media group to score significantly lower than the non-otitis group in production of phonemes and words, production of phonemes in connected speech, the use of combinations of phonemes and word endings, and in varying morphological contexts. She pointed out that the phonological skills that were deficient were necessary for reading skills, and that this fact may account for the educational retardation of the children who have had early otitis media.

A group of middle-class children with early and recurrent otitis media were followed by Sak and Ruben (1982). A control group of the unaffected siblings of these children were also followed. The two groups were given an extensive battery of language tests including the ITPA, the Wide-Range Achievement Test (WRAT), the Detroit Test of Learning Aptitudes, and the WISC. The scores of the siblings with early MEE were consistently lower than those of their matched siblings with statistical significance in four areas of auditory learning. The difference is illustrated in the WISC scores where the verbal scales are significantly lower in the MEE group, although the performance scales are similar. As this population comprised middle class children, both groups performed at superior levels. But the lower scores in the effusion groups showed that even with superior scores these children were not attaining their best potential functioning. One of their most interesting findings was a reversal in the direction of significance in the visual memory subtest of the ITPA, with the MEE group significantly better than the normal group. This finding suggests that children with hearing loss may learn visual compensation for their auditory deficits.

Eight hundred and seventy children were seen by pediatricians at ages 6 weeks, 6 months, and at 1, 1½, 2, 3, and 4½ years (Bax, 1981). A highly significant relationship was found between language delay at 2 years and the reported incidence of MEE in the previous 6 months. At age 3 years, the precentage of MEE among children showing delay was twice as high as among the group of children with normal language development. Although parental report was the source of information, the large numbers involved strengthen a causal relationship.

Early language scales (Receptive Expressive Emergent Language Scale, REEL; Sequenced Inventory of Communication Development, SICD) were given to a group of intensive-care infants who developed documented MEE, and also to a parallel group with normal ear history (Friel-Patti et al., 1982). The results at 12, 18, and 24 months show marked and significant language delays in the effusion group as compared with the controls. The significant fact is that 43% of the MEE group had language delay greater than 6 months, as compared with only 7% in the MEE-free children. There was no language delay in 78% of the intensive-care children—those without any effusion—as against 28% in the effusion group.

A number of other investigators have pointed up the role of minimal auditory deficiencies in lowering school achievement or language skills: Goetzinger et al. (1964), Kodman (1963), Ling (1972), Wishik et al. (1958), Quigley (1970), Eisen (1962), Holm and Kunze (1969), Beratis et al. (1979), Palfrey et al. (1980), Sarff (1981), Burgener and Mouw (1982), Potsic et al. (1979), Thelin et al. (1979), Lehmann et al. (1979), Cass and Kaplan (1979), Zinkus et al. (1978), Bennett et al. (1979), Freeman and Parkins (1979), Menyuk (1977), Hersher (1978), Hook (1979), Davis (1981), Downs (1982), and Zinkus (1982). A useful bibliography of references dealing with communication disorder studies associated with otitis media has been published by Gabbard (1982). The results of all these studies point to minor hearing losses as being responsible for language problems.

The question remains as to whether these language problems will persist and cause irremediable language learning deficits. Only one study suggested that the children might close the language gap with age (Needleman, 1977). But a great many studies of language and developmental delays indicate that the gap will never close, once a language deficit occurs by 2 or 3 years (McKay et al., 1978; Strominger and Bashir, 1977; Schweinhart and Weikart, 1980).

The most numerous data on the prognosis for language have been assembled by the Consortium for Longitudinal Studies (Schweinhart and Weikart, 1980). They show that of all the intervention programs to improve language and cognition in deprived children, the early mother-child intervention programs, birth to 3 years, are the most efficacious and productive of lasting effects. Later programs do not permanently close the language gap. The analogy can be made between studies on environmentally deprived children and children with MEE because the hearing loss from MEE is also an environmental deprivation; or, more pertinently, environmental deprivation is an auditory deprivation. From all the data we have assembled, a realistic and conservative estimate of the prevalence of hearing loss in children is presented in Table 1.5.

What then is a hearing loss? From the above studies it is evident that our definition of hearing loss for children can be defended. It also means that we can define hearing loss in terms other than the decibel hearing level unit. Several of the studies above suggest that mere presence of otitis media is *ipso facto* evidence that a significant hearing loss exists. It may not be possible to specify a 10-dB or 15-dB level as a beginning of a hearing loss for a child, although certainly a generalized criterion might be in the area of 15 dB HL. The diagnosis of a handicapping hearing loss in any given case then, lies in an entire diagnostic process that includes not only ear examinations and hearing tests, but also measures of a child's receptive and expressive language, his vocalization or speech levels, and his behavioral functioning. Such diagnostic evaluations can be made by enlisting other disciplines that will determine if the child is language-delayed sufficiently to warrant educational intervention. The identification of these children, of course, lies in the hands of the family practice physician and the pediatrician, for they are the source of primary care. Therefore they will require directives as to when to apply measures of language competence to determine whether a handicapping hearing loss is present.

IDENTIFICATION AND MANAGEMENT OF THE OTITIS-PRONE CHILD

When a child presents with otitis media and there is an indication that it may be a recurrent problem, a speech and language evaluation screening test must be recommended. Whether or not the child turns out to be otitis-prone the evaluation will serve as a baseline for future references. It is particularly urgent to be zealous about applying these evaluations in the first 2 years of life, for during this period of critical language learning 3 months of poor hearing is an eternity in the development of language skills.

The sequence of management of these children is as follows:

1. MEDICAL INTERVENTION

Medical treatment is the first line of defense in otitis media. The choice of treatment depends on the managing physician. Paradise (1976a) has demonstrated that vigorous medical treatment through tympanostomy tubes is effective in preventing intellectual defects. Gebhart (1981) also showed that tympanostomy tubes is the treatment of choice for otitis media. He observed two groups of children who had had bouts of otitis media. One group received appropriate antibiotics for the infection, the other group was given tympanostomy tubes. Forty-eight percent of the tympanostomy group had no further attacks of otitis media as against 59% of the antibiotic group. Ninety-seven percent of the tympanostomy group had only one further occurrence of the disease as against 48% in the antibiotic group. The latter went on to have more, with 5 or 6 further attacks of otitis media, which did not happen to any of the tympanostomy group.

Even the best medical intervention does not rule out recurrence of MEE in some children. Tos (1980b) has estimated that

Table 1.5.
Realistic Estimate of Prevalence of Hearing Loss in Children

	Percent with Bilateral Loss 15 dB	Percent with Unilateral Loss 15 dB	Total
0–12 mo	4.2	8.4	12.5
12 mo–2 yr	5.2	10.8	16
2–3 yr	4.3	8.6	13
3–4 yr	4	8	12
4–5 yr	4.1	5.1	9.2
6–7 yr	1.7	4.6	6.3
8–9 yr	1.1	3.7	4.8
10–11 yr	1.9	4.5	6.4

Average prevalence:
  10%, birth to 11 yr

about 15% of treated children will have recurrence.

2. SCREENING AND DIAGNOSTIC LANGUAGE TESTS

If the MEE persists for 3 months despite vigorous medical or surgical treatment, or if a hearing loss is present after 3 months, a language screening test should be applied. An example of the kind of screening for expressive and receptive language and for articulation, has been developed by Downs and Blager (1982). If the child is not functioning at age level, referral should be made for a comprehensive language evaluation.

3. EDUCATIONAL INTERVENTION

If the child fails in any item at age level on the language scales, a home language stimulation program should be recommended; if he fails on items below his age level, a hearing aid should also be considered. These are the major educational interventions.

The application of an appropriate educational habilitation program does not supersede the medical treatment. It can be concomitant with any medical or surgical procedures that are prescribed. However, when a child is found on the language assessment to be at risk for educational problems the physician and audiologist together will want to consider the intervention strategies that should be applied.

For an infant under 1 or 2 years of age, one or more of the following intervention strategies can be considered:

Home Language Stimulation Program. The child at risk for any developmental delay, whether it is from auditory deprivation or neurological condition, requires a stepped-up language enrichment environment. Home language enrichment programs such as those offered in child development centers for developmentally high risk children are appropriate for our high risk children. Blager (1982) has published a list of helpful materials available for home language development and language stimulation programs. Although it has never been described, a program of teaching parents how to improve their voice projection may be a possibility. If parents could raise their voices routinely by 10–15 dB, the hearing deficit in their child could be compensated for. Certainly it is worth considering such instruction along with any home stimulation program.

Hearing Aid Placement. A mild ear-level hearing aid, with appropriate limitations on maximum saturation and gain, can be considered even for a young infant. The obvious drawbacks are that it is difficult to convince parents of the necessity for such an extreme antidote, and there are problems in keeping such an instrument on an infant. Hearing aid placement is a feasible procedure only if (a) the parents are highly motivated, (b) continual guidance by an audiologist or speech therapist is obtained, (c) a total support system by doctor, parent and therapist is in effect, and (d) a period of diagnostic therapy with a loaner hearing aid is initiated to judge the effectiveness of the aid.

ECONOMIC IMPACT OF SEVERE HEARING LOSS

We have described the impact of hearing losses on the educational and cognitive future of the child. Another way of looking at the impact of hearing loss is from the economic point of view. Legislators and government agencies are interested in the costs of a handicap to society, compared with the price of prevention or remediation.

An excellent reference text by Schein and Delk (1974) *The Deaf Population of the United States* gives a basis for estimating the costs of deafness to our society. The number of deaf and hard-of-hearing in the United States and in the various states is identified. There is also a breakdown as to the numbers of prevocationally deaf (those whose deafness occurred before the age of 18) and the prelinguistically deaf, whose deafness occurred before the age of 3:

Degree	Age at Onset	Number	% Prevalence
All hearing impairment	All ages	13,362,842	6.6
Significant bilateral	All ages	6,548,842	3.2
Deafness	All ages	1,767,046	0.87
	Prevocational	410,522	0.2
	Prelingual	201,626	0.1

The "deaf" are defined as "those who could not hear and understand speech" (presumably those who could not understand speech even with amplification). The hard-of-hearing are defined as those who "had trouble hearing in one or both ears."

Another Vital Statistics Survey in 1960–1962 (Glorig and Roberts, 1965) estimated 164 per 100,000 (0.16%) with hearing levels worse than 87 dB (ANSI) average.

The direct costs of coping with hearing disorders has been estimated at $410,445,000 per year (Human Communication and Its Disorders, 1969). This annual bill includes costs of:

Public residential schools for deaf	$55,092,000
Private residential schools for deaf	3,883,000
Special day program for deaf and hard of hearing	24,190,000
Special services in regular schools	20,000,000
Preparation of special teachers	2,700,000
Captioned films for the deaf	2,800,000
Vocational rehabilitation	28,000,000
Preparation of rehabilitationists	1,200,000
Compensation for military disability	45,000,000
Audiological services for veterans	1,780,000
Community hearing and speech center	3,600,000
Speech and hearing clinics	6,000,000
Private medical care	80,000,000
Hearing aids and their maintenance	132,000,000
Industrial claims and hearing conservation	4,200,000
	$410,445,000

The educational costs of special education comprise the expenses of educating 55,000 to 60,000 school age children enrolled in special schools and classes for the deaf (Basic Education Rights, 1973).

No attempt is made by Schein and Delk to describe the economics of the hard-of-hearing. They treat only with the deaf, which limits our purview of the cost of hearing loss, but is nevertheless remarkably revealing. In Figure 1.11 are shown the

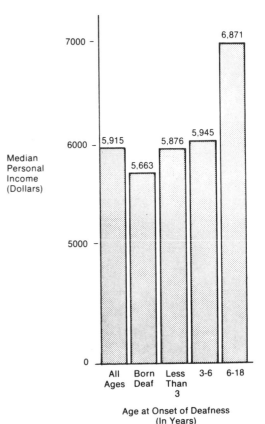

Figure 1.11. Median personal income of employed deaf persons 16–64 years of age, by age at onset of deafness: United States, 1971. (Reprinted with permission from J. D. Schein and M. T. Delk, Jr.: *The Deaf Population of the United States.* Silver Spring, Md.: National Association of the Deaf, 1974.)

relative incomes per year of the deaf, listed by the time of occurrence of the deafness.

If we compare the average income of the deaf ($5915) with that of the normal hearing population ($8188), we find that $2273 per year per person is lost in manpower earnings from deafness. Multiplying by the number of the deaf gives the figure $4 billion per year that is lost to society because of deafness.

But there is another way to look at the economics of deafness. How much could be saved if prelingually deaf children all had the language skills and earning capacity of those who become deaf after 6 years? As Figure 1.11 shows, there is a $1208.00 per year difference between the congenitally deaf and those who became deaf after 6. This difference represents the superior language level of those who had normal hearing for the first 6 years of life. It confirms the importance of learning language during the early critical periods of language development. What would be the result if the prelinguistically deaf were identified early and given language training that would bring them to the level of those who became deaf after 6? It turns out that multiplying the difference in yearly income of these two groups by the number of prelinguistically deaf gives $243 million in manpower earnings per year that might be saved if language levels could be raised.

Other conclusions can be derived from the economic figures in Schein and Delk (1974). For example, each state's economic losses can be similarly estimated. Taking the state of California we find:

Hard of Hearing	Deaf	Prevocational Deaf	Prelingually Deaf
1,427,928	185,708	38,595	19,290

The cost per year in manpower earnings lost to California is $422 million due to deafness; $23 million could be saved per year in California if the language level of the prelinguistically deaf were improved to the level of the deaf at 6.

Almost no cost seems too high to prevent the handicap of hearing loss; the expenses and the manpower wages lost due to learning problems are a drain on the economy that society cannot tolerate.

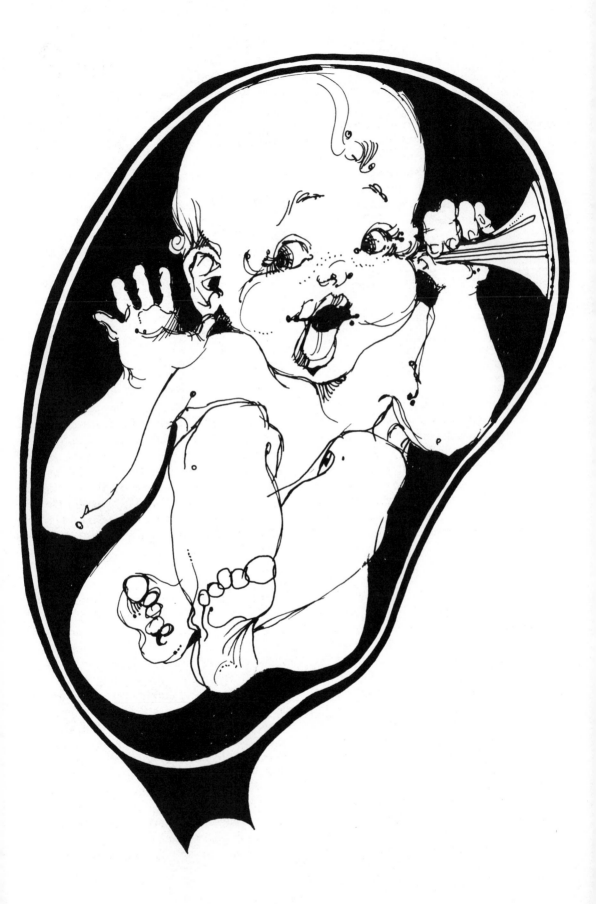

CHAPTER 2

The Auditory Mechanism

The embryologic development of the ear is of more than academic interest to the clinician. An understanding of embryologic relationships helps the physician in his diagnosis and the audiologist in his plan for early identification and management of hearing loss. If one is aware of the timetable of prenatal development and the association of the various structures with each other, the suspicion of deafness and its subsequent diagnosis and treatment become easier. Although the major changes in the development of the ear take place in the mother's womb, first as an embryo and later as a fetus, the baby becomes a more progressively complex structure with time. Several mechanical processes occur concurrently to produce the final structure including enlargements, constrictions, and foldings which are further modified by evaginations and invaginations. However, development of the auditory structure does not cease, nor is it totally complete, at the time of birth.

Knowledge of the origins of auditory structures can be diagnostically significant to the clinician. For example, when an infant presents with a congenital skin disorder, one considers the fact that the skin and the otocyst both originate from ectoderm. It may then be logical to suspect that anomalies of the cochlear structures could have occurred contiguously with the skin disorder and that a search for severe sensorineural deafness is in order.

Similarly, the timing of development of the various organ systems guides us to suspect that a hearing loss may have occurred at the same time that other systems were affected. A noxious influence on the fetus at 2 months of gestation may result in a malformation of the pinna which is developing at that time. The pinna malformation, however, does not necessarily imply malformation of the ossicles of the middle ear. Although the ossicles of the middle ear share partially the same time clock as the pinna in embryologic development, the origins of the structures are different. On the other hand, an insult to one may well result in a related insult to the other.

Principles such as these allow us to look for the occult symptom of hearing loss whenever an overt embryologically related symptom becomes evident. The prognosis for auditory function can then be estimated from what is known of the origin and the expected pathology. A simple review of the embryologic development of the ear and its related structures will clarify some of these principles.

PHYLOGENY

Unfortunately, "ears" and "hearing" are often synonyms to the naive student who may be unaware that the ability to hear is actually a secondary acquired characteristic of the ear. The primary responsibility of the auditory organ is maintaining equilibrium. The study of comparative anatomy confirms that hearing is important only to higher forms of vertebrates, but the basic function of equilibrium remains essentially unchanged in the phylogenetic evolution between fish and man.

In many fish, amphibians, and reptiles the paired internal ears are devoted primarily to functions related to equilibrium. In these creatures the membranous labyrinth of the inner ear is filled with endolymph, and two distinct saclike structures are generally present, the utricle and saccule. An endolymphatic duct extends upward from these two sacs and terminates within the brain case as the endolymphatic sac. A structure known as the lagena, which is actually the forerunner of the cochlea, is formed as a depression pocket in the floor of the saccule. Even in these lower vertebrates, branches of the auditory nerve are associated in the sensory sacs with end organs known as macula.

The macula-type of sensory cell is found in all vestibular systems and is the basic means of transforming equilibrium information into neural codes. These sensory end organs, much like the human cochlear hair cells, have hairlike projections embedded in an overlying gelatinous material, the cupula. In the utricular and saccular maculae, and often in the primitive lagena, this gelatinous material becomes a thickened structure in which are deposited crystals of calcium carbonate. Technically speaking, the very small crystals in the human otolithic membrane are otoconia (Greek = ear dust), while the somewhat larger concretions of some other vertebrates are otoliths (Greek = ear stones). However, the two terms are often used interchangeably (Nolte, 1981).

An interesting equilibrium system utilized by the crayfish is described by Storer et al. (1979). The crayfish has a small sac known as the statocyst located at the base of each antennae. The statocyst contains a ridge of sensory hairs to which sand grains are attached by mucus to form structures called statoliths. The action of gravity on the statoliths causes the sensory hairs to bend, informing the crayfish of his present orientation. Each time the crayfish molts, it loses the statolith lining and must acquire new grains of sand to deposit in the statocyst. The crayfish shows disorientation in an aquarium with no foreign debris particles following molting. When iron filings are placed in the aquarium, the crayfish will pick some up for use in his statocyst and then his equilibrium may be controlled with a magnet held in various positions along the sides of the aquarium.

All vertebrates are, of course, dependent on information concerning turning movements provided by the semicircular canals. In every jawed vertebrate, three such canals arise from each utricle. The three canals are at right angles to each other and represent the three planes of space. Each canal has an enlargement at one end known as an ampulla. Within the ampulla is a sensory end organ, the crista. Displacement of the endolymph in the semicircular canal causes displacement of the cupula which is attached to the cristae, bending the sensory hairs and initiating neural impulses.

Some fish and amphibians have a peculiar sensory system termed the lateral line system. The receptor organ of the lateral line is the neuromast, a generalized name applied to nerve receptors that demonstrate a hairlike projection enclosed in a flexible mass of gelatinous material—the cupula. Neuromasts are generally located on the surface skin of the water-dwelling organism. Evidence of embryonic development of the sensory endings in the human cochlea—which closely resembles the externally placed neuromast organs—may indicate that the internal ear originated phylogenetically as a specialized, deeply sunk portion of the lateral line system.

As animals evolved to become land-dwelling creatures, adaptations in the hearing sense organ were necessitated to process airborne sound waves. Changes were in order to transmit sounds and amplify them to the inner ear which was usually set deeply in the skull. It is now known that a hole exists through the bird's skull connecting both ears and permitting sound localization otherwise not available because of the bird's small head size. The middle ear of amphibians and reptiles is quite similar, in the sense that the hyomandibular bone seen in the fish has changed its function to become a rodlike stapes or columella. The columella crosses the middle ear between the tympanic membrane and the oval window of the inner ear. This columellar-type middle ear ossicle is of particular interest since human middle ear malformations may show this type of deformity. It makes one wonder if this is a throwback to our primitive evolutionary forebears (Fig. 2.1). An abnormal structure reminiscent of normal structures in "lower" animals, such as a cervical fistula or a columella ossicle, is known as a reversion structure or *atavism.*

In the mammals the external ear becomes a prominent structure known as the pinna. A more fundamental change occurs in the middle ear where, instead of a single bone, an articulated series of three ossicles between the eardrum and oval window exists. The middle ear mechanism in man is the result of a 400-million-year evolutionary process in which discarded parts from nearby structures, having lost their original function, became adapted for full use in the hearing apparatus (Himalstein, 1978). According to Romer (1977) the origin of this series of ossicles has been long debated. The question existed as to whether the three ossicles were really due to subdivisions of the columella. Careful study, however, of paleontology, and comparative anatomy led to the conclusion that only the mammalian stapes is related to the lower vertebrate columella. Mammals have developed a new specialized jaw system and the "older" jaw elements have been developed into the other two middle ear ossicles. The reptile eardrum lies close to a jaw joint known as the articular which becomes the malleus in mammals. A second jaw bone, the quadrate, is attached to the articular in the reptile, and to the hyomandibular bone (forerunner of the stapes in the fish). The quadrate retains these primitive connections and becomes the incus in mammals. Thus, these bones which were originally part of the gill structure in fish develop into the jaw structure of reptiles and finally into ear structures in mammals. In Romer's words, the breathing aids of the fish developed into feeding aids in reptiles and finally into "hearing aids" in mammals!

The inner ear in birds and mammals functions from nearly identical physiologic mechanisms—auditory sensory structures vibrated by movements of a membrane located beneath them. Birds and mammals refined their hearing abilities with the advanced development of the cochlea. The number of coils present in the cochlea may vary among mammalian species. As indicated earlier in this phylogenetic discussion, the portions of the inner ear devoted to balance show little change in evolutionary development. Additional information regarding the evolutionary development of the ear may be found in the book *Sound and Hearing* in the Life Science Library (Stevens and Warshofsky, 1965; Stebbins, 1980).

BASIC EMBRYOLOGY

Most audiologists have not had training or coursework in the field of embryology so some basic background information is essential to fully appreciate the development of the ear. The reader is also referred to Zemlin (1981) for a very good discussion of the embryonic development of the facial, head, and neck regions.

All growth is the result of cell division of preexisting cells. Through a process known as mitosis, changes take place in the nucleus of a cell which produce a specific number of double structures. The cell and nucleus then subdivide into two identical "daughter" cells. At the same time "organizers" exist in the embryo which stimulate development of associated areas, and create specific differentiation of cells in the developmental process.

One of the earliest organizational developments in the embryo is the differentiation of cells into three superimposed, cellular plates called germ layers. These germ layers are known as ectoderm, mesoderm, and endoderm. Initially, the cells of each layer are virtually indistinguishable. While all the cells are descendents of the same fertilized egg, chemical changes take place. Ectoderm is generally responsible for development of the outer skin layers, but also gives rise to the nervous system and the

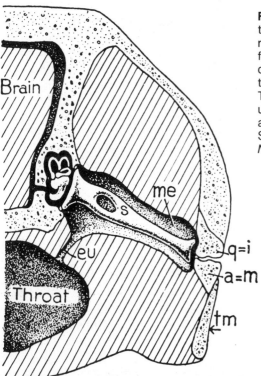

Figure 2.1. Example of an otic reversion structure. (*Top*) Ventricle cross-section of the normal reptile middle ear. (Reprinted with permission from A. S. Romer: *The Vertebrate Body*, Philadelphis, W. B. Saunders, 1977. (*Bottom*) Horizontal cross-section of a human middle ear from a Treacher Collins patient, showing congenital columella-type of stapes with absence of the malleus and incus. (Reprinted with permission from I. Sando and R. P. Wood: *Otolaryngology clinics of North America* (*Symposium*) 4:29–318, 1971.)

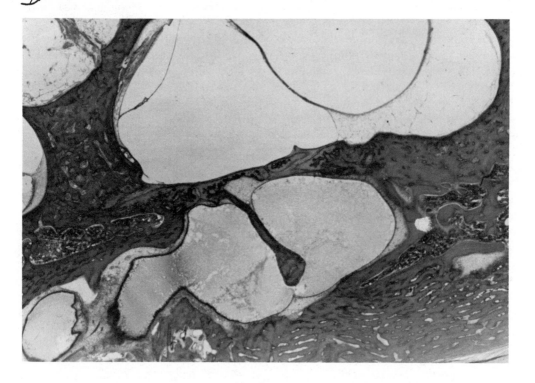

sense organs. Mesoderm is associated with skeletal, circulation structures, kidneys, and reproductive organs. Endoderm creates the digestive canal and respiratory organs. These germ layers are actually not quite so specific in their functions as outlined above; but, as you will see, the outer and inner portions of the ear do indeed develop from ectodermal tissue, while the middle ear ossicles and the bone surrounding the inner ear originate from mesodermal tissue.

A developing baby is known as an embryo (from a Greek word meaning "to swell") during its first 8 weeks of gestation. At the end of the 2nd week a cellular disc exists composed of the three germ layers. By the end of the 1st month of life, the embryo is only about a fourth of an inch long. The embryonic period terminates around the 8th week when the structure assumes a "human" appearance, and is known as a fetus (from the Latin word meaning "offspring") for the remainder of the gestation period.

The ear begins its development during the early life of the embryo, so some discussion of the detailed growth of the embryo itself is worthwhile. The embryonic disc is split by a primitive streak at about 25 hours, which leads the way for development of the ectodermal-lined primitive groove and primitive fold (Fig. 2.2). The primitive groove deepens into a primitive pit, which in turn becomes the neural groove and neural fold (Fig. 2.3). An enlargement exists (the primitive knot) at the cephalic end of the primitive streak which is destined to become the head of the organism. The ectodermal-lined neural folds come together to close off the neural groove, which is now known as the neural tube. It is during the stage of the neural tube that

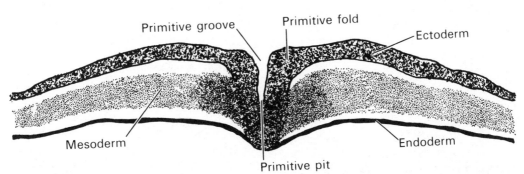

Figure 2.2. Early life of the embryo. The embryonic disc is split at about 25 hours. This drawing is made from a transverse cut through a seven-segment chick embryo. (Modified with permission from L. B. Arey: *Developmental Anatomy*. Philadelphia, W. B. Saunders, 1940.)

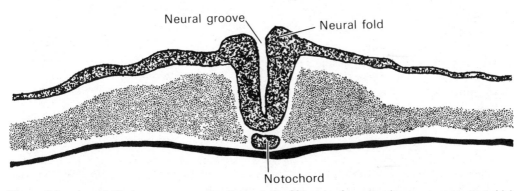

Figure 2.3. A cephalic transverse section through the fifth pair of somites in a seven-segment chick embryo. (Modified with permission from L. B. Arey: *Developmental Anatomy*. Philadelphia, W. B. Saunders, 1940.)

the earliest beginnings of the ear are seen (Snell, 1975).

DEVELOPMENT OF THE EAR

Inner Ear

Only the basic gross essentials of the development of the ear are presented here. Readers interested in an excellent, in-depth presentation on embryology of the ear are referred to Anson (1973).

The earliest demarcations of the ear in the human embryo are seen early in the 3rd week as thickenings in the superficial ectoderm on either side of the open neural plate. These thickenings are the auditory or otic placodes and are obvious by the middle of the 3rd week (Fig. 2.4a). About the 23rd day, the auditory placodes begin to invaginate into the surface ectoderm and are known as the auditory or otic pits. When the mouth of each auditory pit closes on or about the 30th day, it becomes the auditory vesicle or otocyst and appears as an ectodermal cavity lined with epithelium lateral to the now closed neural tube as shown in Figure 2.4c.

The auditory vesicle proceeds to differentiate through a series of folds, evaginations, and elongations and takes on an elongated shape divided into a utricular-saccule area and a tubular extension known as the endolymphatic duct. By 4½ weeks the portion of the auditory vesicle connected to the endolymphatic duct can be recognized as the future vestibular portion of the labyrinth, while the more slender portion of the vesicle begins to elongate from the saccular area as the future cochlea (Fig. 2.5a). At the end of the 6th week, three archlike outpockets are visible and destined to become the semicircular canals. At this same time the utricle and saccule become two definitive areas through a deepening construction of the vestibular portion of the auditory vesicle (Fig. 2.5b).

By the end of the 7th week, the elongated outpocketing of the saccular portion of the auditory vesicle has completed one coil of the future cochlea. During the 8th through 11th week, the two and a half coils of the cochlea are completed. The cochlear duct continues to be attached to the vestibular area by means of a narrow tube known as the ductus reuniens. The cochlear division of the eighth nerve follows the elongation and coiling of the cochlear duct, and fans its fibers out to be distributed along the duct's entire length.

During the 7th week, the complicated convolutions of the otic labyrinth continue to develop, and sensory end organs first appear as localized thickenings of epithelium in the utricle and saccule. Similar localized epithelial thickenings are found in the ampullated ends of the semicircular canals during the 8th week and in the floor of the cochlear duct at 12 weeks. These epithelial thickenings show differentiation into two types of cells including sensory cells with bristle-like hairs and supporting cells at one end. Complete maturation of the sensory and supporting cells in the cochlea does not occur until the 5th month when the entire cochlear duct has shown considerable growth and expansion.

The membranous labyrinth of the inner ear reaches its full adult configuration by the early part of the 3rd month. At this time the otic capsule, which has been encased in cartilage, begins to ossify through a complex system of 14 different endochondral ossification centers in the petrous portion of the temporal bone. The inner ear is the only sense organ to reach full adult size and differentiation by fetal midterm. However, it should be noted that the cochlear portion of the inner ear is the last inner ear end organ to differentiate and mature. Thus, the cochlea may be subject to more possible developmental deviations, malformations, and acquired disease than the vestibular end organs.

Middle Ear

During the period of time that the sensory portion of the auditory system—the inner ear—is developing, the transmission portion of the auditory mechanism is de-

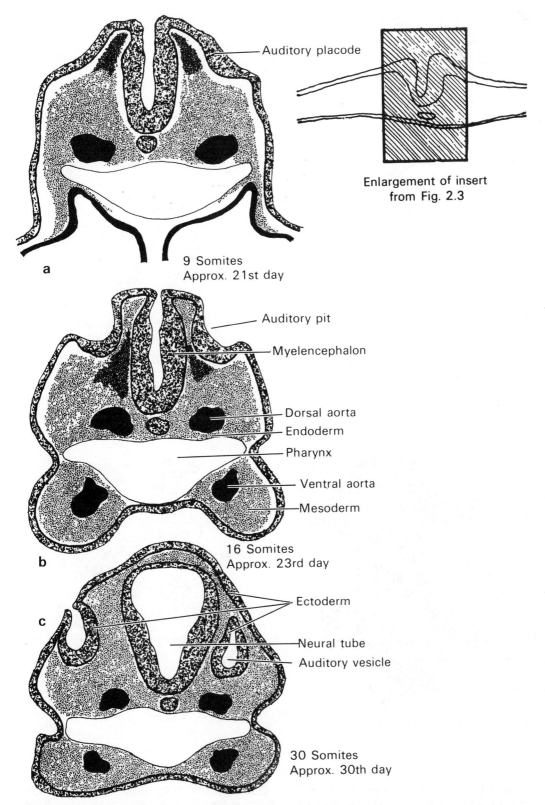

Figure 2.4. Early development of inner ear in human embryo. (Modified with permission by L. B. Arey: *Developmental Anatomy*. Philadelphia, W. B. Saunders, 1940.)

29

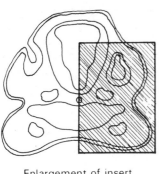

Enlargement of insert
From Fig. 2.4

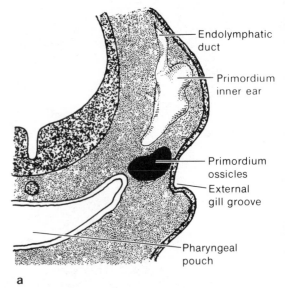

Endolymphatic
duct

Primordium
inner ear

Primordium
ossicles

External
gill groove

Pharyngeal
pouch

a

Approx. 4½ weeks

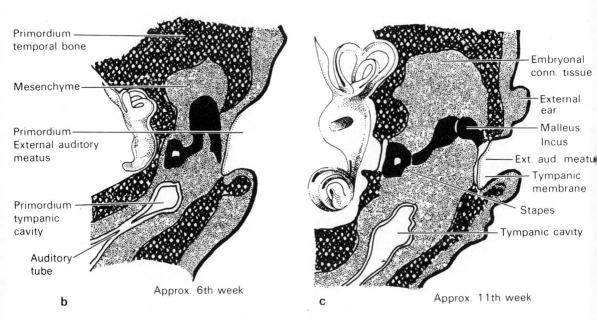

Primordium
temporal bone

Mesenchyme

Primordium
External auditory
meatus

Primordium
tympanic
cavity

Auditory
tube

b

Approx. 6th week

Embryonal
conn. tissue

External
ear

Malleus
Incus

Ext. aud. meatu

Tympanic
membrane

Stapes

Tympanic cavity

c

Approx. 11th week

Figure 2.5. Schematic development of inner and middle portions of the auditory mechanism from approximately 4½ to 11 weeks. (Modified with permission from B. M. Patten: *Human Embryology*, ed. 3. New York, McGraw-Hill, 1968.)

veloping as the middle ear. Unlike the inner ear which originates from ectodermal tissue, the middle ear is an endodermal structure. The middle ear cavity begins its development during the third week while the auditory pit is sinking into the neural plate to become the auditory vesicle. The tympanic cavity and the auditory tube (later known as the eustachian tube) come from an elongation of the lateral-superior edge of the endodermal-lined first pharyngeal pouch. This elongation is called the tubotympanic recess (Fig. 2.5b).

By the time the human embryo is in its 4th week, a series of five branchial grooves or "gill slits" has appeared. These grooves are in the lower head and neck region on the outside of the embryo. On the inside of the embryo a corresponding series of pharyngeal pouches develops and the collective structures are identified as "arches." In the fish these grooves from the outside ultimately meet the corresponding pouches on the inside to form "gills" as part of their respiratory mechanism. In humans, most of the branchial grooves do not form slits with the pharyngeal pouches; however, the embryo's passing through this developmental stage is an example of our inheritance of embryonic structure from aquatic ancestors. It is of interest that in the human embryo one of the gill pouches does actually become perforated, forming a passageway from the pharynx to the outside of the head. This passageway becomes the external ear canal and eustachian tube. The eardrum forms a barrier between these two portions of the passageway, which otherwise would directly connect the pharynx and the exterior as does the gill slit of a fish (Himalstein, 1978). Occasionally an additional opening will occur, forming a cervical fistula or branchial cyst which is an opening on the throat between the pharynx and the surface of the neck. The exact position of the fistula depends on which of the pouches is involved.

During the 2nd month the tubotympanic recess approaches the embryo surface between the first and second branchial arches,

known as Meckel's (or mandi[...] Reichert's (or hyoid) cartilages, resp[...] tively. By the 8th week, the tympanic cavity is present in the lower half of the future middle ear, while the upper half is filled with cellular mesenchyme (Fig. 2.5b). The classical theory of ossicle origin holds that the malleus and incus arise from Meckel's cartilage and the stapes comes from Reichert's cartilage. More recent observations, however, suggest a more complex and dual origin for the ossicles (Pearson et al., 1970). Currently the first branchial arch is credited for most of the body structure in the malleus and incus, while the second branchial arch gives rise to the lenticular process of the incus, the handle of the malleus, and the stapes. The middle ear cavity itself also has a dual origin with the anterior area coming from the first arch and the posterior area coming from the second arch. It is of interest to note that the mandible also arises from the first arch.

By 8½ weeks, the incus and the malleus have attained complete cartilaginous form similar to an adult (Fig. 2.5c). The stapes grows as a cartilaginous structure until the 15th week. By the 15th through the 16th week, ossification begins to occur in the cartilaginous surface of the malleus and incus, which have nearly reached completion by the 32nd week. The stapes does not begin to ossify until the 18th week and continues to develop even after ossification is complete. The stapes develops further during life. Surgeons recognize the stapes in a child to be more bulky and less delicate than the normal stapes seen in the adult.

As the ossicles begin to ossify, the surrounding mesenchymal tissue becomes loose, less cellular, and is absorbed into the mucoperiosteal membrane of the middle ear cavity. When the ossicles are free from mesenchyma, mucous membrane connecting each ossicle to the walls of the middle ear cavity remains to eventually become the ossicular supporting ligaments.

By the 30th week, development of the tympanum proper is almost complete. The middle ear cavity antrum is pneumatized by the 34th through 35th week, and the epitympanum is pneumatized during the last fetal month (36th to 38th week). The air cells of the temporal bone develop as outpouchings from the middle ear cavity during the 34th week. Air does not actually enter the middle ear cavity until the onset of respiration immediately after birth.

External Ear and Eardrum

The auricle develops during the 3rd or 4th week from the first and second branchial arches (Fig. 2.6a). Actually, the auricle is derived primarily from the second branchial arch, and only the tragus seems to originate from the first branchial arch. This is about the same time that the auditory vesicle is formed in the development of the inner ear.

During the 6th week, six hillocks or tissue thickenings form on both sides of the first branchial groove (Fig. 2.6b), arranged as three hillocks on each facing border. The ultimate shape and configuration of the adult auricle depends on the development of these six growth centers; thus many divergent forms of the auricle are within the extremely wide range of normal (Fig. 2.6c). Darwin's tubercle forms in some people as an irregularity in the posterior margin of the helix or outer edge of the auricle as shown in Figure 2.6d. At this time the mesenchymal folds of the auricle are beginning to become cartilage. From the 7th to the 20th week, the auricle continues to develop, moving from its original ventromedial position to be slowly displaced laterally by the growth of the mandible and face. At the 20th week the auricle is in the adult shape (Fig. 2.6d), but continues to grow in size until the individual is 9 years of age.

The external auditory meatus is derived from the first branchial groove during the 4th to 5th week. At this time, the ectodermal lining of the first branchial groove is in brief contact with the endodermal lining of the first pharyngeal pouch. Mesodermal tissue, however, soon grows between the two layers and separates the pharyngeal pouch from the branchial groove. In the 8th week, the primary auditory meatus sinks toward the middle ear cavity and becomes the outer one third of the auditory canal surrounded ultimately by cartilage.

The ectodermal groove continues to deepen toward the tympanic cavity from the external surface until it meets a thickening of epithelial cells known as the meatal plug which has arisen from surface ectoderm. Mesenchyme grows between the meatal plug and the epithelial cells of the tympanic cavity. These three layers of tissue, then, become the tympanic membrane composed of inner circular fibers, the fibrous middle layer of tissue, and the outer radial fiber layer, before the 9th week. The solid meatal plug, however, keeps the external auditory canal closed until the 21st week. By this time the inner and middle ear structures are well formed and ossified. The meatal plug disintegrates and forms a canal, with the innermost layer of meatal plug epithelium becoming the squamous epithelial layer of the tympanic membrane. The external auditory canal continues to develop until the 9th year. At birth the floor of the external auditory canal has no bony portion. In the infant, the external auditory canal is short and straight, while in the adult the canal in longer and curves. This suggests that the infant tympanic membrane might be easier to observe than the eardrum of the adult. That is not the case, however, because the infant tympanic membrane is in an oblique or almost a horizontal position and difficult to visualize. The bony portion of the external canal is not complete until about the 7th year. A summary of major embryologic features and their time sequence is presented in Table 2.1.

A young patient with evidence of multiple congenital anomalies related to first and second branchial arch origins is shown in Figure 2.7. This patient has been diagnosed to have Möbius syndrome, sometimes

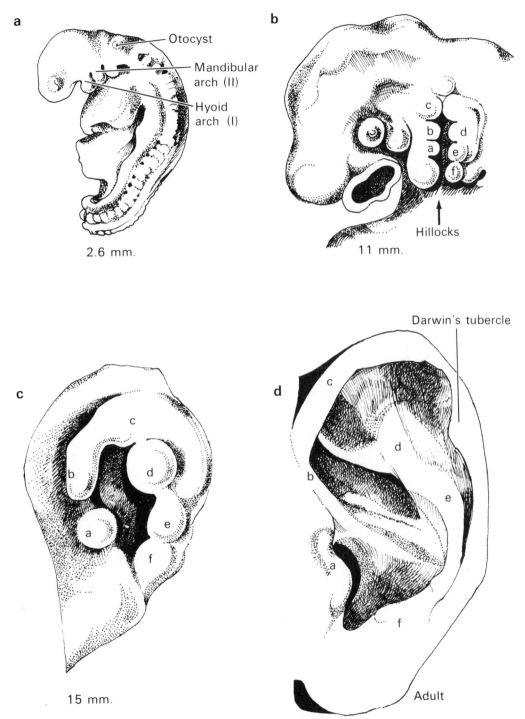

Figure 2.6. Schematic development of auricle from 3rd or 4th week to adult stage. (Modified with permission from L. A. Arey: *Developmental Anatomy*. Philadelphia, W. B. Saunders, 1940; and B. J. Anson: *An Atlas of Human Anatomy*, ed. 2. Philadelphia, W. B. Saunders, 1963.)

Table 2.1.
Embryology Summary of the Ear

Fetal Week	Inner Ear	Middle Ear	External Ear
3rd	Auditory placode; auditory pit	Tubotympanic recess begins to develop	
4th	Auditory vesicle (otocyst); vestibular-cochlear division		Tissue thickenings begin to form
5th			Primary auditory meatus begins
6th	Utricle and saccule present; semicircular canals begin		Six hillocks evident; cartilage begins to form
7th	One cochlear coil present; sensory cells in utricle and saccule		Auricles move dorsolaterally
8th	Ductus reuniens present: sensory cells in semicircular canals	Incus and malleus present in cartilage; lower half of tympanic cavity formed	Outer cartilaginous third of external canal formed
9th		Three tissue layers at tympanic membrane are present	
11th	Two and one-half cochlear coils present; nerve VIII attaches to cochlear duct		
12th	Sensory cells in cochlea; membranous labyrinth complete; otic capsule begins to ossify		
15th		Cartilaginous stapes formed	
16th		Ossification of malleus and incus begins	
18th		Stapes begins to ossify	
20th	Maturation of inner ear; inner ear adult size		Auricle is adult shape, but continues to grow until age 9
21st		Meatal plug disintegrates exposing tympanic membrane	
30th		Pneumatization of tympanum	External auditory canal continues to mature until age 7
32nd		Malleus and incus complete ossification	
34th		Mastoid air cells develop	
35th		Antrum is pneumatized	
37th		Epitympanum is pneumatized; stapes continues to develop until adulthood; tympanic membrane changes relative position during first 2 yr of life	

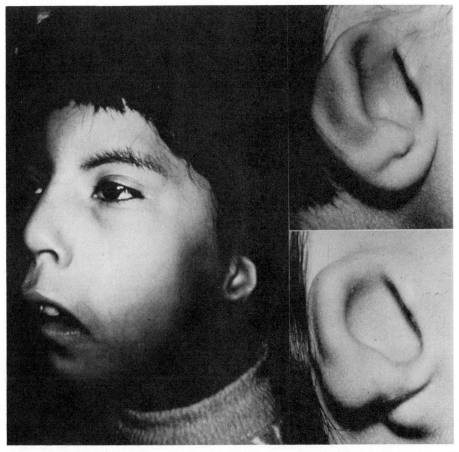

Figure 2.7. A patient with Möbius syndrome, with first and second branchial arch anomalies as described in the text.

termed aplasia of the sixth and seventh cranial nerve (Ford, 1966). Her cranial deformities include obvious malformations of the external ear, bilateral facial weakness producing a consistent masklike appearance, submucous cleft palate with a bifid uvula, and macrostomia or a greatly exaggerated width of the mouth resulting from failure of proper union of the maxillary and mandibular processes. She has no measurable hearing and is a student in a residential school for the deaf. Radiographic tomographic studies reveal symmetric middle ear anomalies including malleus and incus deformities, the absence of the oval window bilaterally, and mastoid dysplasia. The cochlea and semicircular canal system appear normal on the x-ray study, but the

internal auditory canals are abnormally narrow, measuring only 1.5 mm in diameter instead of the normal diameter of approximately 8.0 mm.

A general overview of human development is presented in Figure 2.8.

ANATOMY OF THE EAR THROUGH TEMPORAL BONE STUDY

Knowledge concerning the anatomy of the temporal bone is becoming increasingly more important to the clinician who deals with hearing loss patients. More and more journal articles and oral presentations at meetings include histologic temporal bone sections to demonstrate some aspect of deafness. Many of the significant advances in our knowledge about the etiology of deaf-

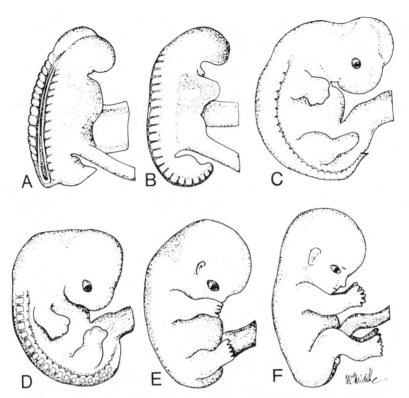

Figure 2.8. Human life and hearing develop together. (*A*) The neural tube, the heart and the brain begin to develop at 3 weeks concurrently with the auditory pit and tubotympanic recess; (*B*) in the 4-week-old embryo, limbs begin to appear and the otocyst develops: (*C*) the embryo is only ⅓ inch in length at the 5th week when the auditory meatus starts to form; (*D*) at 6 weeks, eyes, semicircular canals, and external ear hillocks develop; (*E*) embryonic 7th week includes initial formation of teeth, muscles, genitals, external ear and cochlea; (*F*) now nearly 1-inch long, at 8 weeks the embryo becomes a fetus, and the middle ear ossicles and tympanic membrane begin to form.

ness have come from careful study of temporal bone histologic sections. This new information has influenced many areas of clinical services including hearing aid fittings, educational recommendations and referrals, genetic counseling, and patient progress estimation.

Most speech and hearing training programs have infrequent access to normal or pathologic temporal bone sections. In fact, only a handful of nonmedical clinicians are experienced enough with this technical discipline to teach through the use of histologic sections. Yet this method of instruction enables the student to achieve an understanding of the anatomy of the structures of the ear and vestibular system, as well as an appreciation for the complexity

of the hearing mechanism. An understanding of the anatomy of the normal temporal bone will provide the clinician with new insight into the etiology and pathology of deafness.

The paucity of temporal bone anatomic sections available for the benefit of hearing and speech students has prompted us to include this section of histologic samples from a normal temporal bone. Our own understanding of deafness has been enhanced greatly by careful study of temporal bone anatomy and pathology, and we feel that it is important for students to examine fully the normal temporal bone sections presented in this chapter. These normal histologic samples may be used as a comparative reference for pathologic temporal bone sections shown in other chapters of this book. The clinician can extrapolate from what is known about the pathology of a given ear disease or genetic entity to other similar cases or patients. As example, knowledge of the temporal bone pathology of meningitis deafness can suggest that when little or no hearing can be detected in a child who has had meningitis, the probability of destruction of cochlear structures is quite high. Temporal bone studies of rubella deafness often demonstrate sections of nearly normal tissues that suggest the possibility of residual hearing in a youngster with this disorder, despite clinical failures in obtaining measurable audiometric responses.

Temporal Bone

The temporal bone forms part of the lateral wall and base of the skull, as shown in Figure 2.9. It articulates with other bones of the skull including the sphenoid, parietal, and occipital bones. The petrous part of the temporal bone is the most dense bone of the body, and contains, among other things, most of the structures of the ear. The temporal bone is generally divided into four sections—the squamous, mastoid, petrous, and tympanic areas (Anson and Donaldson, 1967). In general terms, the squamous portion of the temporal bone is superior to the external auditory meatus; the mastoid area is posterior; while the tym-

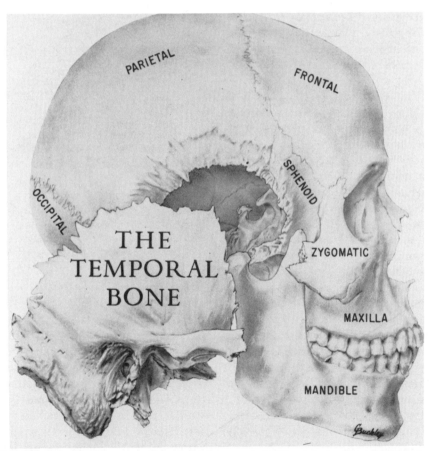

Figure 2.9. The temporal bone section of the human skull. (Reprinted with permission from B. J. Anson and J. A. Donaldson: *The Surgical Anatomy of the Temporal Bone and Ear*, Philadelphia, W. B. Saunders, 1967.)

panic portion forms the anterior, inferior, and part of the posterior walls of the external auditory meatus.

The petrous portion of the temporal bone extends medially from the external auditory canal, and its middle third contains the structures of the middle and inner ear. In the petrous bone it is important to note that the cochlear portion of the inner ear is situated anteriorly and medially to the internal auditory meatus and the vestibular portion of the inner ear. The internal auditory meatus houses the facial nerve (seventh) which lies superior to the auditory portion of the acoustic nerve (eighth) and anterior to the superior vestibular branch of the eighth cranial nerve. The petrous bone is shown in Figure 2.10 as part of the base of the skull as seen from above.

Preparation of Temporal Bone Histologic Sections. The density of the temporal bone and intricacy of the inner ear structures make preparation of suitable histologic slides from the gross bone specimen very difficult. Only a few laboratories in the United States are capable of processing temporal bone specimens into adequate slides for examination.

The processing of a temporal bone into slides is a difficult, demanding, precise, time-consuming, and expensive procedure. Initially, the temporal bone must be removed from the skull of the donor within 24 hours of death or the inner ear structures undergo autolysis. The bone is immediately submerged in formalin for 2 or 3 weeks for fixation of structures. An extensive decalcification process follows for some 5 weeks in an adult bone to remove the dense calcium from the temporal bone. Infant temporal bones that are hours or days old may not show the presence of calcium after the 1st or 2nd week in the decalcification solutions. Excess bone is then pared from the gross structure, and the decalcification chemicals are neutralized and the bone carefully washed.

The temporal bone is then dehydrated with ethyl alcohol solutions, infiltrated,

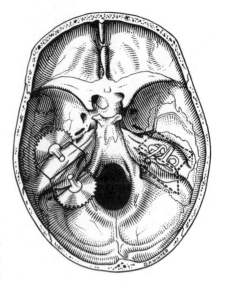

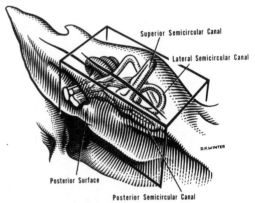

Figure 2.10. Petrous portion of temporal bone shown as part of the skull viewed from above. (Reprinted with permission from J. C. Gallagher: *Histology of the Human Temporal Bone.* American Registry of Pathology. Washington, D.C., Armed Forces Institute of Pathology, 1967.)

and embedded into varying solutions of celloidin for nearly 3 months. The celloidin provides support for the bone tissues to permit sectioning with a microtome.

The temporal bone is sliced into sections of 20 μm thickness, forming some 400 sections from each temporal bone. Only every 10th section is initially stained with dyes, generally hematoxylin and eosin to give the various tissues color for ease in identification. The dyed sections are mounted on microscope slides, ready for reading.

Examination of the stained sections of the temporal bone under high-powered magnification takes expert skills and knowledge gained only through experience and thorough study. The entire procedure involved in preparation of a single temporal bone may involve some 5 individuals, 9 months of time, and is estimated to cost more than a thousand dollars.

Anatomy of a Normal Temporal Bone. An understanding of normal temporal bone structures is necessary before one can appreciate the abnormalities found in temporal bone from patients with various kinds of deafness. Temporal bone study is usually reserved for residents in otolaryngology or physiologists interested in studying mechanisms of hearing, but there seems sufficient reason for all students of hearing disorders to have some

familiarity with anatomy as demonstrated by horizontally cut, temporal bone histopathologic sections.

One must keep in mind the general level of the section under study as it was taken from the inner ear, or temporal bone block. Figure 2.11 shows the general gross structure of the inner ear. Imagine a horizontal line drawn through the most superior portion of the inner ear and you will see that the only structure represented might be the arch of the superior semicircular canal. As the microtome cuts off horizontal sections from a temporal bone block, the superior semicircular canal will be the initial structure to be sectioned. One must then imagine how a horizontal slice of temporal bone tissue will appear when placed on a microscope slide and viewed from above. The student of temporal bone anatomy must

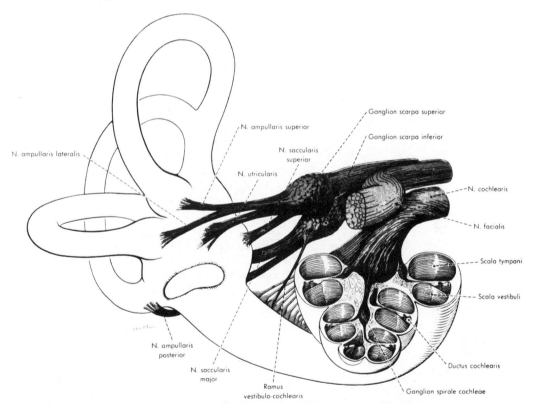

Figure 2.11. The inner ear. Note the position of the facial nerve to the cochlear nerve and to the superior and inferior vestibular nerve. The cochlea is open to illustrate the midmodiolar view as observed in temporal bone sections. (Reprinted with permission from B. J. Melloni: *Some Pathological Conditions of the Eye, Ear, and Throat: An Atlas.* Chicago, Abbott Laboratories, 1957.)

have a draftsman's ability to imagine three-dimensional structures from a two-dimensional picture.

Samples sections from a horizontally sectioned petrous portion of a temporal bone are shown in the next few pages. The sections have been selected because they show specific portions of the inner ear that are of interest to audiologists. Photographs of the midmodiolar section of the cochlear and a single coil, or turn of the cochlear and a single coil, or turn of the cochlea, have been included at higher magnification, so readers can appreciate these interesting structures.

Figure 2.12. Well pneumatized mastoid in the posterior (or left) area of this section. The ampulla of the superior semicircular canal is shown as a nearly round structure enclosing the membranous labyrinth. The crista is noticeable on the anterior edge of the superior semicircular canal ampulla. The facial nerve and its genu are very clearly shown in this slide, which has cut across the superior portion of the internal auditory canal. Immediately anterior to the genu of the facial nerve is the dense bone of the otic capsule which contains the cochlea. The lateral semicircular canal and its membranous labyrinth is also present at the peripheral edges of the structure.

Figure 2.13. This section is approximately 1 mm below the previous slide. The middle ear cavity is now obvious in this section and contains a cross-section view of the malleus and incus joined by the malleoincudal joint. The facial nerve is now encased in the facial canal. The upper portion of the basal turn of the cochlea is now present anteriorly and medially to the facial nerve. The superior branch of the vestibular nerve is visible in the internal auditory meatus, and is shown passing to the macula of the utricle. The endolymphatic duct is also present.

Figure 2.14. A section approximately 1 mm below the section shown in the previous figure. The middle ear cavity shows the malleus and incus with its short process

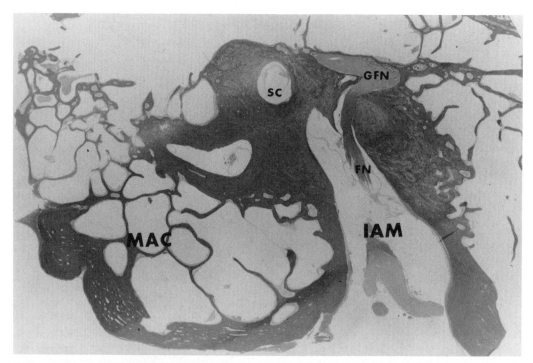

Figure 2.12. Temporal bone horizontal section showing facial nerve genu (*GFN*), facial nerve (*FN*), internal auditory meatus (*IAM*), ampulla of superior semicircular canal (*SC*), and mastoid air cells (*MAC*). (Courtesy of I. Sando, M.D.)

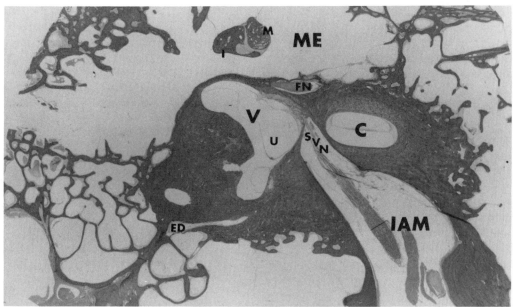

Figure 2.13. Horizontal section of normal temporal bone showing malleus (*M*) and incus (*I*) in attic of middle ear (*ME*), utricle (*U*), basal turn of the cochlea (*C*), and superior vestibular nerve (*SVN*), feeding into vestibule (*V*) from the internal auditory meatus (*IAM*). The endolymphatic duct (*ED*) is seen at lower left corner. (Courtesy of I. Sando, M.D.)

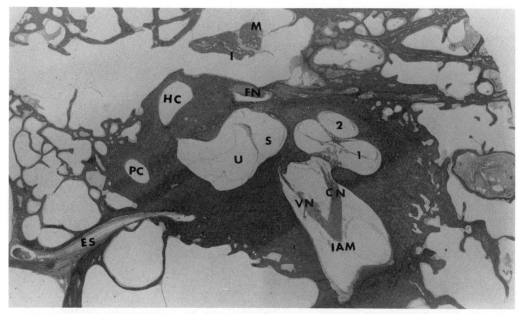

Figure 2.14. Horizontal section from normal temporal bone showing two cochlear turns, basal (*1*) and middle (*2*); vestibular (*VN*) and cochlear (*CN*) portions of the eighth nerve in the internal auditory meatus (*IAM*), the endolymphatic sac (*ES*) is shown at lower left. The uricle (*U*) and the saccule (*S*) may be seen in the vestibule. The horizontal (*HC*) and posterior (*PC*) semicircular canals are also identified. (*M*) Malleus; (*I*) incus; (*FN*) facial nerve. (Courtesy of I. Sando, M.D.).

pointing posteriorly toward the aditus and antrum into the mastoid air spaces. The anterior mallear ligament can also be seen. The large space immediately medial to the facial nerve and canal contains the utricle. This section passes through the basal and middle turns of the cochlea which extend laterally. Reissner's membrane, the basilar membrane, and spiral ligament are obvious, even at this magnification. The modiolus is evident in the center of the basal turn of the cochlea. The inferior division of the vestibular nerve and the cochlear branch of the auditory nerve are shown in the internal auditory meatus. The endolymphatic sac is apparent in the posteriormedial portion of the photograph.

Figure 2.15. This section is about 1 mm lower than the section shown in Figure 2.14. This section passes through the bony modiolus of the basal and middle turns of the cochlea and now includes the final cochlear turn, the apical coil. In the middle ear, the malleus and incus are no longer touching. The large tensor tympani muscle in its canal is very obvious immediately adjacent to the cochlea and running anteroposterior. This section shows the processus cochleariformis extending posteriorly into the middle ear cavity from which the small

tensor tympani tendon can be seen attaching to the anterior surface of the malleus. Part of the stapedial crura can be seen with the stapes footplate in the oval window niche. (An enlargement of the stapes in the oval window with the attachment of the stapedial tendon is shown in Fig. 2.16.) The

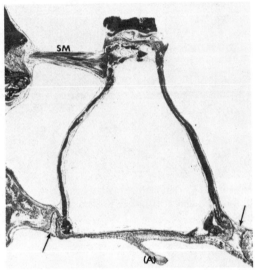

Figure 2.16. Enlargement of stapes in oval window and stapedial tendon (*SM*). Note normal attachment of stapes footplate in oval window by annular ligament (*arrows*). (Courtesy of E. L. Grandon, M.D., Cedar Rapids, Iowa.)

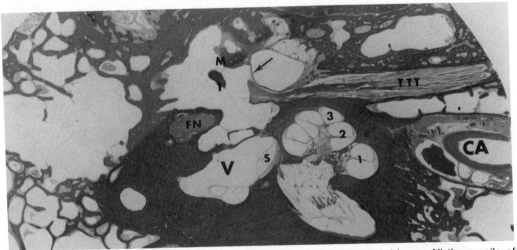

Figure 2.15. Cochlear midmodiolar horizontal section of normal temporal bone. All three coils of cochlea (*1, 2,* and *3*) are evident; the malleus (*M*) is attached to tympanic membrane; the tensor tympani muscle (*TTT*) extends through the processus cochleariformis with tensor tendon (identified by arrow) to malleus. (*FN*) facial nerve; (*V*) vestibule; (*CA*) internal carotid artery; (*I*) incus; (*S*) saccule. (Courtesy of I. Sando, M.D.)

saccule and its innervation can be seen clearly in the vestibule along with the lateral semicircular canal and utricle. The large circular structure at the anterior edge of the section is the internal carotid artery. All three ossicles are difficult to demonstrate on one temporal bone section because they are not lined up equally on a single horizontal plane level.

Figure 2.17. An enlargement of the cochlea as viewed in Figure 2.15. It may be useful to the reader to review the gross view of the inner ear in Figure 2.11 to see how this exposure of the cochlea is obtained. This is a midmodiolar section of the cochlea showing the basal, middle, and apical turns. The nerve fibers are easily seen in the internal auditory meatus, and the ganglion cells of the spiral ganglion may be seen in Rosenthal's canal. The osseous spiral lamina extends radially from the modiolus in each turn. The basilar membrane can be seen extending from the osseous spiral lamina to the spiral ligament and stria vascularis. Reissner's membrane is seen in each coil of the cochlea, separating the scala

vestibuli from the scala media. The basilar membrane supports the organ of Corti which can just barely be seen at this magnification.

Figure 2.18. The classic view of a cochlear turn, emphasizing the structures of the scala media. These structures can be observed on a human temporal bone section by increasing the magnification on a single cochlear turn. The cochlear nerve fibers are shown under the spiral osseous lamina at the left of the photograph. The limbus supports one end of the tectorial membrane, which in its natural position should extend over the outer hair cells. The tectorial membrane, however, is very often seen in distorted position as an artifact of the temporal bone preparation procedure. Reissner's membrane extends from the limbus (crista spiralis) to the edge of the spiral ligament and stria vascularis. The curve between the limbus and the organ of Corti is the internal sulcus. The lower edge of the limbus, pointing and extending toward the organ of Corti, is known as the tympanic lip, which has numerous holes termed the

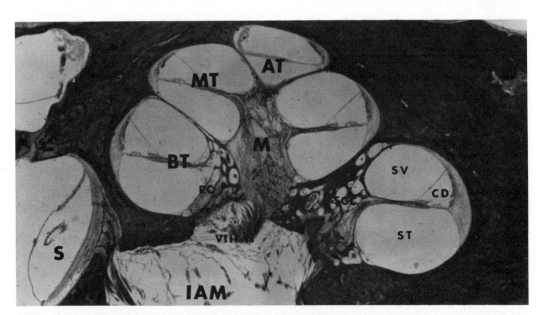

Figure 2.17. Enlargment of cochlea from horizontal temporal bone section shown in Figure 2.15. Note auditory nerve (*VIII N*) in internal auditory meatus (*IAM*) with ganglion cells (*SGC*) in Rosenthal's canal (*RC*). The cochlear basal turn (*BT*), the middle turn (*MT*), and apical turn (*AT*) are clearly shown. Three ducts are seen in each turn, the scala vestibuli (*SV*), cochlear duct (*Cd*), and scala tympani (*ST*); the saccule is also obvious in this view (*S*) with its innervation. (*M*) Modiolus. (Courtesy of I. Sando, M.D.)

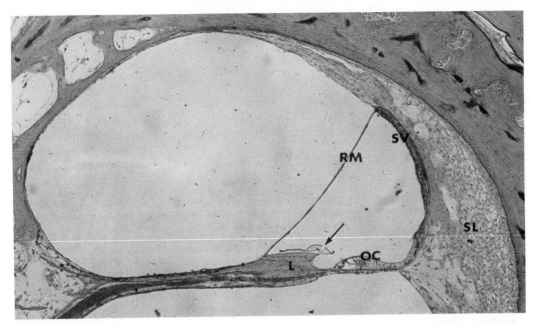

Figure 2.18. Higher magnification of one cochlear duct showing organ of Corti (*OC*), spiral ligament (*SL*), stria vascularis (*SV*), Reissner's membrane (*RM*), tectorial membrane (*arrow*), and limbus (*L*). (Courtesy of I. Sando, M.D., and L. Bergstrom, M.D.)

habenula perforata. The habenula perforata permit cochlear nerve fibers to enter the organ of Corti from below the osseous spiral lamina.

The basilar membrane supports the organ of Corti which includes inner hair cells, outer hair cells, and the tunnel of Corti. The tunnel of Corti is formed by inner and outer pillar cells. Various supporting cells are seen next to the hair cells. Hensen's and Claudius' supporting cells are found between the outer hair cells and the external sulcus formed by the lower curve of the stria vascularis. Nuel's space is between the outer pillar and the first row of outer hair cells. The outer hair cells are supported by outer phalangeal cells (Deiter's cells). Thus, the outer hair cell rests on a Deiter's cell and extends hairs from its upper surface toward the tectorial membrane. The lower portion of the stria vascularis contains a bulge known as the spiral prominence, which contains a blood vessel, the vas prominens.

Our understanding of the anatomy and physiology of the fine structure of the inner ear has increased tremendously since utilization of the electron microscope began in 1951. A newer type of microscope—the scanning electron microscope—is now adding new dimension to our appreciation of inner ear structures. Unlike the conventional electron microscope which transmits an electron beam through the specimen, the image in the scanning microscope is created by secondary electrons emitted from the excited surface of the specimen. The result is a picture similar to the image produced on a television screen. The depth of field obtained with the scanning microscope is about 500 times that of a light microscope. An outstanding monograph has been published by David Lim (1969) featuring three-dimensional views of the inner ear with the scanning electron microscope. A photograph of the organ of Corti taken with a scanning electron microscope is shown in Figure 2.19.

PHYSIOLOGY OF HEARING

In order to fully appreciate the intricacies of hearing impairment, one must under-

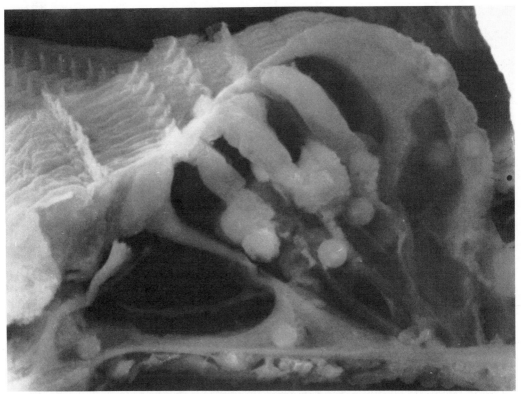

Figure 2.19. Scanning electron microscopic view of the organ of Corti from a guinea pig. (Courtesy of David Asher, Ph.D., University of Colorado School of Medicine).

stand the normal physiology of the hearing mechanism and the nature of hearing loss. These concepts are presented lightly here only as background material so that we may develop discussion regarding the pathologies of hearing impairment in the following chapter.

The phenomenon of hearing is the result of a complex series of events. Sound energy, originating as vibration and transmitted through an elastic medium such as air, impinges on the tympanic membrane causing it to vibrate. The vibrations are transmitted to the oval window of the otic capsule by the three middle ear ossicles. In addition to serving as a conductor to the sound energy, the tympanic membrane and ossicles amplify the sound by two simple mechanical principles consisting of a slight lever action of the ossicles and the areal surface relationship between the surface area of the tympanic membrane and the funneling of

sound energy onto the smaller surface area of the stapes footplate. This middle ear amplification amounts to approximately 30 dB, and may be lost when defects or pathologies inhibit either or both of the amplifying mechanisms (Lipscomb, 1984).

The mechanical vibration transmitted by the stapes to the oval window induces motion in the fluids of the cochlea where the intensity and frequency of the vibrations are faithfully transmitted by traveling waves to the receptor cells for hearing. Perilymph fluid fills two ducts within the cochlea known as the scala vestibuli and the scala tympani. These parallel scalae communicate with each other at the helicotrema in the apical tip of the cochlear coils. When sound vibration displaces the stapes inward into the scala vestibuli, a simultaneous outward motion occurs in the scala tympani at the round window membrane which is termed the round window reflex.

We also can hear by vibrations which bypass the external and middle ear, displacing fluids of the cochlea and resulting in traveling waves which stimulate the hairs of the receptor cells within the organ of Corti.

The organ of Corti is a papillary structure resting on a basilar membrane within the scala media (cochlear duct) and is composed of sensorineural receptors and supporting elements. The organ of Corti is specifically designed to convert mechanical vibrations into electrical events which are transmitted to the central nervous system (CNS).

The vibratory fluid motion in the cochlea ultimately causes a nerve impulse, with the cochlear neural epithelium acting as a mechanical transducer. This cochlear epithelium is composed of about 16,800 hair cells in each ear. According to Bredberg (1968) the hair cells are arranged in an inner row, averaging 3,400 cells (range from 2,800 to 4,000), while some 13,400 hair cells (range from 11,200 to 16,000) are found in three to five rows in the cochlea. The hair cells rest on supporting cells which in turn rest on the basilar membrane, and extend into a third cochlear duct, filled with endolymph fluid known as the scala media or cochlear duct. This third duct is interposed between the scala vestibuli and scala tympani throughout the entire two and a half turns of the cochlea. Hair cells have an orderly arrangement in the cochlea related to sound frequency. Hair cells that respond to high frequency above 2000 Hz are located in the basal turn of the cochlea, while hair cells that are tuned to stimulating frequencies below 2000 Hz are found in the middle and apical cochlear coils.

The peripheral neurons of the cochlear nerve are distributed to hair cells from beneath the basilar membrane and its supporting shelf, the osseous spiral lamina. The fluid motion of the scala tympani displaces the basilar membrane in a traveling wave pattern, due to its physical properties of width, length, thickness, mass and elasticity, producing torsion on the hairlike processes of the cell and creating some type of mechanical-chemical change resulting in peripheral-nerve-ending stimulation (Ryan and Dallos, 1984). Thus, the vibratory energy transmitted by the tympanic membrane is transformed into neural impulse code. Interested readers are referred to Dallos' (1973) text for a more complete discussion of cochlear physiology.

Auditory Nerve

The nerve fibers that innervate the hair cells have their cell bodies in the bipolar spiral ganglion which is located in Rosenthal's canal. Axons from the spiral ganglion cells join in the modiolus and collect as the auditory, or cochlear, branch of the eighth nerve. Just outside the cochlea the vestibular portion of the eighth nerve coming from the semicircular canals, utricle, and saccule, joins the cochlear portion. The two portions of the eighth nerve come together like a rope and pass through the internal auditory meatus toward the medulla. The structure of the auditory nerve is orderly, with fibers from the apical quarter of the cochlea forming the core of the nerve, and around them the fibers from the apex of the cochlea twisting one way, while the fibers from the middle turn of the cochlea twist the other way. Fifty percent of the fibers from the cochlea come from the basal coil, and represent sensory elements that respond to frequencies above 2000 Hz.

Research by Spoendlin (1967, 1969) has shown that most of the afferent neurons come from the inner hair cells, whereas only some 10% of the fibers come from the outer hair cells. Each outer hair cell is, however, innervated by several different neurons, while one neuron innervates a large number of outer hair cells. The inner hair cells are innervated by a large number of different neurons, but each neuron innervates only one inner hair cell.

The eighth nerve divides again, however, before it reaches the medulla. The auditory portion divides into dorsal and ventral branches which go to corresponding nuclei in the brain stem wherein the second-order afferent auditory neuron cell bodies are located.

Experimenters have found that fibers in the eighth nerve are "tuned" to certain frequencies. That is, certain fibers are most responsive to certain stimulating frequencies. This fact is determined by inserting microelectrodes into single nerve fibers and determining the threshold for the action potential "spike" of that nerve fiber for a variety of frequencies, then plotting what is known as the response area for that particular fiber. The threshold sensitivity of a fiber increases gradually and is most sensitive at its "tuned" frequency—which can then be used to name the fiber, such as "7000 Hz fiber." Most of the auditory fibers are high frequency units, usually above 1000 Hz. More recent observations indicate that individual inner hair cells also maintain characteristic responses to "tuned" frequencies, and may actually be more finely tuned than the nerve fibers (Evans and Wilson, 1973). It is remarkable that only a few fibers of the eighth nerve are required to preserve good hearing. The auditory nerve must be sectioned more than halfway to have a measurable effect on hearing, and then, if indeed hearing is left, it is predominantly low frequency hearing (Neff, 1947; Wever and Neff, 1947). To click stimuli, the individual nerve responses, tuned to different frequencies, fire in close synchrony, so that the amplitude of the action potential is representative of the number of fibers that respond (Davis, 1961).

Brainstem Pathways

Much of the brainstem auditory pathway can be seen in Figures 2.20 and 2.21 and is well described by Nolte (1981). The higher auditory pathways are rather complex and often escape significance with students who tend only to memorize the names of the relay stations and major neuronal paths. It is important to realize that although first-order neurons from the cochlea reach the brainstem in the cochlear nuclei, most of the activity that ultimately reaches the cortex is by the way of fourth-order neurons. This seemingly too complex system seldom

breaks down because of alternate paths to the cerebral cortex (Goldstein, 1982; Lynn and Gilroy, 1984).

Two pairs of cochlear nuclei exist, a dorsal and a ventral cochlear nucleus on each side of the medulla, but are referred to collectively as the cochlear nuclei of the medulla. Although some of the neurons of the cochlear nuclei ascend to higher nuclei on the same side of the system, most cross over to the opposite side in the trapezoid body. Auditory units in the cochlear nuclei are also sensitive to specific frequencies as we noted previously with auditory nerve fibers. Inhibitory units have also been reported in the cochlear nuclei, which under certain circumstances actually inhibit response rather than excite the unit under examination. Thus a particular frequency stimulus may excite certain neurons of the auditory system, while inhibiting other units from firing. What starts out in the cochlea as the excitation of the relatively large group of hair cells is narrowed down to a smaller group of neurons through the process of inhibition. In addition, the cochlear nuclei, like the cochlea, exhibit tonotopic organization, or an orderly arrangement of responsiveness to different frequencies. In fact, Rose et al. (1959) reported one unrolling of the cochlear frequency distribution in the dorsal cochlear nucleus and two separate complete frequency patterns in the ventral nuclei. The number of discharges from a single cochlear nucleus unit is apparently related to the intensity of the acoustic stimulus.

The principal terminations of second-order afferent auditory neurons are in the nuclei of the trapezoid body and superior olivary body. The superior olive is the first structure in the medulla which receives fibers from both ears, and may play a role in the localization of sound. From here, neurons originate that course upward in the loosely compacted neurons of the lateral lemniscus to another principal relay station, the inferior colliculus. Collaterals of second- and third-order neurons are given off to the reticular formation which provides an indirect, diffuse, sensory pathway

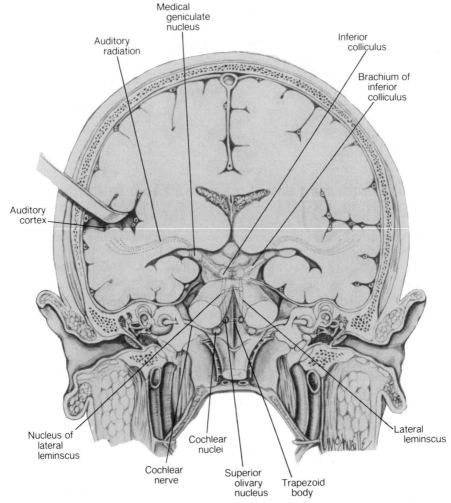

Figure 2.20. The ascending auditory pathway. (Reprinted with permission from J. Nolte: *The Human Brain: An Introduction to Its Functional Anatomy.* St. Louis, C. V. Mosby, 1981.)

to the cerebral cortex. The reticular formation is closely related to arousal and attention during sleep, and may be responsible for the fact that a crying baby may wake only mother, but no one else in the family. Or one may sleep soundly through a barrage of noise but wake suddenly upon hearing a soft familiar voice.

Most of the fibers in the lateral lemniscus pathway terminate in the inferior colliculus, but some may bypass and end in the next relay station, the medial geniculate body. So far as is known, all direct projections to the auditory cortex are relayed in the medial geniculate body. The auditory

cortex is, of course, responsible for the fine discrimination that is necessary in the understanding of speech. The "tuning" function of the higher auditory centers, including the inferior colliculus, the medial geniculate body, and the auditory cortex, has been summarized by Ades (1959): some units at higher levels in the auditory system are frequency specific and some are not; many units respond only to clicks with a complex spectrum and are unresponsive to pure tone signals; many units show spontaneous firing which can sometimes be inhibited by acoustic stimuli; and of the units that are frequency-specific, the response

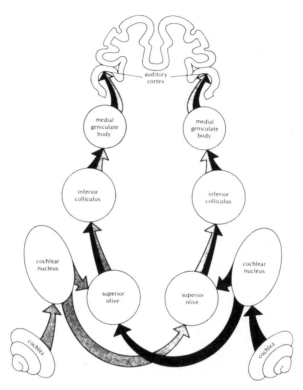

Figure 2.21. A diagrammatic scheme for the ascending auditory pathway. (Reprinted with permission from W. A. Yost and D. W. Nielsen: *Fundamentals of Hearing.* New York, Holt, Rinehart & Winston, 1977.)

areas of the units higher up in the auditory system tend to be narrower than those units found in lower auditory centers. An estimated cell count of each of the levels in the afferent auditory pathway is presented in Table 2.2 (Schuknecht, 1974).

Attempts to map the cortical responses to auditory stimuli have identified the temporal lobe as the responsive area, sometimes further localized as Brodmann's areas 41 and 42. The cortex has at least two tonotopic frequency projections which are the reverse of each other. Kryter and Ades (1943) established a very important fact with significant clinical implication. They showed that, under appropriate conditions, cortical lesions have no appreciable effect on the absolute thresholds of pure tone stimuli. This is true even when extensive bilateral cortical lesions are made. Thus, the ability to respond to tones is not dependent upon cerebral cortex. These

Table 2.2.
Afferent Auditory Pathways and Estimated Cell Count at Each Level

Cochlear nuclei	8,800
Superior olivary complex	34,000
Nuclei of lateral lemniscus	38,000
Inferior colliculus	392,000
Medial geniculate body	364,000
Auditory cortex	10,000,000

same investigators reported that removal of the inferior colliculi created an approximate 15-dB loss in pure tone sensitivity; destruction of the entire auditory system from the midbrain to the cortex created a pure tone loss of about 40 dB. It may be concluded that the most important aspect of auditory sensitivity to pure tones is due to intact neurons below the inferior colliculi, and a nearly normal audiogram may be obtained with a loss of 75% of the neurons of the auditory nerve.

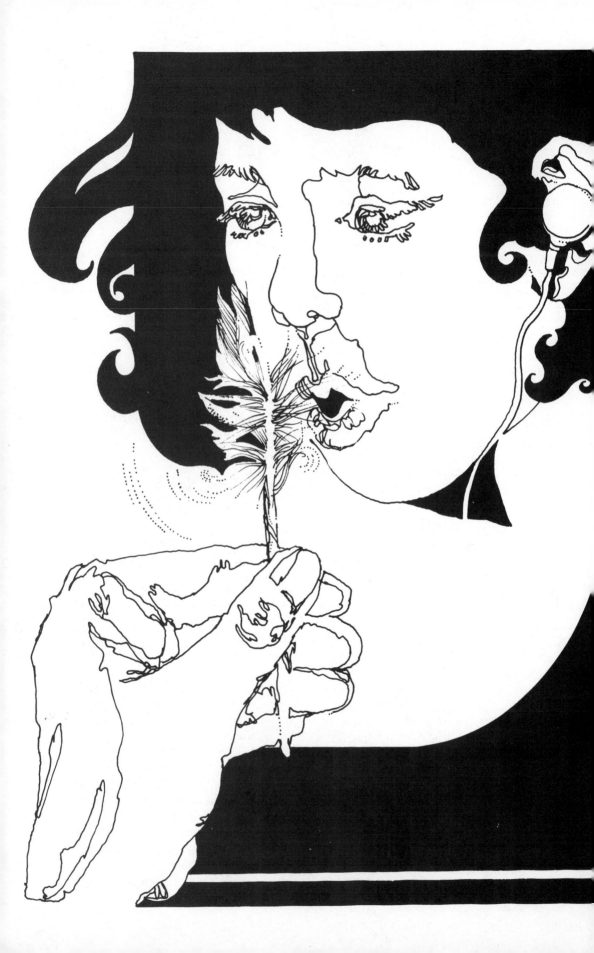

CHAPTER 3

Medical Aspects of Hearing Loss

THE NATURE OF HEARING LOSS

Hearing losses are generally identified as conductive or sensorineural. When a combination of both types of hearing loss occurs, we speak of a mixed type hearing loss. When auditory dysfunction can be shown to exist, yet peripheral hearing mechanisms are within normal limits, the loss is categorized as a central auditory defect.

Conductive Hearing Loss

Interference of any sort in the transmission of sound from the external auditory canal to the inner ear causes conductive hearing loss. The inner ear, in such cases, is capable of normal function, but the sound vibration is able to stimulate the cochlea only with increased stimulus intensity via the normal air conduction pathway (Fig. 3.1).

The conductive-type loss is characterized by a hearing loss for air-conducted sounds, while sounds conducted to the inner ear directly by bone conduction of the skull and temporal bone are heard normally. When the air-conductive pathway is totally blocked as in atresia, stenosis, complete stapes fixation, or ossicular discontinuity, a maximal 60-dB air-conduction hearing loss will exist. Although some conductive hearing losses may resolve spontaneously, frequently some residual of middle ear effusion may remain for long periods of time. Most conductive hearing losses can be corrected through medical treatment or surgery.

Sensorineural Hearing Loss

Hearing impairment occurs when damage has been sustained by the sensory end organ or cochlear hair cells, or the dysfunction may be the fault of the auditory nerve. Traditionally, damage to the sensory end organ is not easily differentiated from neuronal damage, so the resultant hearing loss is lumped under the category "sensorineural." New testing techniques such as electrocochleography and auditory evoked potentials offer promise as an objective means of differentiating between sensory and neural hearing impairment.

In sensorineural hearing losses the air and bone conduction thresholds are nearly the same. Sensorineural hearing losses may easily be overlooked during physical examination since the external auditory canal and tympanic membrane will appear normal. This type of hearing loss is nearly always irreversible.

Mixed Hearing Loss

When both a sensorineural loss and a conductive hearing loss are present, the result is a mixed hearing loss. The audiogram shows less-than-normal bone conduction thresholds which are closer to normal levels than the air-conduction thresholds. A significant air-conduction/bone-conduction gap between threshold levels may exist, which should disappear when the conductive portion of the hearing loss is ameliorated. The mixed hearing loss, however, improves only as much as the degree of air/bone gap, and hearing levels are not likely to return to normal limits.

Central Auditory Dysfunction

This type of impairment is not necessarily accompanied by a decrease in auditory sensitivity but tends to manifest itself in

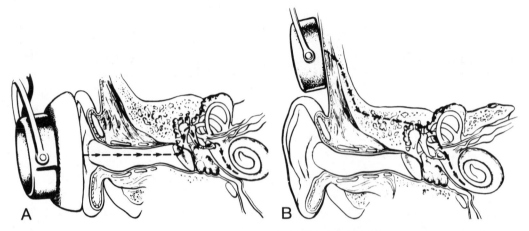

Figure 3.1. *Broken arrow lines* show routes of air-conduction hearing pathway (*A*), and bone-conduction hearing pathway (*B*). (Reprinted with permission from Zenatron Corp., Chicago.)

varying degrees as a decrease in auditory comprehension. For example, the child may have a normal audiogram, but be unable to recognize or interpret speech. Central auditory dysfunction is a complex topic and is discussed more fully in Chapter 4.

Degree and Severity of Hearing Loss

An important consideration of any hearing loss is its degree of impairment. Common descriptive terms used to identify degree of hearing loss include mild hearing loss (26–40 dB), moderate hearing loss (31–65 dB), severe hearing loss (66–95 dB), profound hearing loss (96+ dB), and anacusis or total hearing loss. Sometimes borderline categories of hearing impairment are described with a combination of terms such as "moderately severe" hearing loss.

Additional consideration regarding the severity of the hearing loss must be given to its unilateral or bilateral presence. The child with a totally dead ear on one side but with a normal ear on the other side may function adequately in most situations. He will fail the school screening test, however, and presents special problems to the audiologist who tests his hearing. This youngster's auditory abilities will be lacking in circumstances where sound localization is needed or in instances when noise

exists to compete with the signal of interest. Read management of the child with unilateral deafness (Chapter 5) for more information.

A complete description of a youngster's hearing loss should include its presence as unilateral or bilateral, in addition to a term which identifies its degree of auditory impairment, as well as a statement regarding the type of loss as conductive, sensorineural, or mixed. From the physician's diagnosis a description of the cause of the hearing loss can be made. Samples of hearing loss descriptions might include unilateral, severe sensorineural hearing loss due to mumps, or a bilateral, moderate conductive hearing loss due to middle ear effusion.

DISORDERS ASSOCIATED WITH HEARING LOSS

Detailed descriptions of disorders associated with hearing loss are presented in most textbooks in otolaryngology such as English's *Otolaryngology: A Textbook* (1976), Jaffe's *Hearing Loss in Children* (1977), Goodhill's *Ear Diseases, Deafness and Dizzyness* (1979), and Northern's *Hearing Disorders* (1984). Audiology textbooks may offer material on hearing pathology, but usually in a nonmedical manner so that insufficient information is available to audiologists who work with medical personnel. The material presented below is not as complete as that found in otolaryngology textbooks, but hopefully is more pertinent to childhood disorders than that commonly found in basic audiology books.

Conditions of the External Ear and Ear Canal

The audiologist may have confrontation with various medical conditions involving the pinna and external auditory canal. The fitting of ear defenders for hearing conservation, the making of earmold impressions, and the insertion of impedance probe tips make it imperative for the clinician to recognize disorders of the external ear (Baker and Northern, 1976).

In order to recognize the presence of a diseased state, one must appreciate the normal anatomy of the pinna, the external auditory canal, and their normal variations. The pinna or auricle is an appendage attached to the side of the head, level with the middle third of the face. It is composed of a piece of elastic cartilage with numerous convolutions, covered with thin skin, and fixed in position at the lateral aspect of the external auditory canal by its direct continuity with the cartilaginous canal, auricular muscles, and auricular ligaments. Its major convolutions include the helix, anthelix, tragus, antitragus, and concha. The lobule is unique in that it contains no cartilage and, therefore, has been designated by various cultures as the appropriate place through which, and on which, to hang ornaments for decoration.

An opening, the external auditory meatus, in the concha leads to the external auditory canal which is cartilaginous in the lateral third and bony in the medial two thirds. The cartilage of the external auditory canal is continuous with that of the pinna except in the anterosuperior aspect. Present in the anterior cartilaginous canal wall are several fissures to permit flexibility. Hence, the curved path of the canal can be partially straightened to facilitate inspection by gently pulling posterosuper-

iorly on the pinna. Squamous epithelium lines the external canal and covers the tympanic membrane. This skin is thicker laterally with hair follicles, sebaceous glands, and ear wax-producing glands, but is quite thin over the more medial bony portion of the canal with fewer skin structures present. This skin is unusual because it does not flake as other squamous epithelium, but migrates laterally toward the external meatus, providing a self-cleaning mechanism unique to the ear canal.

At the onset of every clinical evaluation or testing procedure, one should initially note the location of the pinnae and their relationship to the remainder of the structures of the head and face. Normally the superior border of the helix is located at the outer canthus of the eye and the tragus is roughly level with the infraorbital rim (Fig. 3.2). Lowset auricles are frequently associated with other anomalies of the first and second branchial cleft and with abnormalities of the urinary system (Mengel et al., 1969). Even though the pinna may have no abnormality in its location or basic shape, the alert clinician should be aware of any lump, ulcer, or lesion on the pinna.

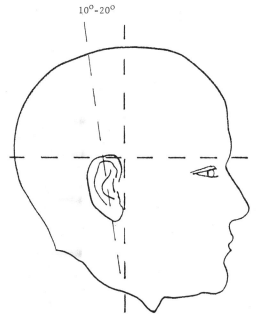

Figure 3.2. Pinna in relationship to structures of face.

After ascertaining that the pinna is located in the normal position, one should observe the size and shape of the auricle. The child with ears that stick out from his head in a prominent fashion may have severe social problems from the ridicule of his peers. Successful surgical treatment of a patient with this deformity prior to the patient's entering school may save a great deal of emotional anguish. About 90% of the time this condition is the result of an excessively deep concha and/or lack of development of the anthelical fold. Correction of these deformities is easily accomplished through an incision of the back of the pinna through which stitches are then used to hold the ear in its new position.

Atresia or Stenosis of the Canal. Atresia is the complete closing off of the ear canal while stenosis is a narrowing of the canal. Atresia or stenosis may accompany microtia, or either may appear in conjunction with a normal auricle (Fig. 3.3). Stenosis may be congenital or acquired. The embryonic atresia plate may be solid bone or membraneous; x-ray examination will help distinguish between these two possibilities. Atresia is frequently observed with cranial, facial, mandibular, or acrofacial dysostoses such as Cruzon's disease or

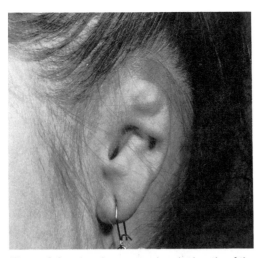

Figure 3.3. Atretic ear canal and microtia of the pinna. See page 85 for additional discussion.

Treacher Collins' syndrome. Aural atresia may also be associated with facial, labial, and/or palatal clefts. Abnormalities of the skeletal system and visceral organs or chromosomal aberrations may also accompany atresia. Children with these defects usually suffer conductive-type hearing losses and may do well with bone conduction hearing aids if medical or surgical treatment is not in order.

Collapsed Ear Canals. In some children the anatomy of the concha-meatal opening is such that collapse of the ear canal occurs during audiometric testing. This situation produces a conductive-type hearing loss from pressure of the earphones against the pinna, tragus and opening to the external auditory meatus (Bess, 1971). Audiometric testing will show an erroneous air-bone gap from supposed conductive hearing loss. The suspected conductive hearing loss will not be confirmed by impedance audiometry or otologic examination of the ear. Such children can be shown to have normal hearing when retested with a hollow auditory canal plug used under the earphone or when tested in sound field conditions (Ventry et al., 1961).

Aural Discharge. The presence of fluid running from the external auditory meatus should give the clinician concern. Fluid from the external auditory canal may be divided in three categories: (1) clear, (2) cloudy, whitish or yellow; (3) bloody.

1. *Clear fluid* may represent cerebral spinal fluid leaking from a temporal bone fracture which offers a ready route for access for infection into the cranial cavity. This condition requires prompt otologic consultation by physical examination, x-ray studies, and perhaps surgical exploration of the ear to confirm and repair the leakage.

2. *Cloudy fluid* usually represents inflammation of the external auditory canal, a condition known as external otitis. Less often cloudy discharge may result from an inflamed middle ear space with existing perforation of the tympanic membrane. Ex-

ternal otitis should be treated before performing impedance audiometry as insertion of the probe tip may cause pain and such evaluation is unlikely to provide additional diagnostic information.

3. *Blood* coming from the external auditory canal frequently results from self-instrumentation of the ear canal to relieve itching or remove ear wax. Blood coming from the ear canal may also be an expression of a fracture of the temporal bone, and as such require immediate medical consultation. Presence of these types of fluid require immediate medical referral.

Cerumen and Foreign Bodies. Cerumen, or ear wax, is a combined product of the apocrine and sebaceous glands located in the skin of the ear canal. Cerumen comes in two varieties: wet and dry. Wet ear wax varies from yellowish to dark brown, even resembles blood at times. Dry ear wax tends to be whitish scales or powdery feathery-like material. Most people's ear canals are self-cleaning of cerumen because of the migratory pattern of the epithelium toward the external auditory meatus. The cerumen may easily be wiped away with a washcloth. People with excessive production of cerumen or inadequate self-cleaning mechanism may accumulate wax in the external auditory canal which can cause hearing loss. These individuals should have the wax removed by a physician who will frequently utilize magnification for improved visibility. The use of a Waterpic, or the use of the infamous Q-tip applicator are to be condemned. Cotton tip applicators, in the hands of an aggressive parent, are a major source of lacerated ear canals, perforated eardrums and occasional sensorineural hearing loss or deafness from displaced ossicles which are accidentally forced into the inner ear.

Children are the leading candidates to appear with a foreign object in their ear canal—objects which may include broken crayons, food, small toys, or pieces of jewelry. Hearing loss is usually not a major concern in such cases unless the foreign object has ruptured the tympanic membrane. Referral to a medical specialist for removal of the object is, of course, mandatory.

Bony Growths. Occasionally bony outgrowths in the external auditory canal may create problems. These come in two forms: (1) multiple growths, termed *exostoses*; and (2) single growths, termed *osteomas*. These are the most common neoplasms of the external auditory canal and appear as smooth, hard, round nodules covered with normal skin. Exostoses do not require removal unless they cause cerumen accumulation, impair hearing, or create canal obstruction. Osteomas usually continue to grow and hence require surgical removal.

Inflammatory Conditions. Occasionally just touching the pinna will cause the patient to wince or react with noticeable discomfort. Conditions most frequently responsible for this phenomenon are: (1) external otitis, (2) perichondritis, and/or (3) furunculosis of the external auditory canal.

1. *Otitis externa* is an inflammation of the skin of the external auditory canal, most frequently due to bacterial infection or fungal infection. The presence of water in the ear canal against the tympanic membrane provides ideal circumstances for bacterial growth. The skin of the canal on acute external otitis is usually red, quite tender, with some form of drainage present. It is of interest that external otitis is frequently found in hearing aid users. The presence of an occlusive earmold results in increased moisture in the ear canal which seems to predispose external otitis. The otolaryngologist may suggest that the patient either switch his hearing aid to the opposite ear or in certain instances go without the aid for a while until the condition clears. The use of open-type earmolds helps prevent this possible condition.

2. *Perichondritis* is an inflammation of the covering of the cartilage of the ear, or ear canal. It is usually secondary to trauma of the cartilage, either accidental or surgical. The pinna is usually red and tender

with generalized swelling. Subperichondrial abscesses may deprive the cartilage of needed blood supply. The resultant lack of nourishment to the cartilage may cause subsequent deformities of the pinna.

3. A *furuncle* of the external canal is a boil or pimple. It is exquisitely tender because the skin of the ear canal is tightly applied to the cartilage.

Each of these conditions is usually quite painful and the patient will usually be most grateful to receive prompt medical attention.

Bullous Myringitis

Blisters occasionally form on the tympanic membrane in association with a coincident upper respiratory infection. The blisters, or bullae, represent an accumulation of fluid between the layers of the tympanic membrane and may appear to the untrained observer as acute otitis media. This disorder is extremely painful and accompanied by a feeling of pressure in the ear. Hearing levels may be within normal limits. According to Roberts (1980), bullous myringitis probably is not a separate clinical entity, but merely acute otitis media with blisters on the eardrum.

Perforations of the Tympanic Membrane

Perforations may occur from some sort of trauma such as a blow to the side of the head, a water-skiing fall, diving, or sudden changes in air pressure, or from middle ear problems such as acute otitis media. The tympanic membrane is about 8 mm in diameter and perforations from acute otitis media are usually much smaller, 1 to 2 mm in diameter. Often these perforations will heal spontaneously.

Conductive hearing loss occurs as a consequence of poor vibration of the tympanic membrane. The degree of loss, however, is variable and dependent upon the size of the perforation and its location on the tympanic membrane. Small perforations may be obvious with hearing levels within normal limits. Impedance audiometry may be

used effectively as described in Chapter 6 to identify children with perforated tympanic membranes. Complications from perforations may be very serious and all such children should be immediately referred to a medical specialist. Parents should be advised to practice aural hygiene by keeping water out of the child's ear when swimming or bathing until proper medical care of the ear has been taken.

Otitis Media

Otitis media is one of the most common disorders in children. Otitis media is defined as an inflammation of the middle ear which may or may not be infectious in origin. A current hypothesis is that the different clinical types of otitis media form a continuum and are dynamically interrelated. At any specific point in the continuum, a definite clinical entity can be identified, and at another time a different clinical entity may be present in the same patient (Paparella, 1976).

The general categories of otitis media are (a) otitis media without effusion, (b) otitis media with effusion, and (c) otitis media with perforation. Each of these categories may be classified by duration into (a) acute, 0–21 days; (b) subacute, 22 days to 8 weeks; and (c) chronic, over 8 weeks. In otitis media with effusion, and otitis media with perforation, the fluid or discharge may be characterized as (a) serous, (b) purulent, or (c) mucoid (Senturia, 1976; Senturia, et al., 1980).

Otitis media is the most common during the first 2 years of life, and decreases in incidence thereafter. The incidence of otitis media has been studied by many investigators and found to be a function of age, sex (more otitis media in boys), race (whites have a higher incidence than blacks); genetic factors, socioeconomic status, season and climate (Teele et al., 1980). According to Teele et al., children living in households with many members were more likely to have otitis media than were children living in households with fewer members, and that children with siblings or parents who had a history of otitis media had a higher incidence of otitis media than children with parents or siblings without a history of the disease. The incidence statistics concerning otitis media are impressive: 76–95% of all children have had at least one episode of otitis media by age 6 years (Howie et al., 1975); approximately 50% of all children have had one episode of otitis media by age 1 and by age 2 the incidence increases to 75%. According to Klein (1979) children may be divided into three general groups with regard to otitis media. Approximately one third of children have no episodes, whereas one third may have an occasional episode, and the remaining third have frequent episodes.

Of particular importance is the "otitis-prone" child described initially by Howie et al. (1975). An "otitis-prone" child has the condition 6 or more times before the age of 6, or whose initial episode of otitis media was due to *Pneumococcus* and occurred before the age of 1 year.

Recurrent tonsillitis and enlarged adenoids were once thought to be the major cause of otitis media. Bluestone (1979) reviewed several studies and concluded that no good evidence exists that tonsillectomy and adenoidectomy reduce the incidence of ear disease.

Eustachian tube dysfunction has long been recognized to be a significant factor in the development of otitis media. The most important function of the eustachian tube is ventilation of the middle ear space. When the eustachian tube dysfunctions from either a mechanical or functional cause, the air trapped in the middle ear cavity is absorbed creating negative middle ear pressure and ultimately, transudation of fluid into the cavity. Paradise (1980) states that eustachian tube function appears less competent in infants than in older children and adults, perhaps because the tubal wall of infants is more compliant and therefore more susceptible to collapse, creating functional obstruction.

The diagnosis of otitis media is based on clinical manifestations, physical examina-tion of the tympanic membrane and possibly impedance testing and routine audiometry. Paradise (1980) categorizes symptoms as either specific or systemic. Specific symptoms include earache, rubbing or tugging at the ears, otorrhea (drainage), hearing impairment, and balance disturbance. Of these, only earache and otorrhea generally indicate active infection. Many cases of otitis media are unaccompanied by significant degrees of hearing loss (Cohen and Sade, 1972). The systemic symptoms include fever, temperament disorders and restless sleep, irritability or low-grade discomfort.

When the diagnosis of acute otitis media is in doubt, or when determination of the causative agent is of question, aspiration of the middle ear fluid is performed with tympanocentesis or myringotomy as shown in Figure 3.4. In patients with an unusually severe earache, myringotomy is performed to provide immediate pain relief.

Considerable controversy and confusion exists concerning the treatment for otitis media. Tremendous benefits would be gained if recurrences of otitis media could be prevented or substantially reduced in frequency. Paradise (1980) summarizes five different approaches to the prevention of otitis media currently under evaluation: (a) adenoidectomy with or without tonsellectomy; (b) antimicrobial prophylaxis (Perrin et al. (1974) have shown a significant reduction in the number of episodes of purulent otitis media in children who were treated continuously with low dose sulfisoxazole); (c) the use of tympanostomy tubes (Gebhart (1981) showed that placement of tympanostomy tubes significantly decreased the number of episodes of acute purulent otitis media); (d) liberal use of myringotomy as an adjunct to antimicrobials; and (e) the administration of polyvalent pneumococcal vaccine.

The complications associated with otitis media are numerous and not uncommon. Complications of otitis media with effusion include hearing loss, perforation of the tympanic membrane with or without sup-

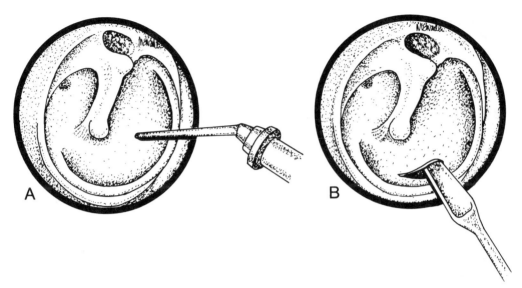

Figure 3.4. View of tympanotomy of surgical puncture of the tympanic membrane often used to aspirate fluid by suction for culture (*left*). Myringotomy, or surgical incision of tympanic membrane, is performed in lower half of tympanic membrane to avoid damage to middle ear ossicles. Myringotomy is conducted to provide instant relief from pain, to drain fluid from middle ear space, and thus help initiate rapid recovery of middle ear disease (*right*).

puration, cholesteatoma, mastoiditis, petrositis, adhesive otitis media, tympanosclerosis, ossicular discontinuity, facial paralysis and labyrinthitis. Intracranial complications include meningitis, encephalitis, brain abscess, sinus thrombophlebitis, etc. Finally, there is increasing evidence that otitis media may impair the development of children's cognitive abilities and detrimentally influence behavior (Stool et al., 1982).

An extremely important finding was reported by Teele and his associates (1980) concerning persistence of middle ear effusion (MEE) following medical treatment. After the first episode of otitis media, 70% of the children in their study still had MEE at 2 weeks, 40% at 1 month, 20% at 2 months, and 10% at 3 months. Pelton and colleagues (1977) also found that approximately one third of unselected children with acute otitis media had persistent fluid in the middle ear for 4 or more weeks. These statistics confirm the importance of careful and thorough medical follow-up for all children identified to have otitis media.

Acute otitis media is generally considered to present suddenly with severe ear pain, redness of the tympanic membrane, and fever. Recent studies by Schwartz et al. (1981a) have attempted to delineate a more precise definition of acute otitis media to include the bulging contour, decreased mobility and color of the tympanic membrane. These studies have confirmed that all three effusion types (purulent, serous, and mucoid) can occur acutely. In 85 infants and children diagnosed with acute otitis media, a poorly mobile, bulging, yellow, opacified tympanic membrane was most typical. The red tympanic membrane was seen in only 19% of the children, 67% had no fever, and 28% had no pain associated with their acute otitis media. In a follow-up study, Schwartz et al. (1981b) noted that approximately 10% of all cases of acute otitis media led to persistent purulent otitis media despite adequately prescribed antibiotic treatment.

Serous otitis media is very common in children between the ages of 3 and 8 years and may be recalcitrant to medical treatment. If pain is present in this disorder, it is usually intermittent and rather mild (Bluestone and Shurin, 1974).

In otitis media with perforation, the tissues of the middle ear intermittently undergo destruction, healing, and scarring during the recurrent infections. The pathology of this disease is characterized by a lack of uniformity among involved ears. The condition is often associated with cholesteatoma.

During healing the middle ear and tympanic membrane may develop tympanosclerosis, which is hyalinized and calcified scar tissue. Tympanosclerosis deposits may cause stiffening of the tympanic membrane or fusion and fixation of the middle ear ossicles. Middle ear granulation tissue, polyps, and monomeric membrane formation are also associated with various chronic otitis media as shown in Figure 3.5.

Adhesive otitis media is a thickening of the fiberous tissue of the tympanic membrane which may be accompanied by severe retraction and negative pressure in the middle ear space. When a retraction pocket forms in the superior portion of the pars tensa of the tympanic membrane, the development of cholesteatoma is probable.

MIDDLE EAR EFFUSIONS IN NEONATES

A number of investigators have shown that MEE occurs commonly in neonates, both in the outpatient population and the intensive care nursery (Jaffe et al., 1970; Warren and Stool, 1971; Bland, 1972; Shurin et al., 1976). In spite of these well documented studies, otoscopy is not routinely performed on neonates because the infant tympanic membrane is difficult to visualize (Fig. 3.6). In an infant, the external ear canal is distensible and often collapsed, and the tympanic membrane lies in a nearly horizontal plane. Balkany et al. (1978) reported results from examining 125 consecutive infants from the neonatal intensive care unit, and found MEE to be present in some 30% of their sample. They felt that this finding was especially important and often overlooked, since unrecognized MEE may act as a focus for dissemination of bacteria into the circulation and/or central nervous system. They also found that na-

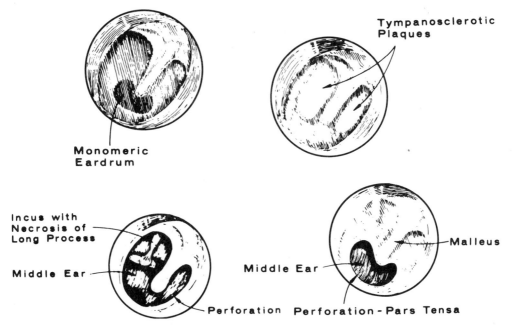

Figure 3.5. Otoscopic views of the tympanic membrane showing some sequelae of chronic otitis media. (Courtesy of Gerald M. English, M.D., Denver, Colorado.)

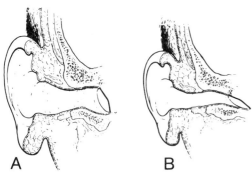

Figure 3.6. Orientation of the tympanic membrane in the adult (*A*) and in the infant (*B*). Note the horizontal plane of the infant eardrum which makes visualization of the tympanic membrane difficult. (Reprinted with permission from T. J. Balkany, S. A. Berman, M. A. Simmons, and B. J. Jafek: *The Laryngoscope, 88:* 399, 1978.)

sotracheal intubation of longer than 7 days is highly associated with suppurative MEE.

Chronic otitis media most often has its onset in early childhood, between the ages of 5 and 10 years. Recurrent otitis media may halt or reverse the process of mastoid pneumatization, or cause mastoid sclerosis. Severe forms of otitis media may, or may not, damage the middle ear ossicles, depending on the severity and duration of the disease. Severe otitis media may produce areas of osteitis in the mastoid septae, resulting in a continuous foul discharge.

Paparella and Brady (1970) reviewed 232 patients with chronic suppurative otitis media and mastoiditis. They found a definite increase in the incidence of sensorineural hearing loss which they suggested was due to a cochlear biochemical change created by toxic materials passed into the inner ear through the round window resulting in gradual destruction of the organ of Corti. English et al. (1973) evaluated 404 patients with various forms of otitis media and reached conclusions in accord with the Paparella and Brady study. English et al. found that bone conduction thresholds worsened with the severity and duration of disease. Post-treatment bone conduction thresholds were unchanged from pretreatment tests, leading these authors to con-

clude that sensorineural hearing loss can be a natural sequela of chronic otitis media.

Cholesteatoma

The continuing maturation and persistent growth of squamous epithelium (skin) often can create problems in the ear. When the growing skin from the ear canal finds its way into the middle ear cavity or mastoid through a tympanic membrane perforation, the material accumulates and forms a cholesteatoma. The size of the perforation may vary considerably from a very small to a large area. Occasionally, the entire tympanic membrane and portions of the annulus may be absent. In some cases, spontaneous growth of squamous epithelium may cover the perforation while invading the middle ear in a medial direction. Retraction pockets on the periphery of the tympanic membrane may also lead to cholesteatoma growth.

A cross-section diagram in Figure 3.7 shows an attic and a middle ear cholesteatoma. Moisture and bacteria may gain access to the cholesteatoma (which is really a deposit of desquamated keratin) and foul-smelling ear drainage may ensue. The disease process may cause erosion of surrounding bone or create meningeal complications or fistulae of the otic capsule.

Tos (1983) reviewed surgical results from 122 children operated on for removal of cholesteatoma. He found recurrent cholesteatoma in 12% of the cases, and remarked that recurrent growth of cholesteatoma is more common in children than adults and develops faster in young people.

Mastoiditis

Mastoiditis is categorized into either acute or chronic stages. The terms represent the degree of involvement of the infected mastoid air cell system (House and Crabtree, 1978). The anatomic continuity between the middle ear and the mucosal lining of the mastoid antrum allows for the coexisting inflammatory process associated

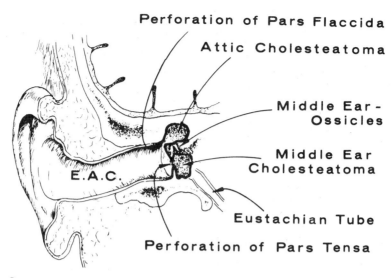

Perforation of Pars Flaccida

Attic Cholesteatoma

Middle Ear - Ossicles

Middle Ear Cholesteatoma

E.A.C.

Eustachian Tube

Perforation of Pars Tensa

Figure 3.7. Cross-section of the external and middle ear showing an attic cholesteatoma through a perforation of the pars flaccida portion of the tympanic membrane: a perforation of the pars tensa portion of the tympanic membrane may lead to development of a middle ear cholesteatoma. (Reprinted with permission from G. M. English, J. L. Northern, and T. J. Fria: *Archives of Otolaryngology*, *98:* 17–22, 1973.)

with these structures. *Acute mastoiditis* is an inflammation of the ciliated mucosa of the antrum. With the onset of edema or insufficient drainage of the mastoid mucosa, pressure is created within the air cells causing localized discomfort. Some of the clinical manifestations of acute mastoiditis are fullness, pain, acute otitis media, tenderness, edema and conductive hearing loss. Other clinical findings may consist of tympanic membrane destruction depending on the status of the typanum or epitympanum.

Chronic mastoiditis occurs with chronic inflammation of the membrane lining the mastoid antrum and ciliated cells. The bone structure is often involved in the infection. Generally, chronic mastoiditis is associated with a history of otitis media, which may be active or inactive depending on whether or not purulent discharge is present. The symptoms of chronic mastoiditis are similar to those of acute mastoiditis, with the exception of the hearing loss, which often takes on a sensorineural component (Ginsburg et al., 1980).

Acute mastoiditis was, until the 1930s and 1940s, a complication of acute otitis media in 25% to 50% of the cases. With the advent of antibiotics such as penicillin, the incidence of acute mastoiditis was lowered to approximately 0.4% by 1955 (Palva and Pulkinen, 1959). However, antibiotic therapy has been attributed to a "masked" presence of mastoiditis, whereby the disease is suppressed enough to reduce the symptoms but not enough to resolve the ongoing destructive process (Holt and Young, 1981).

During the preantibiotic era, some of the most life-threatening complications of mastoiditis were meningitis, brain abscess, and cerebellar abscess. Present complications still include facial nerve paralysis, labyrinthitis, meningitis, and cholesteatoma. Intracranial complications have decreased since the 1930s and 1940s along with a significant decrease in patient mortality (Ballentine and White, 1953). In cases whereby antibiotics have been ineffective in treating acute mastoiditis, a simple mastoidectomy is performed with surgical drainage of the mastoid air cells. Patients with chronic mastoiditis are initially given nonsurgical treatment to dry the ear and prevent complications that would complicate surgical treatment. When medical management fails, a modified or radical mastoidectomy is performed.

Cleft Palate

Deformities of the lip and palate are among the most common major congenital malformations, occurring once in 900 newborns. A substantial number of articles have been published concerning the otologic and audiologic problems of children with overt cleft palate. The incidence of recurrent otitis media in such children is quite high and has been reported from 50% to 90% by various investigators (Holborow, 1962; Graham, 1963; Stool and Randall, 1967; Paradise and Bluestone, 1969).

Paradise and Bluestone (1974) reported the "universality" of otitis media findings in 50 infants with cleft palate. Paradise (1980) commented on 300 additional cleft palate infants examined during the first few months of life. Usually, sterile inflammatory effusions that vary in viscosity are found in the ears of these infants. Paradise recommends infants with cleft palate receive myringotomy and tympanostomy tube insertion at a relatively early age, within the first 6 months if possible, especially if hearing loss seems present or discomfort or infection is present. Physicians should be ready to repeat the myringotomy and tubes if necessary to keep the infant's ears clear and hearing normally.

Complications such as cholesteatoma and adhesive otitis may accompany MEE in cleft palate children. Hearing loss as a secondary problem to the middle ear disorder related to cleft palate is also very common, and may exist in 90% of such patients (Pannbacker, 1969; Yules, 1970). Goetzinger et al. (1960) and Graham (1963) indicate that the incidence and severity of middle ear problems related to the cleft palate decrease as the patient grows older.

Otologic and hearing problems associated with submucous cleft palate have been reviewed by Bergstrom and Hemenway

(1971). The submucous cleft palate is described as an imperfect union of muscle across the soft palate that tends to "tent" when the patient phonates. The area may appear bluish since it is covered by only nasal and oral mucosa. The dehiscence of muscle and bone may be obvious with palpation and is often accompanied by a bifid uvula. From a study of 58 patients with submucous cleft palate, Bergstrom and Hemenway reported an incidence of 39% with recurrent or chronic disease of the middle ear ranging in severity between serous otitis media to cholesteatoma. Conductive hearing loss was demonstrated by 34% of the group, while an additional 25% had either pure sensorineural or mixed type hearing loss. They suggest that the presence of submucous cleft palate indicates the possibility of accompanying middle ear disease, and likewise the presence of persistent or recurring middle ear disease makes the patient suspect for undiscovered submucous cleft palate.

Although numerous ideas have been offered to explain the high incidence of hearing problems associated with overt and submucous cleft palate children, most clinicians agree that the deficiency of palate musculature is the probable cause of poor eustachian tube function (Bluestone and Shurin, 1974). This results in inadequate middle ear ventilation, effusion of fluid, tympanic membrane retraction, and hearing loss. Such disease of the middle ear is most common in children between 3 and 8 years of age which also corresponds to the increased exposure and susceptibility to upper respiratory infections found in this age group (Halfond and Ballenger, 1956; Bennett et al., 1968; Jarvis, 1976).

Clinicians should be sensitive to this increased incidence of hearing difficulty and recurrent middle ear disease in children with cleft palate. The hearing of such patients should be monitored on a regular basis with close medical follow-up. Our experiences with cleft palate children have exposed numerous youngsters with recurrent episodes of otitis media accompanied by significant hearing loss who undoubtedly miss much auditory information at school and home (Keith et al., 1976). Immediate medical treatment is often necessary for these children who may qualify for repeated myringotomy and ventilation tubes. Mild to moderate power hearing aids may be in order for children who do not respond well to medical treatment, especially during the important school years.

The diagnosis of ear disease and hearing loss in the infant with cleft palate is difficult because of the small structure of the external ear and the infant's neurological immaturity (Stool, 1971). Middle ear effusion is often present in cleft palate babies when they are examined in the first days of life (Paradise and Bluestone, 1974). Too often the audiologist, however, is "only a bench-warmer" on the cleft palate team even though the results from hearing evaluations contribute substantially to the total management of these children (Pollock, 1979).

Impedance audiometry is an especially valuable clinical procedure in children with cleft palate. The overt cleft palate is diagnosed within the first few days of life, although the submucous cleft palate may not be diagnosed until years later. Impedance audiometry may identify conductive impairments in even very young infants, not readily amenable to bone conduction testing, and who have sufficient hearing sensitivity to respond well to air conduction hearing tests (Billings and Lowry, 1974; Bess et al., 1975, 1976).

Down's Syndrome (Trisomy 21)

Ear abnormalities such as small pinnae, narrow external auditory canals, abnormal external ear configuration, and a strong tendency to have otitis media (Rigrodsky et al., 1961) are commonly associated with Down's syndrome and suggest the possibility of a high incidence of conductive hearing losses in this population. In addition, it has been suggested that the Down's child may be more susceptible to upper respiratory tract infections than the normal child because of peculiar nasopharynx and eustachian tube development, which can adversely affect proper drainage of the sinuses and middle-ear spaces (McIntire et al., 1965). In early studies, reliable hearing tests were felt to be difficult to obtain due to the mental retardation associated with the syndrome. However, if one considers test procedures suited to the patient's mental age and development, there should be no reason audiometric data are not obtained.

The majority of studies involving Down's patients have been carried out in institutional settings and findings of conductive hearing loss have been quite diverse. The most complete description of hearing impairment in children with Down's syndrome, was published as a monograph by M. P. Downs (1980a). She noted that the Down's child may be treated medically or surgically for persistent MEE, but following treatment the conductive hearing loss may persist. She designed a comprehensive study of 107 noninstitutionalized Down's children and found 78% to have hearing loss in one or both ears. Fifty-four percent had conductive loss, 16% had sensorineural loss, and 8% had mixed-type hearing loss.

Complete otologic examinations were conducted on each of the 107 Down's children. According to Balkany et al. (1978) about 40% of the children with conductive hearing loss could not be explained by MEE or chronic otitis media. On microscopic pneumatic otoscopy the patients had normal appearing examinations, suggesting the presence of middle ear anomalies. Seventeen operative procedures on carefully selected Down's syndrome patients revealed congenital ossicular malformations and destruction caused by inflammation due to chronic infection. Balkany (1980) recommends that children with Down's syndrome and persistent conductive hearing loss be treated aggressively from three perspectives: to normalize hearing, to break the cycle of recurrent suppurative otitis media, and to prevent chronic ear disease.

In the audiologic evaluation of Down's syndrome children, the impedance tests (tympanometry and acoustic reflex measurement) were important to confirm hearing test results. In addition, the high incidence of conductive hearing loss in this population makes impedance audiometry an imperative part of each hearing evaluation (Northern, 1980). Every hearing test on a Down's syndrome child should include some aspect of sound field testing (without earphones) to rule out erroneous "conductive losses" due to collapsed ear canals. An excellent description of the audiometric testing of Down's children has been reported by Downs (1980b).

The results of this study and others (Glovsky, 1966; Brooks et al., 1972; Fulton and Lloyd, 1968; Schwartz and Schwartz, 1978) clearly show that conductive hearing loss in the Down's syndrome population is prevalent in noninstitutionalized infants and children, and often the hearing loss continues in spite of proper medical management. Down's children should not be excluded from vigorous monitoring of middle ear problems and attempts to normalize their hearing by appropriate amplification strategies. In addition, a total team approach, including ENT, audiology, and speech pathology, is recommended for the Down's child in order to provide optimal opportunities for advancement.

Ototoxic Hearing Loss

Ototoxicity is due to the administration of certain drugs and medications that damage the cochlea and/or vestibular portion of the inner ear, causing permanent sensorineural hearing loss and often accompanied by vertigo, nausea or gait instability. Almost any available drug, effective for treatment of certain ailments, has the potential to compromise the human system in some way. Management of illness with chemotherapy becomes a fine-line judgment, weighing the potential benefit to the patient against the risk of adverse side effects.

Antibiotics, diuretics, and antimalarial pharmaceuticals have been implicated as potentially toxic to both the auditory and vestibular systems, as well as the kidney. Kanamycin and neomycin are the worse ototoxic drugs at this time although other members of the aminoglycoside family, including entamycin, vancomycin, amikacin, dihydrostreptomycin, and tobramycin have caused documented auditory problems. Streptomycin is well known to be destructive to the vestibular system. There exists considerable individual suceptibility to these ototoxic drugs, which usually, but not always, cause bilaterally symmetrical hearing loss of varying degree, audiometric configuration, and severity. Aspirin, quinine, and diuretics are the only drugs which produce temporary hearing loss which may recover, fully or partially, when the patient is taken off the medication. Excellent material on aminoglycoside ototoxicity, including information on ototoxicity in children and infants, has been published by Hawkins (1976) and more recently by Lerner et al. (1981).

Ingestion of ototoxic drugs by pregnant women can result in a multitude of congenital abnormalities, including hearing loss, from passage of the drugs across the placenta (Siegel and McCracken, 1981). Apparently, renal failure, concomitant use of diuretics such as ethacrynic acid and furosemide, and a prolonged course of drug therapy are the most important factors in the development of fetal ototoxicity. The evaluation of aminoglycoside ototoxicity in infants is a complex problem since these babies are receiving medical therapy for severe problems including systemic infection which may accompany low birthweight, jaundice, or other health disorders which are themselves associated with deafness.

A 4-year follow-up study of 347 neonates treated with gentamicin and kanamycin was reported by Finitzo-Hieber et al. (1979). Although an excellent study, complete with a control group of nontreated infants, limitations in the study and failure to demonstrate ototoxicity in the experimental group of infants does not completely assure the safety of larger doses of the drugs. Suspect infants require extensive audiologic follow-up and sometimes the mild-to-moderate hearing loss is difficult to verify. Finitzo-Hieber (1981) has advocated the auditory brainstem response as a noninvasive procedure that can be used for measurement of auditory sensitivity in high-risk infants.

The area of vestibular testing in infants and children exposed to ototoxic drugs is even more difficult. The problem is to establish a simple, reliable and noninvasive method of assessing vestibular function that will be tolerated by children. Eviatar and Eviatar (1981) describe a combined evaluation of postural control, developmental reflexes and electronystagmography that provides useful information about the vestibular function in children.

According to Bergstrom and Thompson (1984) epithelial structures in the cochlea and vestibule show the primary damage from ototoxicity. In the cochlea, atrophy of stria vascularis, spiral ligament, sensory hair cells and supporting cells may be seen. The basal and middle coils of the cochlea are more commonly affected than the apical coil, correlating clinically with the high frequency hearing loss typically seen in cases of ototoxic etiology. With increased severity, the apical turn—and accordingly, the low-mid frequencies—can be involved. The outer hair cells in the cochlear duct are more vulnerable than the inner hair cells. In the vestibular system, histopathological studies show damage to the cristae of the ampullae in the semicircular canals.

The incidence of ototoxicity in general figures or for specific drugs has not been accurately established. Thompson and Northern (1981) identify a number of risk factors which may enhance the potential risk of ototoxicity including increased drug serum level, decreased renal function, the use of more than one ototoxic drug simultaneously or in increased daily doses or for an extended period of time, age, health, heredity concurrent noise exposure or in the presence of preexisting problems including severe visual impairment or blindness, or drugs administered in the presence of ear symptoms such as tinnitus, hearing loss and/or dizziness. These factors have been proposed for consideration, but have yet to be verified through research.

Cochlear Trauma

Skull fracture involving the occipital or squamous portion of the temporal bone may extend into the petrous portion of the temporal bone and involve the otic capsule. Should the fracture line cross the external auditory canal, laceration of the skin and bleeding of the external canal may occur with little permanent loss of hearing. More medial fractures may produce bleeding in the middle ear or disruption of the ossicular chain which would create a maximal 60-dB conductive-type hearing loss. Hearing loss due to concussion may recover totally or partially, while hearing loss due to fracture of the cochlea is irreversible (Barber, 1969).

Relatively moderate cochlear trauma to the occiput of the skull can cause a permanent sensorineural hearing loss (Schuknecht, 1974). Numerous animal studies have been conducted with traumatic blows to the head which produce temporary and permanent sensorineural high-frequency hearing loss. Schuknecht (1974) states that a blow to the head creates a pressure wave in the skull which is transmitted through bone to the cochlea just as a pressure wave in air is carried by the conducting mechanism, and the injury must be attributed to intense acoustic stimulation. Meningitis may occur as a late complication of temporal bone fracture.

Noise-induced or Noise-Trauma Hearing Loss

A sound of sufficient intensity and duration can cause injury to the inner ear producing a temporary or permanent hearing loss. The extent of noise-induced or traumatic noise inflicted hearing loss in children is difficult to ascertain, but its presence is relatively common. A most thorough review of the literature concerning noise and children was published by Mills (1975).

A number of devices used by children produce sound levels capable of producing acoustic injury. Devices with sufficiently high sound levels include firecrackers (Ward and Glorig, 1961), model airplane engines tested indoors (Bess and Powell, 1972) as well as toy firearms (Hodge and McCommons, 1966; Marshall and Brandt, 1974). It has been speculated without documentation, that thousands of children have permanent hearing losses which were caused by the acoustic impulses of toy caps (Ruckelshaus, 1972).

The issue of susceptibility of children to temporary threshold shift is still open. This question is critical in the determination of hearing hazard produced by incubators and hearing aids. Fior (1972) presented temporary threshold shift data from children between 3 and 13 years which is similar to data generally reported for adults. It is understandable that data are sparse with regard to experimental evaluation of temporary threshold shift in children because of concern to eliminate any risk of permanent auditory damage.

The hearing loss due to noise exposure typically consists of sensorineural impairment at 4000 Hz in the affected ear, regardless of the type of noise exposure. Often the traumatic noise-induced hearing loss can be related to a single identifiable noise exposure such as the explosion of a firecracker.

Weber et al. (1967) evaluated 1000 children from Colorado with hearing loss and found 249 boys and 51 girls with noise exposure characteristic audiograms. These authors suggest that noise-induced losses are first identified in junior-senior high school boys who have a history of experience with firearms and farm machinery. Litke (1971) evaluated higher frequency hearing among 1516 South Dakota school children. He found high frequency hearing loss in 6% of the population, with an average loss of 58 dB occurring at the highest incidence at grades 3 and 12. Litke found 5 times more boys than girls suffered high-frequency hearing loss with two thirds of the subjects showing 6000 Hz as the most involved frequency.

We are often asked by concerned parents if listening or playing loud rock and roll music can damage the hearing of their children. Although research in the issue of hearing loss and hard rock music is somewhat conflicting, there is little doubt that exposure to loud music can produce temporary threshold shift. Rintlemann and Borus (1968) studied rock musicians and found that only 5% of them incurred noise-induced hearing losses. Jerger and Jerger (1970) reported that eight of nine rock-and-roll musicians, aged 14 to 23 years, showed temporary threshold shift in excess of 15 dB on at least one frequency between 2000 and 8000 Hz, one of whom had a 38-dB shift in threshold at 3000 Hz!

Thorough history questioning may identify unrecognized situations of excessive noise exposure. These youngsters must be carefully counseled regarding the potential hazards of additional noise exposure and fitted with ear defenders as soon as possible.

Tremendous individual susceptibility to hearing loss from noise exposure exists. Some children who hunt, operate noisy farm machinery, or drive motorized vehicles such as snow mobiles or trail bikes, will show evidence of noise-induced hearing loss.

The degree of noise young people are exposed to in daily life was measured by Siervogel et al., 1982. They placed dosimeters on 127 subjects 7–20 years old. The average daily 24-hour log equivalent sound levels ranged from 77 to 84 dB. The noise exposures of the children were the same whether or not school was in session.

NOISE LEVELS IN INFANT INCUBATORS AND THE INTENSIVE CARE UNIT (ICU)

A visitor to the newborn intensive care unit within a hospital is immediately aware of the high noise level. Originally, hospital nurseries were small rooms with four to eight infants in incubators or cribs with virtually no life-support equipment. However, modern technology has created a much noisier nursery environment with the use of machines for life support, diagnosis, and monitoring of baby activity. In fact, one of the greatest problems in the ICU is the multitude of sound sources, respirators, and monitors which generate both background sound and alarm signals (Kellman, 1982).

Noise levels in the ICU may be 20 dB higher than in the well baby nursery, day and night, causing staff aggravation, fatigue, and stress leading to potential patient care errors. Ambient noise levels in ICU have been reported to range from 56 to 77 dBA (Peltzman et al., 1970; Falk and Woods, 1973; Redding et al., 1977). This noise is generally low frequency in nature (most energy lower than 250 Hz), persistent and continuous all hours of the day and night.

Although prolonged exposure to the noise levels characteristic of intensive care equipment and infant incubators may be harmful to the developing neonate, direct evidence for such insult has not been reported. In 1974, the American Academy of Pediatrics Committee on Environmental Hazards recommended that manufacturers of incubators reduce noise below 58 dBA.

Abramovich et al. (1979) examined the hearing of 111 perinatal intensive care survivors of birthweights 1500 g or less at a mean age of 6 years and found no evidence that ambient incubator noise of 65 dB sound pressure level (SPL) had affected their hearing thresholds. However, these researchers warned with the increasing use of noise signals as auditory monitors, attention should be given to ambient noise levels to ensure that potentially damaging levels are not exceeded. Long et al. (1980) recorded 2-hour polygraphic tracings from infants' heart rate, respiratory rate, transcutaneous oxygen tension, and intracranial pressure during the routine ICU schedule. He found that sudden loud noises usually caused agitation and crying in the infants, which led to decreases in transcutaneous oxygen tension and an increase in intracranial pressure, as well as increases in heart and respiratory rate.

A number of concerned investigators have measured the ambient sound level generated within infant incubators. In general, the sound pressure levels of incubators have been reported to be greater than 60 dBA (League et al., 1972; Falk and Farmer, 1973; Blennow et al., 1974; Douek et al., 1976). While these sound levels are not in excess of acceptable damage risk criteria, it must be remembered that infants in such incubators are usually in poor health, may be under treatment with potentially ototoxic drugs, and their noise exposure is continuous, 24 hours per day, 1440 min per day, from several weeks to months (Falk, 1972).

An excellent study was conducted by Bess et al. (1979) of incubator noise with different types of life-support equipment and when impulse noise was created by striking the side of the incubator or by opening and closing the doors of the storage unit. The life-support equipment increased the overall noise levels of the incubators by as much as 15–20 dB with a predominance of high-frequency energy. The impulse signals created by striking the side of the incubator (a common practice of physicians and nurses to forcefully stimulate breathing in apneic infants) ranged from 130 to 140 dB SPL. Opening and closing the storage unit doors created peak amplitudes of 114 dB SPL.

Bacterial and Viral Diseases

Bacterial and viral diseases have long been recognized as causes of deafness. Both prenatal and postnatal infections have been identified as a cause of hearing loss. Maternal rubella has been the cause of large numbers of deaf children, with some 10,000–20,000 children affected by the epidemics of the early and mid-1960s. The sequelae of maternal rubella are discussed further in the appendix "Index of Hearing Disorders." Congenital deafness has also been attributed to meningoencephalitis, chicken pox, and other viruses.

Postnatal viruses and bacterial infections as causes of early acquired deafness commonly result in profound bilateral deafness (Neuman et al., 1981). Infectious meningitis which causes deafness as the result of bilateral labyrinthitis due to extension of infection from the meninges was early recognized as a leading cause of profound bilateral deafness (Vernon, 1967a, 1967b). The infecting agent has been found to pass from the meninges to the inner ear through the cochlear aqueduct and along vessels and nerves from the internal auditory meatus (Paparella and Suguira, 1967). Bacterial postnatal infections known to result in deafness due to meningogenic spread include streptococcus, pneumococcus, and staphylococcus.

Common viruses of later postnatal period known to or suspected to cause deafness and/or vestibular symptoms include mumps, measles, chicken pox, influenza, and viruses of the common cold. Here again deafness results from damage to the inner ear due to direct infiltration via the internal meatus. Disease may be limited to the endolymphatic system with the inflammatory process beginning in the vascular beds (Lindsay, 1967a).

The viral diseases usually cause mild to profound sensorineural hearing loss. Histopathologic effects of viral infections reported have included extensive destruction of organ of Corti, degeneration of saccule, damage of complete destruction of stria vascularis and tectorial membrane, damage or obliteration of vestibular system, and atrophy or destruction of neural pathways (Lindsay, 1976b).

Maternal infections have been demonstrated as the cause of a host of other congenital malformations and abnormalities. However, congenital infections often cause fetal death and miscarriage. Damage to the fetus attributed to congenital viral infections has included congenital malformations such as clubfoot; intrauterine growth; retardation; damage to nervous system including anencephaly, encephalocele, and spina bifida; congenital heart disease; and disease of other organs such as the liver, pancreas, and adrenals.

Residuals of postnatal viral infections include nerve atrophy, notably the optic nerve, cerebral palsy, mental retardation, disturbances of respiration, muscular atrophy or paralysis, convulsions, disturbances of autonomic system, and disturbances of metabolism.

Congenital Syphilis

Congenital syphilis is still one of the most important contributors to perinatal mortality and morbidity in many parts of the world. In Western countries, the disease is now relatively rare, but the recent increase in venereal disease may well mean that congenital syphilis will again become a threat to neonates (Bryan and Nicholson, 1981).

Early manifestations include nasal discharge (snuffles), rash, anemia, jaundice, and osteochondritis. Later manifestations include saddle nose, saber skin, Hutchinson teeth, mulberry molars, and other dental anomalies. Congenital syphilis may demonstrate a multitude of central nervous system abnormalities including vestibular dysfunction, sensorineural hearing loss, and occasionally aortic valvulitis. Possible accompanying mental retardation depends on severity of neurologic damage.

Auditory impairment may not be present at birth. Onset of hearing loss is generally in early childhood, usually sudden bilaterally symmetrical causing severe to profound impairment. The hearing loss is usually not accompanied by marked vestibular manifestations. Poor hearing function and limited use of hearing aid can be expected due to neural atrophy. The general treatment of congenital syphilis consists of prompt treatment of the infant with penicillin. Treatment may be done in utero prior to delivery when an infected mother is identified (Karmody and Schuknecht, 1966).

Cytomegalic Inclusion Disease

The cytomegalovirus causes cytomegalic inclusion disease which is a generalized infection of infants caused by intrauterine or postnatal contraction from the mother. The infection may be contracted by the fetus during passage down the birth canal (Peterson, 1977). It appears microscopically with large easinophilic bodies seen within cells as "inclusions" in certain body fluids (Ward et al., 1965). The viral infection shows little pathogenicity in the mother who may be totally asymptomatic. Bergstrom (1977) states that 10 times as many infants are infected by cytomegalovirus at birth as by rubella.

Some infants, mildly infected with cytomegalovirus, remain asymptomatic with no permanent sequelae and may develop within normal limits. In its most severe form, however, infants usually die during the newborn period. If the disease is clinically detectable at birth, some 80% of infants have sequelae related to the central nervous system. Cytomegalovirus, when transmitted in utero may be associated with a spectrum of problems including varying degrees of mental retardation, spasticity, hyperactivity, microcephaly, and convulsive seizures (Shinefield, 1973). Associated complications may include facial weakness, cleft of the hard or soft palate as well as a fairly high incidence of sensorineural hearing loss (Weller, 1971; Strauss and Davis, 1973). Peterson (1977) states that 25 to 50% of infants with cytomegalovirus infection have been reported to have sensorineural hearing loss, severe enough to be handicapping in 10–25%.

Rh Incompatibility

This condition involves the destruction of Rh positive blood cells of the fetus by maternal antibodies. Complications of Rh incompatibility account for about 3% of profound hearing loss among school age deaf children. Clinical symptoms develop during the immediate neonatal period, and include elevated bilirubin, jaundice, and possible brain damage. Most infants having kernicterus die during the first week with 80% of those surviving having complete or partial deafness. Other common residuals reported include cerebral palsy, mental retardation, epilepsy, aphasia, and behavioral disorders.

The cause of the associated hearing loss is still open to question. Reports are contradictory, indicating pathology in cochlear nuclei, cochlea, and/or central nervous system involvement. Audiometric findings typically show mild to profound sensorineural hearing loss characterized by a "cookie-bite" or "saucer-shaped" curve. Hearing loss is usually sensorineural and bilaterally symmetrical (Goodhill, 1967; Matkin and Carhart, 1966, 1968).

Diabetes Mellitus

Diabetes mellitus is a chronic hormonal disorder of carbohydrate metabolism which is believed to result from insulin deficiency. The exact cause of this problem is unknown but there appears to be a strong genetic predisposition (Lowenstein and Preger, 1976). There are two types of diabetes mellitus: juvenile onset and maturity onset. Juvenile onset is the more severe of the two and usually appears suddenly in childhood or in the teens. Daily insulin injections are required to compensate for a lack of native insulin. The young untreated diabetic is often quite thin, and experiences excessive hunger, thirst, need to urinate, weakness, and weight loss. Diabetics are more susceptible to infection. Long-term complications of this disorder include blindness, kidney dysfunction, and gangrene of extremities. Deafness is not an invariable accompaniment, but when it occurs it is usually a mild to moderate, progressive, bilaterally symmetrical sensorineural hearing loss.

In the normal body system, insulin is produced in the pancreas and is secreted directly into the bloodstream. Insulin's function is to enable glucose in the blood to enter the cells. Insulin also serves to facilitate and expedite the metabolism and storage of glucose in the cells. Fuel for metabolism, heat, and motion is provided by glucose. Any excess is stored by the cells as glycogen or fat, or both. Glucose is also stored in the liver as glycogen and when needed is converted back to glucose and released into the bloodstream. Normally, insulin lowers blood sugar level while glycogen serves to raise it. In diabetics there is insufficient insulin for normal absorption of the glucose by the cells or the liver. The body senses a deficiency of glucose and sends hormonal messages to increase the delivery of glucose. The liver converts glycogen back to glucose, but the glucose still cannot be absorbed by cells without insulin so it accumulates in the blood. The liver also begins breaking down fats and amino acids for metabolism which may give rise to acids which accumulate in blood and ultimately become poisonous to the system. Over many years vascular changes occur and involve the small blood vessels of the body including the capillaries, arterioles, and venules. The diameter of these vessels decreases resulting in less blood flow (microangiopathy).

Morphological and histological studies of the ear generally agree that the etiology of hearing loss in diabetics is damage to the cochlear structures due to microangiopathic disturbance. Cranial nerve VIII and spiral ganglion may also be affected but most auditory tests indicate cochlear disorder. This confusion surrounding etiology of the hearing loss leaves few clues as to the otologic and audiologic symptoms of early diabetes. However, the incidence of hearing loss is higher in diabetics than in nondiabetics of the same age (Axelssen and Fagerberg, 1968; Friedman et al., 1975).

Acoustic Nerve Tumors

Tumors arising from the eighth nerve and extending into the cerebellar-pontine angle have been reported in children. Tumors in this area are usually neuromas originating from the vestibular portion of the eighth nerve. The hearing loss is usually unilateral, progressive sensorineural type and may be difficult to identify, especially in children. The ultimate diagnosis is made from the posterior fossa myelogram which outlines the tumor with dye. Audiometric tests and vestibular procedures may contribute information to the ultimate diagnosis. Cases of acoustic tumors in children, although rather rare, have been presented by Craig et al. (1954), Bjorkesten (1957), Krause and McCabe (1971), and Anderson and Bentinck (1972). The total number of published cases of children with acoustic nerve tumors in 1972 was approximately 10.

MEDICAL REFERRAL OR TREATMENT

It is the audiologist's responsibility to insist that regular medical examinations be obtained for the hearing-impaired child. Until the child is 8 or 10 years of age, an otolaryngologic examination should be insisted upon every 6 months.

An erroneous assumption is that after a child has sustained a hearing loss, nothing more can happen to his ears. Not only is this belief incorrect, but there is some evidence suggesting that even sensorineural hearing impairment may be accompanied by increased susceptibility to other ear disease, to noise-induced loss, or to ototoxity (Falk, 1972). In addition, the demonstrated relationship of progressive sensorineural loss with otitis media poses a threat to the child who cannot afford to lose more hearing (Paparella and Brady, 1970; English et al., 1973). Therefore it is imperative that the hearing-impaired child be monitored more regularly than the normal hearing child. The importance of every dB of residual hearing that the child possesses may be in exponential ratio to each dB of hearing loss.

At the same time an otologic examination is made, a recheck audiologic evaluation should be done. Monitoring the degree of loss pays dividends in information on changes in hearing that are pertinent for the habilitation program. A change in hearing aids, or a revision of the gain-output-frequency response of the aids may be indicated. A more extensive otologic and physical examination may be suggested when deterioration of the auditory threshold or the speech discrimination is found.

The kinds of changes that should be watched for include the following:

Progression of the Sensorineural Hearing Level

Genetic deafness is known to be subject to deterioration, either gradual or rapid. An example of the progression of a recessive hereditary hearing loss is shown in Figure 3.8. The hearing first deteriorated slowly for 4 years, then very rapidly in a period of 2 months.

Progression of the Air Conduction Hearing Level

It should not be necessary to point out that whenever a conductive loss appears, superimposed upon a sensorineural loss, immediate referral should be made to a physician. A problem arises in the case of profoundly deaf children whose bone conduction levels cannot be reached by the audiometer. The air conduction level may not change notably—the fragmentary responses could be tactile—and a conductive element may go unnoticed. For this reason it is always imperative that a tympanogram be obtained at every check-up of the child's hearing. Serious middle ear problems may be prevented by prompt referral of such patients to a physician's care.

Reports of Tinnitus, Dizziness, and Changes in the Quality of Sound

It has been confirmed in children that symptoms resembling those of hydrops can occur with sudden onset (Arenberg, 1980). The child may complain of a ringing sound in one ear, which may or may not be accompanied by dizziness. It is often associated with reports of changes in the quality of the sound perceived in that ear. Whether the physician elects to give treatment, a child presenting with any unusual symptoms should be referred to a physician without delay. Serious ear disease must always be ruled out through the physician's diagnosis. The audiologist is responsible for the child's receiving the proper kind of health care for his ears.

GENETICS

Humans take great pride in identifying distinguishing traits from one generation

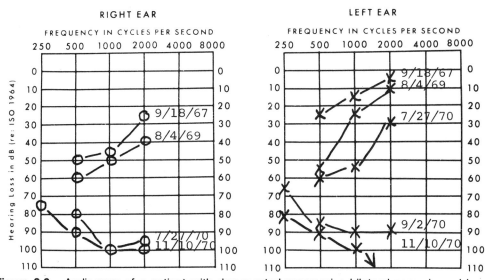

Figure 3.8. Audiogram of a patient with documented progressive bilateral sensorineural hearing loss. This child had normal hearing by observation of responses from birth to age 2½ years.

to the next. We enjoy speculating on the resemblance of children to their parents and question which child has its father's eyebrows or its mother's chin. With such observations begins the study of genetics and the submicroscopic structures known as genes.

Genes are found in the nuclei of the many cells which compose our body. Genes are concerned with the determination of what an individual's characteristics shall be, and they form the hereditary link between one generation and the next. The characteristics of an offspring are, to a large degree, determined by the genes he receives from his parents—from his mother through the ovum, or egg, and from his father through the sperm cell that fertilized that ovum at the time of conception. Genetic factors present at conception are largely unaltered throughout life. The genes are contained in chromosomes which occur in pairs. One member of each chromosome pair is inherited from the father, the other chromosome member is inherited from the mother.

The clinician concerned with hearing disorders should have some basic knowledge of genetics in hereditary inheritance. There is probably some genetic component in almost all disease processes, but the extent of this component varies. Some diseases are almost entirely determined by an individual's genetic constitution such as Down's syndrome, achondroplasia, and other individually rare conditions (Carter, 1969).

Nearly 3,000 genetic disorders have been identified. Of the 3,000,000 babies born in the United States each year, 2–3% have a major genetic or congenital disease. The average person has 4–8 potentially harmful genes—out of a total of 50,000 to 100,000 genes that determine his/her neonatal and physical traits. A number of important technological advances will help reduce these statistics. *Amniocentesis* is a procedure in which physicians withdraw amniotic fluid from the mother's uterus and examine it for abnormal cells that indicate the condition of the fetus. *Ultrasound* techniques bounce sound waves off the fetus to produce pictures. *Fetoscopy* permits the physician to examine the fetus directly with a lighted lens inserted into the uterus.

Of course, the problem of identifying an abnormal fetus may be simpler than the decision regarding abortion. The problem of deciding whether to abort a fetus is complicated by the fact that many genetic disorders present with a wide spectrum of severity. For example, some children born with cystic fibrosis have only minor symptoms throughout their lives, while others die a slow death from respiratory failure. Some mildly involved Down's children may lead useful, productive lives, while others with the same chromosome picture but more severe retardation, will necessarily be institutionalized for life.

The following presentation will include basic information concerning chromosomes and chromosome defects, patterns of inheritance, the genetics of deafness, and genetic counseling. Our goal is to acquaint the clinician who has had little or no formal course work in genetics with the fundamentals of this important aspect of life which contributes to many of the cases of deafness we see commonly in the patient population. We are greatly indebted to Janet Stewart, M.D. (1973), of the University of Colorado Birth Defects Clinic and Pediatric Department, for permission to use her previously published materials on genetic counseling as the basis of the following discussion.

Chromosomes and Chromosomal Defects

All hereditary material, in the form of deoxyribonucleic acid (DNA) is carried as genes on the chromosomes. All human body cells contain 23 pairs of chromosomes or 46 total chromosomes. Twenty-two of these pairs are known as autosomes; the remaining two chromosomes are called the sex chromosomes, two X chromosomes constituting a female (written as 46,XX in genetic nomenclature) and one X and one Y constituting a male (46,XY). The reproduction process of the body (or somite) cells is known as mitosis, while the reproduction of the germ (or sex) cells is called meiosis.

During the process of mitosis, each chromosome becomes shortened and thickened, and splits longitudinally into two chromatids joined at the point called the centromere. This is the form in which most chromosomes are pictured. They are then aligned and split longitudinally through the centromere, separating the two chromatids which then migrate to opposite ends of the cell. Cleavage then occurs in the cell to produce two genetically similar cells. Mitosis is an elegant, yet simple, mechanism for the replication of body cells (Fig. 3.9).

Man, like all forms of life, must reproduce if his species is to continue. An essential factor in the reproductive process is the formation of additional sperm and eggs by a special type of cell division (meiosis) which involves only the germ cells, as shown in Figure 3.10.

In this process the chromosomes again shorten and thicken and split into two chromatids joined at the centromere as described in mitosis. Matching pairs are arranged together and at this time material may be exchanged between paired chromosomes. The paired chromosomes then separate (known as dysjunction) and move to opposite poles of the cell, forming two cells now with 23 chromosomes each (known as the haploid number). Each cell contains either an X or a Y. The next step in the process is simple mitotic division in which there is a longitudinal split at the centromere and migration of the chromatids to opposite poles. In this manner new ova and new sperm are formed, each with 23 chromosomes. At some future time of fertilization, one ovum and one sperm will unite to form a cell, known as the zygote, with a full 46 chromosome constitution.

Abnormalities may occur during meiotic or mitotic division, producing an individual with a chromosomal defect. These abnormalities may involve one of the autosomes or one of the sex chromosomes and consists of either too much or too little total chromosome material. In certain types of tissue, and under certain conditions, chromosomes are readily visible under high magnification. A photographic record of chromosomal constitution of a cell is called a karyotype (Figs. 3.11 and 3.12). The human karyotype is often described in terms of "Denver system," so-called because it was formulated at a meeting of cytologists in Denver, Colorado (Crispens, 1971). In the human karyotype the pairs of somatic chromosomes (autosomes) are identified by number (1 to 22) as nearly as possible in descending order of their length, and also divided into seven groups (usually designated as group A through group G). Each group is composed of chromosome pairs with similar morphologic features. The sex chromosomes are identified by the symbols X and Y.

The most common autosomal defect is known as Down's syndrome, or mongolism. The affected individual has an extra number 21 chromosome (trisomy 21) for a total

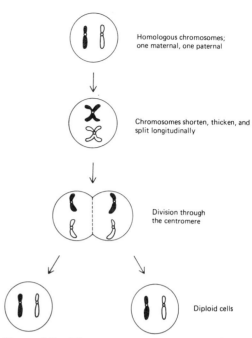

Figure 3.9. The process of mitotic cell division. (Reprinted with permission from J. M. Stewart: Genetic counseling. In *Maternity Nursing Today*, edited by J. Clausen et al. New York, McGraw-Hill, 1973.)

Homologous chromosomes; one maternal, one paternal

Chromosomes shorten, thicken, and split longitudinally

Division through the centromere

Diploid cells

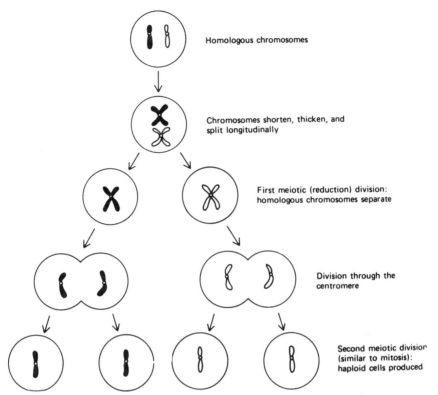

Figure 3.10. Germ cell division, or meiosis. (Reprinted with permission from J. M. Stewart: Genetic counseling. In *Maternity Nursing Today*, edited by J. Clausen et al. New York, McGraw-Hill, 1973.)

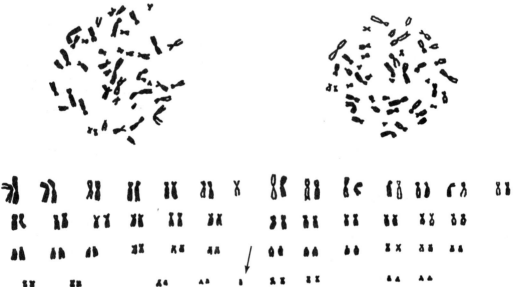

Figure 3.11. Human male karyotype with normal chromosomes. (Courtesy of A. Robinson, M.D., Cytogenetics Laboratory, University of Colorado Medical Center.)

Figure 3.12. Human female karyotype with normal chromosomes. (Courtesy of A. Robinson, M.D., Cytogenetics Laboratory, University of Colorado Medical Center.)

of 47 chromosomes. The clinical features of Down's syndrome are described in the appendix, "Index of Hearing Disorders." Down's syndrome can also occur in another form. An occasional child with Down's syndrome will have only 46 chromosomes, including one large abnormal chromosome which consists of the translocation of the extra 21 to another chromosome. Clinically, the child with the translocation type of Down's syndrome is indistinguishable from the child with the more common form, trisomy 21.

Hearing loss may also occur with trisomy 13 and trisomy 18, as described more fully in the Appendix. These children usually have many severe abnormalities and rarely live beyond a few months of age. The total absence of an autosome is felt to be incompatible with life, although a few exceptions have been reported. For example, a deletion of the short arm of chromosome 5 results in severe mental retardation and a catlike cry in infancy, comprising the cri du chat syndrome.

Unlike the loss of autosomal material, an individual may lose one of the sex chromosomes with surprisingly little defect. Sex chromosome defects do cause disorders usually less severe than autosomal defects, such as Turner's syndrome and Klinefelter's syndrome. About 1% of residents of institutions for the retarded have sex chromosome anomalies (Robinson, 1972).

PATTERNS OF INHERITANCE

The chromosomal defects that have been described above are all grossly obvious in a standard karyotype. Defects involving single genes, however, are much more discrete and invisible by any currently used technique. The determination of the hereditary nature of an abnormality is done primarily by the careful study of an individual's family.

Genes occur in pairs and are located on homologous chromosomes. One gene is maternal in origin and the other paternal. If the two genes have the same effect, the individual is said to be "homozygous" for the gene. If the effect is different, he is said to be "heterozygous" for the gene. The expression of each gene factor depends on its interaction with other genes and the environment. Genetic defects can be inherited in three well known ways and in a fourth less well understood, but commonly occurring, manner.

Autosomal Dominant

A condition or trait is said to be dominantly inherited if it is manifest in the heterozygous state. This is a type of inheritance with an affected individual having a 50% chance of passing the gene on to each of his offspring. Every afflicted individual will have a similarly afflicted parent. An unaffected individual in most cases does not carry the abnormal gene, and all of his offspring will be normal. Dominantly inherited traits have several distinguishing characteristics. They are usually milder, since the gene is passed on by the affected individual who is capable of reproduction. There is much variation in the clinical manifestations of a dominant gene, which is known as "variation in expressivity." In other words, a few individuals are so very severely affected, while those at the other end of the spectrum may be so mildly affected that they have no obvious clinical manifestation of the gene problem. If this occurs, a gene is said to have "decreased penetrance." On occasion, a dominant trait will seem to appear as a spontaneous gene mutation. The parents of such a child are not at an increased risk for future pregnancies, although the affected individual himself would have a 50% chance of passing the trait on to his offspring.

Autosomal Recessive

A condition is said to be recessively inherited if it is manifest only when the individual is homozygous for the defective gene. This is a type of inheritance in which the carrier parents may often be asymptomatic with a 25% chance of producing an affected child. One half of their children will be carriers, like themselves, and 25% will be genetically normal. In many cases, recessive conditions are more severe than dominant conditions, as the abnormality is passed on by the asymptomatic carrier and the affected person need not reproduce. If a particularly recessive condition is rare, there is an increased incidence of consanguinity in the parents. Consanguinity, which refers to a marriage of parents with recent common ancestors, such as cousins, uncle-niece marriages, etc., has genetic significance in that there is a greatly increased chance that two parents who have a recent common ancestor may each have the same recessive gene inherited from that common ancestor. Each partner, then, could give a child this gene, so that it would possess two such genes and be homozygous for the abnormal gene (Brown, 1967). The pattern of this type of inheritance shows a cluster of affected individuals among brothers and sisters, with normal parents. It is not possible to identify such families in the general population until they have produced affected children. An example of an autosomal recessive disorder is Pendred's syndrome, a condition characterized by hearing loss and a goiter which appears in adolescence. Both parents in some circumstances might have normal hearing with no other family history of deafness.

Sex-linked

If the gene for a particular trait or abnormality is located on the X chromosome, the condition is said to be inherited in an X-linked or sex-linked manner. The condition then is X-linked recessive if it is manifest only in the male who is homozygous—that is, the abnormal gene on the single X chromosome is genetically unopposed. The female who has a normal gene on one X chromosome and an abnormal gene on the other is a carrier and usually asymptomatic. The carrier female passes the gene on to 50% of her sons who then manifest the abnormality, and 50% of her daughters who are also carriers but who will not manifest the abnormality. The car-

dinal feature of an X-linked trait is the lack of male-to-male transmission, since the male may pass on his Y chromosome only to his sons. The pattern of father-daughter alternation is characteristic because affected fathers have only one X chromosome, so they must pass the gene to their daughters, and none of their sons, who get the father's Y chromosome and the mother's X chromosome. Sex-linked inheritance patterns have been familiar since biblical times when it was noted that hemophilia, as well as color blindness, seemed to be passed from unaffected females to males (Brown, 1967).

Polygenic

Many of the more common congenital abnormalities, such as cleft lip, cleft palate, and spina bifida are not inherited in one of the manners described above, and yet it is well known that these defects cluster in families. It has been postulated that multiple genes contribute to these defects and that each individual has a threshold above which the abnormality will be manifest. This condition is known as polygenic inheritance. The more severe the defect, the more the predisposing genes must present. Unlike single gene defects, the recurrence risk varies with the number of affected persons in the family.

Genetic Counseling

Genetic counseling is often given to parents who have had one abnormal child and who are interested in knowing the potential for having additional children with the same defect. Genetic counseling may also be offered to siblings of an abnormal individual and to the affected person himself as he approaches marriage age and possible parenthood. Genetic evaluation and counseling may be done in any of some 400 genetic counseling centers in the United States today.

The steps of the genetic counseling vary with the complexity of the problem, but include a careful family, pregnancy, birth, and infancy history to find factors which might explain the abnormality, careful physical examination of the affected individual and other family members, and necessary laboratory work as required. When the evaluation has been completed and the diagnosis reached, the parents return for the actual counseling sessions. Both parents are generally required to attend and the counseling is done in an unhurried and relaxed atmosphere. They are given the final diagnosis and the risk figures for future pregnancies. When possible an attempt is made by the genetic counselors to minimize guilt; however, in situations in which one parent is obviously the carrier of the gene causing the defect, it may be better to acknowledge the guilt and help the parent deal with it. In many instances more than one counseling session is necessary. There is good evidence that parents who seek genetic advice will usually make appropriate and expected decisions about future children.

The field of genetics is old yet it is filled with new discoveries. Only in 1956 were man's chromosomes accurately counted, and in 1959 the first chromosomal abnormality—the trisomy 21 associated with Down's syndrome—was accurately described. Progress has been rapid, however, in the last 25 years, and many of the new techniques are of practical significance in terms of genetic counseling.

The diagrammatic construction of a family pedigree, which is a representation of the family medical history used to determine if the etiology of a disease is indeed familial, is helpful to indicate modes of inheritance. The pedigree may provide evidence to establish whether a trait carried by a single gene is dominant, recessive or sex-linked. Simple pedigrees showing classic types of single gene inheritance are presented in Figure 3.13.

HEREDITARY DEAFNESS

According to Proctor and Proctor (1967) hereditary deafness is a fairly common disease entity, occurring somewhere between

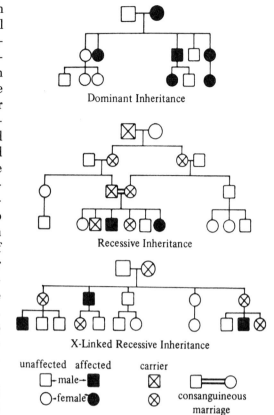

Dominant Inheritance

Recessive Inheritance

X-Linked Recessive Inheritance

Figure 3.13. Family pedigrees showing simple inheritance patterns of single gene factors. (Reprinted with permission from A. Robinson: Genetic and chromosomal disorders. In *Current Pediatric Diagnosis and Treatment*, edited by C. H. Kempe et al. Los Altos, Calif.: Lange Medical Publications, 1972.)

1 in 2000 and 1 in 6000 live births. We use the term "hereditary deafness" rather than "congenital deafness" in this section because we are referring to children with profound, irreversible, bilateral sensorineural hearing loss of early onset. Congenital deafness would include those children with conductive hearing loss due to osseous malformation in the middle ear. Such a condition usually creates a moderate hearing loss, often amenable to surgical intervention, and thus quite a different group of children from those we describe with hereditary childhood deafness (Fraser, 1971). Hereditary deafness is usually a bilateral disease entity (Kinney, 1950). Everberg (1960), researched nearly 200,000 school children in

Copenhagen to conclude that hereditary factors were of importance in only 10%, or 12 cases of 122 patients with unilateral deafness. In studying a child with apparent congenital severe deafness, the clinician must be aware of possible exogenous, or outside, factors that can cause childhood deafness, as summarized in Table 3.1. A major contribution to the study of etiologic factors in deafness has been published by Fraser, *The Causes of Profound Deafness in Childhood* (1976).

A high percentage of congenital deafness is hereditary, according to Fraser et al. (1964), Konigsmark (1972) and Fraser (1976). About 40% of profound childhood deafness is autosomal recessive in origin; 10%, dominant transmission; and some 3%, due to a sex-linked gene. Since deaf persons tend to marry other deaf persons (Schein, 1965; Northern et al., 1971), statistics regarding their potential for producing deaf offspring are of interest. According to Bergstrom et al. (1971), the marriage of two deaf persons gives only a slightly increased risk of deafness in their children because there is small chance that two such persons would be affected by the same exact genetic deafness. Should the same recessive gene be carried by two normal hearing parents, theoretically one fourth of their offspring would be affected and one half of their children would be carriers. However, if both parents are overtly affected by the same recessive type of hereditary deafness, they are homozygous for the trait and therefore *all* their children will not only be affected but also capable of passing the trait on to some of their offspring in turn.

Several modern population studies of deafness have been conducted with rather large samples, and the results have been concisely summarized by Brown (1967) and are presented in Table 3.2. These studies represent data from Northern Ireland (Stevenson and Cheesman, 1956), Japan (Furusho, 1957), England (Fraser et al., 1964) Clarke School for the Deaf in the United States (Brown and Chung, 1964), and Germany (Kittel and Schmoll-Eskuche, 1963). Acquired deafness, for the purposes of Table 3.2, is defined as those individuals in whom a prenatal or postnatal environmen-

Table 3.1.
Summary of Known Exogenous Causes of Prelingual Deafness[a]

Preconception and Prenatal Causes
  Rubella
  Cytomegalovirus
  Ototoxic and other drugs, maternal alcoholism
  Hypoxia (and its possible causes: high altitude, general anesthetic, severe hemorrhage)
  Syphilis
  Toxemia, diabetes, other severe systemic maternal illness
  Parental irradiation
  Toxoplasmosis
Perinatal Causes
  Hypoxia
  Traumatic delivery
  Maternal infection
  Ototoxic drugs
  Premature delivery
Neonatal and Postnatal Causes
  Hypoxia
  Infection
  Ototoxic drugs
  Erythroblastosis fetalis
  Infantile measles or mumps
  Otitis media (acute, chronic, serous)
  Noise-induced
  Meningitis
  Encephalitis

[a] From L. Bergstrom, W. G. Hemenway, and M. P. Downs: *Otolaryngology Clinics of North America*, 4:369–399, 1971.

Table 3.2.
Ratio of Childhood Deafness from Several Population Studies[a]

	No. in Sample	Hereditary Deafness	Acquired Deafness
Northern Ireland	424	.513	
Japan	1561	.502	
England	2355	.517	.578
Clarke School, USA	1222	.512	.544
Germany	2788	.532	.606

[a] Modified with permission from K. S. Brown: The genetics of childhood deafness. In *Deafness in Childhood*, pp. 177–202, edited by F. McConnell and P. H. Ward. Nashville, Vanderbilt University Press, 1967.

tal factor has been claimed as a cause of deafness. One must be impressed at the close relationship of population percentages, across these studies, of deaf individuals with hereditary and acquired deafness.

Another means of identifying the causes of deafness has been accomplished by interviewing large samples of adult deaf persons. The adult deaf, however, are unfortunately poorly informed regarding the cause of their hearing problems. Such analyses are usually obtained through a written questionnaire or personal interview, but in this type of population in which language and communication are problems, such information-gathering techniques suggest caution in data interpretation. We are reminded of the deaf father who told us that he lost his hearing between the ages of 1 and 2. His parents told him that he had cut his finger badly, and the doctor had stitched up the cut without use of anesthesia. The pain was apparently so severe, that his loud crying damaged his hearing. This story from a totally deaf man married to a deaf woman, the parents of three deaf children! A summary of results from two studies of deaf adults who were asked the cause of their hearing loss (Schein, 1965; Northern et al., 1971) is shown in Table 3.3.

Despite the large number of syndromes associated with dominant deafness, the great majority of human inherited deafness (about 90%) is of a recessive rather than dominant type (Proctor and Proctor, 1967). In the case of recessively inherited deafness, both parents must be the carriers of the particular gene, in which event the chance of offspring being affected is only 25%. Most of these patients have no family history of deafness, thereby making the case for hereditary etiology difficult to prove. An exceptional public information booklet is available from Gallaudet College, Washington, D. C., entitled "What Every Person Should Know About Heredity and Deafness" (1975).

CLASSIFICATION OF HEREDITARY DEAFNESS

Childhood deafness associated with other defects has been observed for hundreds of years and cited in journal articles too numerous to count. Konigsmark (1969) indicates that about 70 types of hereditary deafness have been identified in man. Only since the mid-1960s have data been available regarding the relative frequency of various syndrome complexes which include deafness.

The alert clinician is soon aware that malformations and anomalies often "run together." Congenital defects are often caused by prenatal misfortunes which may influence the development of specific body systems or create generalized malformations of all the structures undergoing growth at that time. On the other hand, when multiple congenital malformations appear together frequently, the patient can be described in terms of a "syndrome." The term syndrome is often overused and misapplied. The difficulties of syndrome classification lie in terminology problems, broad spectra of signs and symptoms, and differences in the basis of diagnosis depending on whether the diagnosis is anatomic, histologic, or hematologic. Often experts disagree on the diagnosis of a syndrome, or the youngster may present such a variety of symptomatic signs that clearcut diagnosis is not possible. The definition

Table 3.3.
Etiology of Hearing Loss as Expressed by Manually Communicating Deaf Adults

Etiology	Percentage	
	Northern et al. (1971)	Schein (1965)
Unknown	35.8	32.2
Congenital	25.5	10.5
Meningitis	13.1	12.7
Scarlet fever	9.5	4.6
Result of a fall	8.1	7.7
Whooping cough	3.6	2.3
Measles	2.2	3.4
Pneumonia		2.3
Mastoiditis		1.9
Other	2.2	16.7
N =	137	1132

of a syndrome depends on the level of acuity of observation, and becomes easier the more pronounced the accompanying features are demonstrated.

Many children may likely be candidates for ultimate syndrome diagnosis, but hearing loss will not always be present. In addition, some disorders may manifest progressive-type hearing loss; so that although normal hearing is noted on the initial visit, these children deserve regular reevaluation. The verification of hearing loss is the realm of the audiologist who can substantiate accurately hearing levels in such children with appropriate testing techniques. A summary of communication disorders found in various syndromes has recently been published by Siegel-Sadewitz and Shprintzen (1982).

There are many ways of classifying hereditary deafness. Martensson (1960) suggested a classification system that utilizes the genetic mode of transmission, listing various diseases associated with deafness by their mode of inheritance pattern such as dominant, recessive, sex-linked, etc. Kinney (1950) suggested grouping of deafness disorders by clinical manifestations, while Omerod (1960) classified inherited deafness by the pathology of the auditory system. Black et al. (1971a) presented an excellent summary of hereditary deafness as classified by each of the above mentioned systems. A concise system of classifying deafness was prepared by Bergstrom et al. (1971) ordered around types of hearing loss and body systems as shown in Table 3.4.

CONGENITAL MALFORMATIONS

Congenital Malformations of the Inner Ear

Although wide variety exists in anatomic abnormalities of the inner ear, four classic types exist. These include (a) Michel, complete failure of development of the inner ear; (b) Mondini, incomplete development and malformation of the inner ear; (c) the Scheibe membranous cochleosaccular degeneration of the inner ear; and (d) the Alexander malformation of the cochlear membranous system. A Bing-Siebenmann classification has been suggested by Omerod (1960).

The Bing-Siebenmann anomaly is characterized by a normal bony capsule with malformed membranous components of the cochlea and vestibular mechanism. It has been reported in patients with mental retardation and retinitis pigmentosa. In terms of severity of aplasia, the Bing-Siebenmann deformity would be classified between the Mondini and Scheibe aplasias. These cases generally show profound hearing loss. These four inner ear anomalies have been described by many authors, including notable publications by Schuknecht (1967), Lindsay (1971a, 1971b), and Hemenway and Bergstrom (1972). The question exists whether these malformations are due to embryonic developmental arrest, since in some instances the pathology does not represent any embryonic stage in development of the ear.

Aplasia of the inner ear implies failure of the ear to reach full development. Accordingly, inner ear aplasia is always a congenital malformation. The embryonic time of developmental failure, of course, determines the ultimate structure and appearance of the deformity. According to Schuknecht (1967), an individual may possess different degrees of aplasia in the two ears. Aplasia of the inner ear is a relatively uncommon aberration.

Michel-Type of Aplasia of the Inner Ear. The macroscopic description of this temporal bone anomaly was first described by Michel in 1863. This type of anomaly is represented by a complete absence of the inner ear and auditory nerve. The outer ear may be completely normal with a narrow middle ear cavity. The malleus and incus may be present, but the stapes and stapedius muscle may be absent or abnormal. Maternal thalidomide during pregnancy has been associated with this anomaly, and it has been observed in at least one case of Klippel-Feil deformity (McLay and Marar, 1969).

Mondini Aplasia of the Inner Ear.

Table 3.4.
Classification of Hereditary Deafness

I. **CONGENITAL SENSORINEURAL HEARING LOSS DISORDERS**
Craniofacial and Skeletal Disorders
- Absence of tibia
- Cleidocranial dysostosis
- Diastrophic dwarfism
- Hand-hearing syndrome
- Klippel-Feil
- Saddle nose and myopia
- Split-hand and foot

Integumentary and Pigmentary Disorders
- Albinism with blue irides
- Congenital atopic dermatitis
- Ectodermal dysplasia
- Keratopachyderma
- Lentigines
- Onychodystrophy
- Partial albinism
- Piebaldness
- Pili torti
- Waardenburg's syndrome

Eye Disorders
- Hallgren's
- Laurence-Moon-Biedl-Bardet

Nervous System Disorders
- Cerebral palsy
- Muscular dystrophy
- Myoclonic epilepsy
- Opticochochleodentate degeneration
- Richards-Rundel

Cardiovascular System Disorders
- Jervell and Lange-Nielsen

Endocrine and Metabolic Disorders
- Goiter
- Hyperprolinemia I
- Iminoglycinuria
- Pendred's

Miscellaneous Somatic Disorders
- Trisomy 13–15
- Trisomy 18

II. **CONGENITAL CONDUCTIVE HEARING LOSS DISORDERS**
Craniofacial and Skeletal Disorders
- Apert's syndrome
- Fanconi anemia syndrome
- Goldenhar's syndrome
- Madelung's deformity
- Malformed, low set ears
- Mohr syndrome
- Otopalatodigital
- Preauricular appendages
- Proximal symphalangism
- Thickened ears
- Treacher Collins

Integumentary and Pigmentary Disorders
- Forney's syndrome

Eye Disorders
- Cryptophthalmos
- Duane's syndrome

Renal Disorders
- Nephrosis, urinary tract malformations
- Renal-genital syndrome
- Taylor's syndrome

III. **DISORDERS OF CONGENITAL SENSORINEURAL AND/OR CONDUCTIVE HEARING LOSS**
Craniofacial and Skeletal Disorders
- Achondroplasia
- Crouzon's syndrome
- Marfan's syndrome
- Pierre Robin
- Pyle's disease

Integumentary and Pigmentary Disorders
- Knuckle pads and leukonychia

Eye Disorders
- Möbius syndrome

Miscellaneous Somatic Disorders
- Turner's syndrome

IV. **PROGRESSIVE HEARING LOSS DISORDERS**
Sensorineural Progressive Hearing Loss of Later Onset
Craniofacial and Skeletal Disorders
- Roaf's syndrome
- Van Buchem's syndrome

Eye Disorders
- Alström's syndrome
- Cockayne's syndrome
- Fehr's corneal dystrophy
- Flynn-Aird
- Norrie's syndrome
- Optic atrophy and diabetes mellitus
- Refsum's syndrome

Nervous System Disorders
- Acoustic neuromas
- Friedreich's ataxia
- Herrmann's syndrome
- Myoclonic seizures
- Sensory radicular neuropathy
- Severe infantile muscular dystrophy

Endocrine and Metabolic Disorders
- Alport's syndrome
- Amyloidosis, nephritis, and urticaria
- Hyperprolinemia II
- Hyperuricemia
- Primary testicular insufficiency

Sensorineural or Conductive Progressive Hearing Loss
Craniofacial and Skeletal Disorders
- Albers-Schönberg disease
- Engelmann's syndrome
- Osteogenesis imperfecta
- Paget's disease

Endocrine and Metabolic Disorders
- Hunter's syndrome
- Hurler's syndrome

Progressive Conductive or Mixed Hearing Loss
- Otoslcerosis

Mondini described a temporal bone in 1791 that showed incomplete development of a flattened cochlea which consisted of only a single basal coil. In 1904 Alexander added more detail to this type of anomaly indicating involvement of auditory nerve and the vestibular canals. Characteristic of this anomaly is that it involves both the bony capsule and membranous labyrinth. This anomaly, which often bears both investigators' names, has been associated with Klippel-Feil and Wildervanck syndromes. It has also been found in cases of mental retardation, hydrocephalus, and hydronephrosis. Middle ear anomalies may be present in these cases and atresia of the external canal has also been reported.

Many temporal bone studies have described this deformity which varies considerably from one case to another and may be unilateral or bilateral (Fig. 3.14). Altman (1950) suggested that labyrinthine hydrops might be present in Mondini dysplasia, and a new theory of management has emerged on this basis, utilizing the endolymphatic shunt operation in an effort to relieve the hydrops believed to be causing progressive hearing loss in these cases.

A case of progressive hearing loss beginning at age 37 was reported by Murakimi and Schuknecht (1968). However, there have been reports of Mondini dysplasia in temporal bone patients who had normal hearing throughout life (Polvogt and Crowe, 1937). It has been possible recently to diagnose dysplasia through temporal bone polytomography, leading to more frequent diagnoses of this problem (Illum, 1972; Valvassori et al., 1969). Many patients seem to have fluctuant hearing loss that tends to become progressively worse, and questioning the parents may reveal that the child has difficulty walking at that time. Electrocochleography (ECoG) may contribute to the diagnosis, as Brackmann (1977) described a type of wave form that is a multipeaked or disynchronized acoustic nerve action potential wave form which he

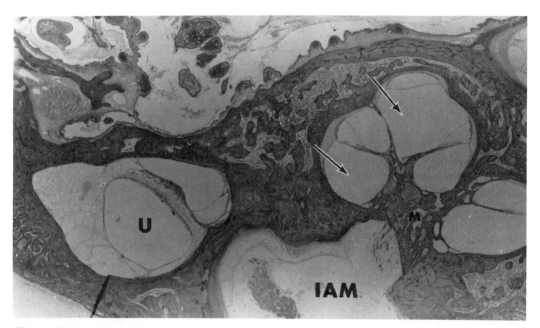

Figure 3.14. Mondini-type of incomplete development with malformation of the inner ear from a patient with trisomy 13-15 syndrome. Note incompletely developed cochlea with absence of the interscaler osseus septum (arrows), and poorly developed modiolus (*M*). Utricle (*U*) and internal auditory meatus (*IAM*) are also identified. (Reprinted with permission from I. Sando, B. Baker, F. O. Black, and W. G. Hemenway: *Archives of Otolaryngology, 96:* 441–447, 1972.)

considered characteristic of Ménière's disease. Mangabeira-Albernaz et al. (1981) found the same characteristic peak wave forms in 12 cases of Mondini dysplasia. These authors also found a suspicion of dysplasia in cases with clearly asymmetrical ECoG thresholds and in those with diphasic action potential responses. It was proposed by House (1964) that an endolymphatic subarachnoid shunt would help to prevent the fluctuation of hearing in Mondini ears and would stop the progression of the hearing loss. The theory is that the progressive loss of hair cells may result from membrane ruptures resulting from endolymphatic hydrops, as the temporal bones that have been studied do show enlarged endoplymphatic sacs and ducts. According to Mangabeira-Albernaz (1981) children with a complete absence of the osseous spiral lamina usually lose their hearing completely about 4 years of age, but in many cases the dysplasia is less severe and the patient continues to have hearing for many years.

As the endolymphatic shunt operations have been done only for a short period of time on Mondini cases it is impossible to predict long-term results. Mangabeira-Albernaz et al. (1981) indicate in 22 ears that surgery does indeed stop the progression of the hearing loss, at least in the 1-year term of their report. This technique does not lend itself to easy investigation, as it is difficult to produce an animal model for it that will permit experimentation. It will remain for the test of time to reveal the efficacy of this procedure.

Scheibe Aplasia of the Inner Ear. The Scheibe abnormality of the inner ear, originally described in 1892, is characterized by involvement of only the membranous portion of the cochlea and saccule. This type of dysplasia is the most common of the inner ear aplasias. Histopathology of these inner ears show atrophy of the stria vascularis, degeneration of the organ of Corti, and rolling up of the tectorial membrane, especially in the basal turn of the cochlea. This anomaly has been identified in cases of Waardenburg's syndrome, the cardioauditory syndrome of Jervell and Lange-Nielsen. Usher's syndrome, Refsum's syndrome, and maternal rubella.

Knowledge of these inner ear anomalies is important for accurate diagnosis, proper treatment of the patient, and genetic counseling for the parents of the handicapped child, as well as for the patient when he (or she) is old enough to become a parent. Therefore, differentiation of the above inner ear problems is crucial in the determination of whether the hearing loss in question is of a genetic or an acquired origin.

The degree of abnormal development that is actually involved in any specific patient may vary considerably from other patients with similar inner ear malformations. Diagnostic considerations must include petrous pyramid polytomography of the inner ear, as well as a complete evaluation of the hearing impairment. Malformations in the bone of the otic capsule can be detected by careful x-ray, and differential diagnosis of the Michel and Mondini aplasias are possible. Some of the membranous labyrinth malfunctions may be inferred from audiometric and/or vestibular testing (Bergstrom, 1976).

Knowledge regarding the residual hearing in children with inner ear anomalies may be of great value in the habilitation of the child so deafened. According to Black et al. (1971a), audiometric patterns in the Michel ear should show no hearing since no true inner ear exists. True hearing is impossible and a hearing aid for such a patient can be of limited value. It is theoretically possible for the Mondini malformed inner ear to have some hearing, since the basal coil of the cochlea may be present with intact higher auditory pathways. The Scheibe ear may show residual hearing in the low frequencies, since in this ear the major damage is in the basal coil of the cochlea. The extent of hearing in the Bing-Siebenmann inner ear is dependent upon the area and degree of malformation present in the membranous portion of the cochlea. The Scheibe and Mondini malformations may be unilateral. Black et al. state that asymmetry of malformation is not uncommon, and the patient may demonstrate one type of inner ear anomaly on one side, and another type of inner ear anomaly on the other side. In such cases, x-ray findings and the degree or pattern of the hearing loss may be quite unlike each other.

More information is needed regarding the presence of these inner ear malformations. As of now, the risk of occurrence and the ratio of male-female incidence has not yet been securely determined. The bony inner ear dysplasias may be diagnosed soon after birth by x-ray, but the membranous labyrinth malformations must be inferred or postponed until the temporal bones can be examined. If the defect is an isolated defect, the individual may live a full life as a hard-of-hearing or deaf person. However, these inner ear defects may be associated with other limiting disorders.

Congenital Middle Ear Malformations

Interest in middle ear anomalies has increased with the advent of microscopic surgical techniques and improved diagnostic capabilities of clinicians. Many patients with abnormal middle ears can have the deformity corrected by surgery. Since the middle ear is largely formed during the first trimester of fetal life, gross developmental anomalies of the middle ear are often related to factors that influence the fetus during that time. An excellent description of middle ear anomalies has been presented by Sando and Wood (1971) and Nager (1971).

Malformation of the middle ear may be due to hereditary factors or to disturbances during embryonic development. Failure in the proper development of the first and second branchial arches may result in the absence of the ossicles or a fusion of the ossicles. A malformation of the stapes footplate, however, is related to the development of the otic capsule. A disturbance in the fetal growth of the first branchial pouch may affect the eustachian tube, middle ear

cavity, as well as the ultimate pneumatization of the mastoid air spaces.

Isolated anomalies of the middle ear ossicles are not particularly rare. Malleus anomalies include fixation or deformation of the malleus head and bony fusion of the incudomalleolar joint or absence of the malleus. Incus deficiencies may exist in isolation or in conjunction with other middle ear ossicular problems and range from total absence to a deficiency of the lenticular process. The incus may have only a fibrous connection to the malleus or be fused to the lateral semicircular canal wall. Stapes anomalies may involve fusion of the stapes head to the promontory, absence of the head and/or crura, the absence of the entire stapes itself, or the presence of a columellar ossicle. Congenital absence of the oval window or the round window may also exist as a unilateral or bilateral defect.

Middle ear anomalies should be suspected whenever other branchial arch anomalies are observed and are often noted as part of congenital syndromes. Branchial arch disorders include atresia of the external auditory canal, cleft palate, micrognathia, Pierre Robin syndrome, Treacher Collins syndrome, as well as low set auricles. Disorders which feature other skeletal defects may also include middle ear anomalies such as Apert's syndrome, Klippel-Feil syndrome, Crouzon's, Paget's, and Van der Hoeve's diseases. Middle ear anomalies have been reported in disorders of connective tissue such as gargolism or Hunter-Hurler syndromes, Möbius syndrome, and dwarfism.

Malformations of the External Ear and Canal

The auricle develops around the first branchial groove as six knoblike protrusions early in embryonic life. These six hillocks soon lose their identity as they coalesce to form the pinna. With six separate growth centers developing at differing rates, it is not surprising that a wide variation exists in final ear configurations that are within normal limits. The shape of the auricle is so different among individuals that European police forces utilize the configuration of the ear much like American police use fingerprints.

Defects of the external ear and canal may be apparent without damage to the middle or inner ear structures. However, severe middle ear anomalies or aplasia of the middle ear may be associated. Supernumerary hillocks, known as "tags" or preauricular appendages, may remain with an otherwise normal-appearing pinna. However, the presence of tags may suggest anomalies of the external and middle ear systems. In cases of the atretic ear canal, occasionally thick soft tissue is found at surgery where the tympanic membrane should be, or more often a bony atresia plate of varying degrees of thickness is present.

External ear and canal anomalies may be visible at birth, but are often overlooked and the defect is not noted until hearing loss is suspected or discovered. Sometimes the auricle and the opening to the external auditory meatus appear normal, but the meatus may funnel down to complete closure lateral to the tympanic membrane. If the atresia is bilateral, the child should be fitted with a bone conduction hearing aid as soon as possible. If the atresia is unilateral and normal hearing can be established in the opposite ear, treatment or habilitation is generally deferred. Aural atresias may accompany other defects of the cranium, face, skeleton, or mandible. The etiology of the aural atresia may be a chromosomal aberration, heredity, maternal thalidomide, or maternal rubella. Nager (1971) and Linthicum (1971) discussed procedures in problems in the surgical intervention for congenital aural atresia and middle ear ossicular anomalies.

Anomalies of the external ear suggest associated middle ear anomalies. Clinicians should be alerted to identify the malformed pinna during initial observations of children as this clue may lead to identification of associated hearing loss.

The Microtic Ear. The microtic ear has always been a problem to professionals as well as to the unfortunate possessor. Fortunately, it occurs only once in 20,000 births (Holmes, 1949), but this is often enough that we see a number of such cases each year in our clinic. The congenitally microtic ear varies from the mildly deformed ear to the conditions of total absence of pinna with no external auditory meatus, or complete atresia of the canal. Unilateral microtia is about 6 times more frequent than bilateral occurrence (Dupertius and Musgrave, 1959), is more common in males than females, and is found predominantly on the right side (Brown et al., 1969).

When a patient has one normal-hearing ear, obviously the problem of unilateral microtia is not so bad. When hair styles are long, the deformity of the auricle is easily covered. Patients, however, who wish to do something about the microtia have a choice between attempted surgical improvement or the use of a prosthetic-type pinna which is attached to the side of the head by special adhesive material. According to Holmes (1949), and supported by our observations, is the statement that regardless of what surgical techniques are employed, the reconstructed ear can never take the place of a normally developed pinna, and the result will never be inconspicuous. For improved hearing benefit, however, as in the patient who has bilaterally stenosed ear canals, surgical intervention may be successful. Schuchman (1971) reported the fitting of a special ear level, bone conduction hearing aid for a patient with bilateral atresia.

TEAM MANAGEMENT OF CHILDREN WITH HEARING IMPAIRMENT

The nature of modern-day hearing losses makes it increasingly imperative that a team of professional people work together to diagnose a hearing loss and chart the management of the child with a loss (Fig. 3.15). The hearing function is not an isolated phenomenon.

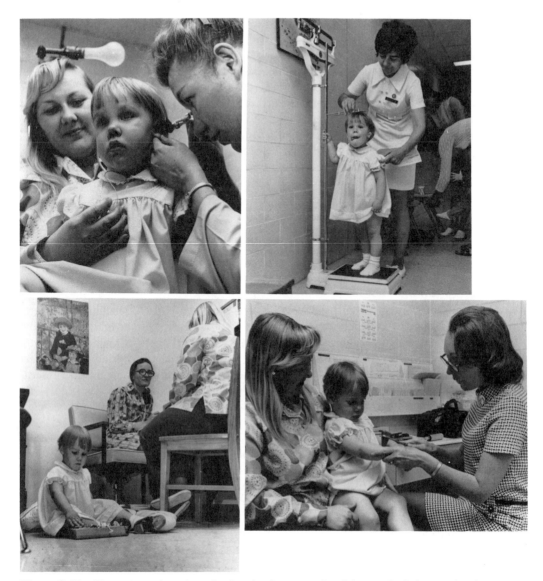

Figure 3.15. The nature of modern-day hearing losses makes it increasingly imperative that a team of professional people work together for the management of the child with hearing loss. In addition to the audiologist's services, the regularly scheduled check-up should include otologic examination (*top left*), physical examination (*top right*), social work interview (*bottom left*), and pediatric evaluation (*bottom right*). (Courtesy of The National Foundation—March of Dimes.)

We have called such a group of experts the Congenital Deafness Team even though the team will deal with hearing problems that may not literally be congenital. The great majority of hearing losses in our present times will be either present at birth or their later manifestation will be present in the genes at birth.

Our emphasis on the team approach to diagnosis in no way minimizes the audiologist's art. The role of the audiologist in decisions concerning diagnosis and management is always a vital one. Not only does he contribute essential information on the degree of loss, the auditory behavior and development, and the auditory functioning of the child, but his familiarity with training methods and their efficacy figures largely in decisions on the placement of the child. Precise audiologic measurements provide the necessary objective data, but the art of audiology weighs strongly in the evaluation. The clinical insight and intuition of the experienced audiologist contribute a much needed element to the decisions that will be made. How does the child relate to the clinician? Is eye contact good? Is the behavior even minimally distractible? Does there seem to be perseveration of auditory behavior? What is the vocal quality and how does he use his voice? How do parent and child relate to each other? These are the questions that can be answered more through intuition than through measure-ments. They are an integral part of the audiologist's art.

A summary of recommended medical workup for the child with hereditary deafness is shown in Table 3.5 Paparella (1977) has stated that every child with a hearing loss or deafness requires a medical diagnosis of the disease resulting in the hearing loss, or a diagnosis as to etiology and pathogenesis of the hearing problem.

Once the audiologist has specified that a certain degree of hearing loss exists, and has delineated the status of the auditory development of the child, a standard protocol of examinations is indicated. Any of these studies, if made in isolation, will fur-

Table 3.5.
Diagnostic Medical Workup of the Child with Hereditary Deafness[a]

History
  Detailed family pedigree
  Maternal prenatal history
General Physical Examination
  Generalized congenital bone disorders
  Congenital absence or sparseness of hair
    and/or nails
  Congenital neurologic deficits
  Ataxia of gait
Concomitant Head and Neck Physical Findings
  Atresia of the external auditory canals
  Malformed external ears
  Facial anomalies, especially of mandible
  Congenital facial nerve paralysis
  Branchial anomalies
  Heterochromia of the irises
  Increased intercanthal distance
  White forelock in scalp hair
Routine Laboratory Tests
  Family audiometry
  Complete blood count
  Urinalysis
Special Laboratory Tests where Appropriate
  (Age 1 year and under)
  Rubella titer
  Cytomegalovirus titer

  Other viral titers
  (Any age)
  Electrocardiogram
  Protein bound iodine
  Syphilis serology
  Serum pyrophosphate and uric acid
  Urine mucopolysaccharide screening

Perinatal and neonatal history
Subsequent medical history

Pigmentary disorders
Congenital heart disease

Hand anomalies

Retinitis pigmentosa
Rubella retinopathy
Congenital cataracts
Dental anomalies
Short neck; neck anomalies
Goiter
Quality of voice and speech

IgM
Viral cultures of urine, throat, and nasopharynx
  for rubella and cytomegalovirus

Dermatoglyphics
Karyotype, buccal smear
X-rays as necessary
Petrous pyramid polytomography
Electroretinography
Vestibular testing

[a] Courtesy of LaVonne Bergstrom, M.D.

nish only a fragment of the total picture of the child and his needs; but when brought together in a team conference, the picture becomes a whole. The team together makes a diagnosis of the etiology, extent, and degree of the problem and decides on the proper management for the child.

After the initial thorough evaluation, it is customary to follow the young child every 6 months to observe his progress and to pick up any loose ends of diagnosis. Not until all facets are put together and the child has stabilized satisfactorily in his program will he be seen only once a year. Such stabilization does not occur until the child is 5 or 6, even if he has been identified in infancy. From then on until adolescence he will be seen once a year, and after that, whenever indicated.

The Congenital Deafness Team should consider itself the monitor of the child's hearing and its function, the advisory group for the family, the judge of the child's potential in relation to his educational program, and the arbiter between the child and the community. Child advocacy is nowhere so effective as when undertaken by a Congenital Deafness Team (Downs, 1981).

Management of the Child

Diagnosis. Diagnosis is a cooperative effort of all the specialists involved, but the pediatrician is the primary manager of the child. The pediatrician can determine the etiology, identify other associated anomalies, and can suggest a myriad of laboratory tests that will contribute to the diagnosis. The pediatrician also assesses the overall development of the child and provide for genetic counseling once the etiology is determined. The pediatrician may seek the otologic expertise of the otolaryngologist who may request other information, such as polytomography, CAT scan, or brainstem evoked potential testing.

The audiologist not only contributes baseline audiometry, but evaluates the relationship of the child's functioning to the degree of hearing loss, thus giving information relevant to the diagnosis (Table

3.6). The speech pathologist provides a baseline speech and language evaluation which will be used to compare later functioning. During the diagnostic workup, the social worker becomes involved in helping determine where parents are in their process of accepting the problem of the deaf child. Are they in the denial stage, the anger stage, the mourning stage—and how can they be helped to an acceptance of the problem which will allow them to best nurture the child? It may be necessary, at any given point, to bring in a psychologist for detailed psychological counseling.

The ophthalmologist is called in for any of the associated eye abnormalities. A renal consultant is obtained in such cases as hereditary chronic nephritis or Alport's syndrome. Cardiologists and neurologists are called in as indicated, and it is found that, in such complex cases as Hunter-Hurler syndrome, the entire roster of specialists at the hospital may be involved.

Placement Counseling. The decision regarding placement of the child in an educational program must be the parents' prerogative. Unless the parents have made the decision, there will be second thoughts and possibly recriminations at a later date. The parents' decision is based on the following contributions from the congenital deafness team: (1) information as to the degree of loss; (2) the results of the speech and language evaluations, if relevant; (3) an introduction to the types of education available in the community. This would include visits to each of the facilities that are offering programs for hearing impaired children; and (4) encouragement to choose freely and to feel comfortable with making a change at a later date if, at any time, it appears that another program will better benefit the child.

It is essential at this point that advice be given by persons who are not involved in the therapeutic process or the educational system. Here the managing physician—the pediatrician—may be the most effective and objective in guiding the parents, but will call for advice from the rest of the congenital deafness team as necessary.

Table 3.6.
Hearing Handicap as a Function of Average Hearing Threshold Level of the Better Ear

Average Threshold Level at 500–2000 Hz (ANSI)[a]	Description	Common Causes	What Can Be Heard without Amplification	Degree of Handicap (If not treated in 1st year of life)	Probable Needs
0–15 dB	Normal range		All speech sounds	None	None
16–25 dB	Slight hearing loss	Serous otitis, perforation, monomeric membrane, sensorineural loss, tympanosclerosis	Vowel sounds heard clearly, may miss unvoiced consonant sounds	Possible mild or transitory auditory dysfunction; Difficulty in perceiving some speech sounds	Consideration of need for hearing aid; Lip reading; Auditory training; Speech therapy; Preferential seating; Appropriate surgery
26–40 dB	Mild	Serous otitis, perforation, tympanosclerosis, monomeric membrane sensorineural loss	Hears only some of speech sounds; the louder voiced sounds	Auditory learning dysfunction; Mild language retardation; Mild speech problems; Inattention	Hearing aid; Lip reading; Auditory training; Speech therapy; Appropriate surgery
41–65 dB	Moderate hearing loss	Chronic otitis, middle ear anomaly sensorineural loss	Misses most speech sounds at normal conversational level	Speech problems; Language retardation; Learning dysfunction; Inattention	All of the above, plus consideration of special classroom situation
66–95 dB	Severe hearing loss	Sensorineural loss or mixed loss due to sensorineural loss plus middle ear disease	Hears no speech sound of normal conversations	Severe speech problems; Language retardation; Learning dysfunction; Inattention	All of the above; probable assignment to special classes
96+ dB	Profound hearing loss	Sensorineural loss or mixed	Hears no speech or other sounds	Severe speech problems; Language retardation; Learning dysfunction; Inattention	All of the above; probable assignment to special classes

[a] ANSI = American National Standards Institute.

Monitoring. In the first year or two, the hearing-impaired child will be seen at least every 6 months for periodic reassessment of the etiology of the hearing impairment. Even when the etiology has been fairly certainly determined, it may be necessary to take another look. Bergstrom (1981) has outlined specific reasons for reevaluation as follows:

1. Repeat audiometry may reveal progression of loss or unsuspected opposite ear involvement;
2. Case history review may reveal overlooked historical items such as early history of disease;
3. Physical examination may reveal overlooked physical findings or newly developed symptoms, such as thyroid problems, renal problems, night blindness, etc.;
4. Repeat family history may show suppressed information. For example, in one case, the father—a physician—was found later to have a hearing loss which he had not reported previously;
5. Repeat family history can reveal false-positive items. For example, a parent's report of childhood deafness in the family was found to refer only to episodes of otitis media, rather than familial deafness;
6. "Red herrings" in the physical and historical evaluation may show up with repeated evaluations;
7. An incorrect initial diagnosis may be corrected by reevaluation;
8. Mental block phenomenon—the human failure to think of all the possibilities in a diagnosis;
9. Progressive concommitant disease may be identified by follow-up evaluations;
10. Completion of the workup, including all the laboratory tests that are relevant;
11. Second thoughts; new information from a consultant; new scientific knowledge; new technology; and, to determine how the child is doing.

Speech and language evaluations are given to monitor the performance of the child in the particular program in which he has been entered. Again, it is important to have someone who is not involved in the therapeutic process evaluate the ongoing improvement of the child or his lack of improvement. Here the policy of flexibility in placement will be useful. If at any point it is obvious that the child is not making reasonable progress in the system in which he has been placed, consideration can be given to looking at a change of program.

Psychosocial reevaluation and monitoring is extremely useful to determine whether or not any help should be given the family in psychological or social matters. It may be necessary to solicit public funds to help the family's finances in supporting the child in the particular program in which he is functioning. At any time in the program, public health support for purchase of hearing aids can be enlisted.

Advocacy. In the team's function as an objective advocate of the child, apart from the methodology of the program the child is in, it may be necessary to arbitrate between the family and the system in the following ways:

1. If parents feel that the school system has mismanaged the child's placement, it may be necessary for the team to represent the family at hearings called to evaluate the disagreement. Federal law now mandates hearings that the parents can request whenever they feel a change is indicated. For example, in a public school system where only total educational programs were available for hearing impaired children, the team sent a representative to present the case for the child's best interests being served by placement in an aural program.
2. When college age is reached, the team may be called upon to support the special interests of the student in obtaining a certain type of education. For example, a very bright, hearing-impaired student wished to attend an

out-of-state college which she felt would be more suitable for her particular skills and goals. However, the social rehabilitation service rules stipulated that the stipend was available only for in-state colleges. It was necessary for doctors, audiologists, and speech pathologists to present the case of students being supported for the out-of-state college placement. The case was eventually decided in the student's favor.

3. The interpretation of new advances, new technologies or new surgeries can better be done by an objective team in which the parent has confidence. For example, our team has saved many a large expenditure for such useless treatment as acupuncture during its heyday; it has prevented expenditures for unnecessary hearing aids that will be urged by unethical salespersons. Further, in this day of microsurgery of the ear and electrical implants, the team must again act as advocate for the child's best interests in helping to determine whether the innovations in surgery and implants may be applicable to the individual child.

It is evident that the work of a congenital deafness team may be never-ending. It will continue until the client is fully achieving and completely comfortable in the environment that has been chosen.

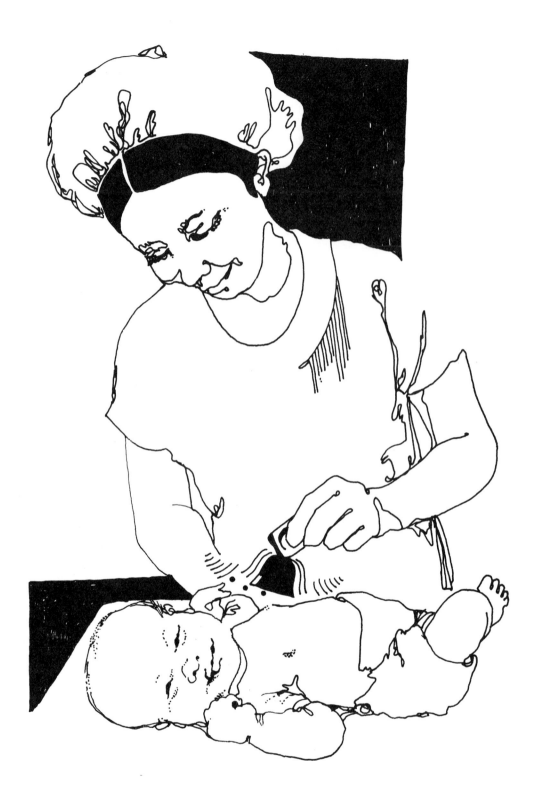

CHAPTER 4

Development of Auditory Behavior

The audiologist has a unique contribution to make to the understanding of how language develops in infants—one which linguists and psychologists cannot offer—and that is the study of the degree to which the acoustic parameters of language learning in the infant are innate, preprogrammed processes, and how they influence language learning. Already there is research evidence demonstrating that there may be special biological predetermined processes of perception for the various acoustic dimensions of speech. These ideas will be reviewed from a number of discipline-specific journals that have made contributions to this field. Once the course of maturation of the auditory response is understood, the hearing testing techniques follow naturally.

PRENATAL AND NEONATAL HEARING

Elliot and Elliot (1964) confirmed physiologically that the human cochlea has normal adult function after the 20th week of gestation. Johansson and his associates (1964) were among the first to report testing fetal hearing. Using high frequency pure tones presented by means of a microphone placed on the mother's abdomen, fetal heart rate increase response to the tones was recorded after the 20th week of gestation. The demonstration of fetal hearing has value in contradicting the theory that the child is born a *tabula rasa* insofar as hearing is concerned. The newborn infant has actually been hearing sounds for at least 4 months—fluid-borne sounds, to be sure—but nonetheless, true auditory signals.

How early does the infant perceive speech and act upon his acoustic environment? There is research evidence for the existence of preadaptive processes of perception for the acoustic dimensions of speech. At birth the infant is able to discriminate its mother's voice and to work to produce her voice in preference to the voice of another female. These capacities were demonstrated by DeCasper and Fifer (1980) utilizing the classic sucking paradigm with infants shortly after delivery. Earphones were placed over the ears of the supine infant and a non-nutritive nipple was placed in its mouth. An assistant held the nipple loosely in place; the nipple was connected by way of a pressure transducer to solid state programming and recording equipment that produced only its or its mother's voice. For five randomly selected infants, sucking bursts produced first only the mother's voice on the tape for a predetermined interval, and then the voice of another infant's mother. For another five infants the conditions were reversed. A preference for the maternal voice was indicated if the infant produced it more often than the nonmaternal voice. It was apparent that the infant soon learned to gain access to the mother's voice, since specific temporal properties of sucking were required to produce the maternal voice.

These data of DeCasper and Fifer show that newborns reared in group nurseries that allow minimal maternal contact can discriminate between their mothers' and others' speech, and moreover, will work to produce their mothers' voices in preference to those of other females. These authors postulated that prenatal, intrauterine influences may be a factor in this early learning.

Is there sufficient acoustic exposure in the uterus to permit such a precocious development? It may be. Bench (1968) has shown that for a 72-dB signal there is the least attenuation of sound going into the uterus at 200 Hz (19 dB); slightly more at 500 Hz (24 dB); more at 1000 Hz (38 dB); and the most at 2000 and 4000 Hz (48 dB). The last two measures were not considered accurate since the strength of the applied signal was not sufficient to overcome the masking of the internal sounds that had been measured at 72 dB. Thus the frequencies of 1000 Hz and below contained the maternal voice which may be heard, if faintly, from the 5th month of gestation when, it has been shown, the fetal ear is capable of analyzing sound.

The Bench study was not made inside the intact amniotic sac and of course did not deal strictly with the sounds available to the fetus. But a study by Armitage et al. (1980) measured the actual sound level inside the amniotic sac of pregnant ewes by means of hydrophones inside the sac, in the normal fluid environment of the fetus. These investigators found that although sounds from the maternal cardiovascular system were not perceived, the sounds of the mothers' eating, drinking, ruminating, breathing and of their muscular movements, were discernable, as were sounds from outside the mother. They found that the attenuation of sounds measured on a C-weighted scale reached a maximum of 37 dB just below 1000 Hz, but it was reduced below and above this frequency, with its higher frequencies attenuated at about 20 dB up to the highest recorded, 5000 Hz. The amount of attenuation fluctuated, however; conversation at normal levels outside the animal could often but not always be understood when transmitted from inside. Raised voices were almost always distinct. If we make the leap from this animal model to the case of the human fetus, then the mother's and even the father's voices would be heard by the fetus. A study similar to the DeCasper and Fifer one, but utilizing the father's voice instead of the mother's would give even more definitive evidence for the fetal hearing of external voices.

Querleu et al. (1981) performed actual intrauterine measures on humans and demonstrated that the fetus could hear the mother's voice and other voices, which were perfectly audible but lacking in tone because the high frequencies were absorbed. When there is no fetal distress the fetus reacts to the sound stimulus by a change in heart rate, often associated with movement. In 1982 Querleu et al. made more careful observations of seven patients during term labor after amniotomy, implanting hydrophones and microphones in the uterine cavity. When external speech was recorded through the uterus, two observers could recognize 64% of the mothers' phonemes and 57% of a male's speech.

An animal model that is relevant is the study of Grier et al. (1980) who transmitted patterned acoustic signals to chick embryos through the eggshell and found that after birth the chicks clapped their beaks and vocalized more often to the patterned signals than did chicks in a nonexposed control group. The authors postulated that prenatal auditory "imprinting" had occurred.

The above studies lend weight to the hypothesis of DeCasper and Fifer that a great deal of auditory experience has preceded the abilities of the newborn to prefer the mother's voice to other voices. But before such early discriminations can be made the infant auditory system would have to be preadapted to various acoustic discriminations. Such discriminations have been shown to be present in the newborn, and, assuming a functional ear and central nervous system, the same capabilities would be present in the 5-month fetus. The innate discriminations that subserve the preference for the mother's voice require the auditory competencies of discriminating rhythm, intonation, frequency variation, stress (suprasegmental aspects of speech) and phonetic components of speech (linguistic aspects).

Supra-segmental Speech Activity

Condon and Sander (1974) reported that neonates move in precise and sustained segments of movements that are synchronous with the articulated structure of speech. Further perception of rhythm in 2-month-old infants was demonstrated by Demany et al. (1977) who utilized varied sequences of time bursts in a habituation paradigm relating duration of fixation on a visual figure. Infants were able to perceive intervals of time as subjective links between sounds. Spring and Dale (1977) showed that 1–4-month-old babies could discriminate linguistic stress as well as location, fundamental frequency, intensity, and duration. Thus the entire gamut of suprasegmental aspects of speech seem to be available to the infant at birth.

Kimura (1964) has shown that the suprasegmental aspects of speech are handled by the right brain. The segmental, linguistic aspects are located in the left brain, according to Studdert-Kennedy and Shankweiler (1970). But this is not to decry the importance of the suprasegmental aspects of speech in learning its intelligibility. Language learning is not confined to the segmental aspects of speech. Rhythm, intonation, duration, and stress are extremely important to understanding multiple meanings of words, as well as to the meanings of homophones. Many words and phrases contain multiple meanings that are made clear only by intonation, rhythm, duration, and stress. This fact explains a part of the problem of a deaf child in understanding some of the subtle parameters of irony, satire, scorn, implied anger, or humor, that convey the sense of multimeaning words or phrases. "You're tired." "You're tired?" are two different sentences depending on the intonation of the rising or falling fundamental frequency. "You drive me up the wall;" "I can't bear it"—make for humorous misconceptions, but it is the kind of thing that is difficult for the concrete-minded deaf child who has not heard the stress and intonations that made the phrases meaningful.

Franklin (1975) showed that there is useful consonant information in the low frequencies. Rosenthal (1972) also showed that when a low frequency band is added to a 1100–2200-Hz high band, there is a significant increase in consonant recognition. So, to return to the prenatal learning that may go on, whether the fetus hears low frequency sounds better than high or not may not matter to the early learning that goes on.

Neonatal Hearing

Stimulus Properties. It has been hypothesized that because the fetus is accustomed to listening to the heartbeat of the mother, he will be quieted effectively by the same sound in his early days in the outer world. Brackbill et al. (1966) found that a tape-recorded heartbeat is no more effective than any other continuous, low frequency stimulus in lowering the arousal level of the infant. Lowered arousal level means a specific reduction of overt behavior and physiological patterns: the infant's heart and respiration rates become lower, they cry less and move about less.

A later study by Brackbill and Fitzgerald (1969) showed that the best pacification is when stimulations by light, temperature, and swaddling are added to the lower frequency sound.

It should be noted that when anesthetics and analgesics are administered to the mother during delivery, one can expect all central nervous system (CNS)-mediated functions to be depressed in the baby for several hours after birth. Stechler (1964) found that responsiveness to visual stimuli is impaired for as much as 4 days after birth when the mother has been given medication during childbirth. Our clinical observations confirm that the same certainly may be true of the auditory responsiveness of the infant who is only a few hours old. The researcher will do well to keep this fact in mind when observing neonates.

Segmental Aspect

Eimas (1975, 1979) and others have given us evidence that the child is also able to discriminate segmental aspects of speech in a categorical and presumably linguistic manner. He chose to utilize differences in voice onset time (VOT). The categorical perception of VOT has been assumed to be a function of the special processing which the sounds of speech undergo and tends to be a special characteristic of perception in a speech or linguistic mode. Eimas (1975) believed that there were special biologically determined processes of perception for this acoustic dimension. In one experiment with 26 infants 1 months old, he employed the classic sucking paradigm in discriminating the differences between the voiced stop /b/ and the voiceless stop /p/ combined with the vowel /a/. His results indicated that infants as young as 1 month of age are not only responsive to speech but are able to make rather fine distinctions in a manner approximating categorical perceptions.

Eisenberg (1970) has demonstrated that most newborns, including those with known CNS abnormalities, can discriminate sound on the basis of frequency, intensity, and stimulus-dimensionality. Thus it is possible that neuronal mechanisms for processing sound pressure levels (SPL) are fully mature at birth.

The processing of frequency differences is described by Eisenberg (1976) as range-dependent. The low frequencies tend to have a soothing, or inhibiting effect on the infant. High frequencies have the property of occasioning distress rather than inhibiting it. However, signals in the range below 4000 Hz are 2 or 3 times more response provoking than those in the very high ranges. The frequency patterns most often used by Eisenberg are matched pairs of ascending and descending total sequences. She states that the effectiveness of pure tones or noise bands can be enhanced by increases in one or more, within limits bearing on the characteristics of spoken language.

What is particularly significant to the clinician is Eisenberg's finding that speech-like signals seem remarkably effective in producing responses in newborns. This fact is certainly true of the older infant, as will be described later, but to find that the newborn already responds selectively to the dimensionality of human speech gives us directions for clinical testing.

It is intriguing to speculate whether speech dimensional signals are more attention-getting because of some preadaptive auditory reactivity, or whether the known frequency-dependent sensitivity of the human ear is operating here. That dependency in itself is intriguing; one wonders which came first, the human ears' greater sensitivity to frequencies in the speech range, or the peculiar properties of the human larynx and resonators to produce speech in that particular range of frequencies. In the area of visual behavior, Fantz (1961) has demonstrated that the newborn infant is more attentive to the dimensions of the human face than to any other visual object, a fact which would argue for a preadaptive response to "humanity."

The newborn's discrimination of intensity was shown by Steinschneider et al. (1966), who recorded increases in the cardiac responses of infants to increases in intensity of a white noise. A similar finding was reported by Bartoshuk (1964), who showed that the relation between the magnitude of the newborn cardiac response and the stimulus intensity was consistent with Stevens' (1961) power law.

Kagan (1972) suggests that stimulus change is another parameter that should be explored. A 2-day-old infant is more attentive to a moving light than to a steady light. The rate of the light change is also important. In the auditory sphere, Kearsley et al. (1962) found that, if an unexpected noise of 70 dB reaches maximal intensity within a few milliseconds, a newborn infant closes his eyes, starts, and shows an increase in heart rate. If the same sound reaches its maximal intensity in 2 sec, the infant opens his eyes, looks around, and is likely to show a decrease in heart rate. The first reaction is a defensive one; the latter displays interest.

Kagan suggests that the attention-getting power of contrast, so evident in the newborn period, diminishes as early as the 2nd month and is succeeded by a different parameter of the stimulus (to be discussed in the section below on "The Older Child").

Later studies by Morse (1972) confirmed the fact that infants respond in a linguistically relevant manner, showing that categorical perception is present in infants before the onset of speech production. Morse investigated 2-month-old infants' abilities to differentiate the voiced stops /b/ and /g/ in a speech context from the same second- and third-formant transitions in a nonspeech context. (The nonspeech context was achieved by eliminating the entire first formant and the steady-state portions of the second and third formants.) Using the sucking paradigm he demonstrated that the experimental infants also recovered differentially from the control group who had heard the synthetic patterns. This, he felt, confirmed the linguistic relevance of their distinctions.

The theoretical considerations of the infant's ability to process a segmental unit of speech have occasioned a great deal of speculation. The arguments revolve around the fact that speech is a very complex code; transformation of the acoustic energy signaling speech to the perceptual event may not be a simple conversion mediated by an auditory decoder. Lieberman (1975) states "The acoustic cues for successive phonemes are intermixed in the sound stream to such an extent that definable segments of sound do not correspond to segments at the phoneme level. Moreover, the same phoneme is most commonly represented in different phonemic environments by sounds that are vastly different. There is, in short, a marked lack of correspondence between sound and perceived phoneme. This is a central fact of speech perception." Lieberman believes that the perception of speech signals is mediated in some manner by central neural events, because infants have had no experience in the consistent articulation of phonetic distinctions. Therefore the ability must be a part of the native endowment of the human organism.

Other theories have been advanced by Stevens and Halle (1967) and Stevens and House (1972), who presented an analysis-by-synthesis model presupposing that an internalized or computed auditory pattern is generated and compared with the stored pattern. But for this theory also the premise is that "perception requires knowledge of phonological rules that can map abstract features into articulatory events" (Eimas, 1975). So all theories lead to the inescapable conclusion that the infant enters this world with considerable knowledge of the phonological component of language.

Eimas (1975) points out that when one compares the degree of categorical perception of the VOT in infants with that of adults the degree does not appear to be age-related and therefore is unaffected by experience with language of either a perceptual or a productive nature. Eimas explains the infant's ability to differentially discriminate VOT differences by assuming these detectors are operative shortly after birth, and may be made functional by merely experiencing speech.

Whether the infants' detectors are activated shortly after birth as Eimas has suggested or whether they have become functional during intrauterine life may be a relevant question to his theory. Four months of listening practice might facilitate in a way the categorical perceptions that are evident at birth. We suspect, however, that if the same kinds of experiments could be made on the unborn fetus at 5 or 6 months of gestational age, categorical perception would be present and would demonstrate that detectors need only be activated by hearing speech in order to be fully functional. It remains for some zealous researcher to attempt to replicate these studies during intrauterine life.

The fact that the infant is able to discriminate the acoustic features of speech means that he can segment an almost continuous acoustic input into discrete elements. This ability to process language into discrete elements is a basis for full language competence. The infant's ability to do this at the very beginning of language acquisition means that he does not have to learn that language is formed by discrete elements. The result is a facilitation of the language acquisition process and indeed the ability to break down discrete elementary language may even be requisite to its formation. The audiologist should note that the capacity to process language in discrete units would not be possible were it not for the damping effect of the structures of the cochlea. Were speech sounds—and indeed, any sounds—allowed to reverberate without hindrance in the ear, the hair cells would not be able to discriminate the frequency components of the speech sounds in a manner necessary to language perception.

State. Bench (1971) describes the relationship between the infant's state and his response, in terms of the law of initial value (LIV): "The magnitude of response change is influenced by the state of the individual before stimulation in such a way that the lower the initial or prestimulus state, the greater is the increase in level of activity on stimulation; the higher the initial state, the greater is the decrease in level of activity." Bench measured the heart rate of 10 normal newborn babies for 10 sec before and after stimulation by a 95-dB broad band noise. The results indicated that the heart rate change to auditory stimulation was dependent on the prestimulus heart rate. The implication of this work for infant audiometry is that any given baby may show an increase or decrease in activity, or no change at all, depending entirely on his prestimulus state. Bench recommends that babies be tested at low levels of activities, in order to obtain a positive response change.

In another study Bench and Boscak (1970) applied signal detection theory to infants' responses to three different stimulus levels of 300 Hz (55, 75, and 95 dB).

The infants' prestimulus states were rated as 1 (deep sleep), 2 (light sleep), and 3 (limb activity). They found that the signal detection is affected by both the SPL of the stimulus and the state of the baby before stimulation. There was a significant trend for the effect of state in the decreasing order of state 2, state 1, and state 3. A light sleep, then, predisposes to the best response to sound.

Bench et al. (1977) found that pure tones and a narrow band centered at 2000 Hz were equally poor signals for eliciting responses in neonates, even at 90 dB. They reported broad spectrum noises as the most effective stimulus, but even here the response probability was of the order of 0.9. They concluded that more than a single presentation of the stimulus is necessary to achieve a high degree of confidence. Responses were best discriminated by the observer when the baby was in a "deep-sleep" state (nonactive, eyes closed).

Taylor and Mencher (1972) also identified infant state as a significant variable in neonatal testing, reporting that light sleep is the optimal state for evaluating a response to auditory stimuli. They applied single and double presentations of different stimuli at 90 and 100 dB to 225 normal newborn infants. The most common response types which they observed were eye movement and arousal responses. Stronger responses occurred more often in the light sleep than in the awake and quiet state. The sleep state was defined by touching the examiner's finger to the closed eyelid of the infant. If eye or body movement resulted, a light state was judged to be present; if there was no movement, the deep sleep state was judged.

Active Response. In addition to responding differently in a passive way to stimulus patterns and intensity, newborns can be active in regulating auditory events in their environment. Butterfield (1968) reported that babies made bursts of contingent sucking responses that controlled the onset and offset of tape-recorded music: classical, and popular, and vocal. An instrumental pacifier nipple operated the musical selections. Four 1-day-old infants were used in his study, and all responded consistently over several tests. This study leaves no doubt but that newborn infants are not passive in their hearing function. Their feedback loop operates actively at as early an age as study is possible. The availability of such an auditory function strengthens the idea of early application of hearing aids to hearing-impaired infants who have sufficient residual hearing to benefit from them. Eimas et al. (1972) used changes in conditioned sucking rates to measure sound differentiation. By 1 month, infants showed, by changes in sucking rates, that they differentiated the onset time distinction between the phonemes "Pah" and "Bah." By 4 months of age the changes were more marked. Differential perception seems to be well established in the first few months of life.

Even suprasegmental aspects of speech such as intonational contour can be distinguished by infants as young as 2 months. Morse (1972) showed that some 25 infants 40 to 54 days old could differentiate changes between phonemes with a falling and those with a rising fundamental contour. This parameter of speech may play an important role in language acquisition.

For the investigator, Eisenberg's (1976) more sophisticated observations on the responses of newborns to sound gives substance to the description of responses:

Overt reactions:
  Arousal
  Gross body movements
  Orienting behavior
    Turning of head
    Wide-eyed "what-is-it?" look
    Pupillary dilatation
  Motor reflexes
    Facial grimaces
    Displacement of a single digit
  Crying or cessation of crying
Cardiac reactions:
  Diphasic (deceleration-acceleration or reverse)
  Longer latency than for constant signals
  Associated with "on"-"off" effects, and with the direction of a tonal sequence.

Eisenberg terms many of these selective reactions as representative of higher and more selective levels of neuronal organization. The peculiar effectiveness of speech-dimensional sounds lend weight to the presence of higher processing of sound stimuli.

To the student of auditory behavior, all of Eisenberg's studies have tremendous significance. It was she who first described differences in habituation to sound as an index of central nervous system integrity. Newborn infants with known CNS involvement failed to extinguish their responses to repeated acoustic signals. Normal infants habituated to the repeated stimuli in a short time. Sometimes called response decrement, this phenomenon is logical for possible use as a screening tool in identifying CNS problems.

Neonates' sensory habituation to a pure tone was shown by Bridger (1961) using heart rate measures to indicate a startle response to pure tones. All the babies who were tested showed a cessation of marked startle to successive stimuli presentations provided the interval between the stimuli was less than 5 sec. Bridger also showed that changing the frequency of the pure tone would renew the startle response after habituation to one tone, showing that babies do discriminate between frequencies.

The hypothesis that CNS-damaged infants will fail to habituate was tested by Shulman (1970a) using heart rate changes as the measure of response. An 80-dB buzzer for 3 sec was used at 20-sec intervals. Heart rate was recorded from a cardiotachometer. Five high risk premature, five low risk premature, and five normal full term infants were compared. All risk children were matched for gestational age. Significant habituation occurred in all three groups, although latency of response was significantly longer in the high risk subjects. Thus Schulman was not able to confirm the lack of response decrement in the AT RISK child that Eisenberg (1970) and Brackbill and Downs (1969) had reported.

It may be that the careful matching for gestational age reduced the differences that others had found in response decrement between the two groups. This fact only points up the hypothesis that response decrement is related to immature central processing.

The Older Infant

The maturation of auditory processing proceeds after birth in ways that have been demonstrated in research designs. Already at 4 weeks the infant can distinguish phonemic contrasts in sound signals, as measured by heart rate changes. McCaffrey (1970) presented 4–28-week-old infants with standard vowel and consonant stimuli which were then changed to contrasting vowels or consonants. At the point of transition from the standard to the contrasting phoneme, significant heart rate changes were found to occur.

A similar study was made by Moffitt (1969) with 20–24-week-old children, utilizing synthesized speech samples generated by Haskins Laboratories, consisting of the consonants "b" and "g." His 20 infants made significant discriminations of the phonemic transition at the end of the seventh and eight trials, or after a 30-sec exposure to the repeated transitions. Other studies by Jusczk and Thompson (1978) showed 2-month-old infants perceiving phonetic contrast in multisyllabic utterances.

Friedlander (1970) terms these reactions "active, critical evaluative processes characterized by creative model-building and formation of hypotheses as to what is likely to happen next." One can conclude that however simple the paradigm, the responses represent some aspect of learning and cognitive processing. This viewpoint is supported by Neisser (1967) who maintains that choices are made of which parts of the incoming information should be attended to. Attending, even in the infant, becomes a constructive, active process rather than an analytic and passive response.

By the age of 3 months, according to Turnure (1969), babies attend better to

mothers' voices on a tape recording than to strangers' voices, even when mothers' voices are modified by filtering. She observed babies' body movements as an indicator of attention in standard time periods during which tape recordings of the mother's natural and distorted voice were played. She also compared their body movements when strangers' voices were played as against mothers' voices in natural and distorted form. Children 3, 6, and 9 months were subjects for the experiment. Turnure reported differences in the way the infants attended to the voices as a function of age level. The 9-month-olds tended to be quieter to the natural mother's voice and progressively less attentive to the distortions. Mehler et al. (1978) later concurred in describing infants' recognition of mothers' voices.

Perception of rhythm in the 2-month-old infant was demonstrated by Demany et al. (1977), utilizing varied sequences of time bursts in a habituation paradigm relating duration of fixation on a visual figure. The infants were able to perceive intervals of time as subjective links between sounds, showing that they apprehend a succession of several sounds as a psychological unit. This ability represents a necessary prelinguistic skill, since language comprehension requires the same kind of process in grasping a semantic unit as a whole despite its sequential character.

Linguistic stress is also discriminated by infants 1–4 months old. Spring and Dale (1977) demonstrated with a high-amplitude sucking paradigm that young infants could discriminate the acoustic correlates of stress, location, fundamental frequency, intensity, and duration. This study completes the number of suprasegmental aspects of speech that have been shown to produce discriminatory responses: intonation, rhythm, and now stress.

Further evidence of the selective listening abilities of infants is given by Friedlander (1970). He devised an ingenious play-test whereby a large pair of response switches are attached to the baby's crib or play pen. The switches regulate a loud-speaker, an electrical control and response recording unit, and a stereo tape player with a preprogrammed selection of two-channel audio tapes. Whenever the baby operates either switch, a record is made of the frequency and duration of his choice, and he turns on one channel or the other of the audio tape. Thus, a record is made of his listening preferences. Babies 9–18 months old were studied over long periods. The findings are summarized as follows:

1. When sounds and voices are placed under the babies' own control, they display phenomenal productivity in listening responses productivity, ranging from one 9-month-old girl's 65,000 sec of responding in 20 days (3000 sec per day) to the average response record of 1200–1500 sec per day of other children. These data indicate that listening to sounds and voices have a hitherto unsuspected potency as a desirable form of activity to babies whose own speech is still very immature.

2. Babies show a great range of discriminative listening to a wide variety of natural, disguised, and synthetic language as well as to other auditory stimuli, as the following examples indicate. (a) A 12-month-old infant preferred to listen to a stranger's voice with bright intonation than to his mother's voice speaking in a flat monotone. (b) A 14-month-old baby could not decide for several days whether to select the stranger's voice or the mother's distorted voice. After several days he made an enormous burst of listening to the mother's voice and after that he ignored completely the switch that turned on the stranger's voice. This choice is regarded as an "aha" effect with the child ultimately recognizing the mother's voice despite its distortion. (c) Another baby was offered a choice between two tape recordings of animated family conversations: one edited to run for 240 sec before it was repeated, the other repeated after 20 sec. The long cycle was considered to have low redundancy and high information; the short cycle had high redundancy and low information. For the first several days, the baby preferred the short tape with high redundancy and low information. After a week he crossed over into a preference for the low redundancy, high information selection. This redundancy study was replicated on 11 babies, 9–18 months, 7 of whom ultimately chose the low-redundancy, high information selection.

Exploring the responsiveness of the 0–6-month-old infants to various stimuli, Bench et al. (1977) found that both younger and 6-month-olds were notably unresponsive to tonal stimuli and even to band widths of 300 Hz. But broad-spectrum noise gave better responses in the younger infants (1 week and 6 weeks). For the 6-month-olds, voice stimuli were most responded to. Moderate intensity signals were not effective for awake 6-month-olds. The younger infants were mostly in sleep states when studied, so stimuli of 90-dB SPL were necessary for response.

Kagan's work (1972) suggests a varied assortment of response parameters for investigation. One of them is the duration of the infant's sustained attention, which Kagan believes is a rough index of how easy or how difficult it is for the infant to understand a new experience. Kagan defines this kind of attention as the duration of sustained orientation that follows the initial orienting response of 2 sec. He believes that during the period of sustained orientation an infant over 30 days old is trying to build a representation of the event. Further study of this phenomenon may add another parameter to the indices of auditory behavior for infants.

What do these studies mean in terms of differential development in children? A study by Irwin (1952) described the early effects of different kinds of auditory input given to infants. He applied both quantitative and qualitative measures to two groups of infants from the time of birth to the age of 1 year. One group comprised the infants of highly verbal, "white-collar" and professional people; the other comprised a low verbal, "blue collar" working and laborer group. The variable was that the first talked a great deal directly to the infant and in its presence; the second group of parents were less communicative both to each other and to the child. The quantity and quality of their vocalizations showed that, at about 3 months, something changed the vocalizations of the two groups. The infants of the highly verbal parents began to increase the number of their vocalizations, as well as the quality of the phonemes used, more rapidly than the infants of the low verbal group. It can be inferred that, by 3 months, the amount and the quality of the auditory input to these infants was already being transformed into commensurate output. The more highly stimulated infants had greater opportunity to select acoustic information and to apply it to their own auditory feedback loop. Active participation and expression resulted, but differentially in the two groups. What more pragmatic proof can there be that infants are active, not passive, in their utilization of incoming acoustic stimuli?

AUDITORY BEHAVIOR AS PRELINGUISTIC ACTIVITY

Concurrent with the maturation of the auditory function are the developing speech and language skills.

The beginnings of language learning occur at birth and—who knows?—possibly before birth. Condon and Sander's (1974) studies showing that the human neonate moves in segments of movements synchronous with the articulated structure of adult speech demonstrate that he is a participant in the rhythm of many repetitious speech structures long before he uses them for communication. These rhythms comprise a prelinguistic activity of the human infant even at birth.

The infant's first use of sounds in a repetitive manner indicates the time at which the auditory feedback loop has become effective. By 2 months he is beginning to put out certain sounds more than others. His selection of which sounds to repeat seems to depend on the nature of the sound. From 2 to 4 months these sounds are vowel-like.

The sequence of use of vowels is presumably from middle (the "schwa" sound /ə/) to front and back vowels (Menyuk, 1972). By 5 months the consonant-vowel sequences begin. Irwin (1947) states that back consonants (velars and glottals) predominant at 5–6 months, with some of the labial (front) consonants entering in. At 9–10 months, the glottal sounds decrease and the alveolar sounds (middle) are frequently used. Menyuk (1972) partially explains this sequence of selection as due to ease of production. It is also possible that the selection is made for them by some differences in the changing vocal mechanism.

Studies of Moffitt (1968, 1969) suggest that the infant responds differentially to acoustic differences between speech sound categories. Perhaps there is a hierarchy of ease of observing distinctions between the acoustic properties of speech sounds. Such a hierarchy might also account for the selection of certain sounds by the auditory feedback loop. Is it related to sound energy? Or to the differential sensitivity of the human ear to various frequencies? Further research will undoubtedly answer these questions. It seems logical that there is an interplay between selective auditory sensitivity and ease of production of sounds, both of which account for the selection of infants' sounds.

Although the infant is able to differentiate various speech sounds in the first few months of life, his production of the sounds does not develop at the same rate. Berko and Brown (1960) describe the lag between the perception of differences in speech signals and the production of those speech sounds. In the newborn period the infant does not produce phonated sounds, only cries and physiologic sounds. Murai (1960) and Lieberman et al. (1971) postulate that the reason for this early lack of phonation is similar to the reason that primates cannot speak: the larynx is positioned relatively high, almost in line with the roof of the palate, limiting the pharyngeal movement that is necessary to speech. In addition, the infants' large tongues fill the oral cavity and prevent them from changing the shape of their superlaryngeal vocal tract by moving their tongues during phonation.

Lieberman (1975) identifies the range of formant frequencies that are necessary to human speech. The well-developed pharynx, with the posterior one third or so of the tongue forming its anterior wall, is the structural arrangment required for a wide range of formant frequencies. In the newborn and in the nonhuman primates, the hyoid bone is high in the throat, so that the tongue lies completely within the oral cavity. There is little or no pharynx. As the larynx and tongue descend, a pharynx is formed and speech sound production becomes possible.

Menyuk (1972) suggests that experimental results comparing primate vocalizations with those of human infants and adults "indicate that speaking is not simply a learned overlaid function on the muscles and structures of breathing and eating, but that man is preprogrammed to develop a vocal mechanism that is specifically adapted to produce speech."

By 1 month typical cooing and gurgling sounds are made in addition to the crying; by 3 months true babbling begins. True babbling consists of the pleasurable repetition of sounds in the parents' absence, and the increase of these sounds in the presence of the parents.

Up to 5 or 6 months of age, the sounds made by the infant do not seem to be related to the speech sounds he hears. His productive capacity for speech lags significantly behind his demonstrated ability to perceive differences. From our observations of otherwise normal deaf infants, their vocalizations are identical with those of normal infants until 5 or 6 months. Furthermore, the deaf infants increase their vocalizations when the parents speak to them, just as normal infants do (Downs and Akin, 1973). It is obvious that the reason for this increase in vocalizations is not the baby's hearing the parent's voice. We postulate that it is a preadaptive, reflexive response stimulated by the presence of the parent's

face, much as is the smile response which appears at the same age. It may be that the increase in vocalization is as necessary a psychic organizer for ultimate communication integrity as the smile response is to ultimate psychic integrity (Spitz, 1965). The phenomenon of increased vocalization may indeed be a milestone that is predictive of eventual communication skills. Certainly the established fact that the auditory feedback loop is present at birth indicates that the elementary babbling sounds have a significant prelinguistic function. The lack of auditory feedback in the deaf child deprives him of early prelinguistic experiences.

Maskarinec et al. (1981) compared the vocalizations of a deaf infant with those of normal infants from birth to 32 weeks. They found that during this time the speechlike sounds increased and the nonspeech sounds decreased in the normal infants, while the deaf child's speechlike and nonspeech production both declined with age, and showed greater variability. One of the normal infants who developed otitis media during the study also had greater variability. These findings corroborated earlier similar results by Mavilya (1969, 1972).

The invariable presence of the babbling responses in both the deaf and the hearing infant seems to us to represent reflexive, preadaptive behavior unique to the human infant. It can be considered as one of the earliest functions in the preprogrammed schedule of linguistic activities that Lenneberg (1967) describes as being innate processes. Its importance in the prelinguistic sequence of activities may be that it reinforces vocalizations by means of rewards. As Bruner (1968) termed it, a code of mutual expectancy is established between infant and parent when the adult responds to some initiative on the part of the child. Thus the child's behavior is converted into a signal initiating an interaction code. Bruner believed that the language channel is dependent on the growth of such codes.

These self-stimulating sounds strengthen

the auditory feedback loop which was earlier demonstrated to be active at birth. The
infant begins early to monitor his own
speech activity, however primitive. The
✳ perception and elementary control of
rhythm, intonation, duration, as well as
frequency range of sounds is evident by 4
or 5 months of age.

By 5 months Chinese children produce
the intonation of the Chinese language.
Also, Polish infants' babbling by 5 months
can be distinguished from English infants
(Weir, 1966). The later skills of linguistic
organization are undoubtedly dependent
upon these early activities.

Menyuk (1972) describes the beginning
of speech from birth on:

Despite the fact that presumably all the possible
speech sounds are produced during this stage
and that the child merely uses vocalizations to
express pleasure or displeasure, all of these studies indicate that the time at which a sound is
first uttered and repetitively used depends on
the nature of the sound. During the early
months of non-cry vocalizations (2 to 4 months)
practically all the sounds are vowels or vowel-
like, and certain vowels are used earlier and
proportionately more frequently than others.
Presumably, the sequence of use of vowels is
from middle (the schwa sound /ʌ/ or /ɘ/) to
front and back vowels. At about 5 or 6 months
the repetitive production of CV sequences begins, and the consonant of these sequences in
terms of frequency of usage varies as the child
matures. Irwin (1947) presents data on the proportionate usage of consonants over the age
range of 1 to 30 months and examines the effect
of place of articulation on proportionate usage.
Back consonants (velars and glottals), and to a
lesser extent front consonants (labials), predom-
inate at the 5 to 6 months period. At the 9 to 10
months period there is less use of glottal sounds,
and the middle of the mouth sounds (alveolars)
are beginning to be used with some frequency.
If we examine the distinctive feature characteristics of the sounds that are used predominately
and more frequently at the beginning of the
babbling period of infants born in American
English-speaking environments (as exemplified
by Irwin's population) and Japanese-speaking
environments (as exemplified by Nakazima's
(1962) population), we find that consonants that
have the features of either +voice, +grave, and
+nasal, or some combination of these features,
are used first and proportionately more frequently than sounds having the features +dif-

fuse, +strident, and +continuant. If we note that
some features appear to be the product of minimal efforts of the vocal mechanism (unmarked
features) whereas others require special adjustments of the parts to produce (marked features),
then the sequence of proportional usage is partially explained. Thus, for example, sounds produced at the lips (p, b, m) are easier to produce
than either alveolar sounds (t, d, n) or velar
sounds (k, g, n), because the tongue is in a
resting position for lip sounds while it has to be
moved to purposefully produce the other sounds.
It is, however, also possible that the infant selects for reproduction the speech sounds that
have acoustic characteristics he can more easily
discriminate. Miller and Nicely (1955) have
found that adults preserved best, when given
nonsense syllables in noise, the features of voicing and nasality in reproducing these nonsense
syllables. This result is some indication that
these characteristics are easier for adults to detect in acoustic signals than are others, but it
may be the case that these characteristics are
also easier for infants to detect in the signals
they hear. Further, since the relationship between production and perception at this stage
of development is not clear, it is possible that
infants are producing certain sounds because of
the nature of the developing vocal mechanism,
while observing distinctions between other and
different speech sounds because of the nature of
the developing auditory mechanism. (Reprinted
with permission from P. Menyuk: *The Development of Speech*, pp. 17–18. Indianapolis and
New York, Bobbs-Merrill Co., 1972.)

Further research will undoubtedly answer these questions. It seems logical that
there is an interplay between selective auditory sensitivity and ease of production of
sounds, both of which account for the selection of infants' sounds.

Reddy and Rao (1977) found that infants
between 12 and 21 days of age can imitate
both facial and manual gestures. Even sequential finger movement (opening and
closing the hand by serially moving the
fingers) was imitated. The infant indeed
enters the world equipped with skills that
appear innate to humans.

Even facial expressions can be discriminated, according to Field et al. (1982). They
exposed 74 neonates (average 36 hours) to
3 facial expressions—happy, sad, and surprised—and observed diminished visual
fixation on each face over trials. The fixa-

tions were renewed upon presentation of a different expression. What was surprising was that the babies made imitative facial movements that clued in observers to the expressions of the model, at greater than chance accuracy.

Measurements of the fundamental frequency of the baby's voice (*fo*) have been made by Kent (1976). He showed that during the first 3 weeks of life *fo* is around 400 Hz; then it increases to around 480 Hz by the 4th month where it stabilizes for 5 months. At 1 year it begins to decrease sharply and levels off at 300 Hz at 3 years. Some interest has been shown in the frequency of the cry of abnormal infants. Vuorenkoski et al. (1971) found abnormally high *fo*'s in the infants with asphyxia, brain damage, and hyperbilirubinemia. A low *fo* was noted in Down's syndrome children. Ostwald and Peltzman (1974) also demonstrated the the distress cries of abnormal infants were higher in pitch than those of the normal baby.

Babbling ceases at about 6 months, and the next few months comprise rather undistinguished progress in vocalizing speech sounds. At this period the mother's feedback of the child's sounds lays the groundwork for his first production of a word. The sounds the child makes are imitated by the mother and additional speech improvisations are added by her. Soon the child imitates the mother's imitations, and speech control is under way. Sometimes the comprehension of the sound sequence precedes the imitation; sometimes imitation precedes understanding of the meaning of the sound sequence according to Murai (1963, 1964).

The infant begins to practice speech as young as 2 months, according to Trevarthen (1975). Films of babies reveal a kind of "prespeech" activity consisting of a rudimentary form of speaking by movements of lips and tongue, with or without sounds. A specific pattern of breathing is noted with prespeech. Even in the 2nd month the baby may imitate a mouth movement of the mother, or a protrusion of her tongue, but this kind of behavior is most often seen

after 6 months of age and only after the act is pointedly repeated in a teacher-like way. Trevarthen states that such embryonic speaking confirms the psycholinguistic theory that language is imbedded in an innate context of nonverbal communciation by which intension and experience are transmitted from person to person. Meltzoff and Moore (1977) have also described both manual and facial imitations in newborn babies.

Bower (1976) described such imitation as occurring at a young age, and has photographed tongue-protrusion imitation in an infant 6 days old. He says this ability disappears early, however, reappearing only near the age of 1 year. Bower describes ear-hand coordination, which he says is present in young infants but is soon lost, sometimes permanently. He ascribes the decline to the fact that hearing is a passive situation—one that cannot be controlled as vision can be. Bower tested this hypothesis by fitting a blind infant with an echo-location device that sent out ultrasonic frequencies and converted the echoes to audible pitches. Within a few seconds after the device was put on, the infant reached for objects and showed that he was making sense of the device. Bower hypothesizes that because auditory stimulation can now be controlled, the hand-ear coordination should not disappear as it does normally at 5–6 months.

More amazing than imitation is the auditory localization of very young infants observed by Aronson (Bower, 1975). Young babies observed their mothers through a sound proof glass screen, with the voices of the mothers coming at various positions of a loudspeaker. So long as the sound came from the place where the mothers were, the babies were quite happy. But when the voices came from a speaker in another position, the infants manifested surprise and upset, indicating not only auditory localization but also an expectation that voices will come from mouths. Adults seem to have lost such localization, being unaware for example that voices in movies come from a place other than the screen.

A bimodal representation of speech is

present in the infant, i.e., the recognition that the sequence of lip, tongue, and jaw movements corresponds to the sounds we hear. Brown et al. (1982) showed that 18–20-week-old infants can detect the correspondence between auditorially and visually perceived speech. They presented the infants with two side-by-side images of a talker articulating, in synchrony, two different vowel sounds and recorded by videotape the infants' visual fixations. The infants consistently looked longer at the face that matched the sound. To determine what characteristics of the auditory stimuli were necessary to the detection of the correspondence, the researchers removed the spectral information from the vowels (formant frequencies) while preserving their temporal characteristics (amplitude and duration). Under these conditions, the percentage of fixations to the matched face dropped to chance, indicating that some aspect of the frequency information of the vowel was requisite to produce the effect. The same phenomenon was reported by Kuhl and Hillenbrand (1979). During the experiments Brown et al. observed that the 10 infants who heard the vowel stimuli produced babbling utterances, whereas only one of those who heard the pure tone nonspectral information, did so. It appears that the intermodal perception of speech is conducive to vocal learning. It follows that 1) communication with an infant should be face-to-face as much as possible, and 2) the intermodal model might well be extended to include tactual information as well as visual for the deaf.

The long period of reception of auditory language symbols is the prerequisite to later language formulation. By the time speech and language emerge, there have been 12–18 months of receiving complex adult spoken language and distilling it into the matrix of the child language structure. This act of refining out of a complex language structure the basic one- and two-word sentences that are the baby's first speech language utterances must rank as creation's noblest day. Chomsky (1966) proposes that

the ability to decode and organize these grammatical structures is an innate function, unique to human infants. Lenneberg (1967) prefers to rely on biological functioning to explain language development. Whichever theory one supports, the important fact is the primacy of reception in the language acquisition of children. Listening to language for a long period of time is essential to the ultimate usage of language. From the studies described above, it is evident that this listening is not a passive process, but one in which the infant participates by acting upon the incoming signals.

By the time the child's first meaningful word is uttered, miraculously full-blown at around 1 year, a whole world of listening activity has taken place. Nothing he will ever achieve is as intellectually complex as what has preceded his first utterance. Lenneberg states. "By the time language begins to make its appearance about 60% of the adult values of maturation are reached."

CRITICAL PERIODS

How early is it necessary for the hearing-deprived child to receive language input, if he is to avoid language retardation? The answer to this question is based on whether there exist critical periods for the development of various functions. The theory of critical periods states that there are certain periods in development when the organism is programmed to receive and utilize particular types of stimuli, and that subsequently the stimuli will have gradually diminishing potency in affecting the organism's development in the function represented. In the case of audition it means that at a certain developmental stage auditory signals will be optimally received and utilized for important prelinguistic activities, but that once this stage has passed the effective utilization of these signals gradually declines. An analogous theory for language development holds that language input must be experienced at a certain stage, or it becomes decreasingly effective for utilization in emergent language skills.

The most vociferous opponent of this

theory has been Bench (1971) who claims that the concept has no more than heuristic value, and that its importance in the field of diagnostic audiology has been greatly overemphasized. Bench requires of the critical period theory that to be thorough, it would demand an irreversibility of the effects. "If a method can be found to change the effects back to normal ('reversing the apparently irreversible'), it is clear that the so-called critical period is not critical after all." He cites the animal studies of Denenberg and Morton (1964), who were able partially to reverse heightened emotional activity in animals caused by deprivation of extrinsic stimulation in infancy, by exposing them to a free environment after weaning.

It is evident that there is a semantic difference between Bench's concept of the critical period theory as demanding a totally irreversible effect, and our interpretation of it as implying an effect becoming more and more devastating with the duration of deprivation following the onset of the period. It can be demonstrated that in the field of auditory perception, total sensory deprivation over a period of time eventually results in an irreversible inability to perceive differences in speech sounds. Downs (1956) undertook a vocational rehabilitation project to determine whether applying hearing aids to deaf graduates of a manual school system could be justified. Four young adults (17–19 years old) with normal or above normal performance IQs who had never worn hearing aids were selected for the study. All had measureable hearing through 2000 Hz, with average losses in the speech range of 75–95 dB (ASA, 1954). This amount of hearing, it should be noted, has permitted children who were given early amplification, to achieve quite adequate speech discrimination. For 2 months the subjects were given 4 hours a day of auditory training and corresponding speech training, on elementary words and sounds. At the end of the period, test results showed that their recognition of simple speech sounds had not developed

beyond random chance. They were able neither to repeat speech sounds accurately nor to identify differences between them. It was concluded that the value of hearing aids to such young people was limited to hearing the difference between noise and non-noise.

It may be argued that the 2-month period was insufficient to demonstrate learning of auditory perceptions, or that another therapy approach may have been more effective. The fact remains that these young people were given every chance to develop gross perception of sound, and did not. It is possible that, in their cases, a lifetime would not be long enough to develop the skills necessary to understanding elementary speech. By postpuberty it appears that the inability to perceive the complex auditory signals of speech is irreversible.

Reviewing the literature on early prelinguistic development, Menyuk (1977) states that during the babbling period the normal infant is making both perceptual and productive categorizations of the speech signal which may be crucially important for later language development. "Therefore" she says, "the term 'early' in early detection turns out to be very early indeed."

The question of whether intervention after age 3 can produce permanent gains in cognitive ability was addressed by McKay et al. (1978) in a large Columbian population of low socioeconomic status families. At ages 43, 51, 63, and 76 months treatment was begun for four different groups. A battery of language tests was given at each age point beginning at 63 months and ending at 86 months. The treatment included nutritional, health, and educational interventions. A matched group of privileged children was given the same battery of tests at each period, but no treatment. The gap between the two groups was dramatically narrowed in the initial period of treatment, but tended to fall off with age, despite continued treatment. There was even a trend toward a larger gap at the end than at the beginning of the study. But the significant finding was that the retardation was less amenable to modification with increasing age, bearing out the need to start interventions during early years of plasticity.

More buttressing of the value of early intervention programs comes from a reanalysis of Bayley's data on 74 children whom she followed for 25 years. Cameron et al. (1967) found that the only items in the Bayley scale that correlated with later IQ were the ratings of vocal behavior of the children. Infant vocalization is a behavior that can easily be increased by reinforcement schedules, so the fact that this predictive characteristic can be changed suggests widespread application of early intervention.

Lenneberg (1967) is of the opinion that puberty marks the last milestone for acquisition of language. With regard to the effects of early deprivation, he cites the difference between the congenitally deaf child and the child who acquires deafness through meningitis after a brief exposure to language. He states that those who lose hearing after having been exposed to the experience of speech, even for as short a period as 1 year, can be trained much more easily in all language arts, even if formal training begins some years after they had become deaf. According to Lenneberg (1967), "It seems as if even a short exposure to language, a brief moment during which the curtain has been lifted and oral communication established, is sufficient to give a child some foundation on which much later language may be based."

A classic case in point is that of Miss Helen Keller, whose great achievements in mastering language skills are rightly admired. However, it must be remembered that Miss Keller acquired her deafness and blindness from meningitis at age 2. One cannot expect equal language achievements from a congenitally deaf and blind child and indeed, one does not see them develop.

Lenneberg (1967) describes in detail the case for the time-locked nature of language learning, and concludes:

The inferences we may draw from this material (animal studies on critical periods) is that many animal forms traverse periods of peculiar sensitivities, response-propensities, or learning potentials. Insofar as we have made such a claim for language acquisition, we have postulated nothing that would be extraordinary in the realm of animal behavior. But at the same time we must sound a warning. Merely the fact that there are critical periods for the acquisition of certain types of behavior among a number of species *does not imply* any phylogenetic relationship between them. Age-linked emergence of behavior may be due to such a variety of factors that this phenomenon by itself is of limited heuristic value when it comes to tracing evolutionary origins of behavior. In the case of language, the limiting factors postulated are cerebral immaturity on the one end and termination of a state of organizational plasticity linked with lateralization of function at the other end of the critical period. (With permission from E. H. Lenneberg: *Biological Foundations of Language*, pp. 175–176. New York, John Wiley & Sons, Inc., 1967.)

By the time language begins to make its appearance, Lenneberg states that about 60% of the adult values of maturation are reached. He assigns the reason for this rapid achievement to the very rapid brain maturation rate during this period.

In the area of language for the sighted deaf, where intensive training has been given the deaf in an attempt to remedy the language lag, only partial reversibility can be demonstrated when training is begun even as early as 2 years. But partial reversibility does not confer on the individual language functioning adequate to our complex life and its demands.

The "Survey of Hearing Impaired Children and Youth" taken in the spring of 1971 by the Gallaudet College Office of Demographic Studies (Series D, No. 9) reports the results of the administration of the Stanford Achievement Test Series to all students in schools for the deaf and hard-of-hearing in the United States. We know from surveys on age of detection of hearing losses that almost all of these children were identified and given beginning training after the age of 2 or 3 years. The highest average reading competence level (paragraph meaning), attained at age 19, was equivalent to grade 4.36. As might be expected, academic reading areas were lowest for those with the most severe degree of hearing loss. Related to the low reading levels of all the students are poor vocabularies and knowledge of word meanings—skills upon which reading ability is built. However, in the nonverbal area of arithmetic computation, the more profoundly deaf students score higher than their better hearing contemporaries. This fact demonstrates that the lowered degree of language and reading skills of these very profoundly deaf students is not caused by lowered intellectual function in this group.

In an expertly designed study, Templin (1966) compares the language skills of deaf children with the skills of matched groups of normal children. In some of the language areas the deaf showed no systematic improvement in their performance beyond 11 years. At that point such skills as understanding of word meanings, sentence construction, and analogies, hit a plateau and remained there without further insights or improvements. The normal hearing went on to achieve to the 14-year language level that was the upper limits of the study. It should be emphasized that there was no substantial difference in intellectual abilities between the deaf and the normal hearing group and that the deaf had had intensive language training in their schools. Their rate of learning up to 11 years was comparable with that of the normal hearing group. But an irreversible language deficit appeared at this age level and precluded further development. The complexity of language forms and of abstract language symbols takes a great leap about this age and leaves the deaf helplessly behind. The blame can be ascribed only to early language deprivation covering many periods critical for language learning.

The reports of animal research supporting a critical period theory of development are numerous.

Reisen (1947) reported that a chimpanzee raised in total darkness for the first 3 months of life never developed adequate vision. But if chimpanzees are raised in light for the first 3 months and subjected to total darkness for the next 6 months, they quickly regain perfect vision when exposed to light. The analogous situation in humans is found in the child born with strabismus of one eye (thrown to a side focus). Ophthalmologists report that unless that eye is forced to be used, through patching the other eye, by the age of 4 no useful perceptions can ever be developed in it despite the fact that organically it is a perfect organ of vision. It is the central perception of vision which, untrained during critical periods, can never regain function. There seems to be no demonstrated reason why auditory perceptions do not fall into the same category as the visual modality. Whether the auditory irreversibility also occurs by age 4 is difficult to prove, but we feel it is probably fairly comparable with vision.

Reisen (1960) also reported that chimpanzees showed a reduction in the efficiency of auditory learning following early sensory deprivation of hearing. In addition he found, in cats deprived of visual sensation, three concomitant manifestations: hyperexcitability, increased susceptibility to convulsive disorder, and localized motor dysfunction. This latter experiment has profound implications for the student of deafness. What are the effects on the central nervous system of early learning deprivation? Many clinicians have described symbolic language disorder, minimal cerebral dysfunction, or other kinds of central involvement in the deaf. Can these disorders be a direct result of the auditory deprivation? If sensory deprivation in animals produces central nervous system disorders, can deprivation have the same result on the human central nervous system?

What has not been considered is the effect of the language deprivation on the deaf infant. If biological theories of language acquisition are correct, then the human infant is just as preprogrammed to develop language skills as he is to develop motor skills. The effect of early sensory deprivation could then be expected to have far-reaching consequences on central nervous system functioning in integrative areas of the brain. The concept of language as a biologically predetermined function thus extends the speculation of early sensory deprivation in humans to another plane where animal research cannot apply. It opens up a whole new area of investigation.

Edwards (1968) has summarized concisely the state of the educator's attitude toward critical periods:

The supremely difficult feat of building language recognition and response which takes place during the first years of life can occur because there is a built-in neurological mechanism for language learning present in every normal human organism. But like the image on the sensitized negative, this potential will not appear as reality unless the proper circumstances develop it. Experience—the right experience—is essential.

Heredity and environment interact. Hereditary possibilities are shaped by the influence that only human culture can provide; they are potentialities that must be developed while the young neurological organism is still rapidly growing, malleable, open to stimulus. If the "critical periods in learning" hypothesis applies to human beings (as we know it does to other creatures—dogs, for instance—and as evidence increasingly indicates it does to us), then the right experience must come at the right time, or the potential must remain forever unrealized (p. 70).

Edwards' solution to this problem is well worth detailing:

We are going to have to make educational stimulation available from babyhood on for the children whose families cannot provide it for them. Whether tutors should go into the homes, whether children should be brought into carefully planned, well staffed *educational* (as distinct from baby-sitting day-care) programs, we do not now know. Experiments going on in several places in the country should help us decide. But however we do it, intervention by the age of 18 months should be the rule for the children of deprived inner-city or poor rural families. (Reprinted with permission from E. P. Edwards: Kindergarten is too late. *Saturday Review*, p. 77, 1968.)

There have been conflicting arguments about the lasting effects of Head-Start programs. The divergent opinions are summarized by Horn (1981) and Darlington (1981). Horn pointed out that the IQ measures taken on the Head Start children showed large initial gains, but that these gains had vanished 5 years after the completion of preschool. He also analyzed Darlington's reports and showed that the beneficial effects of preschool on later school performance past elementary school were no more durable than the preschool effects on IQ. Darlington on the other hand quotes the reports of the Consortium for Longitudinal Studies (1978, 1980) showing that there is no indication that effects last only through elementary school, when the dependent variable is placement in special education classes rather than a more general measure of failure to meet school requirements. Whichever thesis is true, non-enduring effect on IQ has held up, as well as the Consortium's finding that the most long-lasting effect of any preschool program has been the early mother-child-home projects, birth to 2 years, which showed consistent statistical significance of long-term duration of improved functioning (Schweinhart and Weikart, 1980). This latter finding is corroborative of the hypothesis that critical periods for language occur in the birth-to-2 years period.

Although it is difficult to pinpoint the exact age at which it is critical that infants be given language stimulation, a report by Dennis (1973) begins to give some guidelines. In an institution for homeless children in Lebanon, he tested the foundlings at all ages, before and after their adoption into homes. Those who were adopted by or before age 2 soon reached normal intellectual functioning, with a mean IQ jump of 50 points postadoptively. But those adopted after age 2 never overcame their preadoptive experiential retardation. Dennis concludes that there is a period near the second birthday that is critical for complete recovery from the effects of experimental deprivation.

Considered from the physiologic point of view, the infant's auditory system is plastic, that is, it can be modified not only by anatomical alteration but also by variations of acoustic stimuli. Absent or faulty sound stimuli will result in deviant auditory function. According to Ruben and Rapin (1980), the central and peripheral auditory systems exert reciprocal control over each other. As the inner ear matures its input is necessary to the development of at least part of the auditory nervous system. By the time the peripheral auditory system is fully developed, its input seems to be necessary for the maturation and innervations of portions of the central auditory system (Webster and Webster, 1977, 1979, 1980; Clopton and Silverman, 1977). Therefore environmental sounds have the greatest effect in shaping auditory ability from the time the inner ear and eighth cranial nerve first become functional to the time when maturation of the CNS is achieved—roughly from the 5th month of gestation to between 18 and 28 months. The consequences of these findings for intervention programs for the hearing impaired are strikingly apparent. The time for action is early in the 1st year of life.

So far as the deaf are concerned, the most definitive study was done by a group of researchers at Lexington School for the Deaf (Greenstein et al., 1976). Thirty severely hearing-impaired children who had been admitted to the school before their second birthdays were studied. Two groups were identified: those who had been admitted prior to 16 months of age and those admitted between 16 and 24 months. Over a period ending when they were 40 months of age, the children were given repeated measures of language skills including the Receptive Expression Emergent Language (REEL) scale and the Lexington Preschool Oral Language Assessment. In addition, informal measures using observational assessments of Mother-Infant Communication was made. The results indicate that the children admitted prior to 16 months were consistently superior to the later admitted children in all aspects and at all age levels. Regardless of what caused the differences, its occurrence before 16 months

was the variable responsible for the improved speech and language. Here is evidence relating learning ability in the hearing impaired to time of identification of the hearing loss.

It is often hoped that studies of children who have been socially and sensorally deprived since infancy will shed light on the periods necessary to acquisition of language. The 1797 "wild boy of Aveyron" (Lane, 1977) remained mute and incapable of even subtle communication even after Dr. Itard attempted to teach and socialize him. The report of Genie (Fromkin et al., 1974) who was isolated in a closet for 11 years of her life, states that this is "a case of language acquisition beyond the 'critical period.'" However, Genie's history shows that she was exposed to family life for her first 20 months before being placed in isolation until age 13 years 9 months. These early months allowed her to achieve the 60% basic language abilities that Lenneberg states have developed by the age when speech begins. The reported language abilities that she acquired after being rescued from a pitiful situation are actually what one could predict for anyone having had 20 months of normal language input. The really critical periods for language during which Genie had exposure laid the matrix from which her language skills could develop.

CENTRAL ORGANIC AUDITORY DISORDERS

Part of the audiologist's task is to determine whether in addition to a peripheral hearing loss there may be another organic disorder of the auditory system. Chapter 5 details the behavioral clues that should alert the clinician to a possible central auditory problem. In order to understand the central disorders which may produce deviant behavior, it is pertinent to review what is known about the involved pathways and their breakdowns.

The peripheral auditory mechanism extends from the outer ear to the termination of the acoustic nerve in the cochlear nucleus of the brainstem (Goldstein et al., 1972). The neurons leading into the synapse in the nuclei are the auditory input stations for the central nervous system, and we include them functionally in the peripheral system. A lesion at any point along this system results in reduced auditory sensitivity, represented by decreased thresholds for pure tones and speech.

Beyond the cochlear nuclei in the brainstem lie the neurons of the central auditory system, which transmit the auditory information to the brain. Several synapses along the way to the brain begin the coding and analyzing of the information. For example, the neck-turning reflex of the infant to a loud sound is presumed to be mediated at the level of the superior olive. Even at this level and in newborn infants, the reflex can be inhibited by central processing: the normal infant will cease to give a neck turn after several repetitions of the arousing stimulus. The known brain-injured child, on the other hand, once having given this neck-turn response, will be unable to inhibit it on successive presentations of the stimulus (Eisenberg et al., 1966). Even the simple coding system required for inhibiting the reflex will be disrupted by CNS damage.

An excellent historical review of cases of auditory agnosia by Goldstein (1974) shows the sites of lesions that have been reported in autopsies. All lay in the left temporal lobe. In all cases of disordered perception of auditory stimuli the peripheral acuity was within normal range or too slightly reduced to be responsible for the lack of perception.

An example of how long it may take to understand such dysfunction in a child is illustrated by another case history: Brent, a 3-year-old boy, the third of eight siblings, presented with a 60-dB sensorineural loss in the right ear, 85 dB in the left. He conditioned very well, and retests over many years showed the same hearing levels. Mother's pregnancy, labor, and delivery history were uneventful. Brent sat alone at 6 months but at 7 months developed men-

ingitis. He was treated with cholomycetin, sulfa, and penicillin. At discharge he was alert, happy, and at first had no evidence of neurologic disorder. After this disease he did not sit again until 9 months of age, and walked at 11 months. He walks with his left toe turned in and drags it slightly.

At 3 years Brent was fitted with binaural hearing aids and started on an exclusively auditory program. After 6 months he was babbling spontaneously and could localize sounds, but day after day was noted as being "unresponsive to auditory therapy." A Merrill Palmer performance test at this time gave an IQ of 116, and the psychologist noted that although he was visually alert to signs, he had no word comprehension. She felt that there was a specific "auditory comprehension deficit," and noted that "one should not be fooled by his perceptiveness of motor cues and by his perceptiveness of voice inflection into thinking that he understands words."

Six months later the therapist made exactly the same report as before—no meaningful auditory preceptions had been developed in 1 year's time. A psychometric test at that time showed average intelligence on a Leiter scale, and "organic brain damage indications" on a Bender Gestalt test. He could not make simple visual discrimination of forms or perceive and reproduce simple designs.

Brent was then placed in a program emphasizing lipreading and oral training. His teachers reported that he was unable to discriminate any words through lipreading, nor to relate them to reading forms. He mimicked and mouthed words, but only singly. At age 7 he was given an EEG, which was normal, and another psychometric test. "There were indications that mild neurological dysfunction was interfering with his perceptual motor performance. His nonverbal abilities were good, but his lack of language was the main difficulty." At this time the only method of communication he had was by gesture.

At age 9 Brent was finally sent to the state school to learn signing and fingerspelling, where he has had his only success at learning language—but only through signs and reading. He is still at age 16 not able to finger-spell. He still cannot speak more than single words. Auditory communication is so unrewarding to him that that he has not worn an aid for several years. His reading is at the 11-year-old level, and it gives him pleasure, which television listening does not.

This case illustrates one of the fundamental principles in differential diagnosis: that peripheral hearing loss and central disorders are two separate entities, but that they both may exist in the same individual. If tests for auditory acuity show reduced hearing, it is due to a true peripheral lesion, not to a central one. Brent's final diagnosis was "auditory verbal agnosia and visual agnosia for any rapid denotational movements"—all this in addition to a peripheral hearing loss. Each problem must be treated for its own needs, and the combination of problems should, in this case, have been identified sooner. It should be noted that this case, as well as the cases reviewed by Goldstein (1974), had known cerebral insults that accounted for their symptoms.

Goldstein et al. (1972) state, "It is now well established that unilateral, upper level, central nervous system lesions, regardless of their severity, produce no impairment in auditory sensitivity as long as the peripheral auditory mechanism remains intact."

Goldstein (1974) in his classic review of the literature on auditory agnosia has confirmed the fact that such central disorders exist in the presence of normal hearing acuity and are independent of peripheral hearing.

Once this separation between central and peripheral lesions is made clear, one can proceed to test for each problem individually, without confusing the two. In the section on auditory testing we will describe auditory tests on children with central problems, based on this premise.

The evaluation and therapy for organic central auditory disorders is a discipline in itself, and it is not our province to describe

this subject in detail. Experts have written extensively on the subject. If we can demonstrate the differentiation between peripheral and central disorders, we will have fulfilled the requirements of clinical audiology. It is difficult enough to understand all that needs to be known about peripheral hearing loss without attempting another monumental task.

By 4 months the localization of sounds begins. This is a primary skill, and need not be affected by subtle cerebral dysfunction. When localization does not appear at 4 months of age, it may mean a general retardation of the time schedule. It has been our experience that the infant with central neurological problems is more apt to give a localization response at this age than he will at a later age. As such a child grows older, speech becomes meaningless and his responses to it unproductive. He will eventually cease to respond as there is no survival value in his response to speech. Most often, however, he cannot inhibit his reflexive responses to sound, and these responses will be similar to the child with normal hearing. It is extremely rare that both localization ability and auditory reflexes will be absent in a very young, centrally disordered child. Even an anencephalic infant will give large startle reflexes to loud sound. In fact, he will continue to give them ad infinitum as he is not able to inhibit his response because of lack of cerebral control. So testing proceeds much the same for the brain-damaged child as for the normal child, and, if a lack of response is seen, one must believe that it is due to a peripheral lesion. Too many brain-damaged children have had amplification denied because of the erroneous belief that their audiometric loss was due to a central lesion.

By 6 months the infant localizes to very soft speech; by 8 months he imitates some sounds and intonations. To do this, he must have a long period of auditory differentiation, and we know that his skill has been present since birth. Any disruption in the processing of the information disrupts the development of the imitations and of the child's ability to differentiate voice intonations. Usually the 8-month-old child understands the meaning of "no-no" or at least the intonation that accompanies it. When a child is not able to make this differentiation, there begins in his mother the subtle bewilderment that is so often reported by the mothers of centrally involved children. There is a similarity here between the deaf and the centrally involved child: neither shows the milestones of prespeech and prelinguistic skills. The lack of integrity in responding to human communication puzzles the mothers of both such children. The mother-child relationship depends upon an interplay between the two. When this becomes a one-way street, with the child's responses to mother subtly lacking in meaningfulness, a deterioration of the relationship begins. If a problem of peripheral deafness is discovered early, understanding soon reverses the interpersonal breakdown (Greenstein et al., 1976). Once the mother recognizes that the child has a sensory loss, but no other deficit, she is able again to "mother" the child appropriately. Such mothering is difficult for the mother of a neurologically disordered child. Often hyperactive to some degree, these are the children whom nobody understands.

AUDITORY LANGUAGE LEARNING DISORDERS

There are many children who appear to have problems in "the processing of auditory material." They are found today in special classes for "learning disorders," "language dysfunction," or "languaged disabled." A few years ago they were found in therapy classes for "symbolic language disorders"; before that they were labeled as having "minimal brain dysfunction," and before that as the "aphasoid child." Whatever the problem was called, the generic term was "central auditory processing disorder." The only certainty about all this terminology is that it concerns a symptom without a disease. Despite an elaborate system of measuring the symptoms, and a more elaborate treatment protocol, no one has determined the cause or where in the CNS the breakdown might occur.

The type of disorder we are discussing here is not one in which neurological findings are evident from physical examination or can be inferred from a history of brain trauma or insult. The children so labeled may have no known indications of neurological involvement; learning disorders are their only symptoms. The learning problems appear to stem mainly from an inability to utilize auditory input effectively. Inasmuch as this is deemed to be an auditory problem, the onus is on auditory specialists to determine if possible the basis for the symptoms.

Attempts have been made by audiologists to devise auditory tests that will identify children with learning disorders. A sampling of these tests does not, however, give a clear picture of what is being tested: Stubblefield and Young (1975) used the Staggered Spondaic Word Test (SSW) with learning-disordered children. These children made more errors on the SSW than were considered normal for the test. The SSW test purports to identify the integrity of each ear's function. Willeford (1976) utilized a battery of tests on learning disabled children, which included binaural fusion, filtered speech, competing sentences and alternating speech. Great variability was found on the performance of any given test; however, 8 of 9 learning disabled children performed poorly on the binaural fusion test. This test involves brainstem function, and Willeford believes that it indicates that normal relationships between the auditory and visual modalities may be disturbed in these children. Another study, by Hodgson (1966), using low-pass filtered speech tests, found no differences in discrimination between a normal group of children, a high risk group, and a learning-disordered group.

Tests have been devised for the prediction of language learning problems. Martin and Clark (1977) used low-pass filtered speech discrimination tests and a combination of dichotic-diotic speech tests to show differences between a normal group of children and a language-learning-disabled group. Although the low-pass filtered speech did not differentiate between the two groups, the test of the difference between a diotic and a dichotic speech presentation identified the language-disordered children. Those who had higher discrimination scores for the diotic presentation than for the dichotic were predominantly in the problem group. This test procedure entails the Word Intelligibility by Picture Identification (WIPI) Test (Ross and Lerman, 1970) and requires only that the child point to the correct picture.

Barr (1976) found significant differences between children with learning problems and a normal group, on four standardized auditory tests: The Wepman Test of Auditory Discrimination (1958), the Rosner Auditory Analysis Test (1970), the Roswell-Chall Auditory Blending Test (1963), and the Binet Sentence Test. This abbreviated diagnostic battery is believed to identify areas of greatest weakness in auditory perception, and permit planning for a therapy program. (A detailed description of tests for discrete auditory functions is found in Chapter 5.)

All of these tests diagnose symptoms, not disease. Nowhere can one find a correlation between auditory symptoms and an underlying CNS disorder such as one finds in the literature on adults or children who have had demonstrable trauma or insult to the brain as described in the previous section.

In the absence of confirmed lesions in the CNS, there is real doubt as to what is measured in all of the tests for "central auditory processing disorders."

In the area of visual perception and reading there has also been some confusion as to what precisely is measured. Zack and Kaufman (1972) feel that perception is a developmental process, not a unitary event, and state that the evidence that training can alleviate the problem is not overwhelming. Many studies report no real effect on school achievement as a result of special training (Arciszewski, 1969; Jacobs et al.,

1968). And one report shows that special training programs do not seem to influence achievement more than good teaching (Cohen, 1970). Zack and Kaufman (1972) question the method of identification of these children, the definition of their problem, and the techniques of training used. They state, "It would seem that although education begins with an understanding of the strengths and weaknesses of the child, a label derived from a global concept which lacks adequate definition and questionable means for its measurement does not provide a shortcut to good pedagogy."

The tests for auditory learning skills described above, however, do identify the strengths and weaknesses of the child. But the global concept of "auditory processing disorder," without established definition and/or etiology, and with the variable measurements, seems to us to be a tenuous concept. A medical model would eschew labeling a disease without clear and tenable diagnosis of etiology or site of lesion. True, it would treat symptoms, but with the recognition always that a workable diagnosis would permit a more knowledgable application of treatment than mere attention to symptoms. In the realm of auditory learning disorders it may be wiser to attempt to identify etiology if we are to treat symptoms more accurately.

Symptom treatment of auditory learning disorders presupposes that the symptoms have caused the language dysfunction and that isolating the symptoms and treating each one will cure the language learning problem. However, from a developmental viewpoint the specific auditory problems appear to be a result of the language disorder, not the cause of it. Such a developmental approach should certainly be considered. It conforms with the conclusions of Rees (1973a) who reviewed studies purporting to show that various "auditory processing disorders" such as auditory memory, auditory sequencing, etc., are responsible for language disorders. She concludes that what the studies show is that, instead of having an auditory perception problem, the children who were studied had a language disorder.

Rees further points out that the search for the fundamental psychological unit of auditory processing of sentences has led from the phoneme to the underlying sentence itself. Liberman et al. (1967) and Abbs and Sussman (1971) have shown that individual speech sounds follow one another too rapidly in ordinary speech to allow them to be analyzed separately. Therefore, says Rees, speech perception cannot take place one sound segment at a time. Even the discrimination of paired words like *bat* and *pat* rests on a linguistic, not merely an auditory ability. It is the entire sentence that is the basic unit of language, with all its semantic and syntactic implications. Rees agrees with Marquardt and Saxman (1972) that "the importance of any given subskill to speech and language acquisition remains to be demonstrated."

This point of view has been reflected in a Position Statement on Language Disorders, by an American Speech-Language-Hearing Association Ad Hoc committee on Language Learning Disorders (Position Statement, 1982). First, the Committee discounts the view that language-disabled children will succeed in spite of their early manifested problems. Actually, they do not "catch up," but maintain communication problems through adolescence and adulthood (Hall and Tomblin, 1978; Ahram and Nation, 1980; Weiss et al., 1979; Strominger and Bashin, 1977).

Second, the Committee states that language disabilities cannot be viewed only as receptive-expressive breakdowns. Such auditory skills as auditory discrimination, auditory sequential memory, etc., need to be interpreted within the context of knowledge of language and communication systems, e.g., memory is more than memory for sequences of digits. There must be an interaction between linguistic and perceptual factors; e.g., the ability to discriminate sounds is influenced by the knowledge of vocabulary (Atkinson and Canter, 1979; Stark and Wallach, 1980). In addition,

one's ability to remember and comprehend an individual sentence is influenced by the context, one's prior knowledge of the topic, knowledge of linguistic rules, etc. (Bransford and Nitsch, 1978; Wallach and Less, 1983). Thus the Committee acknowledges the complexity of the processing of auditory information.

This approach rejects therapy that is based upon specific disorders in auditory sequencing, auditory blending, and auditory discrimination. It is thus a developmental rather than a unitary approach to auditory processing disorders.

What are the implications of a developmental approach for remediation for auditory learning disorders? Such an approach greatly simplifies the therapy plan, rejecting the training of unitary subskills and concentrating on training language skills rather than isolated functions.

Relevant Research

Many provocative investigations from other disciplines may eventually shed light on the mechanisms involved in organic central auditory dysfunction.

Primacy of Left Hemisphere in Speech and Language, Particularly of the Left Temporal Lobe. Wernicke's area (behind Heschl's gyrus) has been shown anatomically to be larger on the left side in 65% of brains and larger on the right side in only 7% (Geschwind and Levitzky, 1968). The planum temporale is, on the average, one-third longer on the left than the right lobe. This finding correlates with the known specialization of speech and language in the left hemisphere (Penfield and Roberts, 1959; Kimura, 1961; Studdert-Kennedy and Shankweiler, 1970). Right-handedness and right-earedness in most people show the critical nature of the cross-over of sensory messages to the opposite side.

Milner et al. (1968) demonstrated in a dramatic experiment that speech processing in both hemispheres is bound to the left hemisphere. Seven patients with midline section of the cerebral commissures, including the corpus callosum, were given dichotic and monotic competing number tasks. (In dichotic stimulation each ear received simultaneously a different message, usually speech, from a separate channel of a tape recorder, via earphones. In monotic listening one ear is stimulated at a time by any number of related or unrelated signals.) Milner et al. showed that when each ear of their patients was tested individually on the monotic task with competing numbers, the scores were 100% for both ears. However, when the dichotic mode was presented, there was essentially no perception of speech in the left ear. In other words, the right hemisphere has the ability to perceive speech on a rudimentary acoustic level, but when the right hemisphere is disconnected from the dominant left, the messages that are essential to speech interpretation are not transmitted on to the left hemisphere, resulting in an inability to identify and classify the speech material. Speech information transmission seems to be a one-way street, from the right to the left hemisphere, but not in the opposite direction.

A second task was given to these patients, that of retrieving objects through touch alone, when competing messages were given simultaneously in each ear. In this task, the scores for left-handed retrieval were higher for the objects named through the left ear, while through the right ear there was little success in identifying objects. Moreover, when asked to name the left ear items, the subjects commonly gave the names of the items that had been given through the right ear. The specialization of the left temporal lobe for speech in particular, and of the right temporal lobe for tactile identification, seems well demonstrated here.

Berlin and his colleagues (1972, 1973) have thrown further light on the cerebral dominance of the left temporal lobe in children. Nonsense consonant-vowel (CV) combinations (/pa/, /ta/, /ka/, /ba/, /da/, and /ga/) were used in dichotic speech tests on 150 right-handed children 5–13 years

old. Precise alignment was made for the simultaneous presentation of a different CV to each ear at the same intensity levels. The results showed that an advantage for the right ear in giving correct responses was already evident in the 5-year-olds, and did not vary with increasing age. Right-earedness for speech and left temporal-lobedness seem definitely established by age 5, lending strength to Lenneberg's (1967) hypothesis on the age of development of handedness as critical to language learning.

Molfese (1978) and Molfese and Hess (1978) recorded auditory evoked potentials from the left and right hemispheres of 10 adults who were listening to a series of auditory stimuli which varied along linguistic and acoustic dimensions. The brain's electrical responses to these different stimuli were isolated and identified and it was found that phonetic distinctions based on transitional elements occurred only in the left hemisphere. Molfese et al. (1978) also recorded auditory evoked responses from the temporal region of both cerebral hemispheres of human infants, children, and adults in response to forced speech and through nonspeech acoustic stimuli. They found that the left hemisphere of auditory evoked responses were larger in amplitude then the right hemisphere auditory evoked responses to speech stimuli for all groups. However, nonspeech stimuli produced larger amplitude responses in the right hemisphere. Molfese and Molfese (1979) looked at neonates in the same way and found that they showed hemisphere differences due to specialized perceptual systems over the cortex that are sensitive to changes in specific acoustic cues. The second format transitions and format structures were processed by the left hemisphere. They concluded that early laterality effects are due to the presence of mechanisms within the left hemisphere that detect and analyze specific acoustic cues common to the speech signal.

In 1980 Molfese reported that the right hemisphere differentiates tone onset time, allowing it as a result to differentiate between voiced and voiceless stop consonants. He suggests that there are basic acoustic systems sensitive to certain acoustic features common to speech sounds that are responsible for the hemispheric differences found in dichotic listening techniques, and denies the presence of special speech processing mechanisms. The argument may be a semantic one, as one might interpret "basic acoustic systems" as being a part of the speech processing mechanisms.

Sperry (1982) points out that the right hemisphere should not be considered word-deaf or word-blind. The right and left hemispheres do not necessarily have different cognitive modes; rather, the right is primarily "praxic" or "manipulo-spatial" and the left mainly processes higher cognition and self-awareness. This view brings an appreciation of the importance of nonverbal components and forms of intellect. Sperry found, in cases of disconnected hemispheres, that there was a normal and well-developed sense of self and personal relationship along with a surprising knowledgeability in general. It appears that affective components appear to cross at lower brainstem levels and may affect cognitive processes on the other side.

Nagafuchi (1970) also gave dichotic speech tests to young children and found that by 6 years the adult right-earedness was established. At age 3 a sex difference was found: girls were superior to boys in both dichotic and monotic listening tasks. This finding is in line with known earlier development of speech and language skills in girls.

Tests utilizing speech material show even more clearly the breakdown of the auditory system and have more clinical applicability to children. Kimura (1961) presented different digits dichotically to both ears of temporal lobectomy patients. When the left temporal lobe was the involved site, the total number of digits reported from the contralateral ear, as well as from both ears, was greatly reduced; whereas in the case of right temporal lobectomy the scores were higher. Kimura concludes from this finding that the crossed pathways are the stronger, and that the left temporal lobe is more important in the perception of spoken material. This perceptive disruption seems analogous to short term memory dysfunction, but is perhaps dependent upon perception rather than on temporal memory.

Contralateral Strength of the Auditory System and Its Sensitivity to Temporal Sequence. Auditory encephalographic studies have shown objectively the strength of the contralateral temporal lobe in processing auditory stimuli. Rosenzweig and Rosenblith (1953) stimulated observers' ears with single or paired clicks through earphones. When only one ear was stimulated, the observer localized the sound accurately, and his cortical-evoked responses were larger in the contralateral hemisphere. A similar study by Hirsh (1969) used delays between the two signals, and showed that at some frequencies when the contralateral ear receives the leading signal, the amplitude of the evoked response is larger.

Temporal sequencing takes place in the temporal lobe, and is manifested when breakdowns occur due to lesions in the temporal lobe. Sequencing appears to be critical in auditory processing, and has pertinence to children's auditory dysfunction. Efron (1963) tested aphasic patients with high and low tones, and with red and green lights. The task was to determine the order in which the tones or the lights were presented. The intervals between the two tones were varied, as they were for the lights. The aphasics required as much as 500 msec between the two stimuli to make judgments on the order of presentation both for the tones and the lights. Normal subjects require only a few milliseconds to make the same judgment. Normal central processing thus is shown to be crucial in temporal sequencing.

Cat studies confirm the sequencing function specific to the temporal lobe. Neff (1961) and Masterton and Diamond (1964) removed the auditory cortex of cats and found that the cats were then unable to judge sequence and order of clicks; all auditory sequence tasks previously learned could not be retrained. Yet the cats could learn simple frequency difference limen and intensity threshold tasks, and could localize a signal to the correct ear.

Dichotic and monotic speech tests using time lags between presentations of two phonemes (time-staggering listening) demonstrate other parameters of the perceptual process. Lowe et al. (1970) systematically separated their CV nonsense syllables by 15, 30, 60, and 90 msec and presented them to normal listeners. In monotic tests, the lead stimulus was more easily perceived by both ears equally at all time intervals, indicating that the precedence of the first signal suppresses the awareness of the second when one ear is stimulated. However, when a dichotic presentation was given, the right ears' scores for both the lead and the lag signals were consistently better than for the left ear, although the lag syllable was more easily perceived by both ears. Improvement of the lag scores was noted as the time interval increased to 90 msec. By that point the left ears' lag scores approximated the right ears' scores.

The use of time-staggered tests in clinical assessment of recovery after a temporal lobe lesion has been reported by Berlin and Lowe (1972). A patient with a gunshot wound to the superior convolution of the left temporal area was given time-staggered dichotic speech tests. Two months posttrauma there was no lag effect, and the left ear gave the higher scores for both lead and lag positions. One month later the left ear scores were even higher, and the right, lower. Later tests showed further accentuation of the left ear's superiority and the right ear's lowered perception of the speech signals in any position and at any time-staggered intervals up to 500 msec. Berlin and Lowe (1972) identify this progression as demonstrating a growth in perceptual capacity for auditory sequence perception in the left ear, and suggest the use of such

tests in monitoring the growth of the right temporal lobe in perceptual capacity.

These studies have demonstrated that the ability of temporal auditory sequencing is specific to the temporal lobe, and that it has primacy in the left temporal lobe. They also cast some doubts on our traditional definition of short-term memory. Instead of being related to disruption of storage of signals, it may be that it is perceptual breakdowns related to temporal lobe functioning that create what we have called defective short term memory problems.

Specialization of Left Temporal Lobe in Extraction of Linguistic Features of Speech. A group of research reports in which the dichotic listening performance was assessed, indicate in detail the further specialization of the auditory temporal lobe. Studdert-Kennedy and Shankweiler (1970) presented consonant-vowel-consonant nonsense syllables dichotically to their subjects, manipulating only one of the sounds of the CVC, the initial or final consonant, or the vowel. They found that the right ears of their subjects perceived all consonants better than the left ear, but that the right and left ears perceived the vowels equally.

Differences in perception of consonants based on the manner of their production have been reported in several studies. Lowe et al. (1970) and Thompson et al. (1972) found in dichotic speech tests a marked advantage for the unvoiced consonant over the voiced consonant. In an effort to determine whether this advantage is based on some unknown process of selection in the auditory cortex or on an artifact of the test condition, Berlin and Lowe (1972) revised the test condition. They hypothesized that when both bursts of the CVs are initiated simultaneously, the boundary of the unvoiced CVs occurs later in time than that of the voiced onset CVs. They were able, using an electromechanical delay line, to align the onset of the large amplitude vocalic portion of two syllables. When a voiced syllable competed against an unvoiced syllable, the alignment gave the voiced syllable a lag in comparison to the initial plosion of the unvoiced syllable. The results of this test on normal subjects showed that the advantage of voiceless over voiced consonants was markedly reduced.

Even semantic and syntactical levels of information can be subjected to fine research analysis. Lewis (1970) used as his dichotic speech material pairings of words having low associative strength, high associative strength (nonsynonyms) and also low associative strength (synonyms). Lewis' results indicated that the unattended message (low associative strength) is perceptually analyzed and can interfere with the perception of the attended message (high associative strength). He did not report whether there was a right ear advantage, as might be expected.

A dichotic study by Zurif and Sait (1970) did show right-eared laterality effect with nonsense sentences which were either structured or unstructured. The structured sentences were modified from a primary reader, and the connective words were included. These sentences were read with normal intonation. The unstructured list was read without intonation, "like a laundry list." The results showed that the structured material produced the larger laterality effect. Whether this effect demonstrates that it is syntax that is better perceived in the right ear, or that rhythm and intonation are crucial elements in the learning of speech and language, is a moot question.

The bold experiments of Penfield and Rasmussen (1968) of stimulating the exposed cortex with electrical probes give us an idea of the localization of various auditory functions. Their studies show that only the temporal lobe close to the fissure of Sylvius will produce auditory sensory responses. The patients report hearing simple sounds (motor sound, crickets, knocking, buzzing, etc.). The points of stimulation from which responses were obtained are shown in Figure 4.1. Penfield and Rasmussen state that the majority of the responses were found in Brodmann areas 42 and 22, the "auditopsychic" area. When stimula-

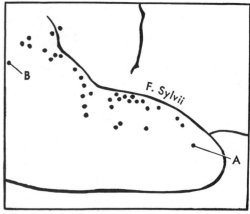

Figure 4.1. Points from which auditory responses were obtained by stimulation of right and left hemisphere shown above as though all stimulation was done on the right side. (Reprinted with permission from W. Penfield and T. Rasmussen: *The Cerebral Cortex of Man.* New York, Hafner Publishing Co., 1968.)

tion was given at point A in Figure 4.1, the patient reported that he felt as if he were singing. At point B another patient heard a quiet buzzing. These points are considered out of the primary auditory area. The "audiosensory" area (41 of Brodmann) lying within the fissure of Sylvius on Heschl's convolution, could be stimulated only once, resulting in a ringing sensation. Whenever sound was produced at any point, it was heard in the contralateral ear in most instances. In general, Penfield and Rasmussen felt that stimulation close to the fissure of Sylvius was more apt to produce simple tones, ringing, etc., whereas stimulation at a distance on the first temporal convolution tended to produce some interpretation of sound. Thus he concluded that interpretive elements are seen in the secondary auditory area rather than the primary area.

Penfield and Rasmussen feel that their studies indicate that there is some degree of intellectual function localized to the temporal cortex. Only in the temporal regions will electrical stimulation (as well epileptic discharge) activate acquired synaptic patterns, not in other brain areas. Therefore they postulate that the organization of the temporal cortex is evidently different from that of other areas of the brain. For the reader's information, Penfield and Rasmussen's chart of the areas of the brain where various functions are considered to be localized is shown in Figure 4.2.

Fedio and Van Buren (1974) have duplicated the Penfield and Roberts experiments, and have described a functional hierarchy in the left hemisphere with memory as a common process. First, immediate memory is affected when there is minor insult, but with severe interference the basic machinery of naming simple objects is disturbed. The primary memory system is considered to be intimately linked with the anterior temporal lobe, whereas the posterior temporoparietal cortex may support secondary memory.

Midbrain's Function as a Binaural Integration Mechanism and the Mediator of Lateralization Phenomena. Two-ear fusion was first demonstrated by Matzker (1959) by means of a dichotic integration test. In one ear of normal listeners he presented a speech signal through a 500–800 Hz band-pass filter and in the other ear the same speech signal through an 1815–2500 Hz filter. Neither band could be discriminated alone, but when both were presented dichotically, frequency fusion occurred and speech sounded normal. When patients with later-demonstrated, postmortem degeneration of ganglion cells through

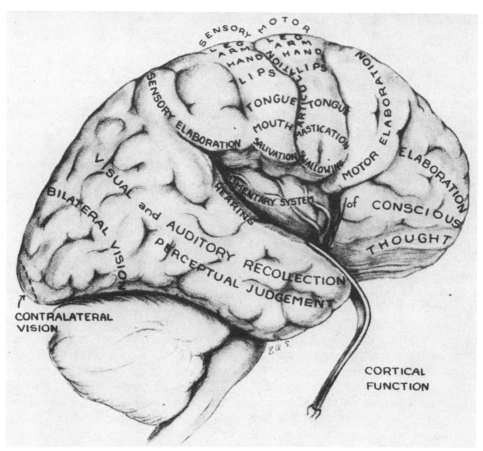

Figure 4.2. Cortical function. This illustration will serve as a summary restatement of conclusions, some hypothetical (e.g., the elaboration zones), others firmly established. The suggestion that the anterior portion of the occipital cortex is related to both fields of vision rather than to one alone is derived from the results of stimulation. (Reprinted with permission from W. Penfield and T. Rasmussen: *The Cerebral Cortex of Man.* New York, Hafner Publishing Co., 1968.)

the olivary regions were given these tests, they made many errors. It appears that integration of binaural signals occurs at a low level in the olivary complex.

The psychophysical judgment of sidedness, or localization of auditory stimuli, is mediated at the level of the accessory superior olivary complex, according to Hall (1965). Hall considers that the superior olivary nucleus can be regarded as a transducer that converts differences of interaural time and intensity into differences of the number of cells excited in the left and right accessory nuclei. On anesthetized cats, he measured the spike discharges in the nucleus as related to click stimuli that were presented in various time and intensity configurations. He found that time and intensity configurations did indeed affect the number of cells excited in the superior nucleus. The manner of excitation was consistent with results from psychophysical experiments in humans on binaural localization (Deatherage and Hirsh, 1959).

It appears, however, that in man the interaction of the auditory temporal lobe is requisite to localization-lateralization ability—or that the transaction required in reporting the sidedness sensation depends on an intact temporal lobe. Sanchez-Longo and Forster (1958) showed that patients with diseased temporal lobes had poor abilities in localizing sound in sound field when it arrived first to the ear contralateral to the lesion. Matzker (1959) demonstrated that accurate lateralization of sine wave pulses, presented dichotically under earphones with time leads, occurred in normal listeners when the time delays were as small as 0.018 msec. But in patients with temporal lobe lesions, the lateralization reports were greatly reduced in accuracy.

Cullen and Thompson (1973) confirmed the site-of-function operative in this test by comparing normal test scores with those of temporal lobectomized patients. They used CNC lists (Peterson and Lehiste, 1962) at 60 dB SPL and filtered noise at 63 dB SPL in the test ear. This combination reduced the normals' discrimination to

40%, and that of the patients to about 33%. (The patients with lesions had poorer discrimination scores in all tests.) But when out-of-phase masking was introduced into the ear contralateral to the test ear, both normals and lobectomized patients showed almost equal gains in discrimination of the CNC words (20–31% in the normals, 20–29% in the patients). Cullen and Thompson propose that this experiment indicates that release phenomena are mediated by two-ear interaction at the subthalamic level, subserved by the same neural mechanisms which play a role in the lateralization-localization phenomena described above. If the auditory cortex were active in suppressing signal pathways for speech, it would be expected that much poorer release scores would be obtained.

Bocca and Calearo (1963) have presented classic studies on the use of distorted speech tests in identifying the level of interruption in the auditory pathway. They applied the following tests to normal subjects and to patients with unilateral temporal lobe tumors.

1. *Low pass filtered speech tests using PB lists of 10 disyllabic meaningful words sent through a low pass filter that eliminated the frequencies above 800 Hz.* The temporal lobe patients showed markedly reduced discrimination scores in the ear contralateral to the lesion. Normals elicited scores of 70–80% whereas the patients with tumors gave scores of 50% in the contralateral ear, 65–75% in the ipsilateral ear. Hodgson (1967) confirmed these findings on a patient with left hemispherectomy after temporal lobe damage. The scores for filtered speech tests were consistently lower in the right ear than the left, both pre- and postoperatively.

2. *Time-compressed speech in which speech is speeded up on a tape recorder, leaving the acoustic spectrum intact.* Although Bocca and Colearo found reduced discrimination scores on this test in ears contralateral to temporal lobe lesions, the results were not as significant as those for frequency-distorted speech.

3. *Interrupted speech in which the speech*

signal is either electronically chopped or blank pieces of tape are interposed between segments of the recorded speech. Bocca and Calearo found no reduction of discrimination scores on temporal lobe patients who were given this task, indicating that the test assesses brain stem function rather than cortical integration. Berlin and Lowe (1972) indicate that, in patients with brainstem lesions, periodic interruption of the speech signal does produce lowered discrimination scores.

It is therefore evident that interrupted speech tests provide another tool for assessing brainstem function, but that frequency distorted speech and time-compressed speech stress the cortical level of the auditory pathways.

Dyslexia

Problems in reading skills seem to be mounting in direct ratio with the escalating demands of our culture for higher learning abilities. Normally functioning children in every other respect are emerging in increasing numbers with deficiencies in reading abilities. An assortment of therapies for reading disorders has proliferated throughout the country, all reporting improvements on the basis of various stategies. None has come forth with the panacea—a permanent cure for the problem.

Few people have made any relation between reading dysfunction and auditory skills, yet the two may be more closely dependent than has been thought. Zigmund (1966, 1973) was able to show that dyslexia may be related specifically to auditory problems. She compared paired associate learning of normal children with that of children with reading disabilities. Her evidence showed that the dyslexic children organized and used psychologic processes in a different way, on the basis of differences in auditory integration abilities.

Evans (1969) found that skill in auditory-visual and visual-auditory sensory integrations were positively correlated with reading achievement; poor readers were significantly impaired in these integrative skills.

He suggests that attention should be paid to auditory function in remedial reading classes.

Can one predict reading dysfunction on the basis of any known auditory tests? Some research suggests that it can be done. DeHirsch et al. (1966) found two auditory perception tasks that made a significant contribution to her predictive reading index: the Wepman Auditory Discrimination Test and the Imitation of Tapped-out Patterns Test. Dykstra (1966) found five measures that contribute to a predictive reading index: (1) discrimination between the difference between initial sounds of words (pat-bat), (2) identification of the rhyming elements in the final sounds of words, (3) identification of correct pronounciation of words, (4) use of auditory clues with context clues to identify unfamiliar words, and (5) discrimination between the differences in final consonants and rhymes.

The Illinois Test of Psycholinguistic Abilities (Kirk et al., 1968) subtests on auditory short-term memory and grammatic closure have been shown to identify reading disabilities.

One must appreciate the direct relationship between previous language experience and the learning of reading. When children come to the reading-learning task with inadequate previous language, as many of the hearing-impaired do, reading becomes a laborious process. As Lenneberg (1967) points out, "... the deaf come in contact with language at an age when other children have fully mastered this skill and when perhaps the most important formative period for language establishment is already on the decline."

How to teach reading to a child who has not had adequate previous language experience? The solution in many schools has been to teach reading through theoretical grammar—the use of sentences learned through the drilling of nouns, verbs, adjectives, and their place in the language structure. Lenneberg calls this "a situation in which the children are on the one hand quantitatively deprived of a large body of examples, and on the other hand are immediately given a metalanguage, a language about the language which they do not have." Although we know the extent of language retardation in the deaf population at large, the wonder is that their level of achievement is as high as it is (Fig. 4.3).

In the neural mechanisms previously discussed that are involved in auditory dysfunction, we may yet find a link with reading disorders. Evidence in the literature on acquired dyslexia points to a relationship between the two.

For example, Geschwind (1962) notes that the brain lesion producing alexia usually destroys color-naming ability, but does not affect the ability to name objects and numbers. He suggests that the reason is that objects are learned through multisensory associations including tactile, auditory, kinesthetic, and olfactory sensations. Numbers are learned originally by using our fingers. But both letter-naming and color-naming involve purely arbitrary connections between the auditioned name and the visualized letter configuration. Objects exist as separate entities in the world; letters do not. In order to make the connection beween letters and a name (audiotoralized), one must proceed from the purely visual

configuration directly to the name—a fairly tenuous pathway from one section of the brain to another. Any slight disruption of this connection could result in dyslexia. But even if the visual-language connections are destroyed, objects can be named because the large numbers of other sensory modes that have been trained allow alternate anatomic routes to be taken.

Confirmation of this theory is found in reports of a few individuals with brain lesions who had formerly been able to read both English and Chinese ideographic language. These individuals, post-trauma, lost the ability to read phonetic English but were able to read the ideographic language. The latter uses symbols related to objects and apparently stimulates more learned sensory and motor associations (Gardner, 1973).

Rozin et al. (1971) applied this theory to therapeutic procedures for severely dyslexic children. They gave English meanings to 30 different Chinese ideograms and were successful in teaching eight second grade children to read them in a few hours. They recommend that these children initially be given characters that represent words rather than sounds, and that a transition be made through a system of syllables each representing a phoneme in one configuration.

Etiology of Auditory Language Learning Disorder

Etiology is of utmost significance in any consideration of auditory language learning problems. A review of the possible etiologies may give further direction to planning for therapy:

Organic Lesions. The presence of one or more of the following factors in conjunction with a learning disorder is the only presumptive evidence that organicity may be present:

1. History of disease with neurological insult: Meningitis, encephalitis, or diseases with high fever producing neurological sequelae that are measurable.

2. History of neonatal trauma, with neu-

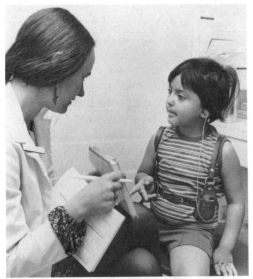

Figure 4.3. Language and speech development is a life-long task for the profoundly deaf child.

rological sequelae: anoxia or birth injury producing CNS symptoms that are measurable.

3. History of head trauma: actual blow or wound to the head resulting in measurable CNS symptoms.

4. Any of the following behavioral symptoms accompanying one of the above histories:

a. *Disordered behavior*. Overactivity that is characterized by lack of clear direction, focus or object.

b. *Short attention span*: Sometimes easily distractible, other times perseverative.

c. *Emotional lability*: Rapid shifts of mood such as sudden tantrums.

d. *Social incompetence*: Clumsiness in games with children and aggressive or withdrawal behavior.

e. *Defective work habits*: Variation in pursuing tasks, either persistently or unevenly.

f. *Impulsiveness and meddlesomeness*: Inability to keep from touching and handling objects, sometimes destructively.

Environmental Deprivation. Several environmental factors may be present singly or in concert, resulting in a deprivation of language experience during the critical period from birth to two years.

1. *Lack of adequate stimulation.* As demonstrated by Heber and Garber (1970), Dennis (1973), Irwin (1952), Uzgiris and Hunt (1966), Wachs et al. (1971), and Uzgiris (1970), exposure to low quality of language or reduced frequency of speaking has the same effect on language skills that auditory sensory deprivation has. Yarrow et al. (1971) reported a careful study that identified the great effect that environmental influences in early infancy have on what they call cognitive-motivational functions. We have shown earlier in our discussion of critical periods that the language deprivation effects of early experiential deprivation appear to be irreversible.

The rat studies of Hebb (1947) confirmed his theory that impaired early experience produces permanent changes in the structure of the cerebral cortex. His studies showed that there is a lasting effect on infant experience in the problem-solving of the adult rat. Forgus (1954) formulated this theory clearly, stating "the organization of adult behavior is largely determined by the quality of infant experience and learning." Hebb further reasoned that such early learning experience produces permanent changes in the structure of the central nervous system, primarily the cerebral cortex. He thus presaged very recent animal studies that demonstrate effects of deprivation on the CNS and imply an analogy to the human condition.

Wachs et al. (1971) stated as a result of a study of cognitive development of underprivileged children, that "infants raised in slum environments will show significantly slower development at a much earlier age than previously suspected ... differences that appear as early as 11 months and which increase from 18 months on." They suggest that programs such as Head Start may be reaching these children 3 years too late.

Similar findings were made by Messer and Lewis (1970) who found that not only did lower-class 13-month-old children vocalize less than middle-class peers, but were also less mobile in the playroom. Understimulation produces apathy and reduced language levels. Such children may end up in language learning classes.

2. *Sensory overloading.* Lest we become too zealous in stimulating young children auditorally there is a warning in some studies that too much stimulation is possible. Wachs et al. (1971) found that high-intensity stimulation from which the infant cannot escape and involuntary exposure to an excessive variety of circumstances are responsible for lower levels of cognitive development on the Uzgiris and Hunt (1966) Infant Psychological Development Scale. In this case, stimulus bombardment rather than stimulus deprivation is shown to be the factor causing developmental problems.

Another study tested children for auditory discrimination (Wepman Auditory

Discrimination Test) and for reading level, and related these scores to the degree of noise levels in their homes (Cohen et al., 1973). Children in the second to fifth grade who had resided in an apartment complex at least 4 years were compared. The apartments in the upper levels (32 floors) were shown to have 14–16-dB higher noise levels than the lower floors, and the children living there had significantly poorer auditory discrimination and reading scores than the children living in the lower levels. The authors stated that "the longer a child must endure noise the more likely he is to ignore all sounds, whether relevant or not. A consequence . . . is a failure to learn to discriminate speech-relevant clues at a time which may be optimal for such learning."

The reason for reduced discrimination abilities may be found in studies comparing children's auditory thresholds in non-ideal testing conditions ("slightly noisy rooms"), with the same tests in sound-treated rooms. Goldman and Sanders (1969) found that high school graduates from low socioeconomic backgrounds seemed unusually unresponsive to the screening test in the nonideal testing condition. They felt that "the presence of high noise levels frequently found in the disadvantaged home environment might interfere with the acquisition by the child of the ability to extract an auditory signal from a competing background." Nober (1973) identified a relationship between reading skills and discrimination in noise by giving the Wepman Auditory Discrimination Test to three groups of children: normal, speech deficient, and reading deficient. The tests were given both in quiet and in 65 dBA of tape-recorded classroom noise. He found that the reading-deficient subjects performed significantly lower in noise than in quiet.

The theme recurs in other studies that children raised in noise environments do not respond as well in a distracting situation as their peers from quiet homes (Deutsch, 1964; Clark and Richards, 1966). In effect, such conditions constitute a sensory deprivation just as surely as do hearing loss and the lack of high quality language stimulation.

3. *Malnutrition.* Three appalling sequelae have been reported from malnutrition during early years and even weeks of life:

a. *Cognitive defects and apathy.* Eichenwald and Fry (1969) showed that chronically undernourished children scored low on the Gesell developmental quotient as well as on measures of visual, haptic and kinesthetic integration The same results were shown in a controlled study of two Mexican child populations by Lewin (1975). A group of severely malnourished infants showed significant lag in language and verbal-concept formation by 6 months as compared with their well nourished peers, a lag which became larger by 3 years. This finding of increasing differences with age seems to be a constant theme in all deprivation studies, suggesting that, if no intervention occurs, the gap between the deprived child and the normal child will continue to widen until adulthood.

b. *Possible CNS effects.* Eichenwald and Fry (1969) state that inadequate feeding of pyridoxal phosphate results in a series of changes in the physiological function of the brain within 6 weeks. If the deficit continues for a longer period, alterations of cerebral function occur, resulting in severe mental retardation. These data suggest that inadequate protein nutrition or synthesis during brain development could result in changes in function. Crarioto (1966) had made experimental observations confirming these facts.

c. *The possible irreversibility of cognitive and CNS effects.* The Mexican study on malnutrition (Lewin, 1975) observed the children after good nourishment, special training and care were instituted. The trend line showed that the underfed children remained behind the control group and were not catching up. The one aspect of intellectual development that proved most resistant to special training was short-term memory. This study also analyzed the effects of stimulating home environments vs. nonstimulating environment. The results showed the effects of poor stimulation on intelligence, with the greatest deficit coming from both malnourishment and poor environment.

	IQ
Well-nourished + stimulating environment	71.4
Well-nourished + deprived environment	60.5
Malnourished + stimulating environment	62.7
Malnourished + deprived environment	52.9

Minimal Auditory Deprivation Syndrome. The impact on language skills of more severe hearing losses is well-known and documented. But the impact of slight hearing loss in early childhood has only recently been recognized. In Chapter I we have described this syndrome and its effect on language skills at older ages. What should be considered is the possible permanent effects on the brain of early auditory deprivation. Just as the animal studies on experimental deprivation showed CNS correlates, so do similar studies on sensory deprivation of hearing. Webster and Webster (1977) created conductive hearing losses operatively in mice at 3 days of age. They also deprived litters of mice of sound by surgically closing the mothers' larynges and rearing them in a sound-attenuated chamber. These two groups, plus a normal control group, were sacrificed at 45 days and their brains were examined. Both the operated group and the deprived group were found to have central morphological defects significantly different from the control group.

Remediation

The question that remains is whether remediation will be effective in restoring or creating CNS connections. Greenough (1975) attempted to answer this question by training adult rats in learning tasks, then comparing their brains with those of matched untrained rats. He found there were significant increases in the outer apical dendritic region in the trained rats, but none in their basal dendritic branching. In comparing these results with the environmental complexity study described earlier, he questions whether "the environment influences basal dendrites only during early development, while apical dendrites continue to be affected?" Although these are only tentative steps toward the understanding of information storage in the developing and adult brain, it does seem that the brain's anatomy can be altered by variety and types of experiences. No studies have shown permanent remediation in these disorders.

What is not indicated is specific teaching of sounds or letters or structures one at a time, for neither phonemes nor words nor phrases are the basic unit of language (Rees, 1973); sentences are the essential unit that should be taught. Nor should linguistic rules be taught formally. Syntactic, morphological, phonological, semantic rules are best facilitated, not learned. These rules seem to be innate in the child, just as pecking is innate in chickens. The child has to hear models and act on them in order to construct infinite utterances from the finite rules. Thus his language needs not to be taught but to be guided. Contrived language lessons are not useful—rather, materials and speech from the real world are preferred.

Most logical is the utilization of techniques which will facilitate the child's construction of his language, such as (Cazden, 1972; Miller, 1975):

1. *Parallel talk.* Using language within the child's ability to talk about what the child is doing.

2. *Expansion.* Taking the child's utterance and expanding it to grammatically acceptable model forms.

3. *Modeling.* Responding to the child's utterance with an unrelated linguistic structure that maintains the stream of thought.

The kinds of language structures that are

used in such a program should be on a slightly higher level than those in the child's repertoire. A sound knowledge of normal language development is requisite to dealing with children on this basis.

Summary

In summary, we have questioned whether language remediation based on an assumption of specific central brain damage in most of the affected children is a valid base of therapy when CNS symptoms are not present. The various measurable auditory subskills appear to be symptoms of language dysfunction, not the cause. What must be considered is the range of possible etiologies of language dysfunction. When etiologies are considered, a developmental approach to many of the problems becomes most logical. The presumptive causes of auditory language learning disorders include diagnosed brain trauma or insult, environmental deprivation, and minimal auditory deprivation in early life. Language facilitation emerges as the appropriate therapy when a developmental theory is accepted.

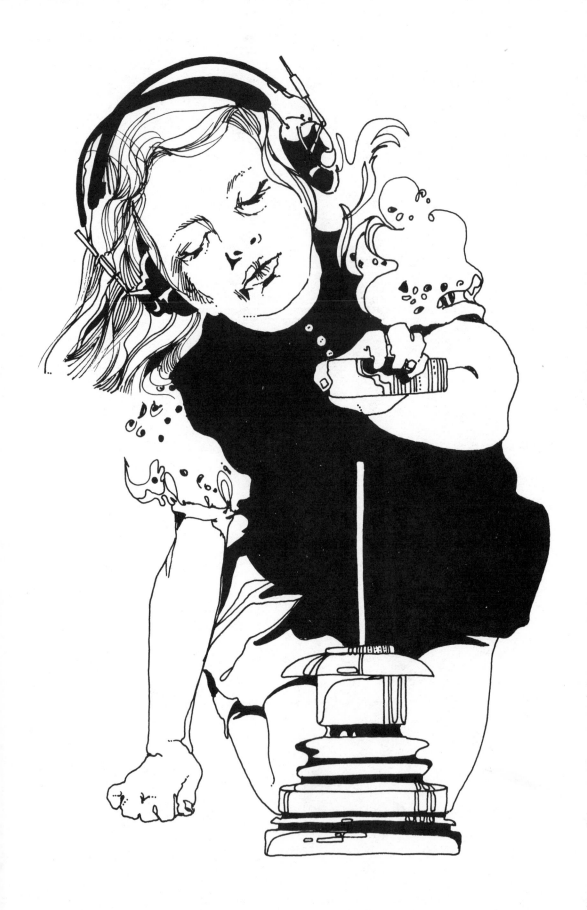

CHAPTER 5

Clinical Audiologic Testing of Children

Modern technology has greatly increased the number of options available to test the hearing of infants and children. However, regardless of how sophisticated testing techniques become, there will always be need for the insightful clinician who can determine which child needs the gamut of test procedures, since some tests will not be cost- or time-effective to administer to every child.

There is available at the present time a logical hierarchy of clinical measurements of hearing, ranging from the technically less-sophisticated observations of behavioral responses of children to the "objective" physiological computer-analyzed responses of evoked brainstem and cortical neuronal activity to auditory stimuli. The lower echelon of behavioral observations can be seen as the initial clinical test procedures to identify those children who need additional levels of testing.

No level of hearing testing is really "better" than any other level. In fact, the experience of the clinician is probably the main key to successful evaluation of the hearing problem in a noncooperative child. A broad test battery approach with children is the best scheme of all, and clinicians who work with pediatric clients must be skilled in a wide variety of testing paradigms utilizing soundfield and earphone measurements. Jerger and Hayes (1976) advocate the Cross-Check Principle in pediatric audiometry, in which behavioral measurements are checked against impedance audiometry and auditory brainstem potentials to confirm hearing levels in difficult-to-test children.

We will try to describe the techniques that have seemed most useful to us, sometimes belaboring the obvious. Most clinical observers are made, not born; and clinical insight to some of us is a matter of seeing so many thousands of handicapped children that it is impossible to ignore the obvious after so many repetitive exposures. Students cannot learn how to evaluate the hearing in children by only reading textbooks such as this one. There is no substitute for experience in testing children. We will try to provide the basics, but the only way to master the techniques is to learn laboriously by repeated application of the observations suggested in the following pages.

QUESTIONING THE PARENTS

The audiologist can contribute, in addition to the actual hearing test, insight into the auditory and oral behavior of the child. No one understands better than he the effect of a certain degree of loss on the child's behavior, nor how the history of auditory development relates to the onset and degree of the loss. The audiologist's time will be most valuable spent in analyzing these aspects of the child's history. Therefore, the sequence of the audiologic session can be as follows:

1. Question the parent as to the chief concern that brought him here. Who referred him? (It may be that this is all the information that is necessary before the audiologic testing, and no details should be pressed.)

2. Administer a pediatric audiology test battery to determine if the child has hear-

ing within normal limits or if a hearing loss is present.

3. If a hearing loss appears evident, query the parent as to the child's auditory and oral development.

At 0–4 Months. When he was sleeping quietly, did sudden noises awaken him momentarily? Did he cry at very loud noises? Did he ever jump to sudden loud noises?

At 4–7 Months. Did he begin at 4 months to turn toward sounds that were out of his sight? Did he keep on making babbling noises of a large variety at 5 and 6 months? By 7 months did he turn directly to sounds or voices that were out of his sight? What kinds of babbling sounds did he make at 6 and 7 months? Could he sit alone at 6 months?

At 7–9 Months. Did he turn to find the source of sounds out of his vision? Did he gurgle or coo to voices or sounds that he could not see? Did he make sounds with rising and falling inflections?

At 9–13 Months. Did he turn and find a sound anywhere behind him? Did he begin to imitate some sounds? Did he have a large variety of different sounds? Did he have a large variety of different sounds, in different pitches? Were some of them consonant sounds (buh, guh, duh)? Did he say "ma-ma-ma-ma," or just "mama"? What specific sounds did he say?

At 13–24 Months. Did he hear you when you called from another room? Did he make a noise in response, or come to you? Did he have any other words or sounds than "mama"? Did his voice sound normal?

From this questioning, and from listening to the child's present voice quality and speech, the audiologist can derive clues as to the onset of the hearing loss and its degree. If the voice quality at the present time is strident, and only vowel sounds are made, an early severe hearing loss would be suspected. If the voice quality is good, in the presence of an evidently severe loss, a later onset would be suspected. Particularly if the child has some words or even sounds in normal intonation, a later onset is suggested. Such clues are helpful in determin-

ing the etiology of the loss. They can only be detected by the intuitive art of the insightful audiologist.

To help in understanding the etiology of the hearing loss, an informal, brief case history may reveal what aspects should be pursued in detail. Table 5.1 contains a list of questions which comprise a basic history that includes the primary items that place a child at risk for hearing loss. Table 5.2 presents a more detailed, medical assessment questionnaire (developed by Nigel Pashley, M.D.) for children with sensorineural hearing impairment.

YOU AND THE CHILD

A word about how the clinician relates to the child. Too often we have heard audiologists say, "I don't like to work with younger children—I can't depend on their responses and they are too inconsistent to be relied upon." Nothing could be less true. Babies do just what they are supposed to do; the clinician often does not. The clinician has to give the right stimulus in the right structured situation in order to get the right response. There are no poorly responding babies—only inadequately prepared clinicians.

What are the general rules about working with children of all ages?

For Infants and All Children. Establish quickly an easy relationship with mother. Speak pleasantly and relaxedly to her; you will find the child looking back and forth between you two, and finally becoming content that all is well, he too will relax. In other words, the child absorbs the cathexis between you and mother and becomes at ease. Many people prefer to work with a child alone and banish the mother from the room. This is fine if you have enough time to establish a relationship with the child. It may be quicker and easier to use mother in the testing situation; there is less apprehension in the child and he stays relaxed during the session. Mothers are usually quite cooperative and entirely rational.

For Play-Conditioning Testing of

Table 5.1.
Audiological Case History Questionnaire for Parents of Children with Hearing Loss

I. *Chief complaint* _____
   When was problem first noted? _____
   Extent of problem _____
   Previous examinations and evaluations _____

II. *Prenatal history*
   Exposure to viral diseases during pregnancy? _____
   Which viral disorder? _____
   During which pregnancy month? _____
   Drugs during pregnancy? _____
   Trauma during pregnancy? _____

III. *Birth history*
   Gestation age at birth _____
   Birth Weight _____ Bilirubin level high? _____
   Asphyxia? _____ Meningitis? _____

IV. *Family history*
   Childhood deafness in family? _____
      Relationship to patient _____
   Birth defect or abnormalities _____
      In any other relatives? _____

V. *Developmental history*
   Age of first smile response? _____
   Age when sat up alone? _____
   Age when first crawled? _____
   Age of "stranger anxiety"? _____
   Age of walking? _____

VI. *Physical history*
   Cleft lip or palate _____ Submucous cleft _____
   Low-set ears _____ Poorly formed ears _____
   High fevers with illness _____ Seizures _____
   Ear infections _____ How many? _____
   Previous treatment for ear conditions? _____

VII. *What do you (parents) really think caused this hearing problem?* _____

   Name of child's pediatrician _____
   Names of other physicians who have seen this child _____

the Older Child. Tell him what he is going to do—do not ask him. In this respect, the very young and the very old are alike, and one handles them both not by asking whether they would like to do something (they never do), but by telling them firmly and plesantly that this is what they are going to do. Children do just what you expect of them, and if you firmly expect them to do what you want them to, they usually oblige. Of course, occasionally, one balks and yells like a banshee anyway—you can't win them all. But, give it a try—children are a great deal easier to handle than you think.

Believe in the Child's Responses. Develop a staunch and fervid belief that, when children hear a sound, they will react in a stereotyped way that is consistent with their level of mental functioning. This holds true for the near-deaf child as well as for the normal child. The child with a threshold of 80 dB for a given sound will respond at 85 dB like the normal-hearing child who hears the same sound at 5 dB. A 2-year-old mentally retarded child with a

Table 5.2.
Sensorineural Hearing-Impaired Child Assessment

Name _____
Age _____
Date of Birth _____
Hospital # _____
Age child identified by M.D. (months) _____
Age suspected of loss by mother (months) _____

Forceps/assisted delivery	Yes	No
Caesarian section	Yes	No
Other	Yes	No
Specify _____		
_____		

FAMILY HISTORY

Were parents relatives before marriage	Yes	No
Family history of kidney disease	Yes	No
Family history of thyroid problems	Yes	No
Family history of progressive blindness	Yes	No
Family history of previous stillbirths or miscarriages	Yes	No
Family history of hearing loss	Yes	No
Another affected child in family	Yes	No

MATERNAL FACTORS

Drugs (inc. antibiotics)	Yes	No
Specify _____		
Exposure to chemicals	Yes	No
Specify _____		
Exposure to radiation	Yes	No
Specify _____		
Amniocentesis	Yes	No
Rh immunoglobulin given Rh or ABO incompatible	Yes	No
Maternal illness during pregnancy	Yes	No
Specify _____		
Bleeding	Yes	No
Anemia	Yes	No
Diabetes	Yes	No
Toxemia	Yes	No
Paternal illness during pregnancy	Yes	No
Specify _____		
Mother worked outside home	Yes	No
Specify _____		
Father worked during pregnancy	Yes	No
Specify _____		
During pregnancy, mother exposed to:		
Measles	Yes	No
Mumps	Yes	No
Chicken pox	Yes	No
German measles	Yes	No
Syphilis	Yes	No
Herpes virus	Yes	No
Influenza	Yes	No
Cytomegalovirus (CMV)	Yes	No
Toxoplasmosis	Yes	No
Other	Yes	No
Specify _____		
_____		
_____		

DELIVERY/LABOR

Full-term pregnancy	Yes	No
Labor induced	Yes	No
Labor less than 3 hr	Yes	No
Labor longer than 24 hr	Yes	No
Premature membrane rupture	Yes	No
Bleeding	Yes	No

INFANT/NEWBORN FACTORS

Small birthweight (<2 kg/5 lb)	Yes	No
Birthweight (lb/oz) _____		
Apgar low at birth	Yes	No
In an intensive care unit	Yes	No
How long (wk) _____		
Breathing problems	Yes	No
O_2 given	Yes	No
How long (wk) _____		
Bilirubin >15 mg/100 ml	Yes	No
Congenital rubella	Yes	No
Defect of ear, nose, throat	Yes	No
Specify _____		
Congenital heart disease	Yes	No
Drugs (inc. antibiotics)	Yes	No
Specify _____		
Exposure to chemicals	Yes	No
Specify _____		
Exposure to radiation	Yes	No
Specify _____		
Paralysis	Yes	No
Seizures	Yes	No
Septicemia	Yes	No

INFANT/CHILDHOOD HISTORY

Eye problems	Yes	No
Specify _____		
Balance/gait/incoordination		
Dizziness problems	Yes	No
Cerebral palsy	Yes	No
Seizures	Yes	No
Head trauma/skull	Yes	No
Ever hospitalized for:		
Meningitis	Yes	No
Encephalitis	Yes	No
Measles	Yes	No
Influenza	Yes	No
Rubella	Yes	No
CMV	Yes	No
Chicken pox	Yes	No
Septicemia	Yes	No
Diabetes	Yes	No
Sickle cell disease	Yes	No
Other (including conductive loss)	Yes	No
Specify _____		
_____		
_____		

mental age of 1 year will respond near his threshold in the way a normal-hearing child of 1 year responds near his threshold. There is no mystique about observing the hearing-impaired child's responses; other than having a hearing loss, he is a normal-behaving child.

The trick, if there is any, is to become confidently familiar with the auditory behavior of normal-hearing children regardless of the integrity of their mental processing or central nervous system functioning.

We would add another principle, at the risk of becoming maudlin—and that is to love every child as a human being. The clinician is often hard-put to develop any charitable feelings toward the wall-climber, the temper tantrum expert, the withdrawn

"Great Stone Face," or in some cases the misshapen, contorted face and limbs of the syndrome-ridden child. The same humanity underlies all these children, the kicker, the screamer, the silent one—all of them humanly acting out their protests at a world that has given them less than it has to others. They too can be loved.

CLINICAL TESTING OF THE INFANT, BIRTH TO 2 YEARS

The intensity levels and the observed responses that will be described for the birth to 2-year-old child are taken from an Auditory Behavior Index used in our clinic since 1966. The Index (Table 5.3) attempts to classify the type of response and the level of the adequate stimulus that will elicit a response at various ages of normal

Table 5.3.
Auditory Behavior Index for Infants: Stimulus and Level of Response[a]

Age	Noisemakers (Approx. SPL)	Warbled Pure Tones (Re: dB HL)	Speech (Re: dB HL)	Expected Response	Startle to Speech (Re: dB HL)
0–6 wk	50–70 dB	78 dB	40–60 dB	Eye-widening, eye-blink, stirring or arousal from sleep, startle	65 dB
6 wk–4 mo	50–60 dB	70 dB	47 dB	Eye-widening, eye-shift, eye-blinking, quieting; beginning rudimentary head turn by 4 mo	65 dB
4–7 mo	40–50 dB	51 dB	21 dB	Head-turn on lateral plane toward sound; listening attitude	65 dB
7–9 mo	30–40 dB	45 dB	15 dB	Direct localization of sounds to side, indirectly below ear level	65 dB
9–13 mo	25–35 dB	38 dB	8 dB	Direct localization of sounds to side, directly below, ear level, indirectly above ear level	65 dB
13–16 mo	25–30 dB	32 dB	5 dB	Direct localization of sound on side, above and below	65 dB
16–21 mo	25 dB	25 dB	5 dB	Direct localization of sound on side, above and below	65 dB
21–24 mo	25 dB	26 dB	3 dB	Direct localization of sound on side, above and below	65 dB

[a] Testing done in a sound room. (Modified with permission from F. McConnell and P. H. Ward: *Deafness in Childhood*, Nashville, Tenn., Vanderbilt University Press, 1967.)

development. The Index was prepared in an effort to replicate an auditory behavior index reported by Dr. Kevin Murphy of Reading, England (1962, 1979). This remarkable observer of infants and children diagrammed the quality of the behavioral responses of children to sounds, chiefly to noisemakers. Our study attempted not only to replicate his findings, but to add to it the level of the adequate signal that would first elicit a response. Comparison of our study with that of Murphy's showed less mature response levels than his, and we used general groupings that indicated an age period at the end of which the response should have developed. At any rate, we found too large a deviation in responses at any specific month of age to make as fine an analysis as Murphy's. Defining the upper limits of the ages at which certain responses can be expected has proved sufficiently useful for clinical judgments.

The value of such an Index lies in its consistency of reproduction in the clinical situation. Particularly reliable are the responses to a speech signal, less reliable are the responses to pure tone signals. This difference was to be expected after Eisenberg's (1969) description of the greater sensitivity of the infant to speech dimensional sounds.

Samples and Franklin (1978) observed the responses of 7–9-month-old infants to speech signals, warble-tones, and noise bands. They found that the intensity level required for a response was lower, and the number of responses were significantly higher to speech signals than to either the warble-tones or broadband noise stimuli. They also confirmed Murphy's (1979) findings that the first maturation of the direct orientation on the lower level was better in the right ear than the left ear, and consistently better (more) responses were noted for the right ear.

Thompson and Thompson (1972) had previously noted that for infants of 7–12 months of age, speech and high-pass filtered speech produced the most behavioral responses over other types of auditory stim-uli. They recommended the use of the high-pass filtered speech signals as a useful stimulus for assessing high frequency hearing in infants. They found that, with 22–36-month-old infants, there is no longer an advantage in one auditory stimulus over another.

The Auditory Behavior Index is used for testing peripheral hearing levels present in all auditory disorders. Where perceptual involvements exist, it is far easier to identify normal hearing in the first year of life than it will be later on. Most normal-hearing, centrally damaged children show excellent reflexive responses to sounds at the expected normal levels. The type of awareness responses they give at a later age may not be consistent, but their startle responses will be normal when they are infants.

A spin-off of the use of the Index has been its unexpected value in identifying mental retardation. As indicted in the Index, not only the level the infant responds to, but also the way he responds, show a maturational sequence (Figs. 5.1 and 5.2). For example, the first localization of the young infant is a rudimentary head turn that may not reach a 90° angle. Later there follows a direct head turn to the side, but only in a lateral plane with the eyes. Direct fixation of a sound source in another plane follows, first on the lower level and then above the eye level; the final maturation is fixation of the source at a higher plane. Although individual differences exist in the rate of maturation, these are indeed guidelines for the kinds of behavioral activity that can be expected at any age.

Thus, if a 6-month-old baby gives only reflexive reactions to sound such as arousal and eye widening, but does not turn his head even rudimentarily, his auditory behavior age is lower than 4 months. If an 18-month-old child gives only lateral head turn and cannot fixate a sound source below or above his eye level, he is behaving on a 6–9-month level.

It is logical that one could correlate auditory behavior with mental age, in view of

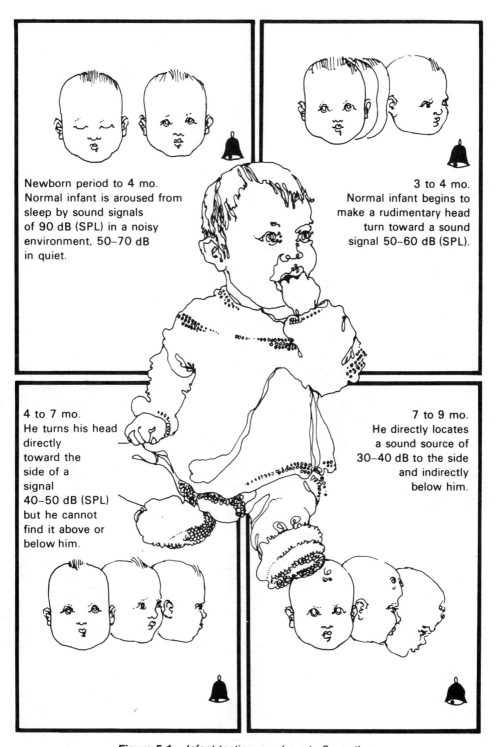

Newborn period to 4 mo. Normal infant is aroused from sleep by sound signals of 90 dB (SPL) in a noisy environment, 50–70 dB in quiet.

3 to 4 mo. Normal infant begins to make a rudimentary head turn toward a sound signal 50–60 dB (SPL).

4 to 7 mo. He turns his head directly toward the side of a signal 40–50 dB (SPL) but he cannot find it above or below him.

7 to 9 mo. He directly locates a sound source of 30–40 dB to the side and indirectly below him.

Figure 5.1. Infant testing: newborn to 9 months.

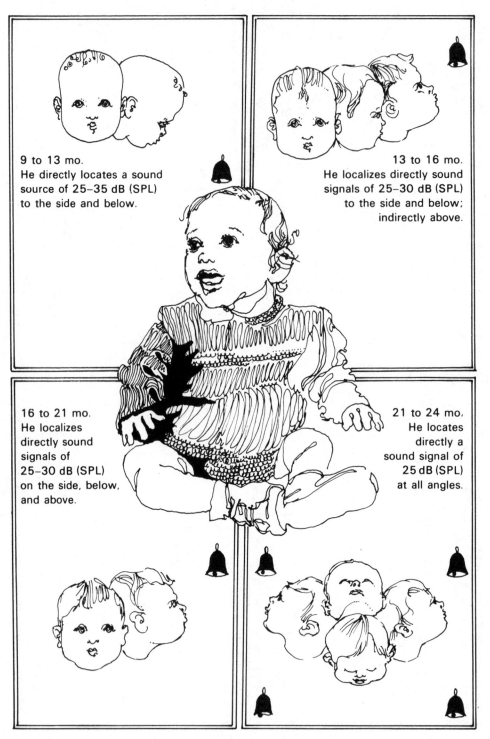

9 to 13 mo.
He directly locates a sound
source of 25–35 dB (SPL)
to the side and below.

13 to 16 mo.
He localizes directly sound
signals of 25–30 dB (SPL)
to the side and below;
indirectly above.

16 to 21 mo.
He localizes
directly sound
signals of
25–30 dB (SPL)
on the side, below,
and above.

21 to 24 mo.
He locates
directly a
sound signal of
25 dB (SPL)
at all angles.

Figure 5.2.　Infant testing: 9–24 months.

the fact that the mentally retarded child behaves consistently in all areas in the normal pattern for his mental age.

One cannot expect a 6-year-old with a 60 IQ to respond to finger-raising techniques in audiometry. If, however, we expect him to behave like a 3-year-old, the application of play audiometry will be as successful as it is with a normal 3-year-old. It is almost always true in mental retardation that behavior remains consistent with the mental age level.

A careful investigation into indices of auditory behavior was undertaken by Hoverston and Moncur (1969). Twenty-one 3-month-old infants and 22 8-month-old infants were given a variety of stimuli at intensities of 30, 45, 60 and 75 dB, and 15, 30, 45 and 60 dB, respectively. Two trained persons observed the babies' responses and recorded their judgments independently. As expected, a voice stimulus produced better responses than did white noise, 500 Hz, music, or 4000 Hz (in that order). For the 3-month group the 50% point of response to voice was reached at 32 dB hearing level (HL); for the 8-month group it was 23 dB. These seem to be excellent threshold levels when one considers that each of the five stimuli was presented twice at each intensity level and that the stimuli presentation order was randomized. The natural inhibition of response to successive stimuli would result in raised thresholds.

Other studies have described the maturation of infants' auditory responses in a comparable way. Watrous et al. (1975) categorized on 60 infants their reflexive behaviors, early attending behavior, and their auditory localization. Reflexive behaviors were noted in the 0–3-month age group; from 3 to 6 months there were changes in activity level toward early attending; at 6 months listening and searching emerged, with localization occurring at 8 months. Localization was at first horizontal but by 10–12 months was found in a vertical plane.

We urge clinicians not to accept our or others' norms for infant auditory behavior, but to generate their own index based on their instrumentation and their clinical style. Such an index should be used only by clinicians who have made the indicated observations on hundreds of normal infants in structured, repeatable situations. Only then can they feel confident in separating the normal from the abnormal.

Clinical Testing of the Newborn Infant

There are three essentials to the clinical testing of newborns: an adequate sound-attenuated room, measured noises, and a sleeping baby. With these given, even the least experienced observer can identify hearing levels as low as 35 dB in an infant.

The Sound Room. Newborns will respond only to very loud sounds when they are in their natural habitat, the noisy nursery. Noise levels of 70, 80, 90, and 100 dB sound pressure level (SPL) have been measured in the usual busy nursery. The newborn has been listening to sounds of 72 dB in utero, so he is accustomed to a background level of noise. We want to place him in the almost total isolation of a good sound booth in order to prepare him to respond to softer signals. It is best to leave him in the nursery crib, which can be wheeled into the sound room. Absolute quiet must be observed once the baby is in the booth. We recommend that two observers be present when an infant is tested in a sound room, in order to increase the reliability of the observations.

The Acoustic Signals. For the kinds of responses we want to observe, toy noisemakers are the most useful signals, largely because of their sudden, rapid onset. They are also more complex than pure tones and include high frequency components that have the best arousal value.

Premeasurement of the noises on a sound level meter is requisite. Note that we do not use the term calibration of the noises; these toys cannot be calibrated like an electronic instrument. They can be measured so their output is known.

A small bell: We prefer the kind of Hindu

bells found in import stores. With careful selection of the highest frequency-sounding bell, we have found some that when rung gently produce frequencies only around 4000 Hz at 25–35 dB SPL at 3 inches. When rung moderately, no more than 45 to 50 dB SPL sould be produced with high peaks at 4000 Hz.

A plastic block or rattle with sand inside that can be shaken suddenly: The sound made should peak at 1000 Hz or above, and with a quick, gentle shake should measure no more than 45–55 dB SPL at 3 inches.

A rubber squeeze toy: This too should be carefully selected to produce the highest pitched and the softest sound that can be found. This sound should peak at 1000 or 2000, at no more than 45 dB SPL.

Tissue paper (or cellophane from a cigarette package): When crushed, this produces 40–50 dB at around 1000 Hz nd higher.

One loud squeeze toy: One is needed which can produce at 50–85 dB SPL (all frequencies).

A commercially available set of preselected noisemakers, with each toy's frequency response and output level measured, is available as shown in Figure 5.3.

The toy noisemakers should be held motionless within 3 inches of the baby's ear for at least 10 sec before making the sound. The waiting period is necessary to obviate any response due the the hand's location in respect to the light source, or to any air movement.

Sleeping State. It is quite possible to observe reactions to sounds in an awake baby. However, as Ling et al. (1970) pointed out, in this condition the chance is too high of observing random responses and judging them to be valid responses to sound. On the other hand, Mencher (1972) reports that the chance of recording a random response in a sleeping baby is 1%. For this reason and in order to recommend the most foolproof method for testing infants, we prefer the sleeping state.

Two states of sleep can be operationally defined: a light state that is demonstrated by an eye or body movement to the flicking of the eyelid; and a deep state demonstrated by the absence of any movement when the eyelid is flicked (Mencher, 1972). Mencher found that the light sleep state is more productive of responses than the deep state. However, because this state of arousal may change from moment to moment, the baby should be tested regardless of which state is present.

Responses and Response Levels. The only response that should be accepted as valid is an arousal from the sleep state. By arousal we mean even a brief, transitory movement that indicates a marked change from the quiet, motionless sleep state. In the clinical situation, where repeated presentations of different stimuli can be made, we can accept the following responses as valid:

1. A definite eye-blink immediately following the presentation of the sound.
2. A slight shudder of the whole body.
3. An opening of the eyes, even briefly.
4. A slight head turn toward the sound.
5. A marked movement of arms, legs, or body.
6. Any combination of these.

The response must be seen within 2 sec of the stimulus presentation in order to be considered valid.

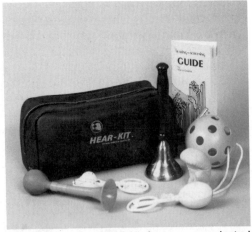

Figure 5.3. The HEAR Kit features preselected and premeasured toys to use in hearing screening of infants and young children. (Courtesy of BAM World Markets, 399 S. Harrison, Denver, CO 80209.)

It is always prudent to present a loud stimulus at the end of the testing period, in order to evoke a large startle response which will reconfirm the observations of movements that have been made.

Procedures. Maintaining complete quiet for at least a minute or two, the observers watch the baby carefully for on-going activity. If there is none, a flick of the eyelid should be made to determine the state of sleep. The fact of a deep sleep will change the judgment that is made of the subsequent responses, for the baby is less apt to give good responses when in a deep state of sleep. If a light state prevails, greater confidence can be placed in the responses or lack of responses that are seen.

A typical testing sequence with stimulus presentations and their intensity levels would be as follows:

1. Small bell rung at 35–45 dB SPL. Wait 20 sec before the next presentation or until baby resumes the sleeping state, if he has moved. Usual response: arousal (body movement, head turn).

2. Soft rattle sound at 45–50 dB SPL. Wait 20 sec. Usual response: eye-blink.

3. Soft rubber squeeze toy sounded at 35–45 dB SPL. Wait 20 sec. Usual response: arousal (body movement, head turn, eye opening).

4. Loud, "squawking" squeeze toy at 85 dB SPL. Usual response: large startle (a sudden rapid movement of arms and other parts of the body; almost a small "jump").

Responses to each of these sounds should be seen in the normal baby. If in doubt, a sound can be repeated after a quiet interval. In a brief testing period, the baby's responses usually do not extinguish when a variety of sounds are presented at different time intervals. The state may change from time to time, however, and one must use clinical acuity as well as the eyelid test to estimate whether he has fallen into too deep a state to test. Shaking of the crib may arouse him sufficiently to test.

If responses are not seen to the softer noisemakers, other sounds should be employed. The crushed tissue paper, voice at 45 dB, white noise and narrow band noise at 45 dB (these last through the loudspeakers), and finally, sudden voice burst at 65–70 dB (re: audiometric 0). We have found that a "buh-buh-buh" at 65 dB usually produces a large startle response at any age.

If no responses are seen to the softer sounds, yet the baby responds to the louder ones, repeat tests should be made at another time. No greater than 5% false-positive (normal-hearing babies who do not respond at a given time) should be found with this technique.

The kinds of responses we see in the infant's arousal from sleep are not high level, integrated reactions. They are rather varying degrees of reflexive responses which can be mediated in the brain stem or even the spinal cord. As such they relate only to the peripheral hearing mechanism, not to central auditory processing.

It has been our experience that at least 95% of the normal-hearing infants—even those AT RISK—can be identified as normal on the first test by the kind of procedure described above. Most of the remainder will be identified in a repeat testing sequence, and only one-half of 1% will require a third visit to the sound room.

So far as warbled pure tones are concerned, the newborn infant requires around 70 dB (re: audiometric 0) before a response can be seen. The esoteric nature of the pure tones does not seem to arouse the infant to the degree that sudden complex sounds do. Therefore, the clinical usefulness of pure tones for newborns is reduced. When such high levels of sound must be used, there is always the possibility of a hearing loss with recruitment, giving the infant a loudness sensation equal to a normal ear.

Testing the Infant, Birth to 4 Months

During the first 4 months of life the infant's gross auditory behavior does not change markedly. In fact, by 3 months of age it may be more difficult to see a baby's response than it was at birth. This is probably because he is apt to be awake during the testing situation, and because he has been exposed at home to a great variety of acoustic stimuli from which he is still learning to select what is meaningful. He obviously has normal hearing, but neither his integrative processes nor his auditory-motor coordination have been well enough established to give the clear-cut responses we want to see. By 4 months he will make a great leap to responding overtly to softer signals than before. Until that time, both parents and clinicians are hard-put to see responses.

The requirements for testing the 0–4-month-old infant are almost the same as those outlined for the newborn baby: the adequate sound room, a quiet state, and measured noises. If the baby is sleeping, the protocol can be the same as described for the newborn.

1. If the baby is awake, seat the mother with the baby in her lap, half reclining in her arm if under 3 months, and sitting leaning against her chest if over 3 months.

2. With a toy in one hand, engage the baby's attention straight ahead. Place your head as close to the toy as possible, so that the baby can look back and forth between you and the toy without much movement of his eyes.

3. With the other hand, hold the noisemaker 3–4 inches from one ear, and behind it enough so that it is out of the baby's peripheral vision. Hold it still for at least 10 sec to be sure he is not aware of the positioning. Extreme quiet is essential.

4. Sound the noisemaker briefly—no more than 2 sec.

5. Watch for immediate responses, which include (a) eye widening—the eyelids raise, and the eyes may turn toward you; (b) quieting; (c) a rapid eye blink; and (d) by 4 months, a rudimentary head turn that may not go farther than looking at you. It may go past you slightly, but until 5–7 months will not be a 90° turn.

Repeat the test with other noisemakers on the other side, as with the newborn protocol, ending with the loud noisemaker to produce a startle.

6. While observing from the instrument room, with the baby still on the mother's lap positioned between two loudspeakers located at 70° angles on both sides and slightly in front, repeat "buh-buh" into the microphone, in a slowly ascending presentation from zero. Keep the instrument room dark so the child will not see the tester. Present the speech signals at 20–30-sec intervals for each ascending 5-dB step. Observe the first awareness response (eyes widening, quieting, eye shift, or beginning head turn), and record the level. Use only ascending 5-dB steps. When a response is seen, do not repeat the test. The speech test is the most consistent of all, but should be repeated only at the end of the testing.

7. Present at 65 dB a sudden speech signal (buh-buh-buh) to produce a startle response. Warn mother not to startle. The child should give a typical Moro's response, almost jumping up at the signal. A startle confirms your previous observations if the infant has given normal responses; if he has a severe hearing loss he will not attend in any way to 65 dB; if he has a moderate loss he may only be mildly aware.

8. Repeat steps 5 through 7 using the bone-conduction receiver pressed firmly by the mother on the midline of the top of the head. The bone-conduction receiver should be calibrated for speech biologically, which usually places 0 dB threshold at 35–40 dB on the dial. Make the same observations of awareness levels to speech as above, but keep in mind that the normal child or one with bilaterally symmetrical sensorineural loss will look to the front for the sound. If there is a conductive loss in one ear or a lesser sensorineural loss, he may lateralize to that side, thus providing a diagnostic clue to the type of loss.

The degree of startle reaction to 65-dB speech is also significant diagnostically (Fig. 5.4). An infant who gives only a mild startle to air-conducted speech at 65 dB, but shows a large jump to bone-conducted speech at that level should be suspected of having an air-bone gap. Infants, even newborns, with middle ear anomalies demon-

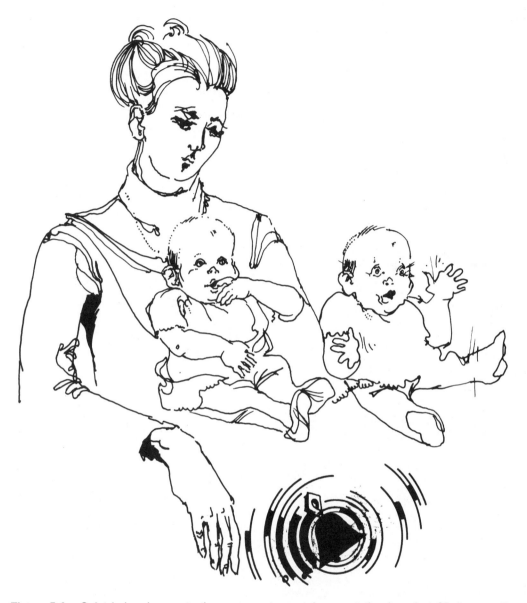

Figure 5.4. Quiet baby shows startle response to sound presentation heard at 65-db sensation level.

strate a dramatic difference between their responses to air- and to bone-conducted speech signals. The fact that their conductive losses muffle their usual reception of air-bone sound makes the contrast between air and bone conduction literally startling.

9. Cross-check audiometric impressions with impedance audiometry (see Chapter 6).

Using the entire battery of tests in the

Index, mild to moderate sensorineural losses become evident even in the first 4 months of life. The speech awareness level usually is consistent with the hearing loss around 500 Hz in cases of severe losses. In milder losses, it is closer to the 1000-Hz level. Care should be taken, however, in estimating the pure tone thresholds from the awareness level for tones.

Table 5.4 shows the rapid development

Table 5.4.
Rapid Developmental Screening Check List[a,b]

NAME: . . . . D.O.B.: . . . .   1st Visit: . . . .

AGE			DATE
1 mo:	Can he raise his head from the surface in the prone position?	Yes	No
	Does he regard your face while you are in his direct line of vision?	Yes	No
2 mo:	Does he smile and coo?	Yes	No
3 mo:	Does he follow a moving object?	Yes	No
	Does he hold his head erect?	Yes	No
4 mo:	Will he hold a rattle?	Yes	No
	Does he laugh aloud?	Yes	No
5 mo:	Can he reach for and hold objects?	Yes	No
6 mo:	Can he turn over?	Yes	No
	Does he turn toward sounds?	Yes	No
	Will he sit with a little support (with one hand)?	Yes	No
7 mo:	Can he transfer an object from one hand to another? . .	Yes	No
	Can he sit momentarily without support?	Yes	No
8 mo:	Can he sit steadily for about 5 minutes?	Yes	No
9 mo:	Can he say "ma-ma" or "da-da"?	Yes	No
10 mo:	Can he pull himself up at the side of his crib or playpen?	Yes	No
11 mo:	Can he cruise around his playpen or crib, or walk holding onto furniture?	Yes	No
12 mo:	Can he wave bye-bye?	Yes	No
	Can he walk with one hand held?	Yes	No
	Does he have a two-word vocabulary?	Yes	No
15 mo:	Can he walk by himself?	Yes	No
	Can he indicate his wants by pointing and grunting? . . .	Yes	No
18 mo:	Can he build a tower of three blocks?	Yes	No
	Does he say six words?	Yes	No
24 mo:	Can he run?	Yes	No
	Can he walk up and down stairs holding rail?	Yes	No
	Can he express himself (occasionally) in a two-word sentence?	Yes	No
2½ yr:	Can he jump lifting both feet off the ground?	Yes	No
	Can he build a tower of six blocks?	Yes	No
	Can he point to parts of his body on command?	Yes	No
3 yr:	Can he follow two commands involving "on," "under," or "behind" (without gestures?)	Yes	No
	Can he build a tower of nine blocks?	Yes	No
	Does he know his first name?	Yes	No
	Can he copy a circle?	Yes	No
4 yr:	Can he stand on one foot?	Yes	No
	Can he copy a cross?	Yes	No
	Does he use the past tense, properly?	Yes	No
5 yr:	Can he follow three commands?	Yes	No
	Can he copy a square?	Yes	No
	Can he skip?	Yes	No

[a] Developed by the Committee on Children with Handicaps, American Academy of Pediatrics, New York Chapter 3, District II.

[b] This check list is a compilation of developmental landmarks matched against the age of the child. These are in easily scored question form and may be checked "Yes" or "No" by a physician or his aide, by direct observation. "No" responses at the appropriate age may constitute a signal indicating a possible developmental lag. If there is a substantial deviation from these values, then the child should be evaluated more carefully, taking into consideration the wide variability of developmental landmarks. (Adjust for prematurity, prior to 2 years, by subtracting the time of prematurity from the age of the child, i.e., a 2-month-old infant who was 1 month premature should be evaluated as a month-old infant.)

check list that is approved by the American Academy of Pediatrics. Care should be taken in interpreting some of the landmarks as indicative of normal hearing. A deaf infant coos and chuckles quite normally at 2–3 months. He laughs aloud at 4 months; he can babble in two sounds before 6 months; he says something like "ma-ma" at 9 months; and by 12 months he may have a vocalization that sounds like "dada." This can be misleading. The parents of one deaf child in our clinic insisted that their boy had normal hearing at 1 year of age because, they reported, he said "mama" and "dada." Yet polytomograms of the child's ears showed congenital gross bony abnormalities of the inner ears that were present at birth and precluded the possibility of any hearing at birth. It is well to view such reports of early speaking with healthy skepticism.

Testing the Infant, 4–7 Months

Around 4 months of age, the infant takes a giant step toward auditory maturity. Not only does he begin to turn his head toward a sound source, but he shows this response to a much softer level of sound than in the first 4 months. From a 47-dB average level of an adequate speech stimulus, he now becomes aware at 21 dB. During this period his muscle strength and his eye and motor coordination also show great improvement; he is out of the newborn period and on the way to becoming an active responder. He laughs aloud, he holds a rattle, reaches for objects and holds them, turns himself over, and sits by 6 months with a little support. By 7 months he can transfer an object from hand to hand and sit without support momentarily.

At this age the clinician should observe the visual acuity of the child: Can he track a bright object visually from one side to the other? Does he have good eye contact with you even for a brief period when he is 4 months and for longer periods of interest at 7 months? Smile and nod your head and say "Hi, Johnny." Is there integrity in the way he looks at you? Observations of many

normal children of this age will give the necessary insight into an abnormal child's behavior.

The improved muscular coordination allows the child at 4 months to begin to turn his head toward a sound, but only on a lateral plane. He is not able to find a sound source below his head level or above it. The head turn at 4 months is a wobbly one which never gets around to a 90° angle. By 6 months the head should come around 90° toward the sound, but the eyes will not fixate the source when it is below or above him on that side.

Procedure. Present the same sequence of sounds as described for the 0–4-month-olds, steps 1 through 9. For the noisemaker tests, the clinician can either kneel at a 45° angle to the child and hold the noisemaker unobtrusively down beside the chair, or kneel behind the baby and present the sound on the side at the lower level (Fig. 5.5, *A* and *B*). The head turn will be evident in this case, but the eye-widening and "aha" effect will not be seen.

For speech audiometry the baby should be held seated in his mother's lap, facing forward toward the window.

A small, not-too-attractive toy can be given the mother to hold in front of the baby on his lap. She should be instructed not to talk to him or to make any undue noise. Both loudspeakers are used. Present the speech first on one side until a head

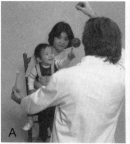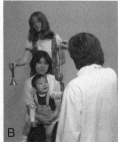

Figure 5.5. Demonstration of behavioral observation audiometry (BOA) with screening noisemakers: (*A*) Shows the testing technique with one tester, while (*B*) shows the utilization of a two-tester team. (Photographs courtesy of BAM World Markets.)

turn is noted. Then quickly switch to the other loudspeaker and note whether the head turns back. The average level of the lowest speech which is responded to at this age is 21 dB.

At this age the speech testing should include saying the baby's name: "Hi, Johnny"; "Hello, Johnny." Always find out which name the parents are using for the baby at home. It does not help to say "Hi, Johnny" to John Edwin who is called "Eddie" by his family.

As he approaches 7 months the infant may become responsive to "bye-bye" and that sound should be included in the speech reception battery with his name.

The entire battery of audiological and impedance tests should always be used. One test confirms the other. Particularly, the startle to 65 dB should always be included at the end of each test period. Be sure to sit the child as far forward on mother's knees as possible, with little support except for mother's hands. If reduced hearing has been suspected, the lack of a startle or the reduced quality of the startle will confirm the previous findings.

Testing the Infant, 7–9 Months

In the 7–9-month period, the improvement in motor coordination allows the infant to sit steadily by himself and to change his position without falling. He manipulates two objects simultaneously, and transfers objects hand-to-hand and hand-to-mouth. This is the "explore-everything-in-the-mouth stage"—a good way to supplement information about the environment. We often see this stage represented in older mentally retarded children who are functioning at this mental age level.

He is able to play peek-a-boo, and may begin to learn pat-a-cake. He begins to be initially shy with strangers. He may be able to respond to bye-bye with a wave of his arm and a cupped hand. "Dada" and "mama" may be heard, but not with specific referents. He should imitate gross speech sounds nicely by 9 months.

Auditorally, the infant is now able to find a sound source below his eye level and to the side, but only by looking first to the side and then down. This is what is referred to as the "indirect fixation" of a sound source at a lower level. The transitional stage of his fixation ability becomes evident here. He is not yet ready to find the sound when it is above his eye level.

The level of an adequate speech signal now drops to a 15-dB average, showing the gradual maturation of the auditory response.

Procedure. 1. With the child seated on his mother's lap, let her hold a toy in front of him to play with—a small doll or a fuzzy animal. Usually he will be content to sit in his mother's lap and be mildly amused.

2. Present the same sequence of tests as before (steps 1 through 8). The noisemaker test again can be done by kneeling in front of the child at a 45° angle, being very careful not to let him see the noisemaker in your hand. Observe carefully the direction of his head turn. At 7 months it may only be to the side but by 9 months, he should turn to the side and then look down.

3. For the speech awareness level, begin by saying "Bye-bye Johnny." As in all the tests, you should develop a feeling for the moment when the child will be the most responsive. If he is still exploring his environment, wait until he settles down. If he is too engrossed in the toy in front of him, wait until his enthusiasm dies a bit.

Present the speech through one loudspeaker; if his head is turned toward one side, choose the loudspeaker on the opposite side. Once a head turn is noted, switch to the other loudspeaker and repeat the signal. At this age, you can begin to manipulate the head turn like that of people watching a tennis match, if you want. Not for long, however. It is not an interesting enough activity to sustain his interest.

At this age also, there may be a vocalization response to the speech signal. After listening to the voice, he may gurgle or respond with a questioning "eh" in a rising inflection. He may even imitate an "oh-oh" with inflection. He is a usually happy, outgoing baby, not fearful of anything. He will submit to the impedance meter probe tip without complaint. Only at a later age does fear arise.

Testing the Infant, 9–13 Months

It is normal by 9 months for the baby to be afraid of strangers if they come too close or attempt to hold him. "Strangeness" is one of the psychic organizers described by Spitz (1959). The child who will come to the arms of a complete stranger at this age may suffer a lack of psychic development. One should observe carefully the eye contact the child gives at this age. He should relate to you with interest, even if it becomes negative interest. Let mother handle him exclusively for the test. The advantage of testing from a dark sound room is evident at this point. It takes you out of the picture and allows the baby to relax and feel secure with mother. Normal babies do not mind the silence and confinement of the sound room. Occasionally an older child with cerebral dysfunction will object violently to the sound room, but will usually settle down and enjoy the quiet.

By 11 months the baby is on his feet, cruising around his playpen or walking holding on to furniture. He is expected to say "mama" and another speechlike sound, but do not count on it. It may not be meaningful to him if he does make the sound. And remember that deaf children have been reported to say "mama" and "dada" by their hopeful parents.

The baby knows his own name now, and by 12 months can wave bye-bye. So we will now use "bye-bye Johnny" as our speech signal. It is an added premium if, as you present the phrase on an ascending threshold, he waves bye-bye to the loudspeaker at 5 dB. It is the best speech reception threshold obtainable.

The auditory behavior in this period progresses from the indirect to the direct localization of the sound source on the lower level. At the end of this period the baby should be localizing indirectly on the upper level; i.e., he will first look laterally and then shift his gaze upward. He is very interested in strange sounds in his environment, and will orient rapidly to the sound.

Procedure. 1. Go through the entire auditory and impedance measurement sequence as before. Include in the noisemaker test the presentation of a sound above and behind the baby's head, out of his eyesight.

2. In the speech sequence, the use of "bye-bye" will very often produce a hand wave in the direction of the sound. Another useful signal is "no-no," for by a year of age the child will stop what he is doing when he hears this signal, however faint. "Oh-oh" may produce an accurate imitation. The average threshold of response to speech at this age is 8 dB.

Testing the Infant, 13–24 Months

Once the child has reached 13 months, his orientation response is fully mature. After 2 years he may begin to inhibit his responses because of the strange social situation, but up to that time his reactions are still pure and untouched. In this period (by 15 months) he learns to walk—a skill that occupies him intensely for a while. He should be combining two words and be able to say three words other than mama and dada, but by 2 years it is not too alarming if he does not. He should, however, be using his voice meaningfully and in many variations. Up and down intonations, phonetic "grunts" of all sorts, and speechlike pauses in his vocalizations should be part of his repertoire if his hearing is normal. At this age in the deaf child the strident voice and the limitation of vocalization to the back vowels becomes evident. Once heard, the raucous "a-ah" of the deaf child can never be forgotten.

By 18 months he may know a few simple objects well enough to look for them. This ability can be used in testing. "Where's the meeow?" may elicit a quick look at the toy cat, or even a hit at it. By 2 years it is often possible to have him pick up toys on command during the testing session. So some simple speech audiometry can be added to the protocol. However, it is always well first to go through the testing sequence as for the younger infant, in order to have some information on his hearing level in the event he does not choose to cooperate.

Procedure. 1. Go through the audiological and acoustic impedance test sequence as before. The average level of response at this age is very close to 0 dB.

2. After the observations have been made of his orientation levels, try for some identification of speech in an ascending presentation: "Bye-bye." "Where's your nose?" "Where's mama?" "Where's the bow-wow?" "Want to go bye-bye?" As he becomes older he can pick up a few toys on command and give them to mama: "Give mama the airplane"—or the baseball, or the baby, or the kitty. Find out from mother which are his favorite toys, and use them in the presentation. In order to keep his attention on what you are saying at soft levels, you may have to set the carrier phrase ("Give mama the. . .") at 20-dB level and quickly shift down to the level you want to test, for the key word. Do not be alarmed if suddenly he stops responding. After a certain time you lose him to the game. Know when to give up—when you have exceeded the limits of his interest in what you are doing. This is true even of the 3-year-old during play audiometry. Every child has a limit to his period of interest. You must either change the game or give up testing when the limit is reached.

Remember that the speech games are just as effective using bone conduction as they are in free field. Although the child may not tolerate the earphones, the differences between his free-field threshold and his bone-conduction threshold are significant. He will usually tolerate the bone-conduction receiver held at the midline or behind his ear.

The use of the darkened instrument room is still indicated up to 2 years of age. The purity of his behavior includes an unquestioning response to the voice signal. At a later age he will be confused by the voice without a visible speaker, and it may interfere with the actions one wants to stimulate.

CLINICAL TESTING OF THE CHILD AGED 2–5 YEARS

In this period the child grows into the independence of early maturity. He begins to separate from mother without much fuss; to dress himself, first with supervision and then without; and to understand his own identity. He becomes a wanderer, so do not turn your back on him or you will lose him. He begins to understand some abstract words like "cold" or "hungry," and can give his full name when asked. He becomes an eager beaver, happy to please you, and as a result gives the clinician a hard time in testing. Once he knows his cooperation in the play-conditioning pleases you, he may forget what he is supposed to listen for, in his eagerness to be praised. (Strangely enough, this attitude is often found in older deaf children—even in teenagers—who will give false responses in order to please, or to give a "good" test.)

The learning of play-conditioning techniques starts at 2 years. But do not be deceived by the bright, talkative 2-year-old who appears certain to be able to learn the procedure. Play safe, and first get all the information obtainable from the observations of his behavior described for the younger child. Then when you draw a blank you have some valuable information as a basis for future tests or for a medical examination.

He may protest, however, when it comes to impedance audiometry. All of the audiologist's skills are called on to complete this test. Chapter 6 provides some suggestions for dealing with children and impedance measurements.

Until the child is 4 or 5 years old, all the ingenuity the audiologist has must be brought forth; however, do not traumatize him so much that he will be frightened the next time. There is always another day.

The darkened instrument room should

not be forgotten even for these older children. A shy, immature child of 2½ may learn play-conditioning techniques easily, but the odd situation of a stranger's face in the window is too much for him to handle. The bodyless voice over the speaker can be coped with. It takes the stranger out of the situation. All the necessary instructions can be given through the speech circuit without being seen. So occasionally it will be useful to keep the instrument room darkened.

The description that follows of testing this age group is primarily related to double sound room testing. When the audiometric test is done in the same room with the child, the procedure can be easily adapted. The choice of audiometric testing in a double sound room or in a single seems to rest on personal preference. Whatever suits the individual's style should be elected. The speech reception tests (SRT) will always have to be done with the clinician outside of the testing room.

The armamentarium of the child tester should include a carefully selected array of toys, the names of which approach spondaic principles as closely as possible. However, in order to present children with easily recognizable toys, some compromise may be necessary. It is more important that the child knows and enjoys the toy than that it confirms to equal-stress-on-each-syllable principle.

Spondaic Words
  Airplane
  Baseball
  Toothbrush
  Hot dog (from the pet department)
  Cowboy
  Fire truck
  Birthday (a play cake with candles)
Nonspondaic Words
  Baby (a small baby doll)
  Kitty
  Doggie
  Horsie
  Car
  Truck
  Hamburger (pet shop)

No more than 4 of these need be selected for the 2–3-year-old, and 6 for the 4- and 5-year-olds. These items may be presented on a picture board, although actual toys are much more interesting to the child. Small toys may be wired to picture board material.

Procedure for Behavioral Play Audiometry

1. Placement. Place the young child in his mother's lap, with a table of toys in front of him. The older 4- or 5-year-old may prefer to sit alone with his mother in another chair, but mother's closeness may be important even at the older age.

2. Initial Rapport. Sit down and talk to mother first, developing an easy rapport with her. "What seems to be Johnnie's problem?" Let her tell you briefly why she is here, but do not belabor the history. Johnnie is the chief target. Turn interestedly to him and ask him how old he is, or comment on something he is wearing or has brought along. Little girls like their hair to be noticed. Ask him if he would like to play with your toys. "What is this?" If he does not answer, say "It's a big airplane, isn't it?" Try with other toys, and eventually he may tell you the name, or just ask the child to point to each toy as you name it. Proceed to find out whether he can identify the toys. Eliminate those he is not familiar with, and select those he seems to know best and enjoy.

During this period many observations can be made. Listen to his voice quality and how he articulates the words. Does he substitute for the high frequency consonants? If he omits or substitutes for the unvoiced consonants, either a mild sensorineural or a conductive loss can be suspected. If he misses the voiced consonants and some of the vowel sounds in addition, a more severe sensorineural loss may be predicted. Is he able to repeat words readily, but not to identify the corresponding toy? This is common in two types of children: those with sensorineural loss who have been given too much formal speech therapy or speech stimulation without sufficient experiences in hearing the word in connection with the object; and those with an auditory receptive disorder which allows them parrot-like imitation but no higher integration of the auditory-visual relationship. It may be difficult to decide which factor is present until diagnostic therapy reveals the degree of learning potential.

3. Introduction of Speech Test Procedure. Tell him what he is going to do. (Never ask him if he will do it.) "Now we're going to play a telephone game. You are going to put on the telephone like this, and I'm going to telephone to you. I am going to tell you which toy to show me. Won't that be fun? Now we'll put the telephone on you, and you can say hello to me. Hello!" Put the earphones gently but firmly on his head, saying "Hello, how are you? Now wait and I'm going to telephone to you from the other room." Try to get out before he balks at the phones, but if he does, do not fight it. Take off one phone and have mother hold it to his ear "like a real telephone." With the very young and shy child it may be preferable not to start with earphones at all. Do a trial run in sound field first, allowing him to become familiar with the situation. Then the earphones' placement may be attempted (Fig. 5.6).

4. Speech Test Procedure. In the instrument room, set the speech level at 40 or 50 dB (or as indicated) and say "Hello, Johnnie. Can you show me the airplane?" If he does, praise him and clap your hands. Then descend in 10-dB steps, asking him to show you a toy at each level. When he no longer responds, ascend 5 dB, but set the carrier phrase "Show me . . ." at a 10- or 15-dB higher level and switch quickly to the lower level. Too long a silent period will lose him to the game, so when searching for threshold the louder carrier phrase should be given. Accept two valid responses on the ascending presentation, and switch quickly to the other ear. Listening at low levels is not a child's cup of tea, and one must sacrifice some accuracy for the sake of holding his attention. If any discrepancies appear later, a recheck can always be done. It need hardly be said that the tester's

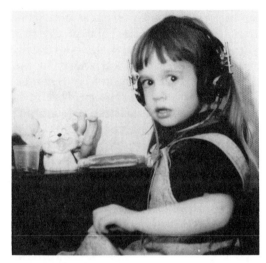

Figure 5.6. Speech audiometry measurement using earphones and toys.

mouth should be covered while giving the words.

Note that the speech reception threshold is obtained first in order to obtain information that will guide the clinician in the audiometric test. Too often a clinician will begin by training a child in audiometric techniques, starting at 40 or 50 dB, when the child has a 60-dB loss at that frequency. A complete, normal audiogram will then be recorded because the child plays along with the clinician's silly little game of responding when he thinks he is supposed to. *Never*, never presuppose a level of hearing in a child. It is better to obtain an awareness level as in the younger child and confirm it with a startle response at 65 dB, than to enter blindly into a test with a young child. The greatest number of misevaluations occur because of this failure.

Masking must be used if the SRT in one ear is 40 or 50 dB worse than the potential bone-conduction thresholds of the opposite ear. At this age masking is more productive of valid results in speech reception tests than it is in pure tone testing. The esoteric nature of pure tones may confuse the child when a masking noise is present. Always prepare the child for the noise. "Now we're going to be on an airplane, and you can hear the airplane noise. See if you can hear me over the noise and show me the toys." It is rare that masking will interfere with speech reception once the child has learned the technique.

By 4 or 5 years, simple speech discrimination tests can be given. The challenge is to select a test on the basis of the child's present receptive language level. Even if his language level has been identified on the basis of previous language tests, there are no children's discrimination tests which will fit the language shortcomings of every age and of every degree of hearing handicapping condition.

5. Introduction of Pure Tone Test. Now begin the instruction for the pure tone test. Take the earphones off the child (he is bored with them by this time) and put them on yourself. Have available a number of sets of motivational toys geared to different ages: plain blocks for building a tower; a graduated ring tower; beads to throw into a container; a peg board with colored peg (put a horse or a car in the center and build a fence or a garage. Girls prefer the horses; boys prefer the cars); and a piggy bank with pennies to put in.

Other motivational games can be devised by the ingenious audiologist. Usually one is sufficient to accomplish the task, but you must be ready to switch to another one at the first sign of boredom. It is largely the enthusiasm of the clinician that keeps the child attending, but occasionally novelty must be employed.

Show the child what the game is about, "We're going to hold this peg (or block, etc.) up to our ear and listen for a little bell. Oh! I hear it, so I can put the peg in the board. Now I'm going to listen for a little one. Oh! I hear it, so I put the peg in. Now you can do it, and build a fence for the horse." In the case of the 2- and 3-year-old, instruct mother to hold his hand with the peg up to his ear, and to guide his hand to the peg board when the sound is heard. Then practice it through sound field so the mother will hear it. Three or four trials should be sufficient for the child to learn.

6. Pure Tone Procedure. Now tell the child he is going to do it all alone and switch to the earphone. Present the tone at 40–50 dB above the expected threshold. Praise him for a correct action by switching to the speech circuit. Instruct the mother to have another peg ready to give him the moment he has responded accurately by placing the peg in the board. Descend as rapidly as possible from 40 or 50 dB in 10- or 15-dB steps, indicating that he is to listen for a "tiny little baby bell." Again, work quickly to obtain threshold, accepting two responses on the ascending presentation.

Select 2000 Hz as the first frequency to be presented. It is the most important one so far as a sensorineural loss is concerned. If the SRT has not been normal, be sure the initial practice tone is loud enough to cover a possible high frequency commensurate with the SRT or the awareness level. Sometimes a child will seem to be cooperative at first, but soon forgets what he is supposed to do. In this case, recondition him with the mother's help, at levels you are certain he can hear. Several reconditioning periods may have to be run during a test. *Do not give up* until it is quite apparent that he is not about to stay with the task.

The next frequency will be 500 Hz, significant in a conductive loss. Then switch to the other ear and obtain thresholds at 2000 and 500 Hz. If by this time you have lost the child, at least you have some valuable information. If he stays with the task nicely, fill in the 1000- and 250-Hz thresholds, and then 4000 Hz. Know when to stop, because the bone-conduction test is still to be done, and there must be some reserve of attention to carry him through it. It should be noted that when the child persistently refuses to wear even one earphone, sound field audiometry should be resorted to. Warbled pure tone, or narrow bands of noise, precalibrated to the location where the child is sitting, should be presented utilizing the play-conditioning techniques. The thresholds will represent the hearing in the better ear only, but will give the most essential information about how the child is hearing.

7. Now Repeat the Above with the Bone-Conduction Receiver. "We're going to use another kind of telephone— one that goes behind the ear. But you can hear the sounds just like the other telephone. That's like airplane pilots (or astronauts) use!"

Repeat the test as above, doing the more important frequencies first, and filling in with the others where possible. If there is any doubt about the bone-conduction thresholds, give an SRT through the bone-conduction receiver just as for the air conduction. It is assumed that the bone-conduction SRT has been precalibrated on normal-hearing people. The average normal threshold is generally around 35–40 dB on the dial of most instruments. Merely switching to the "microphone" input and the "bone conduction" output puts the speech circuit into the bone-conduction receiver on most audiometers. If SRTs are all that can be obtained on a child, the differ-

ence between air- and bone-conducted speech threshold gives significant information. In addition the bone-conducted speech can be masked effectively in the opposite ear without affecting the validity of the child's responses. The bone-conducted speech test is one of the most useful of the audiologist's tools. At the end, praise him or reward him with some token. This is insurance for future cooperation. You may have to see this child many times, so lay the groundwork for a happy return visit.

8. Verify Audiometric Impressions with Impedance Audiometry. The impedance test battery consists of tympanometry, acoustic reflex measurement, and physical volume measurement. See Chapter 6 for an explanation.

Speech Discrimination Testing in Young Children

Speech discrimination testing (Table 5.5) in children is an area that has yet to be fully developed, although research is cur-

Table 5.5.
Selected Pediatric Speech Audiometric Procedures[a]

Test[b]	Materials	Message Set; Response Mode	Task Domain	Minimum Age (yr)
SERT	30 environmental sounds (train, telephone)	Closed; picture identification	Unrestricted: 4 alternatives	3
ANT	Numbers 1 through 5	Closed; picture identification	Restricted: 5 alternatives	3
NU-CHIPS	50 monosyallabic words (food, school)	Closed; picture identification	Unrestricted: 4 alternatives	3
PSI	20 monosyllabic words (dog, spoon)	Closed; picture identification	Restricted: 5 alternatives	3
PSI	10 sentences, 2 syntactic constructions (Show me a bear brushing his teeth.) (A bear is brushing his teeth.)	Closed; picture identification	Restricted: 5 alternatives	3

[a] From S. Jerger: Speech audiometry, in J. Jerger, *Recent Advances in Speech, Hearing, and Language, Hearing Disorders*. San Diego, College Hill Press, 1983.

[b] SERT = Sound Effects Recognition Test (Finitizo-Hieber et al., 1980); ANT = Auditory Numbers Test (Erber, 1980); NU-CHIPS = Northwestern University—Children's Perception of Speech (Elliot and Katz, 1980); and PSI = Pediatric Speech Intelligibility (S. Jerger et al., 1980, 1981).

rently underway to rectify this situation. As Olsen and Matkin (1979) point out, the selection of receptive vocabulary competency, the designation of an appropriate response task, and the utilization of reinforcement are primary factors that may affect the reliability and validity of pediatric measurements. The results obtained during speech discrimination measures may actually be more a reflection of the child's interest and motivation for the task at hand, than a real indication of higher auditory speech discrimination abilities.

There is no well accepted standard technique or test of auditory discrimination in children. Although numerous tests have been developed for this purpose, apparently none of them "fits the bill" well enough for all clinicians to generally agree on which is most suitable for clinical work. One major problem with most current speech discrimination procedures is that the data base underlying the development of the test has not been standardized well enough on a broad spectrum of children of varying ages and backgrounds, and few implications can be generalized between the normal-hearing and hearing-impaired children.

Many children are too shy to speak in the test room environment, and, of course, articulation problems are common in children so it may be difficult for the audiologist to score speech discrimination tests as we do with adults. The most practical method of testing auditory discrimination in children has been to use some form of picture identification task. The child hears the test word, and attempts to identify an appropriate picture.

Susan Jerger recently published an excellent discussion and review of current speech audiometry materials for children. She points out in her paper (1983) that two basic principles have been important in the history of speech testing in children—vocabulary restriction in the selection of test material, and limited response set definition. She adds to these basic tenets, two more important considerations necessary in pediatric speech test development and administration, (1) the need to control the influence of receptive language ability on test performance and (2) the need to consider the effect of extra-auditory (cognitive) factors on children's performance.

Probably the most widely used speech discrimination test for children currently is the three-list phonetically balanced word lists selected from the spoken vocabulary of kindergarteners developed by Haskins in 1949. This is an open-ended set of stimulus words usually administered live-voice or via tape recording, and known as the PBK-50 word lists. It must be kept in mind that these words are from a kindergarten level vocabulary, and, without task-oriented or play techniques, children younger than 4½ years may not do well. Smith and Hodgson (1970) did show that tangible reinforcement (i.e., candy, toy, pennies, etc.) was an effective method of maintaining the interest of young children in the PBK-50 test. In fact, token reinforcement created significant improvement in speech discrimination scores from these children aged 4–8 years. Olsen and Matkin (1979) recommend that clinicians use caution with this test unless there is relatively good assurance that the receptive vocabulary age of the youngster under evaluation approaches at least that of a normal-hearing kindergartener.

One of the earliest attempts was the Discrimination by Identification of Pictures (DIP) test developed by Siegenthaler and Haspiel in 1966. Their test consists of 48 cards with two pictures on each card. One can quickly surmise that chance selection would produce fairly high scores since only two choices were involved in each presentation. Of interest is the fact that these investigators selected test words on the basis of contrasting acoustic dimensions rather than the traditional phonemic balance approach. The test was standardized on 295 normal-hearing children, between the ages of 3 and 8 years, and was administered at sensation levels of 0, 5, and 10 dB.

Ross and Lerman (1970) developed a picture identification test for hearing-impaired children known as the WIPI (Word Intelligibility by Picture Identification). They evaluated the test on 61 hearing-impaired children of ages 5 and 6, and caution about the use of the test with children younger than 5 years of age. The test consists of 25 picture plates with six pictures per plate with only four of the pictures on each plate used as test stimuli. The test is thus a closed-response set. The lists are reported to have high reliability coefficients, and the tests are simple and rapid to administer.

In 1976, Sanderson-Leepa and Rintelmann compared the speech discrimination performance of 60 normal-hearing children on the WIPI test, the PBK-50 test, and the Northwestern University Auditory Test No. 6 (NU-6). The children were in groups by age, 3½, 5½, 7½, 9½, and 11½ years. They found that the WIPI test yielded the highest discrimination scores, the PBK-50 intermediate scores, and the NU-6 the lowest scores. Their inclusion of the NU-6, although an adult speech discrimination test, was to determine the lowest chronological age for its appropriate use. They recommended that the WIPI was the test of choice for the 3½-year-olds, the WIPI and the PBK-50 were appropriate for the 5½-year-olds. For children 7½, 9½, and 11½, the NU-6 test was more difficult than the PBK-50 test. Clinicians must be cautioned that this study was conducted on normal-hearing children, and the same age recommendations might not be appropriate for hearing-impaired children.

Erber (1980) noted that the traditional speech discrimination tests developed for children are often inadequate for real diagnostic purposes, or too difficult for children with severe hearing impairment. He developed a simple auditory test to determine whether a young hearing-impaired child can perceive spectral aspects of speech or only gross temporal acoustic patterns. Known as the Auditory Numbers Test (ANT), this live voice test required the child to identify counted sequences and individual numbers. The ANT requires only that the child be able to count to five and be able to apply these number labels to sets of from one to five items. Picture cards are used which are color-coded and depict groups of one to five ants with the corresponding numerals. Erber recommends this test for rapid evaluation of speech perception in young severely and profoundly hearing-impaired children to aid in the planning of auditory training and habilitation activities.

The Northwestern University Children's Perception of Speech (NU-CHIPS) test developed by Elliot and Katz (1980) uses 50 monosyllabic words that were documented to be in the recognition vocabulary of normal children older than 2½ years of age. The test includes 65 word pictures, and interchanges 50 words as test items and foil items. Simple words, such as "food" and "school" are represented in a four-alternative picture set. The NU-CHIPS test is commercially available and appropriate for children as young as 3 years of age.

Finitzo-Hieber et al. (1980) described the development and evaluation of a Sound Effects Recognition Test (SERT) to use in the pediatric audiologic evaluation. They point out that such a test may be the only available standardized measure of auditory discrimination in children with limited verbal abilities. The test is comprised of three equivalent sets, each containing 10 familiar environmental sounds (such as a dog barking, a toilet flushing, a mother singing, hammering, a cat meowing, a baby crying, etc.). The authors indicated that the SERT is not intended to be a substitute for traditional speech discrimination tests but rather to supplement them, especially when the child has very limited verbal abilities.

In a review article regarding the effects of noise on perception of speech by children, Elliot (1982) points out that quite young children have poorer-than-adult levels of performance when listening at low levels in quiet, to words that are well within their receptive vocabularies. Using the NU-CHIPS test, in order for normal hearing 3-

year-olds to perform with nearly 100% accuracy, the words had to be presented at levels more than 10 dB greater than the level at which 5-year-olds reach 100%, approximately 15 dB greater than the 10-years-olds, and nearly 25 dB greater than the level needed by adults to score 100%. These differences occurred even though the words and pictures had been developed to be well within the receptive vocabularies of 3-year-old children when presented at comfortable listening levels. Her data warn that environments for children, such as classrooms, etc., need to be designed for very low ambient background noise.

S. Jerger et al. (1980, 1981) recently described their use of realistic speech materials to control the receptive language factor in children by incorporating the actual responses of normal youngsters between the ages of 3 and 6 years in the new Pediatric Speech Intelligibility (PSI) test. The children composed both monosyllabic word and sentence test items elicited by picture stimulus cards selected from lists of words and actions comprising children's early vocabularies. The PSI test is composed of 20 monosyllabic words and a 10-sentence procedure. The word lists include simple nouns such as "dog" and "spoon," and two types of sentence construction identified as Format I and Format II. An example of a Format II sentence is "A bear is brushing his teeth." The different sentence formats represent the different speech patterns of normal children between 3 and 6 years of age. The test materials are applicable for children as young as 2½ or 3 years old.

Although the PSI is still under development, the Jerger group has worked long and hard to establish a strong data base and to evaluate a number of influencing variables that control a child's performance on speech discrimination/intelligibility tasks. Their carefully designed approach to the PSI test development has documented information regarding the utilization of the test items in the presence of a competing message, and the definition of performance-intensity functions for children of varying chronologic and receptive language age groups. Their results hve confirmed the ability of children to perform these tasks that were previously applied only to adults. They have focused attention on the importance of variables such as predetermination of receptive language ability and cognition skills, rather than considering only chronological age. The PSI test is still undergoing evaluation and refinement, but should soon be commercially available (Figs. 5.7 and 5.8).

TESTING THE CHILD AGED 5–16 YEARS

By 5 years the child of normal intelligence can cooperate in the standard adult pure tone techniques and can repeat simple words. He will attend for fairly long periods of time to the hand-raising technique, given sufficient praise and encouragement. Not too much encouragement, though, as he may begin to give false responses in order to please. He will repeat the speech discrimination words willingly, but a few errors should be expected even in the normal-hearing child.

The pure tone audiometric technique that is chosen is a matter of preference, so long as it fulfills the requirements of the descending-ascending technique that is a modification of the method of constant limits. Newby (1964) and Carhart and Jerger (1959) described the most commonly accepted techniques for obtaining thresholds. In addition, a method proposed by Berlin and Catlin (1965) has some real advantages over the traditional procedures. The initial tone presentation is given at 0 and ascends in 10-dB steps until the level is reached where the subject responds. Another signal is given at 5 dB above that level to confirm its validity, and then another presentation is given at 10 dB below the last one. An ascent is then made. If a response is given, the next tone is presented at 10 dB below that level and the next tone ascends 5 dB. Three no-responses must be found at 5 dB below the level of "threshold" and three responses at 5 dB above. Two or three

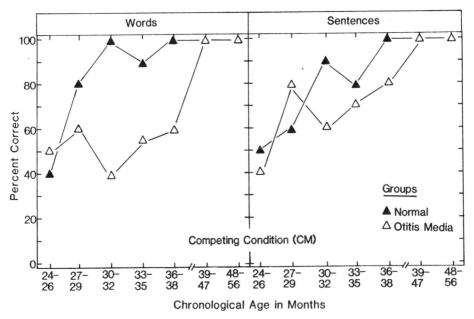

Figure 5.7. Data from the Pediatric Speech Intelligibility (PSI) test with a competing message condition for a group of normal-hearing children and a group of children with otitis media. Note the disparity between the two groups shown with the word materials. Although the sentence materials also bring out perceptual differences between the two groups, the poorer performance by the otitis media group is especially evident with the word test. (Courtesy of Susan Jerger, Baylor School of Medicine, Houston, Texas.)

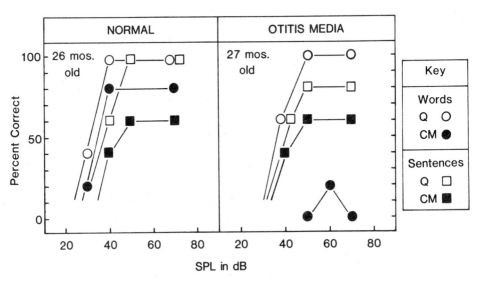

Figure 5.8. Pediatric Speech Intelligibility (PSI) data from two children of equivalent chronological age and receptive language ability. PSI performance-intensity functions in quiet look quite similar between the two patients, but note the performance-intensity function for the otitis media child when words are presented with a competing message background. (Courtesy of Susan Jerger, Baylor School of Medicine, Houston, Texas.)

responses must be seen at "threshold." Advantages to this method are: (1) it structures the bracketing of threshold; (2) it confirms the first response on the ascent by obtaining a response at a higher level; (3) it eliminates the taking of false responses as the threshold, by confirming the lowest response level through a 5-dB higher level; (4) it accustoms the subject immediately to listen for softer tones rather than louder tones; and (5) in the case of a functional hearing loss, it minimizes the "measuring stick" of the subject by the presentation of lower hearing levels at the start.

Whether this precise method is used, the experienced clinician will routinely employ the confirmatory procedure of presenting a 5-dB higher level than the presumed threshold. False responses can be rapidly spotted through this maneuver.

Modifications of Standard Testing Procedures for This Age Range

Age 5–10 Years. The younger child in this age group requires motivation to keep his attention on the test. Usually this can be done by social approval: smiling, nodding the head, clapping the hands, etc. It is rarely necessary to resort to bribery (commonly known as reinforcement technique). However, when the clinician has not enough resources or energy for social motivation, reinforcement can be used in the form of money, candy, etc.

The speech reception tests should be kept fairly simple at this stage. Usually 10 or 12 spondee words are sufficient to obtain threshold. Always familiarize the child with the words before the test. This can be done while sitting and talking to the child in an initial get-acquainted period.

The time spent in gaining rapport with the child is worth the effort. Talk to him about his clothes, his interests, his toys. Display a real interest in him. During this time you will make many useful observations about his voice quality, his articulation, the extent of his vocabulary, and the degree of cooperation you can expect.

Explain to him exactly what is going to happen, telling him this is what he is going to do—not "will you do this for me?" Be sure particularly to explain that he is to raise his hand (or finger) even when the tone sounds very faint and far away. He will have to listen hard for these little tiny sounds, because they are a long way off.

Always make certain of the mental age of the child. If a 5-year-old has a known IQ of 70, he should be treated like a 3½-year-old, not like a 5-year-old. The methods described for that age should then be used. Many children over 5 are labeled "untestable" merely because the clinician failed to apply the test procedure appropriate for the mental age level represented.

Age 10–16 Years. Very few modifications of the standard audiometric procedures are ever required for this age group. The development of rapport, the complete explanation of the test procedure, and the use of mild motivational techniques are usually sufficient for a valid test. However, there are a few precautions to take at this age, given below.

If the clinician has been presented with an audiogram from elsewhere showing a 30–60-dB loss, yet the child responds perfectly well to soft speech levels, be prepared to conduct the hearing tests very carefully. In this case, always start with a slow, ascending presentation of both pure tones and speech. Time will be saved in arriving at an understanding of the child's problem.

The deaf or hard-of-hearing child of this age must be handled carefully. Often he will attempt to respond when he does not hear, in an attempt to appear to have more favorable hearing than he actually has. It is best never to let such children see you during the test presentation. Face them completely away from you, because they can catch even a raised eyebrow out of the corners of their eyes. During the test, give them long periods of silence occasionally, and if they respond falsely, reprove them from the false response. Perhaps the clinicians who have tested such a child have been overeager to motivate him, and he is merely trying to please. Gentle reprimands are sometimes necessary to counteract this behavior.

At this age, and also at younger ages, the child has a right to understand what it means if he has a hearing loss, providing he had any receptive language at all. Too often we tend to "talk over" the child to the mother, in words that he does not understand. In the meantime, he is sitting there, wondering what it is about and worrying over what is wrong with him. The clinician should take time to explain to him in words that he can understand, just what kind of a loss he has, how severe it is, and what is going to be done for him. Often the clinician's explanation of the problem will ease the way toward his accepting the amplification and habilitation that will follow. Parents may be unable to explain these things to him, or may try to gloss over the facts, leaving the child bewildered and sometimes antagonistic. The child may be worried over what the other children will think of him in school. Explain that he is going to be a little different from the others, but only in this one respect. Otherwise he is just like everyone else, a good baseball player, a good game player, or a pretty girl who can play with the other girls. But in addition he will now hear his friends and his teacher better, and they will like that.

Operant Reinforcement Audiometry

In behavioral observation audiometry (BOA), the testing of infants and young children is accomplished without reinforcement of responses, and rests on the subjective observation of responses under structured conditions. The major advantages to BOA are efficiency in time required and the lack of need for specialized equipment or additional observers. The disadvantages of BOA include the fact that it is difficult to eliminate tester bias, the responses of infants and young children are quick to reach extinction without reinforcement, and a wide variance of responses are noted in such youngsters. Critics of BOA argue that the technique is useful for initial hearing

screening, but some form of operant reinforcement audiometry should be used in the establishment of specific hearing threshold data.

Wesley Wilson of the University of Washington has developed operant conditioning in children as a technique to establish hearing levels (Wilson et al., 1976). He points out that the use of reinforcement for responses made to audiometric stimuli strengthens the test paradigm, maintains the child's responses longer, reduces habituation to the stimulus often noted in BOA, and thus allows for a more precise estimate of hearing thresholds in young children.

Wilson describes two modes of operant conditioning which he terms *operant discrimination* and *conjugate procedures*. In operant discrimination the stimulus precedes the responses and acts as a discriminative signal that reinforcement is available. In the conjugate procedure the stimulus follows the response as a consequence. The intensity of a continuously available reinforcing stimulus varies as a function of the rate of the response. Since the stimulus is a consequence of the response, in the conjugate procedure the stimulus must have in itself reinforcing value to the child. Since auditory threshold determination is a discrimination task (presence or absence of signal), Wilson uses the operant discrimination paradigm in hearing testing.

An example of a conjugate reinforcement technique is high amplitude sucking (HAS) in infants originally developed by Siqueland and De Lucia (1969). This procedure relies on a natural newborn response and capitalizes on the reinforcing properties of the stimulus. The spontaneous behavior (sucking) is brought under stimulus control through the use of response-contingent stimulation. The auditory stimulus is then made contingent upon a criterion-level sucking response, and the auditory stimulus itself takes on reinforcing properties for the infant. Disadvantages to the high amplitude sucking response is the heavy physical demand placed on the infant, a baseline criterion level of 20–40 sucks per minute so that criterion level changes may be noted, and the fact that the general length of time required to complete studies is substantial. Eisele et al. (1975) generated threshold hearing data from 100 infants by observing the rate of sucking as a function of stimulus intensity.

Aslin et al. (1983) summarize four versions of the BOA head-turning technique that have been used to evaluate auditory abilities in infants. The first version is a simple auditory threshold procedure in which the infant's task is to respond to any just detectable sound emitted from a single loudspeaker. In a second version, the same task is involved for the infant except that two soundfield speakers are used. The infant is centered between the speakers and silence is interrupted by a signal presented from one of the two speakers. The first directional head-turn response is scored and correlated with the location of the sound source.

A third technique is somewhat more complex as it involves the addition of a background stimulus that is interrupted by the presentation of a different (or target) stimulus. This is then a discrimination procedure to evaluate an infant's ability to differentiate between two suprathreshold auditory stimuli. A "catch trial" is essential in this technique, which consists of informing the observer that a scoring interval is occurring, but not letting him know if the target stimulus was included in this tone interval. This is done as an attempt to eliminate experimenter bias. A fourth version of the head-turning technique involves the addition of a trial-to-criterion measure to the basic discrimination response procedure. These discrimination techniques have been used to evaluate speech perception in early infants by Kuhl (1979) and Kuhl and Miller (1982).

Tester-Observer Bias. Response bias by testers and observers is one of the most difficult errors to avoid in the clinical hearing evaluation of children. Several studies have confirmed that there is a tendency for judges to score responses when no auditory signals were presented (Moncur, 1968; Weber, 1969; Ling et al., 1970; Langford et al.,

1975). These studies have all dealt with the specific problem of observer bias involved with infant testing. Mencher et al. (1977) felt that the problem of observer bias was reduced if the infant was sleeping lightly and only "yes-no" judgments were made for arousal responses.

Recently, Gans and Flexer (1982) investigated observer bias in behavioral observation audiometry with profoundly involved multiple handicapped children. Their findings implicated clear observer bias in 85% of the children. At low test intensities, observers aware of the stimulus events tended to score fewer responses than those judges unaware of stimulus intensity. In cases of high sound intensities, judges tend to "see" more behavioral changes to sound than actually occur. Gans and Flexer were disappointed that, even when observers were told that they exhibited biased scoring responses, this information did not influence the observer's subsequent scoring tactics. The investigators concluded that the estimation of hearing thresholds during BOA with handicapped children should be made by observers who do not have access to the sequence of stimulus presentations.

Weber (1969) described an equipment design for behavioral observation audiometry to reduce tester bias. Using two persons to test the child, one observer is in the room with the child while the tester operates a tape recorder in the control room. The operator selects a randomized stimulus schedule with 20 stimulus presentations—10 of which are heard only by the child. The observer wears earphones and hears all 20 stimulus presentations but cannot tell which sounds are presented to the child under evaluation. The operator and observer each make judgments about the responses of the child which are compared to the stimulus presentation schedule following the test session.

Visual Reinforcement Audiometry

Liden and Kankkonen (1961) first coined the term "visual reinforcement audiometry" (VRA), based on a technique described by Suzuki and Ogiba (1961) and termed by them "conditioned orientation reflex" (COR) audiometry. This procedure as currently used employs lighted transparent toys which are flashed on simultaneously with the presentation of the auditory signal during a conditioning period. During the testing phase the light is flashed immediately following a response (looking toward the light). Liden and Kankkonen used interesting pictures on a slide projector to reinforce any response from the child, whether the responses were merely awareness, eye blink, orientation, or smiling. Matkin (1973) reported success using any of these responses as indicative of the child's hearing of the tone. Matkin also found that the technique is useful with earphones, and that VRA is successful with 90% of both normal-hearing and hearing-impaired children between the ages of 12 and 30 months. Furthermore, he stated that speech stimuli are as effective as the warble tones usually prescribed. The VRA technique can also be used to test the child's responses with hearing aids.

In sound field it is apparent that VRA audiometry will test only the better ear in some children, even when loudspeakers on each side of the child produce the signals and the lights for localization. Hodgson (1972) stated that the child with a severe hearing loss will not have learned to localize sound. He suggested that where there is confusion in localization, it is best to use only one loudspeaker in testing. In order to distract the child from looking constantly at the loudspeaker, an animated toy can be activated in another direction.

Fisher and Freedman (1968) simulated unilateral losses in normal children by plugging one ear, and found that they gave accurate sound localization. Thus, even with unilateral loss and one normal ear, such a child may locate the sound source. We feel that the localization skills depend upon the age of the child and upon the stimulus used. Warble tones are difficult for many infants under 12 months to localize consistently, whether the children are normal or hard-of-hearing. Matkin's suggestion for using speech as the stimulus would seem to be more productive of results for infants before 12 months of age.

Haug et al. (1967) described a procedure to overcome the problem of testing only the better ear. Their "Puppet in the Window Illuminated Test" (PIWI) was successful in obtaining thresholds in children under 3 years of age. With two loudspeakers, localization responses were reinforced by the appearance of a puppet behind a lighted window. After a conditioning period, earphones were placed on the child and the puppet again was illuminated every time the child responded to the tone by looking toward the window.

Moore et al. (1977) affirm the success of VRA in eliciting responses in infants as young as 5 months. A complex noise centered between 1000 and 4000 Hz and maintained at 70 dB was used by them as a stimulus. Each of 60 infants between 4 and 11 months of age were given this stimulus 40 times, reinforced by a toy animal that moved in place. A control trial was also given. The 2–5-month-old group and the 7–11-month-old group responded significantly more frequently to the signals that were reinforced visually than to the non-reinforced signals. The authors believe that this technique may eventually be effective in establishing reliable thresholds on many infants under 12 months of age. In other investigations by Moore et al. (1976), 6-month-old infants were shown to give 35-dB SPL thresholds for complex noise when a descending VRA technique was used.

In testing Down's syndrome infants with VRA, Wilson et al. (1982) found that they did not achieve a high success rate until 10 months BSID (Bayley Scales of Infant Development) equivalent age.

In a previous study, Moore et al. (1975) had determined that the rank order of signals according to their effectiveness in producing VRA localization responses in 12–18-month-old infants was: (1) an animated toy, (2) a flashing light, (3) social reinforcement, and (4) no reinforcement (Fig. 5.9).

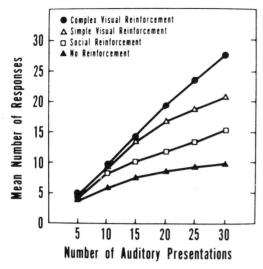

Figure 5.9. Response curves for operant conditioning audiometry. (Reprinted with permission from J. M. Moore et al.: *Journal of Speech and Hearing Disorders*, 42: 328, 1977.)

The signal used was a complex noise at 70 dB.

In the same laboratory Wilson et al. (1976) searched for auditory thresholds with their predetermined techniques. Ninety infants between 5 and 18 months of age were divided into groups of 15 according to age. Threshold level was first obtained using behavioral observations of responses to a complex noise signal. The VRA protocol was begun at that level, with a protocol of attenuating the signal 20 dB after each positive response and increasing it 10 dB after each failure to respond. Threshold was described as the lowest presentation level at which the infant responded at least 3 times out of 6. The results showed the VRA responses to be significantly better than the behavioral observation. Even for the 5-month-olds, the 10th and 90th percentile points were 20 and 40 dB SPL; for the 6–18-month-olds they were 20 and 30 dB SPL (Fig. 5.10A–C).

Eilers et al. (1977) utilized VRA techniques in a speech discrimination paradigm designed to show developmental changes of discrimination ability. They demonstrated that 1–3-month-old infants as well as older infants could discriminate certain easier phonemic contrasts such as sa-sa, sa-va. But other contrasts are more difficult for very young children than for older infants as they approach 14 months, e.g.: fi-θi, sa-za. Thus the use of VRA techniques is

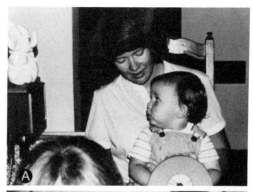

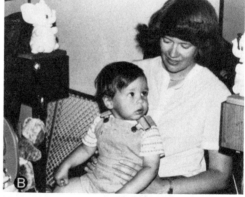

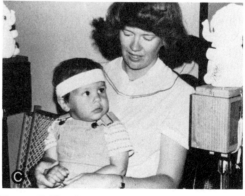

Figure 5.10. Visual reinforcement audiometry. Note head localization to either side when auditory stimulus is heard. Head turn is reinforced by flashing lighted toy. Bone-conduction testing can also be conducted with this technique following the Weber localization concept.

extended into the study of the development of auditory prelinguistic skills.

VRA, however, should be considered a routine part of any clinical assessment of infants over 5–6 months old. Even when VRA audiometry is to be used, we prefer first to make observations of behavioral responses on an ascending threshold as described previously. In this manner one takes out insurance against the possibility of failing to obtain consistent information with VRA techniques.

Tangible Reinforcement Operant Conditioning Audiometry (TROCA)

Lloyd et al. (1968) described a technique of systematic reinforcement audiometry for use with mentally retarded children. The technique has also found favor among clinicians for testing normal young children (Matkin, 1973). TROCA procedure uses positive reinforcement (candy, cereal, or a trinket) for appropriate responses and a mild punishment (time out) for false responses. The child's behavior is conditioned until he pushes a response button on a feeder box whenever he perceives a sound. Lloyd et al. employed continuous reinforcement in their initial study of the technique. Others have used a fixed ratio scheduling (Bricker and Bricker, 1969).

Another operant procedure was reported by Spradlin et al. (1969). Their project demonstrated the use of escape avoidance and conditioned suppression procedures in searching for threshold.

Using a Tester Assistant

Although many audiology clinical settings require that the audiologist work alone, the hearing testing of children is often enhanced by the use of an extra observer, or an assistant to the tester. This tester assistant remains in the test room with the child to help control the test paradigm, to monitor and direct the behavior of the child under evaluation, and communicate with the tester as necessary. Guide-lines are in order so that the tester assistant can be of maximum use in the audiological evaluation.

To be a successful team, the tester and the assistant must have clearly defined roles and areas of responsibility understood before the testing begins. One person is identified as the "tester" and typically is the person responsible for the task at hand. The other person is the "assistant" and follows the directives of the tester. Both are in continuous contact by earphones and the talkback circuit of the audiometer, or through the soundfield system, or even by closed-circuit video. The designated responsible person has the task of all major communication with the parents. It is very disruptive to the situation to have both the tester and the assistant talking to the parents at different times during the test session appointment.

The assistant is in charge of the test room in as much as possible, and maintains the behavior of the child and the parents. It may be appropriate for the assistant to briefly talk to the parents during the session to warn them of what is about to happen in the test sequence, or to guide their communication with the child, or to caution them about influencing the responses of the child unless specifically asked to do so. The team must often make an educated estimate about whether or not to include the parents in the soundroom during the test session based on a number of observations including the behavior of the parents, the relationship between the parents and the child, the number of accompanying relatives, friends, neighbors, and siblings.

Prior to the start of the test session, the soundroom environment needs to be well-organized. Toys must be kept out of sight until they are ready to be introduced to the child, one at a time, under control of the assistant. The test room should be as visually bland as possible to keep distraction at a minimum. Careful consideration must be given to the arrangement of chairs, tables, soundfield speakers, visual reinforcers, position of the parent(s), assistant, and child, all with thought so that the tester will also have an unobstructed view of the child under evaluation.

The parent's chair should be oriented so that the infant or child is at a 90° angle to the visual reinforcer. The infant must be held, or the child seated, in such a way that if they turn to "find" the parent for reassurance, that the head turn will be away from the reinforcer. The situation should be organized so that when the child seeks the reinforcer light and/or toy, a clear head-turn response will be required.

The test session should be started when the infant or child is showing a moderate amount of interest in a quiet toy used as a distractor. The timing of the test signal presentations, and the time interval between signal presentations is very important to the success of the test session. Generally, the initial test presentations are slow, and as the child's performance improves, trials can be generated with much shorter intertrial intervals. "Time-out" may be utilized following false responses from the child, allowing the youngster to "settle down" again. One of the most common errors made by inexperienced testers is to run through the test session too quickly too soon. Well-trained infants and children can perform quite well with rapid trial presentations, but the tester must be sure that the desired response relative to the stimulus presentations has been adequately shaped.

The assistant's task is to keep the child in a moderate state of alertness—not so absorbed in the toys that he/she will not be responsive to the auditory stimulus, yet not so uninterested that he/she will continuously visually search the room or fixate on the reinforcer. It is to be expected that there is tremendous variability among children's behavior in the test room environment. There is also wide variation in the child's attention level during the test session. The real challenge is for the assistant to precisely judge and anticipate the state of the child, and have an ability to manipulate and maintain the child's state at the desired level.

Obviously, the choice of toys is important. Toys vary in how much attention they demand from children. Sometimes a child will have no preconceived idea of what a specific toy is supposed to do, so the imagination of the assistant has much to do with how successful a toy can be during the test session. Beware of toys that generate noise and action toys that become too intriguing. Introduce only one toy at a time, and keep all other toys out of sight. Put finished toys also out of sight and out of reach. Toys in use should be kept directly in front of the child to eliminate false head turns. The manipulation of the toys by the assistant is very important to the timing and the eventual success of the hearing evaluation.

CENTRAL AUDITORY TESTING

The emerging area of testing children for central auditory problems due to either organic lesions of the central auditory pathways or auditory perceptual dysfunction, will be a major area of concern during the 1980s. A complete discussion of this topic is beyond the scope of this textbook, but as more professionals become concerned and better data are generated through research, the clinical value of central auditory testing will take its place as a necessary skill of each clinician. The interested reader is referred to a number of recent textbooks replete with copious references including Barr's *Auditory Perceptual Disorders* (1976), Katz' *Staggered Spondaic Word Test* (1982), *Central Auditory Dysfunction* (1977a), *Auditory Perceptual Problems in Children* (1980a) and *Central Auditory and Language Disorders in Children* (1981) by R. W. Keith.

A number of problems exist which continue to make the topic of central auditory testing somewhat "fuzzy." One of the major problems is the lack of data on the cause and effect relationship of auditory-perceptual deficits and language, reading, and learning disorders. The lack of standardized terminology and diagnostic techniques raises doubt about the validity of remediation for such "problems." Central auditory processing, testing, and treatment raises more questions now than we have answers. Another cause for concern is that no professional specialty seems interested in stepping forward to claim this area as their own—which may only imply the multidisciplinary nature of the problem.

On the other hand, educators agree that central auditory processing of various sorts exist in their students, and the classroom teacher eagerly awaits each new development with hope that answers wil be forthcoming. Keith (1982) hypothesizes that some basic auditory-perceptual skills exist in every child, e.g. appreciation of frequency, intensity, and duration of sounds, that serve as building blocks of audition leading to language development through imitation. As language skills are acquired, children also acquire other linguistically dependent auditory-perceptual skills such as memory, discrimination, closure, blending, etc. In addition, as the child's neuroanatomic pathways mature, the ability to cope with higher level auditory tasks such as dichotic listening, binaural release from masking, and other nonlinguistically based listening skills begin to improve.

Keith (1982, pg. 1018–1019) defines the most common central auditory abilities that test developers attempt to measure, and presents examples of these tests in Table 5.6.

Localization. The ability to locate auditorily the source of a sound. This ability requires binaural stimulation.

Binaural Synthesis. The ability to integrate centrally incomplete stimulus patterns presented simultaneously or alternately to opposite ears.

Figure Ground. The ability to identify a primary signal or message in the presence of competing sounds. Auditory figure-ground can be a monaural or a binaural task.

Binaural Separation. The ability to listen with one ear while ignoring stimulation of the opposite ear. Dichotic listening, as a binaural separation task, requires the listener to attend to and report back different signals presented simultaneously to two ears.

Memory. The ability to store and to recall auditory stimuli, including length or number of auditory stimuli, and sequential memory, or the ability to recall the exact order of auditory stimuli presented.

Blending. The ability to form words out of separately articulated phonemes.

Discrimination. The ability to determine whether two acoustic stimuli are the same or different. In speech, auditory discrimination is the ability to recognize fine differences that exist among phonemes.

Closure. The ability to perceive the whole (word or message) when parts are omitted.

Attention. The ability to persist in listening over a reasonable period of time.

Association. The ability to establish a correspondence between a nonlinguistic sound and its source.

Cognition. The ability to establish a correspondence between a linguistic sound and its meaning. Cognition is the highest level of auditory perception and results from a summation of all auditory (and all sensory) tasks.

NONORGANIC HEARING LOSS IN CHILDREN

The child who presents with a nonorganic, or functional, hearing loss is a quite different problem from the adult with a nonorganic loss. He is a much less sophisticated feigner of poor hearing than the adult, and his underlying motives, whatever the impelling factor, are sometimes more obscure. The needs which drive him to give an inaccurate hearing test are probably more honest, more unrecognized by him, and certainly engender more sympathy than in the adult.

Table 5.6.
Examples of Tests That Attempt to Measure Certain Auditory Abilities in Children[a]

Auditory Abilities	Test
Localization	Sound Field Localization
Binaural Synthesis	Rapid Alternating Speech Perception
	Binaural Fusion Test
Figure Ground	Goldman-Fristoe-Woodcock Test of Auditory Discrimination (GFW)
	Flowers-Costello Test of Central Auditory Abilities
	Kindergarten Auditory Screening Test (KAST)
	GFW Selective Attention Test
	Composite Auditory Perceptual Test (CAPT) Figure-Ground Test
	Kindergarten Figure Ground Tests
Binaural Separation	Willeford Competing Sentence Tests
	Dichotic CV Identification Test
	Staggered Spondaic Word Test
Memory	Illinois Test of Psycholinguistic Abilities (ITPA): Auditory Sequenctial Memory
	Wepman Auditory Memory Span Test and Auditory Sequenctial Memory Test
	GFW Auditory Memory Test
	Lyness Auditory Perception Test
Blending	ITPA Sound Blending Test
	KAST
	GFW Test of Sound Blending
	Rosewell-Phall Auditory Blending Test
Discrimination	KAST
	Wepman Auditory Discrimination Test
	GFW Auditory Discrimination Test
	Lyness Auditory Perception Test
Closure	Flowers-Costello Test of Central Auditory Abilities
	Filtered Speech Subtest: Willeford Battery
	Time Compressed Speech
	ITPA Test of Auditory Closure
Association	Competing Environmental Sound Test
Cognition	Wechsler Intelligence Scale for Children (WISC)
	Carrow Test of Auditory Comprehension of Language

[a] From R. W. Keith: Central auditory tests, in *Speech, Language and Hearing*, Vol. III. Philadelphia, W. B. Saunders, 1982, p. 1031.

The differences between the dynamics of simulated hearing loss in adults and those in children are striking. Under the age of 16 the secondary gains are never monetary, and the children are rarely consciously dishonest; i.e., the child is not often aware of the fundamental "wrongness" of his actions. He is impelled by such great needs that acting them out becomes a necessity to him.

Any child who presents with a functional hearing loss has a problem, whether it be a minor transient difficulty or a deep-seated permanent disorder. It is a symptom of something, just as a runny nose or a fever is a symptom of something. It should never be disregarded or passed off as a temporary foible. It may represent a cry for attention, an apology for poor performance, or a rebuff to a hostile world. The child is saying "Help me, please." He is a lucky child, because the symptom he has chosen is the only one out of a host of possible physical and personality symptoms that can be accurately measured and definitely identified as being nonorganic and emotionally based.

Children who have some basic need that is unfulfilled may choose from a variety of symptoms that are available to them, ranging from the conscious to the psychosomatic. They may complain of stomachaches, headaches, poor vision, poor hearing, or specific pains. They may act out their needs in aggressive behavior or in withdrawal. Their symptoms may enter the psychosomatic realm, with disorders like eczema or chronic stomach disorders. Even psychosis may be present. When their behavior becomes outwardly aggressive and approaches delinquency, their disturbance becomes a threat to their families and to society. If in this chain of symptoms just one symptom is found that can be measured and identified as being purely emotional in origin, the progression of the symptoms can be halted by proper management. Hearing loss is such a symptom. Although not always serious, the problem is the only one which can be recognized for what it is, and its specific treatment outlined.

The clinician can recognize a possible "nonorganic child" by the exaggerated behavior—exaggerated either in being too withdrawn, uncommunicative and lacking in affect, or in being overtalkative, brash, and manipulative. Both types are already acting out the individual personality dynamics that will be evidenced in the audiometric test. Most often they will understand what is said to them even if it is spoken low and out of their vision. The brash one will think to say "what?" occasionally, but will forget to do it when sufficiently interested. Even if these behaviors are not dramatically obvious, the clinician will intuitively feel some hostility in the child. Often the clinician is hard-put to control his own hostility, and may not understand why he feels it. One must keep reminding oneself that the child's behavior is not malicious and requires sympathy, not a reflection of the hostility.

The symptom of nonorganicity in children can often be said to be man-made, in that the opportunity for it has been created by the presence of audiometric screening programs. The large majority of children who present with such problems are referred because of failure on the screening test in school. Johnny sees that Joe, who has failed the hearing test, is given special treatment: he is excused from school to have further examinations, and he is given special seating and attention in school. It is like having headaches or stomachaches— it gives an excuse for poor performance and a chance to bid for sympathy. Thus there is added another symptom to the choices possible to an upset child, and this time it is a man-made choice.

It should be recognized that this discussion of nonorganic hearing loss does not include those children who did not understand the instructions given them during a previous test. It should be obvious when the child has responded only to the loudness level of the first tone he heard. However, this is also the strategy used by the child with true nonorganic hearing loss, so care should be taken to ensure the fact that the child has completely understood the directions.

Leshin (1960) reported a screening program which identified a number of cases of nonorganicity in children. He investigated the social dynamics of each case, and instituted a remedial program which would fulfill the children's needs that impelled them to a symptom such as hearing loss. Such a program can be highly recommended.

From the above discussion, we can list briefly the presenting symptoms, the recommended test procedure, and the management suggested for each personality type.

Presenting Symptoms

1. Exaggerated behavior: withdrawal and lack of affect, or verbosity and brashness.

2. Exaggerated straining to hear the sound.

3. Inconsistent intratest results: thresholds varying 15–20 dB with presentations at the same frequency.

4. Variable intertest results, depending on initial orienting tone level.

5. Speech reception thresholds normal or markedly better than pure tone responses.

6. Better thresholds, usually normal, given on retesting with slow ascending technique.

Recommended Test Procedure

It is extremely rare that any of the classic auditory tests for nonorganicity need to be used on children. Their naiveté in giving normal threshold responses to the ascending technique and to speech reception tests usually renders further testing unnecessary. Occasionally in the case of a monaural feigned loss, it is useful to give the Stenger test to verify the true threshold level.

Once the inconsistencies above have been noted, apply the following procedure:

1. Inform the child (in the sound room, not over earphones) that this time the test will be different. This time he will hear the tone coming from miles away, and it will be a tiny "beep-beep." He is to tell you as soon as he hears it from far away.

2. Start presenting the signal at—10 dB, and keep it pulsing for at least 30 sec. Look questioningly at the child as if you expect him to hear.

3. Repeat the same at—5 dB, and then at 0.

4. If the speech reception has been normal, make a special effort at 5 dB: while the tone is being pulsed, point first to one ear and then the other questioningly, to see if he will identify the ear where the tone is present. Usually he will respond in some way.

5. Repeat if necessary at 10 dB, but if the speech reception has been normal, stop at that level.

6. Proceed to another frequency and repeat the technique.

If the speech reception threshold has not been quite normal, the same steps as above can be taken with spoken spondees, again

"waiting him out," and looking quizzical when he fails to respond even at below threshold levels.

Observers of this technique have voiced their concern over the child's worrying briefly about whether he really can hear. Such critics can be assured that the gains accruing to the child from the information obtained will far outweigh any temporary discomfiture he may have.

General Management Recommendations

The continuum of the severity of emotional causes of nonorganicity runs a gamut from mild, transient problems to severe psychosis. Keep in mind that there will always be an overlapping between the ratings that are made.

Transient. If in the judgment of the audiologist and the managing physician the parents have sufficient insight to fill any needs represented by the nonorganic symptom, and if there appear to be no obvious psychologic problems, the treatment should be entrusted to the parents. A report should be sent to the school indicating the estimate of the transient nature of the problem.

Mild. If the parents report other evident behavioral problems and recognize a justifiable familial or environmental situation, referral can be made to the school psychologist, with the parents' full knowledge and acceptance. Report should be made to the managing physician.

Moderate. In the presence of other identifiable symptoms or deep-rooted familial problems, psychiatric counseling should be advised. If such referral is rejected, the parents should be told that a report will be sent to the referring school and the managing physician, as a routine procedure.

Severe. Given truly bizarre behavior and parental bewilderment over the cause, psychiatric counsel should be urgently advised, with the agreement of the managing physician.

The cry for help that is inherent in the

presentation of nonorganic hearing loss in a child should not be taken lightly by the audiologist. Listen to the sound of his need.

TESTING THE DIFFICULT-TO-TEST CHILD

The judgments the clinician makes on children's hearing abilities often necessarily involve a differential evaluation. In the presence of other disorders the child's behavior or his level of functioning may be so erratic that standard techniques of audiometry cannot be used. In order to apply appropriate tests for hearing, the clinician must be able to recognize the dysfunction that is present and to adjust the tests to it. The classical disorders that are to be differentiated are mental retardation, cerebral dysfunction, and autism (Myklebust, 1954). More than one of these may be present in one child. If the clinician has been trained in evaluating any of these disorders, he may also test the child's functioning in that specific area, as well as in the hearing area. But at the very least he has the responsibility of recognizing the disorder that exists. He must be able to apply the proper tests for hearing and to make referral for diagnosis and treatment of the other disorder.

In discussing the entities which must be recognized, it is necessary to reiterate an important fact—that neither cerebral dysfunction nor central auditory disorders nor mental retardation nor autism result, in themselves, in a decrease of auditory acuity as represented by the audiogram. The responses which can be elicited certainly require more ingenuity to obtain. But when credible responses reveal reduced hearing for pure tones and speech, a peripheral hearing loss is present, in addition to any central disorder that may exist (Goldstein et al., 1972; Kleffner, 1973). The clinical audiologist's task is to choose the appropriate test procedures that will reveal the presence or absence of peripheral hearing loss. It is not always a simple task to make this distinction.

To guide the clinician in fulfilling his charge, we will attempt to describe the salient features of the various disorders and to suggest appropriate tests that may be chosen.

Mental Retardation

One principle should be kept in mind when dealing with the mentally retarded child. If generalized developmental retardation is his only disorder, he will behave in all areas at the level of his mental age. This principle will hold up in all cases except those in which autistic behavior or cerebral dysfunction is superimposed upon the general retardation. Then the testing problem is further compounded, but is not insoluble. Of course, this group of difficult-to-test children are prime candidates for auditory brainstem evoked potential (ABR) measurement described in Chapter 6.

Age 0–5 Years. Infancy is an ideal time to test the retarded child's hearing. He has not yet developed the social behaviorisms, the self-stimulating activities, or the inattention patterns of the older retardate. In the first few months of life he sleeps a great deal, giving an opportunity for good observations of his responses in a sound room. Until 4 months the quality of his auditory responses cannot be distinguished from those of the normal child.

After 4 months we begin to identify the retardate through his auditory behavior as well as through the developmental landmarks present. If by 5 months he is not making even a partial head-turn toward the sounds, determine whether he can reach for and hold objects, and if he laughs aloud. He may not even be holding his head erect, or be able to follow a moving object—behavior which would place him below the 3-month level of functioning. In this case one can expect only the auditory responses that are listed for the child under 4 months old. If he then responds to all acoustic stimuli like a child under 3 months old, his hearing is judged to be normal.

The same observations of auditory behavior and developmental behavior should be made of the older child, referring to the developmental landmarks. If all behaviors are consistent for a certain age level, and the auditory indices are within the normal limits listed for that age level, the hearing level is judged to be normal. For example, if a 15-month-old child's behavioral landmarks are at the 8-month level, a speech awareness level of 15–20 dB and pure tone awareness of 45–55 dB are considered to be normal hearing.

If previous developmental scales or IQ test results are available, the clinician will have no difficulty in correcting the auditory test results for mental age. It is when the intellectual status is unknown that the clinician must apply his own observations of developmental landmarks. If these are not consistent at a certain age level, another disorder should be suspected. The 5-year-old who has normal motor coordination and good personal-social adjustment for his age, yet is unable to identify all of a group of familiar toys, should be evaluated further, providing that his hearing test is normal.

The behavioral responses previously described for infants (response to 45-dB speech level, and startle to 65-dB speech), however, have been shown to yield a high percentage of successes in severely mentally retarded children. Knight (1973) studied 100 mentally retarded institutionalized students from 2 to 35 years of age, and applied to them this technique and the related criteria, as suggested by the authors. The functioning levels of the students were classified predominantly as severe to profound retardation levels. Of these, 25 were designated as untestable for mental age.

Among the audiologic and otologic studies on the prevalence of hearing loss and ear disease in institutions for mental retardation, the percentages of loss range from about 10% to 45% or greater. Lloyd (1970) presented a review of the literature on the audiologic aspects of mental retardation in which a summary of the various reported incidences is given. Each percentage is affected by the chronologic and mental age of the population tested, by the testing procedures used, and by the criteria for failure which are applied.

The objection may be voiced that 45 dB is too high a screening level and that it may miss milder hearing loss. But if we estimate the intellectual functioning level of these severe retardates as equivalent to the first 4 months of infancy, then response to a 45-dB speech signal is the normal threshold level for this group. True, some with mild sensorineural loss and recruitment may respond at the 45-dB level but these would be very rare. We feel that at the present time the procedure of behavioral responses, acoustic impedance measurement, and if necessary, ABR testing, offers the most practical means of testing this group.

Dahle and McCollistar (1983) have reviewed all of the procedures for evaluating mentally retarded children, including an appropriate review of the physiological tests of hearing. They point out that normal ABR tracings in this group of children gives valuable information about their auditory peripheral sensitivity. However, when the ABR is abnormal, and a central nervous system abnormality is obvious, the ABR results are ambiguous (Worthington and Peters, 1980).

Age 5–16 Years. The very severely retarded in this age group can be tested as discussed above. A large number of these children, however, will have a level of functioning that permits behavioral conditioning or speech audiometry tests to be used. If their mental age is over 2 years, the tests described for children of that age can be applied. Play-conditioning techniques often are successful with the older retarded child when standard techniques fail.

A period of pretest observation will reveal what can be expected of the child. Present him with toys and see how familiar he is with them. Can he hand them to you on a command? If he recognizes most of the toys and can give them to you on command, he is probably able to give both a speech reception threshold and play-conditioned thresholds. If not, the routine observations of behavioral responses can be made.

When precise thresholds are desired in such a borderline functioning child, the techniques of visual reinforcement audiometry, impedance audiometry and ABR should be used in accordance with the Jerger-Hayes cross-check principal.

The Centrally Disordered Child

The suggested techniques for testing the brain-damaged child rest on two basic assumptions.

1. That any reduction in auditory acuity for pure tones, speech, or other signals is caused by lesions in the peripheral auditory system, not in the midbrain or higher pathways (see our discussion in Chapter 4 on "Disorders in Auditory Learning"). No real evidence has ever been presented that lesions central to the cochlear nuclei result in reduction in auditory sensitivity.

2. That only in the extremely severe centrally damaged child with gross motoric involvement will we see the complete absence of all of the four basic auditory reflexes: head turn, eye blink, startle response, and arousal from sleep.

The first rule in testing such a child is to determine his level of behavior. Pretesting will show what he can and cannot do. Sit and talk quietly and play with him in the sound room. Can he attend for any length of time to anything that you say or do? Can he give his name, age, or other appropriate information? Can he hand you toys or repeat words on request? In the case of a very young child, as well as an older one, is his eye contact steady and does it have integrity? Can he sit still for any length of time? Is he hyperactive and does he throw things around?

The child who has auditory perceptual dysfunction may be able to sit quietly and attend to visual stimuli but not be able to repeat words or to pick up objects on com-

mand. Such a child may, however, be perfectly able to do play-conditioned audiometry with pure tones and speech signals. Do not give up on formal testing unless it is proved to be ineffective.

If it is evident that formal testing techniques will not be successful, it is best to start at the lowest level of testing procedure, as has been described for the infant from 4 months on. The entire battery of observations should be made, from localization procedures to startle reactions. Remember that this child may be inconsistent in his responses to various stimuli, and at various times. A clear-cut response to one stimulus at 5–10 dB can be relied upon, even when responses to other stimuli cannot be seen at that level. The startle or the eye blink response will always confirm the observation of some reactions to soft levels.

It is rare for all of the auditory reflexes to be absent in a child. The reflexes are mediated at the level of the brainstem and are usually intact in the presence of higher cortical dysfunction. Auditory reflexes only tell us about the integrity of the peripheral auditory system through the brainstem. They tell us nothing about the higher orders of perception and integration.

Only in the presence of degeneration of the brainstem at the olivary complex can the absence of the head-turn and eye-blink reflexes be expected. Even then, the startle reflex, mediated at a low brainstem level, should be active, unless there is widespread motoric damage that prevents the muscular system from coordinating. Although the startle or eye-blink reflexes to a 65 dB (SL) signal do not eliminate the presence of a mild sensorineural loss, one may be sure that the loss is not of a degree that would produce the severe degree of symptoms found in a child whose only testable avenue is the reflex. Often the audiologist's task is to identify the primary disorder; a hearing loss may be only secondary to the major problem. The startle reflexes will enable him to do so. When reporting on such a case, the audiologist can say with confidence: "Hearing loss is not the primary problem in this child's communication dysfunction." Where the clinician is equipped to apply tests for central auditory dysfunction, he will be able to include the type and degree of the disorder.

The Autistic-Like Child

It is seldom that one sees the purely autistic-like child; but when one does, the bizarre behavior he displays can be recognized almost immediately: refusal to meet any person's eye gaze, disregard of all human speech stimuli, long-term fixation on some object, and refusal of physical contact with humans. He will consistently fail to attend to any speech stimulus, yet he will attend to some other acoustic signals. One such child will look for pure tone signals at low intensities, another will search for a cat "meow" at soft levels, and another will localize a white or a complex noise signal at normal levels. All will startle or eye blink to 65 dB voice in a structured sound room situation if hearing is normal. All the stimuli described for testing from birth on should be tried. Something is guaranteed to produce a response if the hearing is normal, even if it is only a startle reaction.

The real testing problem arises when autistic behavior is superimposed on central dysfunction. Indeed, one wonders whether all brain damage is not accompanied by some degree of autistic behavior. The symptoms are often so similar that they defy separation. In addition to the behavior described above, there may be the heightened activity and lashing out at humans. If such a child is difficult for the neurologist and psychiatrist to understand, so too is he for the audiologist.

The testing procedures described for mental retardation and for central nervous system disorders are applicable here. Keep in mind the fact that autistic symptoms are sometimes found in the deaf child, so do not let anything mislead you in the search for peripheral hearing loss. The audiologist's task in identifying the hearing level is unique, and no other discipline can lend guidance here. One must simply remember that the auditory reflexes cannot be suppressed even in an autistic child when the properly structured sound room condition prevails. If one is lucky, a stimulus may be found that will confirm perfectly normal hearing, aside from the reflexes. Acoustic impedance tests may provide valuable information.

Freedman and Kaplan (1967) list the four chief identifying features of autistic-like children.

1. They exhibit aloneness, and will occupy themselves for long periods of time without attention to anyone.

2. Some fail to use any language or communication; others may show precocious speech with scholarly words that have no real meaning to the child.

3. They show an obsessive desire for the maintenance of sameness. Fearing new patterns, they endlessly reiterate old patterns, almost as rituals.

4. They have a fascination for objects in place of interpersonal relationships, and will occupy themselves endlessly with a familiar object.

The autistic-like child is different from the mentally retarded or the brain-damaged child in that he usually has a high intellectual capacity, as indicated in IQ tests when they can be performed.

The Deaf-Blind Child

Except for the eye-ear syndromes described in the Appendix, most of the etiologies for deafness-combined-with-blindness fall at the present time into the maternal rubella category. These cases are most often confounded by central nervous system damage which makes it difficult to structure the testing situation properly.

In severe cases of multiple involvements, we have found it most expedient to rely again on the auditory reflexes, on orientation responses, and on quieting responses. In the absence of speech and language, one must apply the tests as for the infant proceeding to the upper limits of the auditory abilities present.

An excellent report on the neurological handicaps, degree of hearing and visual disability, as well as level of language and developmental characteristics of a young deaf-blind population was published by Stein et al. (1982). These authors reviewed data from 141 deaf-blind children evaluated at their clinic between 1972 and 1979. Although many of their patients were victims of the rubella epidemic of 1964–1965, now between 14 and 16 years of age, a large proportion of the deaf-blind children in their study were less than 14 years of age, suggesting that the major causes of deaf-blindness have not been eradicated.

Of the 141 "deaf-blind" children seen for diagnostic evaluation, 38 were found to have normal or near-normal hearing and, therefore, were technically not "deaf." The diagnosis of normal hearing in most of these difficult-to-test children was accomplished only through the use of the ABR technique (Stein et al., 1981). The previous diagnosis of deafness given these children was based largely on behavioral testing— and these children simply failed to respond behaviorally to sound. This finding is not uncommon in groups of "deaf-blind" children.

Stein and his co-authors summarize the findings in their study as follows:

1. A high incidence of neurological handicapping conditions are associated with congenitally deaf-blind children, including neuromuscular disorders.

2. Severe hearing disability was more common than severe vision disability in their sample of deaf-blind children. Sixty-eight percent of the children had so little usable hearing that the potential benefit of wearable amplification is minimal at best.

3. Many of the "deaf-blind" children referred for evaluation proved to have normal peripheral hearing without normal behavioral responses to sound. The use of the ABR as part of the audiological evaluation is thus an absolute necessity with these children.

4. The combination of hearing and visual problems together with neurological handicapping conditions has a profound effect on the language level, cognitive skills and general development of these children.

5. The severe hearing loss and neurologic problems will require that most, if not all, these children will require supervised care for the rest of their lives.

It is the audiologist's responsibility to make the decision about the blind child's hearing abilities. It must, perforce, be a bold decision, for any equivocation is not useful to the child. The conservative hearing aid trial with careful observations by all concerned during a diagnostic therapy period will not hurt the child. Hesitance may deprive him of critical time for learning auditory skills and thus do him a disservice.

MANAGEMENT OF THE CHILD WITH UNILATERAL DEAFNESS

Unilateral deafness has always been common among children, and its prevalence does not appear to be lessening. Chiefly due to mumps, it develops with a suddenness that often baffles both the child and his parents. Audiologists and otolaryngologists are not usually concerned over such deafness, other than to identify its etiology and assure the parents that there will be no handicap. Seldom is he able to express his bewilderment, yet the occurrence is more traumatic to him than adults can appreciate. He is infinitely relieved if someone takes the time to explain to him what has happened, how it will affect him, and what he can do to compensate for it. In addition, the vestibular mechanism can occasionally be affected by mumps, as well as the cochlea being involved, and this poses another problem that needs to be understood.

Until recently children with unilateral deafness have not been considered educationally handicapped. Studies by Bess (1982) and his associates at Vanderbilt University, however, have brought renewed attention to the child with only one normal hearing ear. They identified 60 children with unilateral hearing loss who were enrolled in the Nashville Metropolitan School System and closely examined their educational records. They found that approximately one third of this group had *failed* at least one grade during their school years, and nearly 50% of the group needed special resource assistance in the schools! In a series of research studies conducted by Bess, with 25 of the unilaterally hearing-impaired children matched with 25 normal-hearing children, the children with unilateral hearing loss performed much poorer on localization tasks and syllable recognition tasks. Based on his studies Bess concluded that children with unilateral hearing loss experience considerably more difficulty in communication and in education than was previously supposed. Perhaps there is a significant need for us to reexamine our basic assumptions underlying the identification and management of this unique population of hearing-impaired children?

The following points should be made in interpreting the problem to the child.

1. Assure him that he will be able to go through school and learn just like any other child.

2. Explain what has to be done to compensate for the monaural loss: special school seating, using the eyes to find the sound source, and placing oneself with the good ear toward the speaker.

3. If there is vestibular involvement, ask the doctor if some things like scuba diving or scaffold climbing should be done.

4. Give hearing conservation rules to protect the good ear: (a) stay away from loud noises; (b) get prompt medical care for any ear infection; (c) avoid putting anything into the ear; (d) avoid oxotoxic drugs unless absolutely necessary; (e) take special care of general health, especially during flu seasons; (f) have an otologic and audiologic check once a year; and (g) do not get advice on treatment from anyone but qualified otolaryngologists and audiologists.

5. Inform the patient that a CROS hearing aid is available if he ever is in a position where it may be needed.

PARENT MANAGEMENT

Often it is the audiologist who must inform the parents that they have a deaf or hard-of-hearing child. It is always best to have the parents observe the child's responses in a free-field situation so that they can see for themselves that the child does not hear normally, and what he can and cannot hear. It will be an extremely traumatic situation for them. Whether they show grief openly or contain it within themselves, you may be sure that they will be deeply disturbed over the knowledge. The audiologist must find ways to help them over this initial shock.

Stein and Jabaley (1981) have published an excellent chapter on parent counseling in their textbook, *Deafness and Mental Health*, in which they describe their conclusions based on 15 years of talking with parents of hearing-impaired children. They state that the two most common factors in the environment of deaf children that can account for their emotional or behavioral differences are (1) the lag in language development and its effect on family communication and socialization, and (2) the psychological response of parents to the diagnosis of hearing handicap in their child. Stein and Jabaley describe three stages of parental responses as initial expression of anger toward the professionals who diagnose the deafness in their child, followed by expressions of anger toward the child as they find it increasingly difficult to deny the existence of the hearing loss, and finally the third-stage response centers on the acceptance of hearing-impaired children by their parents which marks the transition from sadness and anger to the development of adaptation and coping behaviors. They urge the development of a working relationship with the involved parents to reduce the high prevalence of emotional and behavioral problems, while helping to establish the important parent-infant bond.

It is the usual tendency of parents to want to find out immediately everything that concerns the future of the child and his functioning. One must resist the temptation to go into great detail about the prognosis for the child's development. Whatever is said will be only half-absorbed and largely distorted on the first visit. One should limit the amount of information to the relative degree of loss that seems to be present—mild, moderate, severe, or profound—and concentrate on the implications of the loss and what is going to be done for the child. If the parents press the question as to whether the child will speak, what kind of school he will go to, or whether he will ever communicate, assure them that you will be able to answer these questions, but only after a period of diagnostic therapy. No one can ever guarantee what a child will be able to do with training; only the results will demonstrate that.

There is perhaps no way to cushion the shock of finding out that a child is hearing impaired. Any attempt to minimize the problem would be a disservice and would avoid the reality of the situation. But a sympathetic attitude and an understanding of the parent's feelings will help as much as possible; "You probably feel pretty upset about this news," or "It's perfectly natural for you to feel badly about this." Let them air their questions and fears. Allot sufficient time for them to express their feelings. Offer to be available for any questions that they might have and let them feel that you will work with them closely on finding out what their child can do with his loss. Emphasize that he is a child first, and has a hearing loss only secondarily. He is just as lovable as any other child.

Wherever possible, parents' groups under qualified psychologic counselors should be organized, in order to provide on-going guidance. If further help seems indicated, psychiatric or psychologic counsel should be sought for the individual parents. The audiologist should be aware of his limitations in providing psychotherapy for parents who cannot handle their problems.

In his relationship with the parents, the audiologist's responsibility includes the following points.

1. A complete explanation of what the audiogram means, and what the child can and cannot hear.

2. A description of the type of loss, whether conductive or sensorineural, and what it means in terms of whether medical treatment may or may not be possible.

3. A thorough explanation of the educational programs that are available for the child: auditory, oral, or total. The parents should be directed to visit each program so that they may participate in the decision as to which program will be chosen. With proper guidance, they should be able to make this decision themselves.

4. Psychologic support. This may take the form of a one-to-one relationship, or the parents may require group programs or even individual psychiatric counseling. The audiologist should remember that in this difficult role he can and should seek counseling for himself and for the parents if he feels unable to cope adequately with the situation.

All students of audiology, as well as practicing clinicians, should read the excellent book written by David Luterman, Ph.D., *Counseling Parents of Hearing-Impaired Children* (1979).

THE AUDIOLOGIST'S UNDERSTANDING OF HIMSELF

In the audiologist's zeal to help the hearing-handicapped child and his parents, he often overlooks his own motivations and how they will affect his relations with the parents. These relations may be critical to the parents' acceptance of the problem. Quite without meaning to, he may leave the parents with fears and with pent-up emotions that can adversely affect the habilitation process. At some point the audiologist must look at himself introspectively to see that his own feelings are in relation to the way he gives information to the parents, and how he handles them. If he has gone into the audiologic profession with an emotional zeal for "do-gooding," he may see himself as the authoritarian figure who directs the lives of people. He will not permit the parents to express themselves because he is in charge of operations. If he has gone into the field through an objective interest in the scientific manifestations of hearing, he may shrink from becoming emotionally involved and committed to the parents' problems.

So the audiologist too may have problems in feeling comfortable in his role as protagonist in the drama of the parent-clinician interplay. This subject deserves extensive coverage because it is vital to the ultimate emotional health of the child. A most meaningful exposition of the subject has been written by two experts in parent management, Dr. Brian Hersch, a psychiatrist, and Carol Amon, an instructor of deaf children. We are indebted to them for permission to use their analysis of the dynamics of the parent-clinician relationship (Hersch and Amon, 1973), presented below.

To parents who are anxious to hear that their idealized child is perfect, the statement that "Your child has a hearing impairment" may be painful words. Those words can cause many emotions ... shock, bewilderment, depression, anger, guilt, or anxiety. If these emotions are outwardly expressed by the parents, the audiologist, too, will experience feelings which may also be painful.

In order to avoid this uncomfortable experience, many audiologists today choose a painless method of reporting the diagnosis—a way that, although it is painless for themselves, may have devastating effects on the parents and their child. After listening to many parents relate their experiences and frustrations, we began to realize that the act of reporting the diagnosis was not only of paramount importance, but also that it was the beginning of a process that would include the habilitation and education of the child as well as the crucial involvement of the parents. This process could be enhanced or interfered with, by the interpersonal relations of the initial contact.

An approach toward lessening the trauma of the initial contact is proposed. It is an outgrowth of an idea that an interdisciplinary approach to understanding hearing-impaired infants and their families (the disciplines being audiology, deaf education, and psychiatry) is far superior to an isolated fragmented approach of one profession (Schlesinger and Meadow, 1972).

Schlesinger and Meadow describe three ineffective professional stances which are often seen today in the reporting of the diagnosis:

1. *The "hit-and-run" approach.* The diagnosis is reported very quickly and matter-of-factly in passing. "Your child didn't respond too much today ... his hearing loss is probably severe to profound. I'll see you in 6 months for another evaluation." The parents are left with their feelings of bewilderment as to what to do next. The reporting of the diagnosis appears to be a dead end with no source of help.

2. *Minimizing the problem.* The clinician infers that there is really nothing to worry about. "In this day and age, deaf children can be given hearing aids and go to regular school just like any other child." These words give false hope to the parents, but the audiologist says them in order to make the parents feel better.

3. *The objectivity approach.* Many audiologists are hidden behind objectivity, using the "big word" technique. In 1 hour's time, they report the diagnosis, explain the audiogram and the hearing mechanism, and how their child differs from normal, describe methods of habilitation, demonstrate the use and maintenance of a hearing aid, and schedule the child for the first habilitation session. The audiologist does most of the talking, often using professional jargon which leaves parents confused and feeling lost. The audiologist avoids listening.

4. *The action-oriented approach.* This fourth approach is also a popular one. The audiologist states the problem, and almost before he completes the reporting of the diagnosis he tells the parents what they are going to do to take care of the problem. The action part is essential, but only if there is adequate provision for exploring the feelings of the parents.

Such approaches by the audiologist greatly interfere with the process of acceptance of the handicap. A lack of acceptance prohibits the parents from helping their child grow both emotionally and educationally. The parents may deny the information and shop around for a professional who will tell them that their child is normal. Beck (1959) and Meadow (1968a) have pointed out that parents are more likely to listen and to integrate painful and unpleasant information from interested and "feeling" individuals.

The ineffective approaches used by the audiologist stem from a number of complex variables. First, he may lack knowledge and understanding of the habilitative process, and of the effect of his initial report. Second, he may be uncomfortable with the range of emotions that these parents may feel. Often audiologists state that they simply do not have the time to devote to reporting. This reasoning, however, may actually be a way of avoiding a more significant factor ... that is, the audiologist has not yet worked out in his own mind what it means to him to tell someone some painful news. It is natural for people to avoid pain. The audiologist and the parents in a way become secretly and jointly involved in an agreement to avoid dealing with feelings.

There is no painless way to inform parents that they have a child with a hearing loss. However, pain does not have to be regarded negatively. It is part of a process that facilitates and encourages a family's involvement. Even though there is no way of softening the blow, there is a way to help parents accept the realities of the situation and to make use of the resources available to them. The goals of this important first discussion of the diagnosis are multifold.

1. *Statement of the facts.* Initially, it is important to state the facts as clearly and as emphatically as possible. These parents want up-to-date and accurate scientific information about their child's problem presented to them authoritatively, but in language they can understand. If an alliance is going to be created with these parents, it is most important that the audiologist admit any lack of information or knowledge about the problem that he has, doing so confidently and without strain. Throughout the giving of this information, the audiologist must convey a true interest in this family. The tone of voice and non-verbal behavior of an audiologist can convey callousness, or it can convey concern. It is essential to convey concern rather than the idea that you are just doing your job.

2. *Support through listening.* Perhaps the most important goal is to provide support through listening. By listening patiently and nonjudgmentally, you may be able to bring some of the parents' feelings out into the open—feelings of which they may not have been aware. Many parents have indicated during the initial conference that they had been anxious about their child for a long period of time, but had never shared that anxiety with anyone, not even the spouse. This may be the first opportunity they have had to express what they have been feeling for months.

In order that these feelings be expressed by both parents together, they should both be present to discuss the diagnosis unless it is physically impossible. During this discussion, we can begin to assess the parents' interactions and begin to decide whether they have the kind of relationship that will provide support to one another or whether they will require some help from outside. It is important that the audiologist note and report his initial impression of the parents, as these notes may be valuable to others involved with the family.

3. *Giving the parents a role.* Another important goal of this first contact is to convey to the parents that they have a great deal to offer, even though they may have little formal knowledge about hearing loss and child development. Focusing on the parents' interaction with their child during that initial contact can give them some confidence. "You seem to sense Joey's needs very well." "That's beautiful, you called Joey's attention to that sound." "That's one of the most important ideas you will learn and you already appear comfortable with it." You can provide initial reinforcement of attributes that the parents are already equipped with, that will help their child's development.

During the initial discussion, the parents need to be made aware of the resources available to them—not only resources for habilitation and educational programming, but also resources available to help with emotional needs. Ideally, the audiologist will remain in contact with the family periodically, in order not only to give repeated evaluations, but also to act as a coordinator of professionals working with this family. It is vital that there be an interface between the person delivering emotional supportive services and those people primarily responsible for the habilitation program. This interaction will provide an opportunity to share and be aware of mutual concerns and will prevent the traditional approach of professionals working in isolation of each other.

In order for these goals to be realized, four criteria need to be present: First, the clinical audiologist must have some knowledge of the rehabilitative process; second, he must be comfortable dealing with feelings; third, adequate time must be provided for the reporting; and fourth, an atmosphere of mutual respect must be created.

For many years the clinical audiologist has accumulated experience in diagnosing and fitting hearing aids, but has known little about the habilitation process. There is a trend today to provide audiologists with more information about habilitation, a trend which we see as positive. Perhaps as audiologists become more familiar with rehabilitative methods, they can objectively direct parents toward programs suited to their child's needs and alleviate the emotional controversy of the deaf.

Many audiologists are sensitive and concerned about their role in helping these families, but this does not necessarily mean they they feel comfortable in dealing with feelings. Sensitivity in raw form can potentially be a valuable tool and an asset for the audiologist, but just because the potential is there does not mean that it will automatically be used in a facilitative way. To learn how to use one's sensitivity effectively is a delicate process and cannot be taught. This exemplifies the necessity for an interdisciplinary approach where the audiologist who is uncomfortable in this area may take advantage of the mental health professions that deal with feelings routinely.

A seemingly minute detail in the criteria for effective reporting of the diagnosis is the allotment of time; however, this is probably an essential factor in reporting. One of the most consistent complaints of parents in their dealings with audiologists initially is that the situation was regarded lightly and not enough time was devoted to this important problem. It is our feeling that the audiologist must allocate a minimum of 45 min to this initial reporting. Should this not be possible, or should both parents not be available during this initial session, it is critical than an appointment be scheduled within the next 24 hours to discuss the problem thoroughly. As was indicated earlier, parents may experience a number of feelings at the outset, the most frequent being shock. Then may come anger, guilt, or depression. It is very important not to tell parents what they may feel because people experience different emotions. It is important to provide an open-ended approach, however, such as, "Today I have told you about your son's hearing loss. Over the weeks and months to follow, you may or may not experience some uncomfortable feelings as many parents naturally do. We will be available to you to discuss whatever feelings you may be having. Let's plan to talk again in a month or anytime before that, should you desire."

The approach to effective reporting of the diagnosis is not only dependent upon the audiologist's knowledge, his comfortable feelings and the allotment of adequate time but also upon the atmosphere created. It is the universal observation of those who have constructed programs for special groups of young disabled children that unless the parents' emotional needs are adequately dealt with, the programs themselves have limited benefit for the children (Mindel and Vernon, 1971). Thus, it is critically important that an atmosphere of mutual respect and honesty be created—an atmosphere which allows the expression of feelings in nonjudgmental and accepting ways.

Often the atmosphere of mutual respect is interrupted when the parents' depression explodes into external anger which sometimes is directed at the audiologist. If the audiologist does not understand that this expression of anger is only an indication of the parent's internal struggles, he may become defensive. The parents will be aware of his defensiveness even if it is only conveyed nonverbally, and thus the climate of mutual respect is destroyed.

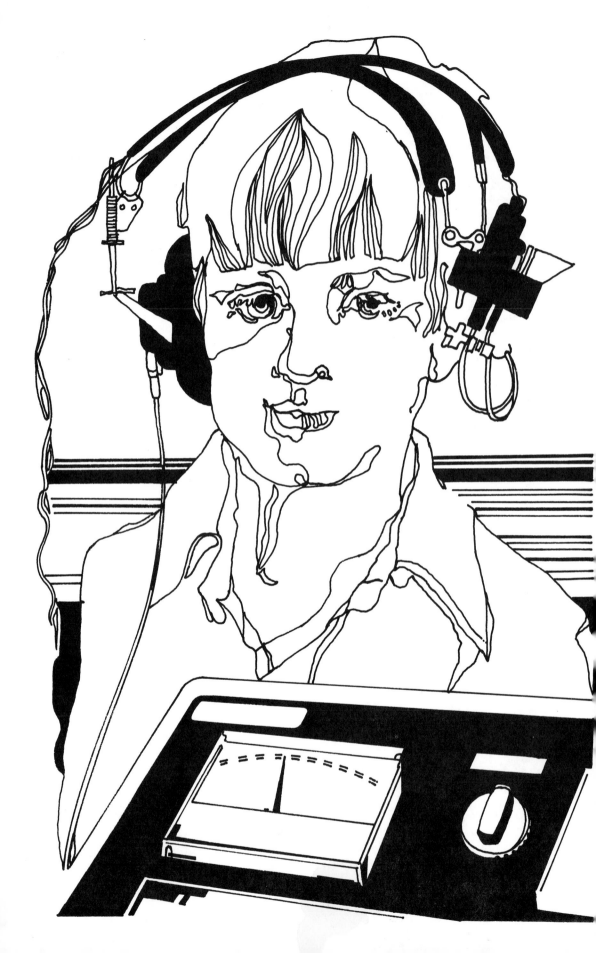

CHAPTER 6

Physiological Hearing Tests

Nothing can be more frustrating to an audiologist than to work with a 2-year-old child who needs to have his hearing evaluated, but who refuses to cooperate with any of the testing procedures. It seems impossible that a youngster who sat quietly and politely in the patient waiting area can suddenly turn into a crying, yelling, totally uncooperative subject as soon as he enters the sound-treated booth. And what causes a child, who has been happily playing while waiting for his hearing test, to suddenly become an overly self-conscious, introverted, and unworkably shy patient? How does a clinician establish rapport with a youngster who is hidden in his mother's skirt or wrapped around his father's leg? Every clinician ultimately faces the child whom he just cannot test. There are, indeed, means of handling such children, but the skills necessary to evaluate the hearing in uncooperative children are gained only through experience and insight.

One may expect the behavior of "normal" children to occasionally be obstinate. What about testing the hearing of a hyperactive, mentally retarded child? How does one elicit cooperation and establish play-conditioning techniques with an autistic or mentally disturbed youngster? Can you fit earphones on a child with hydrocephaly? Play-conditioning techniques are obviously not possible with a patient who will not even sit down! Just when the audiologist thinks that he has seen every conceivable situation, a child will show up who once again baffles every attempt to evaluate his hearing. Audiologists continue to seek a simple and accurate objective hearing test that can be used with any uncooperative child much like the early Spanish explorers continued to hunt for the Fountain of Youth! Almost no other aspect of audiology stimulates interest in the same manner as a new report describing a promising objective hearing test to solve problems associated with testing the hearing in difficult-to-deal-with children.

To deal with these difficult-to-test patients, the field of audiology has worked long and hard in the development of "objective" tests of hearing. An objective hearing test is one which defines a patient's hearing ability without the patient's active participation or cooperation. In the case of children, many factors may influence his ability to cooperate. He may not have the mental or physical capabilities to fully cooperate or to attend the hearing test task set before him by the clinician. The child's interest span may be too short. A clinician's skill in evaluating the hearing of these children often depends on his ability to establish rapport with the youngster and, at the same time, make an accurate evaluation of the child's capabilities in performing some task. A false start with these children may alienate them toward the testing situation, making additional test sessions necessary, and possibly more difficult.

Many "objective" hearing tests, usually related to an autonomic physiologic response, have been suggested and reported. Waldon (1973) proposed the term "audioreflexometry" as the method of measurement of hearing levels through the observation of involuntary responses resulting from presentation of acoustic stimuli. The Ewings of England in the early 1940s (Ewing and Ewing, 1944) observed eye blinks, squinting, involuntary jumping, and sound localization with body or head movements while testing young children. Froeschels and Beebe (1946) evaluated the cochleopalpebral reflex (also known as the auropalpebral reflex)—defined as the involuntary closing of eyelids due to acoustic stimulation—in children and infants.

Unfortunately, new objective hearing tests are formulated with older children or cooperating adults, and these results are then generalized to young children. Another common means for new objective procedures is initiated with nonorganic hearing loss adults. Somehow, the generalization that such procedures which work well with adults, therefore should apply also to children, comes to a sudden lack of credibility when the clinician comes face to face with a screaming, wall-climbing, mentally retarded, 2-year-old patient!

Nonetheless, with the advent of each new "objective" hearing test, the inevitable flurry of excitement passes among audiologists, pediatricians, and otolaryngologists. We should pause to reflect that the presence of some physiologic response, seemingly related to the presence of an auditory signal, does not ensure that the child does indeed "hear." Hearing, in this sense, implies meaningful interpretation of the sound so as to produce thought and language with verbal or nonverbal encoding and decoding. The toughest test for a new clinical procedure is to withstand clinician criticism by proving itself to be reliable, quick, easy to administer, inexpensive, and worthwhile over a long period of time.

IMMITTANCE AUDIOMETRY

The clinical application of acoustic impedance measurements has come to be known as immittance audiometry. The terms "impedance" and "immittance" are used interchangeably. The testing techniques are especially well-suited for children since they are objective, accurate, quick, easy to administer, and create little discomfort to the patient. Often children who will not cooperate with conventional audiometric techniques will not object to the immittance test battery. Immittance audiometry results are of special benefit to the physician who is unable to perform adequate otoscopic examination on a youngster, as well as to the audiologist who has difficulty in establishing valid hearing thresholds on an uncooperative child.

Vast numbers of children have been tested with the immittance technique and a wide variety of normative immittance test values are available. Studies by Brooks (1968, 1971), Jerger (1970), and Robertson et al. (1968) have validated the tremendous benefits of immittance audiometry in children.

Northern (1978c, 1980c) published comprehensive reviews of the use of impedance audiometry in special populations including profoundly deaf children, the retarded, deaf-blind, cleft lip and palate, children with Down's syndrome, and children with craniofacial disorders.

The clinical impedance technique in the evaluation of the auditory mechanism was originally proposed by Metz in 1946 and has been used routinely in Scandinavia since that time. North Americans, however, were slow to accept the clinical utility of this testing procedure until Alberti and Kristensen (1970) and Jerger (1970) independently published articles exhalting impedance audiometry as a valuable routine procedure for assessing the nature of hearing loss in patients. Jerger succinctly stated the significance of impedance audiometry by commenting, "We frankly wonder how we ever got along without it." Immittance audiometry is now included as routine testing technique in many otologic and audiologic clinics, and we have found it to be particularly useful in the evaluation of hearing in children.

By definition, immittance audiometry is an objective means of assessing the integrity and function of the peripheral auditory mechanism. The electroacoustic immittance meter may help determine existing middle ear pressure, tympanic membrane mobility, eustachian tube function, continuity and mobility of the middle ear ossicles, acoustic reflex thresholds, and nonorganic hearing loss. The electroacoustic immittance meter is equally practical for private office work and institutional clinics.

The electroacoustic impedance technique is based on the principle that sound pressure level (SPL) is a function of closed cavity volume. A diagram of the impedance meter is shown in Figure 6.1. An air-tight seal is obtained with a small probe which is inserted into the external auditory canal of the patient. The probe has three small holes. From one hole a 220-Hz probe tone is emitted; a second hole is an outlet for an air pressure system which is capable of creating positive, negative, or atmospheric air pressure in the cavity between the probe tip and the tympanic membrane; the third hole leads to a pick-up microphone which measures the sound pressure level of the 220-Hz probe tone in the canal cavity.

The SPL of the 220-Hz tone in the ex-ternal auditory canal cavity is determined by the compliance of the tympanic membrane and integrity of the middle ear system. The pick-up microphone quantifies the SPL of acoustic energy that is reflected back into the external auditory canal. A high amount of reflected energy is measured when the middle ear system is stiff or heavy as in such pathologic conditions as ossicular fixation, otitis media, or cholesteatoma. In contrast, discontinuity of the middle ear system creates a flaccid tympanic membrane which absorbs most of the probe tone sound energy and reflects very little sound back into the external auditory meatus (Northern, 1971a; Northern and Grimes, 1978).

The immittance test battery includes tympanometry, static compliance, the ear canal physical volume test (PVT), and acoustic reflex threshold measurement. Although each of the test procedures can provide significant information, their diagnos-

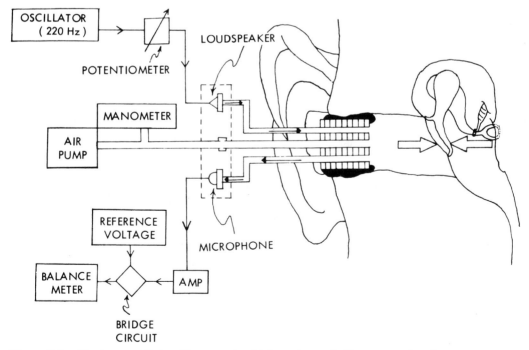

Figure 6.1. Electroacoustic immittance meter. Note probe sealed into external auditory meatus with three holes for (a) 220-Hz probe tone from oscillator; (b) air pressure system from air pump and manometer; and (c) pick-up microphone to compare sound pressure level in the cavity between the eardrum and probe tip with the reference voltage of impedance bridge. (Reprinted with permission from J. Jerger: *Archives of Otolaryngology 92:* 311–324, 1970.)

tic capabilities are strengthened when results from all three procedures are considered together (Table 6.1). The entire battery of three tests can easily be administered by an experienced person in 60–90 sec per ear.

Clinicians using immittance measurements must learn to follow three general rules: (1) recognize overall patterns in the tests of the impedance audiometry battery, (2) pay little attention to the absolute value of any of the immittance test battery results, and (3) beware of the implicit diagnostic conclusions based only on the immittance test battery (Northern, 1980b).

Tympanometry

Tympanometry is an objective technique for measuring the compliance, or mobility, of the tympanic membrane as a function of mechanically varied air pressures in the external auditory canal. The general term, tympanometry, refers to methods and techniques for measuring, recording, and evaluating changes in acoustic impedance (or resistance of the auditory mechanism) with systematic changes in air pressure. The compliance of the tympanic membrane at specific air pressures is plotted on a graph known as a tympanogram.

Table 6.1.
Summary of Immittance Audiometry Applications in Children

Tympanometry
   Objective measurement of tympanic membrane mobility
   Measures middle ear pressure
   Identifies perforations of tympanic membrane
   Confirms patency of ventilation tubes in tympanic membrane
   Estimates static compliance
Static Compliance
   Differentiates middle ear fixation from disarticulation
Acoustic Reflex Threshold
   Objective measure of cochlear pathology
   Validates nonorganic hearing loss
   Validates conductive hearing loss
   Differential diagnosis of conductive hearing loss
   Objective inference of hearing sensitivity

Tympanic membrane mobility is of particular interest since almost any pathology located on or medial to the eardrum will influence its movement.

Children with middle ear effusions are typically identified by physicians through an otoscopic examination. Physicians vary in their ability to visually examine the tympanic membrane (Stool and Anticaglia, 1973). Otologists teach that pneumatic otoscopy is an absolute necessity to identify the presence of middle ear effusion, yet only 25% of physicians use the pneumatic otoscope (Howie and Ploussard, 1974). In a study of the accuracy of otoscopic diagnosis, 15–20% of ears in children under 3 years of age with effusions were missed clinically (Paradise, 1976a).

Tympanometry, however, is more objective than the otolaryngologist's eye, and the air pressures involved with the technique are very small compared with the air pressures created with a pneumatic otoscope. Often, eardrums noted to have normal mobility by pneumatic otoscopy examination can be shown to have abnormal mobility with tympanometry.

The compliance of the tympanic membrane is at its maximum when air pressures on both sides of the eardrum are equal. That is, the eardrum achieves its best mobility when the air pressure in the external auditory canal is exactly the same as the existing air pressure in the middle ear (Fig. 6.2). The electroacoustic impedance meter permits the compliance of the eardrum to be evaluated under systematic variance of air pressure which is controlled by the clinician. Thus, when the clinician finds the air pressure value where the eardrum reaches its maximal compliance, he can then infer that the middle ear pressure is the same as the ear canal air pressure. The air pressure at the point of maximal compliance is also the middle ear air pressure. This fact has been shown experimentally by Eliachar and Northern (1974) and Eliachar et al. (1974).

The knowledge of middle ear pressure is important clinical information. When the

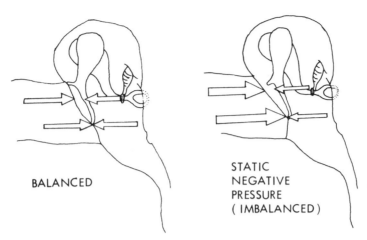

BALANCED

STATIC
NEGATIVE
PRESSURE
(IMBALANCED)

Figure 6.2. Compliance of the tympanic membrane is at its maximum when air pressure is equal on both sides of tympanic membrane as shown on the left. When air pressure on either side of the eardrum is unequal, as shown on the right, the tympanic membrane does not move well and a conductive-type hearing loss can often be noted.

process of aeration in the middle ear is halted, as in closure of the eustachian tube, the now static air in the middle ear space is absorbed by the blood vessels in the mucosal lining. This situation produces negative air pressure in the middle ear space causing transudation of fluid and retraction of the tympanic membrane (Magnuson, 1981). If the aeration process of the middle ear cavity is blocked for an extended period of time, fluid may totally fill the middle ear space. Thus, the early identification of negative middle ear pressure may permit the physician to practice preventive medicine and avoid the condition of otitis media.

The presence of unequal pressures on either side of the tympanic membrane usually occurs when negative pressure exists in the middle ear space. This may be sufficient to cause a retraction of the eardrum accompanied by mild conductive hearing loss in spite of the fact that no fluid may be observed in the patient's middle ear. The most explicit example of this occurs when air pressures are changed in the passenger cabins of commercial aircraft. A normal-hearing passenger will first experience discomfort due to unequal air pressure in the middle ear cavity and external ear canal. When the passenger forces open his eusta-

chian tube in order to alleviate this discomfort, he will also notice that, when the air pressures are equalized and the eardrum is again in a most compliant condition, the environmental sounds in the aircraft become suddenly louder. This may be a practical explanation of the numbers of children seen by audiologists to have mild conductive hearing loss, and they are found by the examing physicians to have no evidence of otologic problem. Audiologists are quick to blame the patient or the audiometric test condition for this "unexplainable" conductive loss which may be due to the presence of negative middle ear pressure.

Jerger (1970), Liden et al. (1970), and Paradise et al. (1976) have described basic tympanogram patterns and related them to conditions of the middle ear. Jerger's classification system of tympanometry curves, which he also calls "pressure-compliance functions," is summarized in Figure 6.3. For simplicity, Jerger ascribed alphabetical letters to each type of curve. This classification is convenient, but it may be more explicit to describe each tympanogram in terms of its dynamic compliance and the air pressure at which maximal compliance is noted.

Tympanogram Type A. Type A curves are found in patients with normal middle

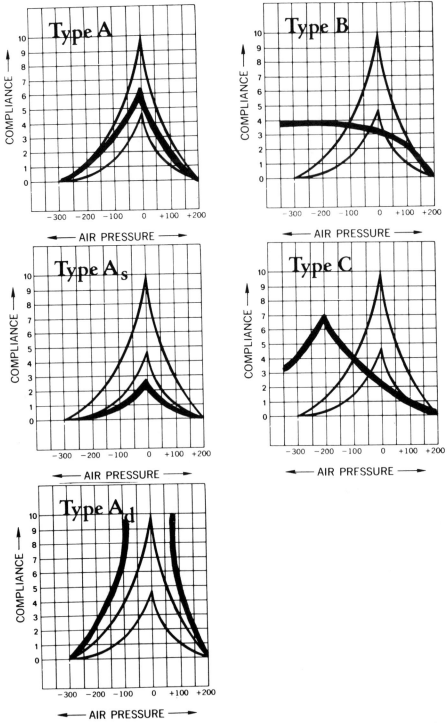

Figure 6.3. Classification of tympanograms according to Jerger (1970). See text for clinical significance of each type of tympanogram.

ear function. The curve shows adequate relative compliance and normal middle ear pressure at the point of maximal compliance. Some controversy exists concerning the limits of normal middle ear pressure values. Alberti and Kristensen (1970) recommended the use of ± 50 mm H_2O as normative values, but we have noted many instances of negative middle ear pressure as great as -150 mm H_2O in patients who demonstrated normal audiograms and normal otoscopic examination. Brooks (1969) evaluated 1053 children in England and determined "normal" middle ear pressure from a statistical distribution to be from -170 mm H_2O to 0 mm H_2O. Decisions regarding "limits of normal" in terms of middle ear pressure will undoubtedly vary depending on the clinical situation and circumstances.

Tympanogram Type A_S. This pressure-compliance function is characterized by normal middle ear pressure and limited compliance relative to the mobility of the normal tympanic membrane. This type of curve may be seen in cases of otosclerosis, thickened or heavily scarred tympanic membranes, and some cases of tympanosclerosis. The subscript "S" nomenclature is indicative of "stiffness," or "shallowness" of the tympanogram.

Tympanogram Type A_D. This curve is represented by large changes in relative compliance with small changes of air pressure. The A_D curve is noted in middle ears where discontinuity of the ossicular chain has occurred, or the eardrum demonstrates a large monomeric membrane. The significance of this curve is its representation of an extremely flaccid eardrum, with the subscript "D" indicating "disarticulation" or a "deep" tympanogram curve.

Tympanogram Type B. The type B tympanogram is characterized by a function representing little or no change in compliance of the middle ear as air pressure in the external ear canal is varied. Often no point of maximal compliance is observable with air pressure as low as -400 mm H_2O. This curve is seen in patients with serous and adhesive otitis media and some cases of congenital middle ear malformations (Northern and Bergstrom, 1973). This curve is also noted in patients who have perforations of the tympanic membrane, ear canals totally occluded with cerumen, or with a patent ventilating tube in the eardrum.

Tympanogram Type C. This tympanogram is represented by near normal compliance and middle ear pressure of -200 mm H_2O or worse. This curve may or may not be related to the presence of fluid in the middle ear, but one can conclude that the eardrum still has some mobility. Bluestone et al. (1973) reported a very low incidence of middle ear effusion in children with type C tympanograms upon whom they performed myringotomies. Paradise et al. (1976) published an impressive set of data dealing with the use of tympanometry and detection of middle ear effusion in infants and young children. They report that a poorly compliant negative pressure tympanogram is approximately 3 times more likely to be associated with middle ear effusion than a negative pressure tympanogram that is highly compliant.

Persistence of the type C tympanogram infers poor eustachian tube function in the presence of an intact tympanic membrane. Sometimes patients can be instructed to "pop their ears" or perform the Valsalva procedure (patient holds his nose and forces positive air pressure into the middle ear cavities). If the patient can open his eustachian tube, a repeat tympanogram may show that the type C curve has changed to the type A curve. Youngsters, however, with upper respiratory infections seldom can alleviate the type C tympanogram with the Valsalva maneuver.

A major drawback to the use of such categories to classify tympanograms is that the clinician inevitably comes across a tympanogram that does not clearly fit into one of the expectant categories. Such tympanograms may be few, but they do exist. In addition, various categorical systems do not always agree on the same nomenclature for the tympanogram patterns. The clinician should describe the mobility of the eardrum in terms of compliance and middle ear pressure, or draw a simple picture of the tympanogram if possible. Margolis (1979) suggested that we express acoustic immittance clinical results in quantitative physical measurements rather than in arbitrary units.

The technique for obtaining a tympanogram is quite simple. The eardrum is put into a position of known poor mobility with an air pressure of +200 mm H_2O pumped into the cavity created by the meter's probe tip and the patient's tympanic membrane. Then the positive air pressure is removed and relative changes in the compliance of the eardrum are noted. The compliance change is actually measured by the electroacoustic meter as a decrease in the SPL of the enclosed cavity. When the compliance of the eardrum is permitted to increase, with the release of air pressure, more of the sound energy is transmitted through to the middle ear creating a decrease in the sound pressure level of the enclosed cavity.

As the air pressure variation approaches the point of maximal compliance, the mobility of the tympanic membrane increases. Maximal compliance is, of course, achieved when the air pressure in the external auditory canal equals the existing air pressure in the middle ear space. The clinician continues to reduce the air pressure in the enclosed cavity, which unbalances the equalized air pressure on either side of the tympanic membrane, and therefore creates a decrease in eardrum compliance again (Harford, 1980).

Clinical uses of tympanometry are many. The type B tympanogram quickly and easily identifies children with stiff middle ear systems even when the presence of the conductive problem is not sufficient to cause hearing loss. The diagnosis of otitis media, for example, does not pose a problem for the trained otolaryngologist as long as the eardrum can be clearly visualized. Tympanometry resolves many of the disadvantages of conventional audiology and otologic assessment. It requires only passive cooperation from children, total visualization of the tympanic membrane is not necessary for accurate tympanometry, thereby eliminating the need to remove cerumen from every patient's ear (Northern, 1978b).

Tympanometry can be used to follow the entire progression and resolution of serous otitis media in children. Typical tympanograms obtained under such circumstances are shown in Figure 6.4. Imagine a 2-year-old youngster who demonstrates a type A tympanogram under healthy conditions. As the otologic disease process begins with a closed eustachian tube, negative pressure is created in the middle ear space which produces a type C tympanogram. As fluid develops medial to the tympanic membrane, the compliance of the eardrum is decreased, and a type B tympanogram will be demonstrated by the child. If prescribed medications are effective and the fluid condition of the ear begins to resolve, we would expect to once again see the type C tympanogram, and finally the type A tympanogram when the middle ear is back in its normal healthy condition.

Tympanometry is also useful in monitoring recovery of the middle ear following surgical procedures. Tympanoplasty grafts, for example, are thick and heavy immediately following surgery and produce a type B tympanogram. As the graft heals and becomes thinner with improved mobility, the tympanogram approaches the type A pattern. Resolution of Gelfoam in the middle ear can be followed with tympanometry. And, of course, this technique is valuable in evaluating postsurgical ears in which the air-bone threshold gap persists or reappears following the surgical procedure.

Paradise (1982) published an editorial retrospective review of tympanometry in which he states that tympanometry has instructional, practical, and intellectual value for the physician. Tympanometry serves the primary care provider in three ways: (1) separating infants and children not easily examined otoscopically into two

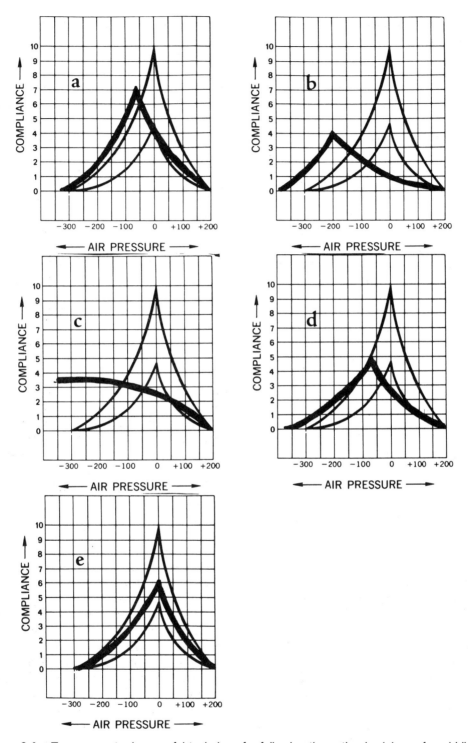

Figure 6.4. Tympanometry is a useful technique for following the pathophysiology of a middle ear effusion. A near normal tympanogram is represented in (a); negative middle ear pressure and reduced compliance often accompany an upper respiratory problem (b); middle ear effusion is present in (c); return of the middle ear to its proper normal control condition is shown in (d) and (e).

subgroups, those with suspected or nearly certain disease who require careful examination, and those virtually certain to be free of disease; (2) in refining and clarifying doubtful otoscopic diagnoses; and (3) objectifying the follow-up evaluations of patients with diagnosed middle ear disease. However, Paradise indicates that it is for the clinical researcher that the value of tympanometry has become most firmly established, since in investigations that in any way involve otitis media, diagnostic accuracy is critical to the validity of the findings.

Studies have been conducted to show the influence of negative middle ear pressure (identified with tympanometry) to elevate hearing thresholds. Cooper et al. (1977) examined 1133 children with middle ear pressures between −150 and −400 mm H_2O and found their hearing thresholds to be elevated as much as 25 dB. An orderly relationship exists between the degree of negative middle ear pressure and hearing threshold shift, with approximately 8-dB shift in the speech frequency range and middle ear pressure of −100 mm H_2O, increasing to at least 20 dB shift when middle ear pressure is −400 mm H_2O.

Static Compliance

Static compliance has traditionally been known as acoustic impedance, particularly in the United States. Compliance refers to the mobility, or springiness, of a system while impedance refers to the immobility or resistance of a system to movement. The choice of terminology between compliance and impedance is much like the old adage of describing a glass of water as either half full or half empty. We have chosen to orient our thinking in terms of mobility of the middle ear system; since this compliance measure is made during resting conditions of the system, we use Jerger's suggested nomenclature, "static compliance."

The concept of acoustical impedance, or static compliance, is a direct outgrowth of applications made by electrical engineers and physicists to describe the willingness of an electrical system to permit electron flow, and the ease with which a mechanical system moves.

The impedance of any mechanical system involves a complex relationship between three factors—the mass, friction, and stiffness of the system. In the middle ear mechanical system, mass is represented primarily by the weight of the three ossicles. The weight of the three ossicles, however, as is immediately obvious to one who has ever held the ossicles in his hand, constitutes very little mass. Friction in the middle ear is due primarily to the suspensory seven ligaments and two muscles which support the ossicular chain. This intricate suspension of the ossicles, however, lends to ease of mobility; thus friction as a factor in mechanical impedance constitutes meager influence in the impedance of the middle ear. The third element of impedance, stiffness, has a much more prominent role in the middle ear. The stiffness element has been identified as occurring at the footplate of the stapes, where a large resistant component must be overcome to move the fluids of the cochlear ducts. Thus, the impedance of the middle ear mechanical system is stiffness-dominated (Zwislocki, 1963).

Acoustic impedance is traditionally expressed in acoustic ohms; acoustic compliance is measured in equivalent cubic centimeters (cc) of volume. The measurement of compliance with the electroacoustic impedance meter is based on the fact that sound pressure level is a function of volume cavity size. That is, for a given probe tone of known intensity and frequency, the sound pressure level of the tone will increase as the cavity size is decreased, or the sound pressure level of the probe tone will decrease as cavity size is increased. Thus a specific relationship exists for a tone of known frequency and intensity (measured in dB sound pressure level) and cavity volume (measured in cubic centimeters). The electroacoustic impedance meter uses a pick-up microphone to measure the intensity of sound energy within the cavity created by the airtight probe tip and the tympanic membrane. This intensity in dB is read in cubic centimeters of equivalent volume for ease and clarity of measurement.

Compliance is technically the inverse of impedance. A system with a great deal of mobility, or high compliance, has very little resistance to motion, or low impedance. Likewise, a poorly mobile system has low compliance and high resistance. This small equivalent volume in cubic centimeters of compliance is equal to a large impedance in acoustic ohms, and vice versa. In the middle ear pathologies, serous otitis media, for example, creates a middle ear system of very low compliance or very high impedance. On the other hand, a disarticulated ossicular chain in the middle ear creates a condition of high compliance or low impedance.

Static compliance is actually tested by making two equivalent volume measures with the tympanic membrane under specific conditions. The first volume measurement (C_1) is made with the eardrum clamped with +200 mm H_2O pressure. The second volume measurement (C_2), which is really an equivalent volume measure, is done with the eardrum in its most compliant air pressure condition. The two volume measures have little actual significance individually because they include the volume of the external ear canal. However, simple subtraction of the two volumes, C_2-C_1, cancels out the contamination of the ear canal from both measures and gives an answer equal to the static compliance of the middle ear.

One of the major weaknesses of static compliance is its wide variance in values related to specific pathologies of the auditory mechanism. The central tendencies of small sample populations may reflect significant differences among various ear pathologies which make the measure look quite valuable. However, in clinical patient populations, the variation in static compliance values create considerable overlap among normal middle ears, otosclerotics, and ears with discontinuity shown clearly by Alberti and Kristensen (1970). Jerger (1970) showed that differential diagnosis based only on static compliance measures may be difficult (Fig. 6.5).

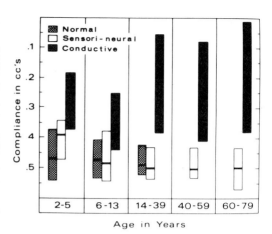

Figure 6.5. Static compliance distribution from Jerger (1970) as a function of age and nature of hearing problem. Static compliance should separate conductive, or middle ear disorders, from normal and sensorineural loss ears. Considerable overlap may be noted especially in 2–5 and 6–13 age groups. Numbers of normal-hearing patients in the 40–59 and 60–79 age brackets were too small to be included. Each vertical box encompasses semi-interquartile range, and solid horizontal stripe is the median value for the group.

Jerger et al. (1972) have shown normal static compliance to vary as a function of age and sex. Men show higher acoustic compliance than females at all ages, while both men and women show a general overall decrease in compliance as they grow older. These facts caution against attempts to construct norms for static compliance. As a guideline, however, the middle ear can be considered abnormally stiff when the static compliance is less than 0.28 cc of equivalent volume and abnormally flaccid when the static compliance is greater than 2.5 cc of equivalent volume. Serous otitis media often creates poor compliance of 0.1 cc of equivalent volume or less. Jerger et al. (1974a) found static compliance to be the least informative test of the impedance battery in children under 6 years of age.

Physical Volume Test (PVT)

Since the immittance meter is able to measure volume in cubic centimeters, information about the absolute cavity size medial to the probe tip can be quite significant. The immittance meters rely on the physical principle that the intensity of a sound trapped in a closed cavity is a direct function of the cavity size. Thus, a signal of fixed intensity introduced into a large cavity and into a small cavity will produce two different sound pressure levels in the two cavities. The larger cavity will have a lower sound pressure level while a higher sound pressure level will be measured in the smaller cavity.

In the presence of an intact eardrum, the typical enclosed ear canal cavity between the probe tip and the tympanic membrane should be 1.0–1.4 cc in an adult, or 0.8–1.0 cc in a child. In infants the PVT value may be as small as 0.5 cc. This value may vary depending on how far the probe tip cuff is inserted into the ear canal, or how large or small the diameter of the external canal might be (Fig. 6.6).

When the physical volume size is considerably greater than these norms in light of an hermetically sealed probe tip and cuff, the clinician can reasonably assume that the cavity includes the external ear canal, middle ear space, and possibly even the mastoid air cells and entrance to the eustachian tube orifice. In circumstances of a nonintact tympanic membrane, and PVT value may be three or four times greater than normal volume values, often exceeding 5.0 cc. We use the PVT as a means to rule out a nonobservable perforation behind an exaggerated anterior canal wall overhang or beneath an adherent crust on the eardrum. The PVT can be used to identify obstruction of ventilation tubes as well as blind attic retraction pocket perforations.

Knowledge of the physical volume in cubic centimeters will help clarify the etiology responsible for B-type tympanograms. Nonmobile tympanic membranes with volumes larger than 2.0 cc in children are usually indicative of a perforation or patent ventilation tube; B-type tympanograms with normal volume measurement are indicative of a nonmobile intact tympanic membrane; abnormally small physical volumes may be related to cerumen occluding the external canal or probe tip, or perhaps the probe tip is pressed against the canal wall (Table 6.2).

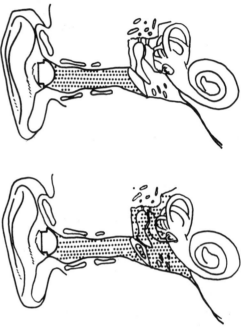

Figure 6.6. Diagnostic representation of utilization of the immittance meter to measure absolute volume size. *Top* scheme shows volume between probe tip and intact eardrum; *bottom* view shows greater volume measurement when eardrum is perforated or has a patent ventilating tube in place. (Reprinted with permission from J. L. Northern: *Clinical Impedance Audiometry*, Ed. 2, edited by J. Jerger and J. L. Northern. American Electromedics Corp., Acton, Mass., 1980b.)

Table 6.2.
Tympanometry and the Physical Volume Test (PVT) in Children

Tym-panogram	Physical Volume	Etiology
Type A	0.8–1.0	Normal middle ear
Type B	<0.3	Cerumen or canal wall
	0.8–1.0	Serous otitis; middle ear congenital anomaly
	>2.5	Tympanic membrane perforation or patent ventilation tube
Type C	0.8–1.0	Negative middle ear pressure; inadequate eustachian tube function

Acoustic Reflex Thresholds

The acoustic reflex test in the immittance battery is the determination of the signal threshold level at which the stapedial muscle contracts. Metz (1952) and Jepsen (1963) reported that, in normal-hearing individuals, a bilateral stapedius muscle reflex can be elicited by stimulating the subject's test ear with pure tone signals between 70 and 100 dB hearing threshold level (HTL) and approximately 65 dB HTL for white noise. The lowest signal intensity capable of eliciting the acoustic reflex is recorded as the acoustic reflex *threshold* for the *stimulated* ear. Under some circumstances the clinician is interested in the presence or absence of the acoustic reflex in the probe ear; for other purposes, the ear of interest is the earphone, or stimulated ear. Regardless of which ear is under examination, it is standard practice to *record* the acoustic reflex for the stimulated ear.

The function of the stapedial muscle is still open to question, but the classical interpretation offered by Wever and Lawrence (1954) is that the stapedial muscle reflex is responsible for protection of the inner ear from loud sounds. Anatomically, the stapedial muscle is attached from the neck of the stapes to the posterior wall of the middle ear cavity. When the stapedial muscle contracts, it pulls posteriorly on the ossicular chain, thereby decreasing the compliance of the middle ear system and attenuating the intensity of the sound which actually reaches the cochlea.

Much emphasis has been placed on the clinical value of the acoustic reflex measurement, particularly by the Scandinavians. Since the acoustic reflex is mediated by loudness, it is a sensitive indicator of cochlear pathology. The acoustic reflex threshold level in patients with cochlear pathology may often occur at sensation levels less than 60 dB above the auditory pure tone threshold. The patient with cochlear pathology hears the test signal as though it were much louder, due to abnormal appreciation of loudness. Thus, the acoustic reflex threshold provides an objective, simple technique to identify the site of pathology to the cochlea.

The ability to establish the presence of the loudness recruitment phenomenon permits the clinician to localize the site of auditory lesion to the cochlea. Anyone who has ever attempted the traditional psychophysical loudness balance procedures on a youngster under 6 years of age to identify a cochlear site-of-lesion, will immediately appreciate the simplicity and objectivity of this technique.

Klockhoff (1961) states emphatically that a recordable stapedius reflex is proof of the absence of a conductive or middle ear component to a hearing disorder. Anderson and Barr (1967) obtained distinct acoustic reflex responses in 16 of 19 children with subsequent surgical intervention for ossicular malformations that exhibited conductive hearing losses. It may be that the acoustic reflex is indeed contracting in the presence of a conductive hearing loss, but generally the mechanism that is altering the conduction ability of the middle ear system is also inhibiting the tympanic membrane from showing a change in compliance as the muscle contracts.

The informed audiologist can achieve considerable diagnostic information through the subtleties of acoustic reflex interpretation (Northern, 1984). For example, the acoustic reflex sensation level shows a "decibel for decibel" inverse relation to the degree of sensorineural hearing loss. The acoustic reflex sensation level decreases from approximately 70 dB for patients with a 20-dB sensorineural hearing loss to approximately 25 dB for patients with a 85-dB sensorineural hearing loss. Jerger et al. (1972) concluded that as long as the cochlear hearing loss is less than 60 dB, there is a 90% likelihood for the presence of the acoustic reflex being observed when the *earphone is over the ear with the hearing loss* with a normal tympanogram in the opposite ear. As the sensorineural loss increases above 60 dB, chances of observing the acoustic reflex grow less. With 85 dB hearing loss, the chances are only 50% of observing the acoustic reflex; if the loss is 100 dB HL, only a 5–10% chance exists of the reflex being present. Thus, the presence of acoustic reflex thresholds in the earphone ear at 100 dB or less, in light of hearing loss, provides a powerful indication for sensorineural diagnosis. In patients with unilateral cochlear hearing loss less than 85 dB, the acoustic reflex should be easily observable bilaterally.

In children with conductive hearing problems, the contralateral acoustic reflex can be observed only in mild *unilateral* conductive hearing loss. When the unilateral conductive hearing loss exceeds 30 dB HL the acoustic reflex is typically obscured bilaterally. Thus, when the stimulating sound is presented to the conductive hearing loss ear, the 30 dB+ hearing loss is sufficient to prevent the signal from being perceived loudly enough to elicit the acoustic reflex. Then when the earphone is on the normal ear, and the probe is in the unilateral conductive loss ear, the mechanism causing the conductive loss prevents the eardrum from showing a change in compliance. Naturally, in a bilateral conductive loss, the acoustic reflexes will be absent bilaterally because the pathology in *each* ear prohibits the probe from noting a compliance change when the opposite ear is stimulated with sound. This acoustic reflex result proves to be a tremendous asset in the evaluation of unilateral conductive hearing loss in children less than three years of age.

Since conductive-type pathology precludes tympanic membrane compliance change, the acoustic reflex can be expected to be absent when the probe tip is in a conductive loss ear regardless of how small an air-bone gap exists. The presence of a small air-bone gap of only 10 dB is sufficient to obscure the reflex to the probe ear nearly *80%* of the time (Jerger et al., 1974b). Conversely, if acoustic reflexes can be noted in the probe ear, it is virtually impossible for a conductive hearing loss to exist in that ear. Thus, even a *very mild*

bilateral conductive hearing loss will obscure the acoustic reflex bilaterally. In a group of 154 patients with unilateral conductive loss Jerger et al. (1974b) showed that the amount of air-bone gap necessary to abolish the stapedial reflex was approximately 25 dB with the earphone on the bad ear, and approximately 5 dB with the probe tip in the bad ear.

Other types of unilateral hearing loss do not obscure the stapedial reflex bilaterally. A unilateral sensorineural hearing loss with a contralateral normal-hearing ear will usually show bilateral acoustic reflexes as long as the unilateral hearing loss does not exceed 80 dB HTL (Jerger, 1970). A unilateral "dead" ear with a contralateral normal-hearing ear, however, will show absence of the acoustic reflex unilaterally when the stimulating earphone is on the "dead" side. Thus interpretation of acoustic reflexes in unilateral hearing losses can be diagnostically important, and of particular value when the patient is a youngster in whom audiometric masking for unilateral hearing loss is impractical or impossible.

Clinical Application of the Immittance Battery with Children

While tympanometry, static compliance, and the acoustic reflex threshold each provide some information about the function of the auditory system, their results become more meaningful when relationships between the three tests are considered. Diagnostic judgments and patient referral are made with greater authority and assurance when the over-all pattern is considered. Jerger (1970) indicated that tympanometry alone is useful to only a limited degree, static compliance norms are too variable for accurate diagnosis, and the absence of the acoustic reflex may occur from several factors. When considered together, however, the limitations of each test are reduced while their combined implications are enhanced (Table 6.3).

Examples of the immittance test battery and its relation to clinical diagnosis are shown in Figures 6.7 and 6.8. Immittance test results from a case of negative middle ear pressure in a youngster's right ear are demonstrated in Figure 6.7. The audiogram shows a mild hearing loss with a 20-dB air-bone gap on the patient's right ear and normal hearing in the left ear. The audiogram gives no clue as to the etiology of the unilateral conductive hearing loss. The tympanogram for the left ear is superimposed on the normal tympanogram pattern, while the tympanogram for the right ear shows slightly reduced compliance and middle ear pressure of −200 mm H_2O. Static compliance is reduced in the right ear suggesting stiffness, thereby corroborating the reduced compliance noted in the tympanogram. Static compliance in the left ear is within the normal range. The acoustic reflexes are present, but show elevated

Table 6.3.
Use of Immittance to Help Confirm Audiometric Impression in Evaluation of Young Children[a]

Tympanometry	Static Compliance	Acoustic Reflex	Confirm Behavioral Audiometric Impression
Type A bilaterally	Within normal range, bilaterally	Normal bilaterally	Bilateral normal hearing or bilateral mild-moderate sensorineural hearing loss or unilateral mild-moderate sensorineural hearing loss
Type A in one ear; type B or C in other ear	Normal in A ear; low in B or C ear	Absent, bilaterally	Unilateral conductive loss
Type B or C bilaterally	Low bilaterally	Absent, bilaterally	Bilateral conductive loss

[a] From J. Jerger: Clinical experience with impedance audiometry. *Archives of Otolaryngology*, 92: 311–324, 1970.

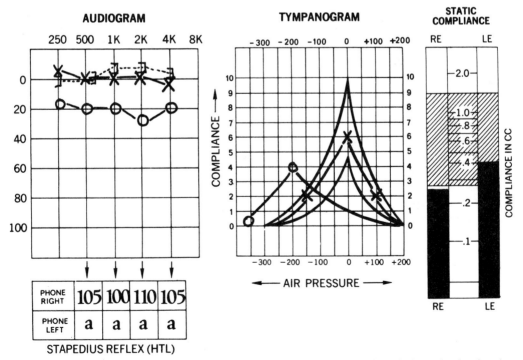

Figure 6.7. Audiometrics and immittance results accompanying a right-sided conductive hearing loss caused by significant negative middle ear pressure. See text for full explanation.

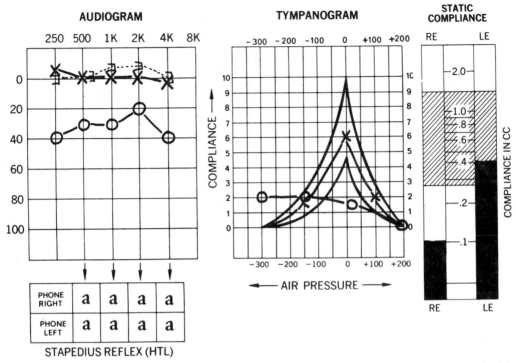

Figure 6.8. Audiometrics and immittance results in a unilateral conductive hearing loss of otitis media etiology. See text for full explanation.

thresholds when the stimulating earphone is on the involved ear. The 20-dB air-conduction hearing loss in the right ear is not severe enough to prohibit loudness from eliciting the acoustic reflex when the earphone is on this ear. When the earphone is placed over the normal-hearing left ear, the acoustic reflexes are absent. The probe tip is now in the involved conductive loss ear, and the conductive loss element prohibits compliance change in the right tympanic membrane. Knowledge of only the immittance test battery results, accompanied by experience in test interpretation, would permit a close estimation of this patient's audiogram if audiometry could not be successfully accomplished.

Figure 6.8 demonstrates findings in a patient with unilateral otitis media. The audiometric results show a stiffness-type air conduction curve with an approximate 30-dB air-bone gap in the right ear. Hearing in the left ear is normal. The tympanogram on the involved right ear shows a type B pattern, substantiated by a rather low static

compliance measure. These results insure the presence of a stiffness component to the etiology of the right conductive hearing loss. The fact that the stapedius reflex is absent bilaterally, in view of a unilateral hearing loss, confirms that the loss must be conductive in nature. This overall pattern could also represent cerumen packed in the right ear canal, a perforation of the right tympanic membrane or otitis media. Diagnosis is in the realm of the physician, but these impedance test findings, even without the audiogram, would suggest referral of this child to a physician.

Robertson et al. (1968) were among the earliest investigators to utilize impedance measurements in children. They suggested several applications for impedance measures in children including validation of air-bone gaps in conductive hearing loss and demonstration of invalid air-bone gaps by observation of strapedius reflex measurements. They suggested that children who have problems accepting amplification with hearing aids may have tolerance problems resulting from loudness recruitment which can be identified with the acoustic reflex. A further application suggested by these authors is consideration of the acoustic reflex as an index of residual hearing in children who offer no response to sound or speech in any form.

Bluestone et al. (1973) compared air-conduction audiometry and tympanometry in 84 youngsters with concurrent or recent middle ear disease to determine which procedure could better predict the presence of middle ear effusion. They concluded that tympanometry is far more sensitive than air conduction audiometry for detecting common conduction defects in children. They caution, however, that tympanometry cannot detect sensorineural hearing loss and thus cannot be substituted for pure tone audiometry as a screening technique. They suggest that tympanometry in combination with air conduction audiometry appears to constitute the best method available for detecting middle ear disease and hearing impairment in large groups of children.

S. Jerger et al. (1974) reported an extensive evaluation of impedance audiometry in 398 children less than 6 years of age who were seen for routine clinical audiometric evaluation. Complete impedance results were obtained with 77% of the group, while satisfactory audiometry on the initial visit could only be obtained from 55% of the group. Immittance findings offered supplementary information not available from behavioral audiometric testing in 67% of these patients. They reported that the unsuccessful impedance results were generally found in children less than 3 years of age, who could also not be tested by standard audiometric techniques.

Impedance and Infants

There is contradictory evidence in the literature regarding the merits of performing acoustic immittance measurements in infants. Margolis (1978) described the situation with a statement that impedance measurements in infants have provided results that are ". . . both promising and perplexing." In an effort to determine whether immittance could be effectively used with newborns, Keith (1973) tested 40 healthy infants from the newborn nursery between 36 and 151 hours of age. Keith reported normal tympanograms in 33 of the infants and a "W-shaped" tympanogram in 7 infants. Keith also examined stapedial reflex measurements in these 40 infants with stimulus presentations of 100-dB HTL at 500 and 2000 Hz. He reported that stapedial reflex responses were often contaminated by behavioral movement of the infants. In fact, from 160 stimulus presentations, only 33% resulted in clear stapedial reflex responses. No acoustic reflex responses was noted in 26% of the stimulus presentations, and 4 of the 40 infants showed no acoustic reflex in either ear initially, although all 4 babies were later confirmed to have normal hearing responses.

In a later study, Keith (1975) investigated the middle ear function of 20 neonates younger than 36 hours of age. The tympanometry results were similar to those reported in his previous study of infants older than 36 hours of age. Keith concluded that tympanometry could be used as a simple, reliable measure of middle ear function in normal neonates.

Immittance data from 18 infants between the ages of 3 and 11 months were reported by S. Jerger et al. in 1974 (Fig. 6.9). They reported a systematic increase in the number of acoustic reflexes present with the increasing age of the infants, a finding consistent with observations reported previously by Robertson et al. (1968). The number of missing reflexes decreased from 20% at ages 0–35 months, to only 5% at ages 60–71 months. The authors offered two explanations for the absence of acoustic reflexes in very young children: (1) it is possible that the acoustic reflex arc undergoes maturation during the early years of childhood, and/or (2) the reflex arc is complete in the neonate but there may be a relatively high incidence of undetected middle ear

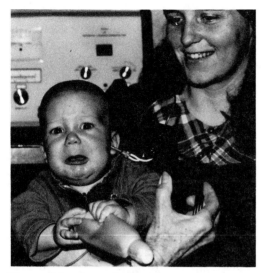

Figure 6.9. Acoustic impedance testing is an essential part of every pediatric hearing evaluation.

abnormality in very young children. The authors concluded also that the impedance technique offered the single most powerful tool for pediatric evaluation. They warned, however, that impedance findings cannot stand alone, and that impedance should only be interpreted in combination with some independent assessment of hearing sensitivity level. Unfortunately, this warning has been largely unheeded.

Immittance utilization with infants seemed to be a reasonably well accepted clinical tool until the publication of an article by Paradise et al. (1976). Their evaluation of 280 children ranging in age from 10 days to 5 years showed a high positive correlation (86%) between tympanometry and otoscopy for subjects over 7 months of age. Poor correlation, however, was found between the two measures in infants less than 7 months of age. In fact, from 43 infants less than 7 months of age, 40 of 81 ears had confirmed middle ear effusion (determined by myringotomy), yet 24 of the 40 abnormal ears displayed *normal tympanograms*. The authors concluded that although the use of tympanometry had much to offer in the diagnosis of middle ear effusion, its use (tympanometry) was not rec-

ommended in infants less than 7 months of age.

Howie et al. (1976) with outspoken disbelief of the Paradise et al. findings in infants less than 7 months of age, quickly set out to replicate the study with their own comparative evaluation of tympanometry and otoscopy in neonates. Howie and his colleagues found that from 59 ears with confirmed middle ear effusion (by myringotomy) 26 showed normal tympanograms and they, thus, emphatically stated that the results and conclusions of the Paradise group were accurate and should not be questioned or challenged.

Reichert et al. (1978) examined 878 3-month-old infants with otoscopy and tympanometry. All infants were examined tympanometrically while being held in their mothers' arms and being comforted with a pacifier or bottle. The authors concluded that tympanometry produced a low diagnostic specificity (accuracy in identifying nondiseased individuals) with a high number of false-positive results—16 "flat" tympanograms were found in ears that were otoscopically normal. In their discussion, Reichert et al. recognized that inclusion of the measurement of the acoustic reflex may have provided different results than were obtained only with the use of tympanometry.

Jerger (1970) has long cautioned clinicians against the use of any single immittance measure to reach a diagnostic conclusion. He has repeatedly pointed out that "tympanometry alone is useful to only a limited degree" in making diagnostic judgments.

Keith (1978) summarized the situation by stating it is imperative that tympanometry and stapedial reflex testing always be done together. To do less, according to Keith, results in erroneous statements that "... tympanometry is neither accurate nor reliable for use in screening infants." Keith expressed concern that such statements will be interpreted by some as indicating that the immittance *battery* is not valid or reliable for infants under 7 months of age.

This misinterpretation is unfortunate in that it may result in reluctance to use a valuable diagnostic tool with a population of individuals who are difficult to examine both otoscopically and audiometrically. Jerger and Hayes (1980) state that in the "diagnostic application of impedance audiometry there are no absolutes; . . . the results of any single impedance measurement are usually ambiguous and have little individual value."

Studies published by Orchik et al. (1978a, 1978b) clearly show that prediction of middle ear effusion on the basis of tympanometric data alone is difficult at best, unless the tympanogram is a flat, nonmobile pattern where a 90% occurrence of effusion is present. Orchik's studies proved that tympanometry with acoustic reflex threshold measurement show the highest correlation to surgical findings relative to the presence of middle ear effusion. That is to say, the combination of tympanometry and measurements of acoustic reflex threshold are superior to the use of either impedance component alone as a predictor of the presence of middle ear effusion.

Schwartz and Schwartz (1978a, 1980) published data which supported the combined use of tympanometry and acoustic reflex measurement to identify middle ear effusion in infants. They conclude that while a normal tympanogram cannot be considered evidence of a mobile tympanic membrane or effusion-free middle ear, the presence of an acoustic reflex with a normal tympanogram supports normal middle ear function. Freyss et al. (1980) also found that the presence of the acoustic reflex provided a higher sensitivity than tympanometry for separating normal dry middle ears from middle ears with fluid.

Abahazi and Greenberg (1977) measured acoustic reflex thresholds in 62 normal infants between 1 month and 12 months of age. They used pure tones (500, 1000, and 2000 Hz), broad-band noise, low-pass noise and high-pass noise to elicit the reflex. Only 23 of the 62 infants showed acoustic reflex responses to all stimuli, while the remaining 39 infants had acoustic reflexes, but to less than the total number of stimuli. The findings suggest that as the age of an infant increases, less stimulus intensity is required for the acoustic reflex threshold. Keith and Bench (1978) showed that the acoustic reflex is clearly present in all normal infants by 3 weeks of age.

McCandless and Allred (1978) produced an extensive study of the emergence of the acoustic reflex in 53 infant subjects tested daily in the hospital nursery and tested weekly following their hospital discharge. These researchers evaluated two probe-tone frequencies, 220 and 660 Hz, and established acoustic reflex thresholds with a bracketing procedure for stimuli of 500, 1000, 2000, and 4000 Hz. The tympanometry results showed an average middle ear pressure of +26 mm H_2O from birth to 48 hours of life. The infant acoustic reflex thresholds showed a range from 70 dB to 100 dB HTL with no significant threshold change over the first 6 weeks of life. The average infant acoustic reflex threshold was 94 dB HTL at birth, with only an average decrease of 3 dB during the initial 6 weeks of age. With the 660 Hz probe-tone and the 500-Hz eliciting stimulus, 89% of the infants showed acoustic reflexes during the initial 48 hours of life. The 220-Hz probe-tone with a 500-Hz eliciting stimulus showed acoustic reflexes in only 4% of the infants during the same 48-hour period. The acoustic reflex was noted in some infants as early as 4 hours after birth. Although the 220-Hz probe-tone was superior for tympanogram tracings, the 660-Hz probe-tone was clearly better for acoustic reflex measurements in infants.

In contrast to the studies which question the efficacy of tympanometry with infants, successful tympanometric results with 91 infants between 4 weeks and 17 months were reported by Groothuis et al. (1978, 1979). These clinicians used otoscopy and tympanometry in 549 evaluations to study the pathogenesis of acute and chronic otitis media. Normal tympanograms and normal otoscopy findings correlated highly in 92%

of the evaluations; flat tympanograms and abnormal otoscopy findings were correlated 93% of the time. However, the intermediate negative pressure tympanograms and otoscopy correlated only 59% of the time. Groothuis et al. reported that the tympanometric examination took about 45 sec. Crying infants were given a bottle to suck during the test. The test was relatively unaffected by the sucking behavior. Finally, the authors reported that *no* flat tympanograms were found in otitis-free infants.

The Groothuis studies provide some especially interesting findings: (1) because of the report of Paradise et al. regarding the shortcomings of tympanometry in infants less than 7 months of age, Groothuis et al. examined their data separately for infants older and younger than 7 months. They found that the high correlation of tympanometry and otoscopy findings were similar in infants *above* and *below* 7 months of age; (2) when a nonmobile tympanogram appeared in an asymptomatic infant in the study who had not previously had otitis media, acute otitis media developed within one additional month; and (3) the resolution of otitis media was often prolonged as long as 6 months in 60% of the infants. The authors concluded that tympanometry is a most useful tool and may be utilized for the earlier identification and more accurate follow-up of acute otitis media in infants.

The cause of the false-negative tympanograms is unclear. Although misdiagnosis is possible with tympanometry and infants, increased accuracy should result by utilization of the impedance test battery by clinicians well-experienced in testing infants. Howie (1979) suggested that the position of the infant during the impedance test may provide the answer to the false-negative tympanogram. Thus, fluid-filled middle ears may show normal tympanograms if the neonate is on its side with the test ear pointed up, permitting fluid to settle toward the medial aspect of the middle ear space and "freeing" the tympanic membrane to move normally. A comprehensive review of studies of impedance in infants was published by Northern (1981).

Practical Pediatric Impedance Considerations

Nearly anyone can be trained to turn the dials and read the meters of an immittance meter. And most clinicians have little difficulty testing cooperative adults. But the real challenge occurs when the clinician is face-to-face with a screaming, uncooperative youngster! A prime requisite for impedance clinicians faced with a screaming youngster is *confidence*. Persistence has its reward when working with children and impedance; so do not give up easily if difficulty is encountered—a second, third, or fourth effort may yield important results. The clinician who manages each child with a matter-of-fact attitude of self-assurance will often triumph!

On occasion, the clinician must be willing to compromise the entire test battery for less than optimal information. While it is desirable to complete the immittance test battery whenever possible, with some difficult to manage children the clinician may have to settle for a quick tympanogram and a single acoustic reflex measurement in each ear. Clinicians must be prepared to work rapidly and efficiently; a smooth, effective initial effort is often surprisingly successful.

The main limitation of immittance measurements in young children is that the test battery cannot be completed while the youngster is vocalizing—speaking, crying, yelling, or any combination of these noises. Stapedial muscle reflex contraction and eustachian tube changes during vocalization, cause the compliance of the tympanic membrane to alter wildly, thereby making impedance measurements impossible. The clinician's most challenging task is to make the youngster stop vocalizing for just the few necessary moments to obtain impedance data. Each clinician must devise his own techniques to momentarily distract the screaming child. Impedance skill with children requires the highest competency in both manipulating the equipment and the child.

The information presented below includes a number of practical suggestions pertinent to immittance measurements in children. Although these techniques are especially good with children under 2 years of age, we have also found them useful in working with other difficult-to-test pediatric patients including the mentally retarded, the deaf-blind, the congenitally deaf, and other children with multiple handicaps (Northern, 1980c).

For children less than 3 years of age it is also helpful and essential that a second or even third person be utilized for obtaining impedance measures. Practice and coordination of these personnel are helpful and they must be in constant communication during all aspects of the test to ensure rapid and reliable results. It is difficult for one person to manipulate the ear insert while at the same time operate the pressure pump and other dials on the immittance devices. It is preferable to have one person operate the impedance instrument while a second stabilizes the child's head and inserts the probe tip. This latter person must be appraised at all times as to whether or not a seal has been obtained or the pressure manometer must be in a position to be observed directly by him. Sometimes it works well to hold the probe tip in place by hand after insertion and the head stabilized by the assistant during the entirety of the test to prevent a loss of pressure seal due to head movement.

A suggested technique in handling the head piece is to remove the head phone and hold it over the contralateral ear. The head piece itself can be placed over the wrist and the insert placed into the ear canal. In younger children it is helpful to have a parent cradle the child with their arm passively immobilizing him, then place the headband over the parent's shoulder and insert the ear probe into the child's ear while holding the head phone on the contralateral ear.

The age range between 2 months and 12 months presents one of the most difficult periods in which to obtain immittance tests. The children are not old enough to understand the test or to respond to verbal enticements, yet they are old enough to react (sometimes decisively!) both to the test situation and to the insertion of the probe tip in particular. We have found that it is most effective to employ a distractive technique to redirect the youngster's attention from the test. The form of distraction is relatively unimportant so long as it is sufficiently novel to compel the infant to disregard the insertion of the probe tip. The external stimuli can be visual, tactile, auditory, or in combination. Prior to assuming a distractive procedure to be essential in immittance testing, one should try to first place the probe tip quickly, but gently, in the ear. Frequently this takes the child by surprise, and further games are not necessary. Often, the entire impedance battery can be completed before the child really has time to react or respond; however, at the first hint of reaction from the child the clinician should be prepared to present a visual distraction. If habituation to one mode of distraction occurs, instantly alter or introduce other diversionary tactics. If the diversions fail, it may be possible to apply passive restraint of the child's body, head, or hands to complete the test.

Distractive or diversionary tactics are most effective if the headset is not used. Instead, rely on an assistant to insert the probe tip while holding the head piece over the wrist or over the mother's shoulder with the child in the parent's lap. When using visual distraction keep the diversionary object well within the child's field of vision to prevent undue head movement which produces artifacts.

The following are examples of the many possible distractive techniques which can be used with children under the age of 3 years. The number and type of devices are limited only by the ingenuity of the examiner. (The authors are indebted to Geary McCandless, Ph.D., University of Utah

Medical Center, for permission to use material from his NIH sponsored project. "Manual for Impedance Testing in Children," which describes some pediatric impedance techniques developed at the University of Colorado Medical Center.)

Animated Toys. Introduce animated toys only as required at critical times necessary to complete the test. Avoid movement artifacts by keeping the toy well out of the reach of the child.

Cotton Swab. Gently brush the back of the child's hand, arm, or leg in a slow even motion. Make the distraction visual as well as tactile by making oscillatory or exaggerated movements of the swab.

Pendulum. Using a bright and unusually shaped object, make a pendulum with about an 18-inch string. This technique is highly effective if the examiner will swing the pendulum about in various motions within various areas of the infant's vision. Swing the pendulum rather slowly in short excursions, permitting easy visual following. Frequently stop or alter the swinging motion to provide novelty to the pendular action.

Mirror. To an infant less than 1 year who is capable of reacting and attending to faces a large mirror is sometimes irresistible, at least for a period sufficiently long to place a probe tip and to perform the impedance test battery.

Toys Which Produce Sounds. Toys or other devices which elicit intense sounds should be avoided if at all possible, since they may evoke an acoustic or other reflexive response from the child. Toys which produce softer sounds in no way interfere with the test and can therefore be used effectively, especially if the sound is somewhat novel.

Food. Children, like adults, seem to enjoy sweets and, although swallowing and sucking movements are notorious for producing artifacts in the tympanogram and reflex measures, food can still be used as a distractive technique. Flavored jello powder in water, honey, Kool-Aide, or sweetened lemon juice can be dropped into the child's mouth at intervals during the test. Avoid taking measures until the reflexive sucking action has subsided. Administering small amounts of liquid well spaced can keep the children occupied for many minutes.

Watch. In front of the child, simply remove one's wrist watch, manipulate or wind it well out of reach of the child, or point to it.

Shoe. A simple, yet effective, technique is to begin lacing and unlacing a child's shoe either on or off his foot. This should be carefully timed to coincide with the insertion of the test tip into the ear. Move slowly and methodically and do not appear to have any objective in mind except to lace and unlace or tie and untie the shoe.

Action Toys. A variety of toys are available which perform repetitive actions such as a monkey which climbs down a stick pole. Often these are not the best distractive devices because children 1 year and older often wish to handle or manipulate this type of toy.

Wad of Cotton or Kleenex. A cotton ball or pledget can facilitate effective passive attention by balancing the cotton on the hand, arm, or knee of the subject or on the hand of the assistant. It can be squeezed or otherwise manipulated; it can be blown or allowed to fall repeatedly from the hand. A Kleenex can also be used as a parachute, torn slowly into strips, rolled into small balls and be placed in the child's hand, waved, punctured, etc.

Tape. A roll of adhesive or paper surgical tape has been found to be one of the most effective distractive devices available in the clinic. Bits of tape can be torn off or stuck on various parts of the child's or examiner's anatomy. The child can be allowed to pull the tape off, objects can be picked up with the adhesive side of the tape, fingers can be bound together, links can be made with small strips, rings can be formed, fingernails covered, and innumerable other totally nonmeaningful manipulations can be performed. Tape works wonders for the few seconds necessary for obtaining impedance measures.

Lollipop. A lollipop can be utilized when the child is cradled and partially immobilized in the examiner's or parent's arm. The examiner can stroke the child's lips or tongue with the lollipop. Careful spacing of the lollipop permits completion of the entire impedance test battery.

Miscellaneous Devices. Tongue blades, cotton swabs, colored yarn, or similar devices are all effective as distractive devices. They are best utilized when manipulated or "played with" by the examiner. If the child insists he can be allowed to manipulate tape or string, etc. But care must be taken to permit only passive action so as to reduce movement artifact while the test is proceeding.

The audiologist should beware of a too-elaborate array of toys or gadgets because the child may want to play with the toys and not be bothered with the test procedure. For impedance testing extensive entertainment is usually not warranted.

There is no way to predict the behavior or reaction of children between 1 and 3 yers of age. Their reaction to the test situation is influenced by past exposure to other tests, to "doctors," by their age, their personalities, and by their general evaluation of what they see is about to happen to them. In many instances they are most concerned whether or not the procedure will be painful. For these reasons some general rules apply when testing children in this age group: first, never ask a child for permission to perform impedance tests; calmly assume you are going to administer the test and proceed to do so. Second, avoid undue explanation regarding the test procedure. Instructions to the subject contribute nothing to the test results unless it helps reduce physical movement. Besides, the child would not understand explanations even if given. It is sufficient to say something like, "here, listen to this," or "hold still," or "listen to this radio," then proceed with the test. Most often it is better to say nothing unless the child reacts to placement of the headset or insert. Explanations usually take longer than the test itself!

For most children older than 3 years of age, no special distraction is required when applying immittance measures unless the child is particularly apprehensive in an unfamiliar clinical situation. Only a few children in this age category will demonstrate adverse reactions to immittance testing. Where necessary one can reduce anxiety by saying simply, "we are going to test your hearing, please hold still," or other uncomplicated statements of reassurance. Most 3-year-olds can be tested with a single examiner. Allowing the child to observe other children or adults being tested helps to allay any fears that a pain will occur. With these children as with the younger group refrain from asking permission to perform the test. Distractive techniques are viewed with suspicion so treat this age category essentially as you would adults except for mild and occasional words of instruction or encouragement (Fig. 6.10).

Impedance Audiometry with the Mentally Retarded

The evaluation of hearing in the mentally retarded patient presents a most difficult

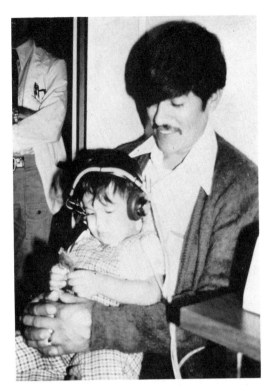

Figure 6.10. Successful acoustic impedance testing in children requires a perceptive and experienced clinician.

task. The problems are vast and an entire book devoted to audiometry for the retarded has been published (Fulton and Lloyd, 1969). Many retarded children do not condition well to pure tone play audiometry. They may not have sufficient maturation to perform auditory localization tasks or may lack consistent startle response. They may be too hyperactive to cooperate or too lethargic to be aware of changes in the environment (Fig. 6.11). Incidence studies have established that there is a higher incidence of hearing impairment among the retarded than among the nonretarded (Lloyd, 1970; Rittmanic, 1971). Yet the retarded are excluded from traditionally recommended screening techniques because of their limited capacity for responding.

Brain damage in these children often makes physiological auditory responses unreliable. Yet, accurate assessment of hearing function or middle ear status of these

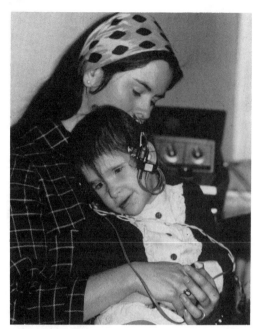

Figure 6.11. Immittance testing can be accomplished with difficult-to-test patients as shown above with this mentally retarded rubella youngster.

children may be critical for educational placement or medical/surgical treatment. Sometimes even a tympanogram or acoustic reflex measure can be a valuable result since the clinician can then make reasonably accurate assumptions regarding the presence or absence of middle ear problems and the need for medical referral. Immittance measurements are also valuable in the evaluation of the severely mentally retarded "mattress care" children, who are virtually impossible to test with any other testing procedure. These institutionalized youngsters are certainly at high risk for developing chronic middle ear disese.

The earliest acoustic impedance studies with retarded children were published by Lamb and Norris (1969, 1970). They compared acoustic reflex thresholds in 15 mentally retarded children and 15 children of normal intelligence. All subjects had normal hearing, and the acoustic reflex thresholds for both groups were at similar levels. Although it was reported that considerable variability in reflex thresholds was noted

among the mentally retarded subjects, the authors note that the retarded subjects were easily tested, and they recommended that the impedance technique should be included as a part of the audiometric test battery. Fulton and Lamb (1972) reported normative results from a retarded population with tympanometry, and demonstrated that tympanometry can be of use to help differentiate etiology of hearing loss.

Borus (1972) used impedance measurements in a group of 23 young retarded children to establish the value of impedance audiometry in determining the nature of hearing loss. She concluded that impedance measurements "offer great promise" in quickly determining normal hearing in a retarded, difficult-to-test child, identifying cases where there is clearly a conductive component, and singling out retarded children who do have some auditory anomaly requiring further evaluation.

Jordan (1972) pointed out that even a mild degree of hearing loss may have a disproportional impact on the mental retardate because he is less capable of compensating cerebrally with the aid of his other senses. Mentally retarded children now considered to be educable were "mattress cases" 25 years ago. Standards set forth by the Accreditation Council for Facilities for the Mentally Retarded in 1971 require that all new residents of institutions, and all other residents, at regular intervals must be given audiometric screening. Audiologists in such facilities find themselves faced with great numbers of retarded patients of all ages and functioning levels, for auditory screening. We see no alternative for auditory evaluation of such patients without impedance audiometry.

The Deaf-Blind Child. In our opinion, evaluation of hearing in deaf-blind children is the most difficult task faced by the audiologist. The task is even more formidable when mental retardation accompanies the deaf-blind handicap. Audiometrically we are limited to observation of basic behavioral auditory orientation responses, the acoustic startle reflex, and quieting behavior to brief introduction of various interesting sound stimuli. When severe visual motor, or other neurological deficits are present, the primitive reflexive auditory behavior responses may be inhibited or absent. The audiologist must be prepared to perform, or refer such patients for, auditory evoked potential evaluation.

It is the audiologist's responsibility to make the decision about the blind child's hearing ability. Little textbook information or standardized developmental scales are available regarding techniques for evaluating the hearing response in these children. It is often useful to the audiologist to discuss the hearing potential of deaf-blind children with the parents and or teachers who are with the child for long periods of time. Sometimes the peripheral reflexive hearing mechanism seems within normal limits but the child is "functionally deaf" since sounds are seldom imitated, little vocalization occurs, and response to verbal cues is inconsistent.

Immittance with the Congenitally Deaf Child

The workup of patients with substantial sensorineural deafness will usually not identify superimposed middle ear anomalies. Impedance audiometry provides a useful means of evaluating the conductive hearing mechanism in patients with sensorineural hearing loss (Northern, 1980c).

Children attending schools for the deaf are not routinely evaluated by otolaryngologists. These deaf children seldom complain about their ears or of changes in their hearing sensitivity due to otologic pathology. Bone conduction measurements are of limited usefulness in this special population with severe-to-profound sensorineural hearing impairment. Only a few published articles are available describing impedance measurement results from children attending schools for the deaf (Rubin, 1978; Ruben and Math, 1978; Rood and Stool, 1981).

Rossi and Sims (1977) reported the use of acoustic reflex measurements in the severely and profoundly deaf in an effort to evaluate the validity of audiometrically determined air-bone gaps. They conducted impedance studies of 35 deaf students showing that some 80% of the "air-bone gaps" produced by audiometry were, in fact, invalid. They recommend the use of impedance measurements of the acoustic reflex to resolve the ambiguity of responses due to probable tactile-vibratory stimulation with the audiometric bone oscillator from true conductive components.

These studies show that immittance provides a useful means of evaluating the conductive mechanism in patients with profound deafness. The Brooks (1975) study brought out an important additional fact about the increase in hearing loss which accompanies middle ear problems. In deaf children this additional hearing loss may have significant deleterious effect on hearing aid performance. If the child is mature enough to recognize the need to turn up the hearing aid gain, problems may be created with distortion and feedback; if the child is too young to note the change in hearing, poor performance with the hearing aid may also result. Impedance audiometry should, by all means, be a routine procedure for children attending schools for the deaf.

Sedation and Immittance

On occasion it may be necessary to consider the use of sedation to quiet down an uncooperative youngster for acoustic immittance evaluation. Chloral hydrate or secobarbital are often used because of their ease of administration and general effectiveness. The action of chloral hydrate and secobarbital is such that drowsiness, quieting and sometimes deep sleep is achieved within an hour. Following the immittance evaluation, the youngster can be aroused and taken home. The major disadvantage to chloral hydrate and secobarbital is that both drugs are long-acting sedatives. Acoustic reflexes can be observed in patients sedated with chloral hydrate or secobarbital, but researchers have shown the acoustic reflex thresholds to be elevated (Borg and Moller, 1968; Gicomelli and Mozzo, 1965; Robinette et al., 1974; Mitchell and Richards, 1976).

Clinicians must be aware, that a child's reaction to such medication is not always as expected. Children vary considerably in their response sensitivity to sedatives and the recommended dosages may not be sufficient to induce the desired effect. The same dosage in other children may actually increase activity and excitement levels so that the desired impedance study is still not possible.

Mentally retarded children are often maintained on medication for management of behavioral or convulsive disorders. Thus, the absence of acoustic reflexes in this population may be drug related. Richards et al. (1975) evaluated impedance findings in 10 functionally retarded normal-hearing children on phenobarbital. These authors reported that low-level amounts of phenobarbital have no effect on the acoustic reflex threshold.

Immittance evaluation under conditions of general anesthesia is usually unsuccessful. Results are influenced by the anesthesia technique and drug agent. Middle ear pressure is increased under inhalation of some gases such as nitrous oxide, thereby decreasing the compliance of the tympanic membrane and obscuring the acoustic reflex (Thomsen et al., 1965). Researchers have shown that nitrous oxide collects in closed gas-filled body spaces, so middle ear pressure measurements taken during endotracheal inhalation anesthesia showed increased middle ear pressures as great as $+450$ mm H_2O with nitrous oxide, while no pressure elevation was noted with halothane or ethrane (Patterson and Bartlett, 1976). The use of sedation or anesthesia, in our opinion, is seldom worth the trouble (Northern, 1980b).

Hearing Loss Prediction by the Acoustic Reflex

A revolutionary application of impedance audiometry was developed by Niemeyer and Sesterhenn (1972) to determine air-conduction hearing thresholds from stapedial reflex measurements. They noted that the acoustic reflex threshold for white noise was lower than the acoustic reflex threshold for pure tones, and that the difference in decibels between the two thresholds is related to the degree of sensorineural hearing impairment. They verified their results on a large group of normal-hearing and hearing-loss subjects, and concluded that their technique provided an objective means to predict hearing levels within 10 dB in just a few minutes without extensive equipment expenditures.

Two years later, Jerger et al. (1974b) simplified the procedure into a test he called SPAR (Sensitivity Prediction with the Acoustic Reflex). SPAR is an attempt to ascertain sensorineural hearing loss within four categories of impairment (normal hearing, mild loss, severe loss, or profound loss). The Jerger technique calls for establishment of pure tone acoustic reflexes at 500, 1000, and 2000 Hz and broad-band noise threshold difference to predict the degree of hearing loss. In addition, the *slope* of the audiogram is predicted by establishing reflex thresholds for a low pass band of noise and high pass noise band. In a series of over 1000 patients, Jerger et al. (1974b) reported that the predictive error of SPAR was clinically insignificant in 63% of the group, moderate error in 33%, and serious error in only 4% of the patients.

Jerger et al. (1978) have subsequently published a modified version of the SPAR including the abandonment of the high-low pass noise stimuli to predict audiogram slope. The success of these SPAR procedures and their clinical utility have inspired a number of innovative approaches to predict hearing loss with acoustic reflex measurements. Hall and Bleakney (1981) divide these approaches into three general categories—SPAR, regression equations, and the bivariate plot system. All depend, in one fashion or another, on the noise-tone difference in acoustic reflex thresholds and have been reviewed in detail by Hall (1980) and Popelka (1981).

In general, the regression equations predict hearing threshold level by assigning acoustic reflex threshold data for pure tones and noise in differentially weighted equations. These formulas are based on statistical regression techniques. The bivariate plot coordinate system simply differentiates those patients with normal hearing from those with sensorineural hearing loss. According to Hall and Bleakney (1981), the SPAR methods, regression equations, and bivariate plot system all appear to estimate, or identify, hearing loss with accuracy rates in excess of 60%. None of the methods, however, invariably predict hearing loss without error.

Hearing loss prediction from the acoustic reflex is apparently influenced by a number of variables including chronologic age, minor middle ear abnormalities, and audiometric configuration (Jerger et al., 1978). Fortunately, for those of us involved in pediatric audiology, predictive accuracy with the SPAR test is more successful in children (ages 0–10 years) and grows less accurate in older children and adults. Jerger et al. (1978) conclude that the best approach to predicting the presence of hearing loss of any degree is to rely on the broad-band noise and pure tone acoustic reflex difference, whereas the absolute acoustic reflex threshold level for broadband noise stimuli is used to predict the degree of hearing loss. In the Jerger et al. (1978) study, 100% of the children predicted to have normal hearing did, indeed, show normal audiograms. Severe hearing loss was accurately predicted in children 85% of the time. Prediction of moderate hearing loss in children was somewhat less accurate (54%).

The prediction of hearing loss with the acoustic reflex is a valuable asset to those clinicians involved with hearing evaluations in children. Objective prediction of hearing loss in children has numerous applications in daily clinical testing, and all clinicians should be familiar with, and able to implement the technique when appropriate. Reports of successful use of these procedures with children have been re-ported by Jerger and Hayes (1976), Keith et al. (1976), Keith (1977b), Niswander and Ruth (1977), Abahazi and Greenberg (1977), and Hall and Weaver (1979). According to Hall (1980), there is reason for optimism about the potential of acoustic reflex-hearing level predictions. In very young children, acoustic reflex prediction methods clearly offer the most rapid objective measure of hearing sensitivity—even with the "difficult-to-test" child.

Ipsilateral Acoustic Reflex Measurement. Some immittance meter designs have improved the ability to measure the acoustic reflex in an ipsilateral mode. In ipsilateral reflex measurement, the eliciting acoustic stimulus is presented through the probe tip and the reflex response is monitored in the same ear. Major advantages of ipsilateral reflex measurement is that confusion is eliminated regarding which ear is being tested. Utilization of ipsilateral reflex techniques virtually eliminates the need for the cumbersome headband-earphone arrangement which is typically used in contralateral reflex measurement. Thus a whole new family of hand-held probe tips, without headband, are appearing on portable impedance meters. The use of ipsilateral reflex measurement and the new hand-held probe tips should encourage the use of impedance measurements in mass screening programs. Research reports which compare acoustic reflex threshold sensitivity between contralateral and ipsilateral stimuli have been published indicating that ipsilateral thresholds are 3–6 dB more sensitive than contralateral thresholds (Moller, 1962; Fria et al., 1975).

HEART RATE RESPONSE AUDIOMETRY

Change in heart rate response to presentations of auditory signals is a well established feature of electrocardiac measurements. Zeaman and Wegner (1956) noted that upon presentation of a brief, moderately loud tone, the human patient will display a temporary wave-like alteration of the electrocardiogram. This is an unconditioned response often used by psychophysiologists in cardiac conditioning experiments (Zeaman et al., 1954; Zeaman and Wegner, 1956).

The early evaluations of heart rate change due to auditory stimulation did not attempt to use the technique to establish auditory thresholds. The physiologic measurement is based on the fact that, immediately prior to each cardiac contraction, an electrical impulse is initiated and travels through the heart. As this electrical impulse passes through the muscle of the heart, small electrical currents spread into the tissues surrounding the heart. Some of this current reaches the surface skin of the body and is measured with sensitive electrodes. With the electrodes placed on either side of the heart, the potentials are recorded with an electrocardiograph.

Zeaman and Wegner (1956) established that changes in the heart rate patterns of adults were specifically related to the intensity of the auditory signal. Bartoshuk (1962a, 1962b, 1964) examined cardiac responses to acoustic signals in some 100 neonates. His cardiac recording technique (1964) utilized an electrode on the infant's left leg and the second electrode on the head in the frontal area. A cardiotachometer was used to determine stable heart rate, and ancillary recordings included electromyograms from the right forearm extensors, bipolar EEG electrodes on the left frontal and parietal area, respiration, and body movement measurements. The analysis of results was done by comparing the five or six cardiac beats immediately prior to stimulus onset with the initial five or six beats following termination of the stimulus. His results verified that cardiac acceleration to auditory signals was reliably observed in all neonates; that cardiac acceleration was greater in 4-day-old infants than 1-, 2-, or 3-day-old infants and that repeated stimulus presentations created cardiac response decrement exhibited by a shortened period of acceleration. Keen et al. (1965) tested 40 infants and found consistent heart beat acceleration following auditory stimulation of moderate intensity

which showed response decrement to long, 10-sec stimulus presentations.

In a clinical study of heart rate change in infants, Schulman and Wade (1970) tested 30 high risk babies between 6 weeks and 9 months of age. A computer program was used to present auditory signals and average responses over trials. Heart rate change was measured by sampling the cardiac record at each 2-sec interval during a prestimulus period until 2 sec before the onset of the next stimulus. Each trial period was composed of 10 sampling points which were averaged across trials to compare prestimulus and poststimulus heart rate. Since gross motor movement can influence test results, the infants were tested during quiet sleep or following feeding. Under the conditions of their evaluation of the 30 infants, cardiac rate responses were obtained in 27 subjects at 34 dB SPL. The other three subjects appeared to have elevated auditory thresholds, even with repeat testing.

Schulman (1970a, 1970b) tested a hypothesis proposed by Luria (1963) and Eisenberg et al. (1966) that infants with central nervous system damage fail to habituate to repeated stimulation. Schulman used 80-dB SPL stimuli presented for 3 sec at 20-sec intervals. Examination of heart rate change averaged across time for trials 1–5 and trials 26–30 showed significant habituation for both the experimental group of high probability CNS-damaged babies and a matched control group of normal full term infants. Butterfield (1962) was unable to obtain positive heart rate responses in three retarded patients, although normal patients were easily tested. She reported difficulty in finding mentally retarded patients who could cooperate with the testing procedure.

Schulman attempted to use the heart rate response in audiologic evaluation of children. In a study of 24 children, ranging in age from 3 weeks to 13 years, heart rate change, cortical evoked potentials, and conventional audiometry results were compared in the assessment of auditory response levels. Heart rate responses were obtained at approximately normal-hearing levels, and agreed closely with other test results in subjects with documented hearing loss. The authors concluded that heart rate change is a sensitive measure of auditory function, and is within clinical feasibility.

Eisenberg's chapter on "Cardiotachometry" (1975) is a most thorough description of efforts to study cardiac behavior. In her laboratory work with heart rate measures, she has focused mainly on suprathreshold responses to speech-like stimuli. Eisenberg (1974) stated that cardiac measures of audition are potentially important, but future research programs are needed to further define the parameters of testing technique.

Gerber et al. (1976, 1977) and Mulac and Gerber (1977) contend that heart rate response has value in audiometric evaluation of children, especially infants. Borton and Smith (1980) recently published a review article on the status of heart rate audiometry.

EVOKED AUDITORY RESPONSE AUDIOMETRY

Nearly 45 years ago Davis (1939) noted that the electrical activity of the brain as indicated by electroencephalographic recordings showed a change when the subject heard a loud sound. This led numerous clinicians to attempt to use the standard EEG technique as a test for hearing acuity. Results, however, were disappointing. The electrical response in the cortex to auditory stimuli is so small that it is difficult to see in the normal ongoing electrical activity of the brain, particularly when the stimuli are low intensity pure tones.

In the early 1960s a number of special purpose computers appeared on the commercial market. These computers, known generally as signal-averager computers, utilized a summation technique to cancel out random on-going background physiologic "noise," which created an improved signal-to-noise condition, which in turn enhanced specific, time-locked potentials of small magnitude. These computers store and av-

erage potentials which are related in time to the onset of a stimulus, while "random" noise which consists theoretically of an equal number of positive and negative electrical potentials, is averaged out to be of zero value. Thus, only the wanted potential activity summates in the computer (Fig. 6.12).

The cortical evoked response results from generalized electrical activity on the cortex due to the presentation of various sensory stimuli including light, vibrotactile stimuli, and sound. In fact, the presentation of any sensory stimulus of sufficient intensity, or the abrupt change of any stimulus, produces a widespread evoked potential from the human brain during the 300 msec following the stimulus presentation. By the mid-1960s, evoked response audiometry was being hailed as "the answer" to audiometric testing problems and the difficult-

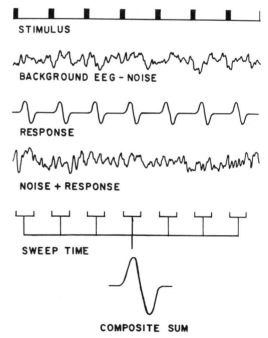

STIMULUS

BACKGROUND EEG - NOISE

RESPONSE

NOISE + RESPONSE

SWEEP TIME

COMPOSITE SUM

Figure 6.12. Signal-averager computers utilize a summation technique to cancel out random on-going background physiologic "noise," which creates an improved signal-to-noise condition to enhance specific, time-locked potentials of small magnitude. (Courtesy of Laszlo Stein, Michael Reese Medical Center, Chicago.)

to-test patient. Unfortunately, this did not prove to be the case for "late" potentials measurement. Technical problems, equipment expense, and time-consuming clinical testing arrangements made routine use of cortical evoked response audiometry impractical for most clinical facilities.

During those years, clinicians attempted to use what we now call "late" cortical evoked potentials (occurring at latencies longer than 80 msec post-stimulus), but clinical results were difficult to interpret. Efforts to use late cortical potentials in clinical measurements were largely abandoned in the early 1970s.

The average evoked response is not a unitary response, but rather a composite reflecting general cortical activity. An idealized response is characterized by a multiphasic wave having fairly consistent latencies. The negative and positive peaks and valleys in the classic waveform have been labeled P_1, N_1, P_2, N_2, and P_3. Goldstein (1973) presented an idealized evoked response that separates the peak components into early (50 msec or earlier), late (50–400 msec), and contingent negative variations (later than 400 msec). The amplitude of the cortical evoked response is generally related to the intensity of the stimulus; the more intense the stimulus, the larger the average evoked response to a certain point. The growth in amplitude of the wave is accompanied by a decrease in latency of the peak components. As the stimulus signal is decreased toward threshold levels, the presence or absence of the averaged evoked response becomes difficult to separate from the biological baseline activity.

Auditory Brainstem Evoked Responses (ABR)

In 1967 an important discovery was reported by two Israeli physicians, Sohmer and Feinmesser, who used click stimuli to evoke a polyphasic response recorded with electrodes on the vertex of a human subject. This evoked potential was of very short latency, within the initial 12.5 msec post-stimulus and consisted of a specific pattern with five positive-direction waves. In 1970, Jewett noted seven positive peak wave forms, occurring within the initial 10 msec post-stimulus, which had remarkable stability and consistent wave-form latencies. These studies were the beginning of a tremendous change in the field of physiological evoked potential measurements. Improvements in equipment and computer technology have helped clarify the various evoked potentials in humans, and in turn, have influenced greatly the field of audiology.

The evoked potential literature has absolutely grown by leaps and bounds during the 1970s, and this avid interest in the electrical activity of the brain for sensory functions will no doubt continue during the 1980s. Most audiology and otolaryngology textbooks now include complete materials devoted to descriptions of auditory evoked potentials. Our task will be to present a current overview of the early evoked potentials and their application in the clinical evaluation of hearing in children. Our discussion has drawn heavily from the materials of Fria (1980), Jerger et al. (1981), and Beagley and Fisch (1981).

The advent of the early latency auditory brainstem response (ABR) has had a tremendous impact on the field of audiology. The clinical applications of ABR measurements are extremely varied and include auditory, visual, and somatosensory evaluations. Auditory ABR measurements provide information regarding the identification of site-of-lesion in the auditory brainstem pathways including acoustic nerve tumors, assessment of auditory function in patients with stroke or trauma, infant hearing assessment, predicting hearing sensitivity in difficult-to-test children, evaluation of aided versus unaided auditory performance, neurological disease and/or dysfunction, as well as central auditory processing information. ABR measurements are utilized by audiologists as well as other medical specialists such as otolaryngologists, neurologists, ophthalmologists, neurosurgeons, anesthesiologists, and orthopedic surgeons. In fact, ABR potentials are so widely used now, that the prestigious *New England Journal of Medicine* published an outstanding two-part review on the use of ABR in clinical medicine (Chiappa and Ropper, 1982).

Jewett and Williston (1971) systematically recorded the early ABR human responses to varying stimulus and recording parameters. They labeled their seven positive peaks from I to VII as shown in Figure 6.13. Waves VI and VII have subsequently been found to be not always readily apparent, and general clinical interpretation has focused on waves I through V. Wave V has proven to be the most prominent component of the response pattern, and is often seen combined with wave IV to form the "IV–V complex." The normal latency of each wave is about 1 msec longer than its designated number, so wave I has a latency of about 2 msec, while wave V latency is about 6 msec, as shown in Figure 6.14. Although the amplitude of the waves is easily influenced by numerous variables, the latency of the peaks is very stable.

The neural generators for the ABR were postulated to be the peripheral acoustic nerve and the various nuclei of the ascending auditory pathway. Experimental studies in animals, and studies of ABR in human patients with confirmed lesions, have led to the general conclusion that wave I represents the auditory nerve site, waves II and III are associated with the medulla and

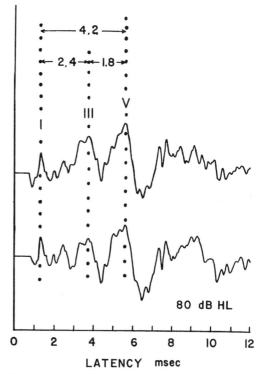

Figure 6.14. Typical latency measurements, and interwave latency measurements for a high-intensity auditory brainstem evoked response. (Courtesy of Laszlo Stein, Michael Reese Medical Center, Chicago.)

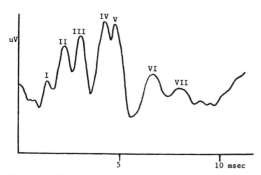

Figure 6.13. An idealized example of the peaks in the early component evoked response according to Jewett and Williston (1971).

pons, specifically the cochlear nucleus and superior olivary complex. Changes in the wave forms of IV and V are associated with lesions affecting midbrain auditory structures, the lateral lemniscus and the inferior colliculus (Fig. 6.15). A number of investigators have contributed to this scheme of interpretation including Sohmer and Flinmesser (1973), Starr and Anchor (1975), Starr and Hamilton (1976), Stockard and Rossiter (1977), etc. Although controversy exists over the exact specification of origin sites for each wave of the ABR, Picton et al. (1974) suggested that waves I through IV represent activity from the auditory nerve and brainstem auditory nuclei, but the total wave pattern is also influenced by the composite contribution of multiple generators. J. Jerger et al. (1981) point out that, with such a "far-field" recording technique with electrodes on the scalp, it is too

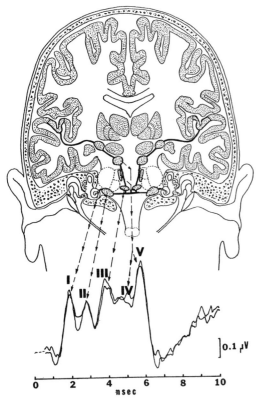

Figure 6.15. Diagrammatic representation of the auditory brainstem response waves and their generator sites. Wave I is associated with the auditory nerve, wave II comes from the cochlear nucleus, wave III comes from the superior olivary complex, wave IV is thought to come from the area of the lateral lemniscus and wave V from the inferior colliculus. (Courtesy of Laszlo Stein, Michael Reese Medical Center, Chicago.)

vous system state, and the replicability of the wave-form pattern. In fact, the validity of an ABR tracing is usually verified by repeating the test and comparing both runs. Shimizu (1981) also points out that the technique with children is attractive because the ABR is relatively unaffected by the physiological state of the patient, the measurement is accomplished as a nonsurgical test, with excellent results in both awake and sleep stages.

RESPONSE PARAMETERS OF ABR

The ABR is optimally recorded differentially from the vertex scalp to either mastoid with an electrode on the contralateral mastoid serving as ground. The ABR is usually evoked with click stimuli, repetitively presented ($N = 2000$) at 30 per sec and summated by computer analysis. Click stimuli provide a sufficiently short rise time to ensure a synchronous neural burst from the auditory system (Hecox et al., 1976). Therein, however, is the main shortcoming of the ABR technique—the lack of frequency specific information about the hearing of the patient. The spectral energy of the transient click stimulus is shaped by the earphone resonant characteristics and the duration of the click. Because clicks fail to allow frequency specificity in the auditory system, the ABR reflects predominantly the basal turn of the cochlea, or hearing information between 1000 and 4000 Hz.

Stockard et al. (1979) have shown that stimulus factors can have an interactive influence on the ABR wave form, but varying individual parameters of the stimulus will also exert modification of the wave pattern. Increasing stimulus intensity influences the ABR wave form by increasing the amplitudes and decreasing wave latencies. The relationship between stimulus intensity and wave peak latencies is used to plot "latency-intensity functions" for each of the waves. Figure 6.16 shows typical latency-intensity functions as used in differential diagnosis of hearing losses com-

simple to assume site-specification of each wave to a unique generator. It is more reasonable to assume the ABR represents a "complex interplay and interaction of evoked potential activity from multiple overlapping dipoles involving all the structures of the auditory system."

The clinical attributes of the ABR were summarized by Davis (1976) to include wave-form consistency, easy recordability with proper equipment and technique, and optimal latency—slow enough to avoid confusion with the cochlear microphonic, yet fast enough to avoid being masked by muscle reflexes. The ABR is widely known for its freedom from the effects of central ner-

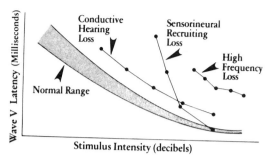

Figure 6.16. Characteristic latency-intensity functions obtained with normal listeners and various types of hearing loss patients. (Courtesy of Nicolet Biomedical, Madison, Wisconsin.)

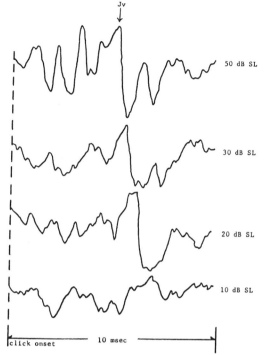

Figure 6.17. Summed brainstem evoked responses at decreasing intensities. Each response represents 2048 click presentations. (Courtesy of Steven Staller, Ph.D., Denver Ear Institute.)

pared to the normal range of latency-intensity responses.

The latency-intensity function is usually plotted for waves I, III and V, and it is important to know that the pattern of all three functions is approximately parallel. This also indicates that the interpeak intervals (sometimes called interwave latency intervals) are relatively constant over the entire intensity range. Thus, the interpeak intervals (i.e., I–III, III–V, or I–V as shown in Fig. 6.14) can be measured at any intensity level without concern that the measurement will be affected. In general the I–III interpeak interval is about 2 msec, the III–IV interpeak interval is approximately 2 msec, and thus the I–V interval is about 4 msec.

At high stimulus intensity (80 dB HL or greater) all five waves are usually seen with clarity in normal subjects. As stimulus intensity is decreased, below 60 dB HL for example, waves I, II, and IV tend to become difficult to identify with certainty. Rome (1977) reported that when stimulus intensity nears auditory threshold, wave V is often the only remaining landmark in the response tracing. In this fashion, as shown in Figure 6.17, ABR is used to estimate auditory threshold. The tester must keep in mind the lack of information provided from traditional audiometric test frequencies below 1000 Hz. Likewise, the ABR is very sensitive to peripheral high-frequency hearing loss and central auditory pathway disorders. These conditions, either singu-

larly or together, can make the ABR wave form difficult to interpret.

An increase in the stimulus click rate increases the latency and reduces the amplitude of the ABR waves. The amplitude of wave V is constant up to 30 clicks per sec, although the peak latency of wave V may change about 1.0 msec as stimulus click rate is increased from 10 to 100 clicks per sec. These technical considerations make it mandatory that all clinical facilities that wish to perform ABR establish their own norms for their particular test parameters and procedures prior to testing patients.

Another important variable in the interpretation of ABR tracings, especially in premature infants, is the effect of maturation on the wave forms. The effect of maturation in infant populations is significant, and without proper normative standards, misinterpretation of peak wave latencies can easily occur. However, between the ages of 18 months and 25 years of age, the ABR shows little change in latency or amplitude. Figure 6.18 shows the general maturation of the ABR from newborn to adulthood (Jacobson et al., 1982). More information on the maturation effect in premature infants may be found in Chapter 7 (ABR in infant screening).

Binaural stimulation is often useful when testing children. Binaural stimulation with clicks produces wave forms that are about 1½ times greater in amplitude than noted with monaural stimulation of either ear. The latencies of the waves are essentially the same for monaural and binaural stimulation. The binaural stimulation tech-

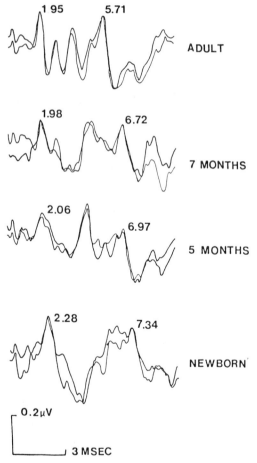

Figure 6.18. Maturation of the auditory brainstem response from postnatal newborn period to adulthood. (Reprinted with permission from K. Hecox and J. Jacobson: *Hearing Disorders*, edited by J. L. Northern. Little, Brown & Co., Boston, 1984.)

nique is good for approximating auditory threshold, since the response to binaurally presented clicks is the same as the response to monaurally presented clicks in the better hearing ear.

A major disadvantage in ABR with children is that most children between the ages of 12 months and 4 years of age must be sedated for the duration of the testing session. This requires the use of a professional medical staff to be on hand during the session. We allow a minimum of 1 hour for each test session, although we are always prepared to carry on longer if necessary to obtain adequate information about the hearing of the patient. Most children older than 4½ can be entertained during the session, or will sit fairly quietly until the test is completed.

Jerger and Hayes (1976) have brought out the value of the cross-check principle in young children who may yield a behavioral audiogram, but whose validity is under question because of conflicting speech audiometry results or impedance audiometry findings. No ABR study should be undertaken without first attempting behavioral audiometrics and impedance audiometry. Shimizu (1981) warns that ABR is only a part of the whole diagnostic process for clinicians whose responsibility must cover history taking, traditional audiometrics, evaluation of the patient's overall communicative abilities, parent counseling, and overall case disposition. Fria (1980) states emphatically that the ABR cannot test "hearing" in the perceptual sense, nor can it identify a specific neurologic lesion at a given location (Table 6.4). Consequently, the ABR results cannot stand alone and must be interpreted in the context of other clinical information. J. Jerger et al. (1980) cite overinterpretation of ABR as the most common error made by clinicians and/or failure to consider other test findings in the whole clinical picture.

AUDITORY MIDDLE-LATENCY EVOKED RESPONSES

The auditory middle-latency evoked responses, so called because their latency lies

Table 6.4.
Candidate Pediatric Populations for Auditory Brainstem Evoked Response (ABR) Tests

Age Group	Definite Candidates	Possible Candidates
Newborns (0–2 mo)	Conditions leading to intensive care nursery admission Conditions leading to high risk register enrollment Failure of behavioral hearing screening in normal nursery Meningitis	
Infants (3–23 mo)	Meningitis Congenital atresia Persistent otitis media with effusion Sepsis and ototoxic drug therapy Delayed speech Parental suspicion of hearing loss	Recurrent apnea Failure to thrive Infantile autism Developmental delay
Children (24 mo+)	Mental retardation Emotional disturbance Learning disability Suspicion of retrocochlear lesion Meningitis	Autism Developmental delay Sudden and progressive sensorineural hearing loss

[a] From T. Fria: *Monographs in Contemporary Audiology*, vol 2. Maico Hearing Instruments, Publishers, Minneapolis, Minn., 1980, p. 37.

between that of the early or brainstem evoked responses and the late cortical evoked responses. The latencies of the middle-latency evoked response peaks are found between 12 and 60 msec post-stimulus. The discovery and major investigation of auditory middle-latency evoked potentials is associated with Goldstein and Rodman (1967), Mendel and Goldstein (1969), and Mendel (1980).

Actually, the middle-latency responses have received little attention and are used in only a few clinical facilities. The site of generation has not been identified precisely, although Beagley and Fisch (1981) believe it to be situated in the auditory radiations in the thalamic region, and in the primary auditory cortex in the temporal lobe.

Hood (1975) describes the nature of the middle-latency response to be two major positive peaks, P_o with a latency of 12 msec and P_a with a latency of 32 msec, and three negative trough, N_o, N_a, and N_b, occurring at 8, 18, and 52 msec, respectively. Hood suggests, based on the works of Goldstein and associates, that with the finding of close agreement between middle-latency re-

sponse thresholds and behavioral thresholds for the same stimuli, the middle-latency evoked response may serve to be an indicator of auditory sensitivity.

Recently, Ozdamar and Kraus (1983) published a study of auditory middle-latency responses (MLR) and ABR in the same subjects. They found that mild sedatives did not appear to affect either MLR or ABR, that MLR differed from ABR in their stimulus-related properties, implying that the neuronal mechanisms underlying their generation are not the same. In contrast to previous studies (Mendel et al., 1975), they found that the MLR wave components were not as readily identifiable at low stimulus levels as the ABR wave V, and concluded that the ABR appears to be the test of choice when hearing sensitivity is in question. And finally, they suggest that MLR are likely to be most clinically useful in patients with neurological or central auditory processing disorders.

ELECTROCOCHLEOGRAPHY (ECoG)

Investigators have long been intrigued by the electrical potentials generated within the auditory system. Clinicians have made many efforts through the years to utilize these auditory potentials in some form of clinical procedure. These measurements were termed "electrocochleography" by Lempert et al. (1947). The most important cochlear potential is the cochlear microphonic which originates from the hair cells in the organ of Corti, originally described by Wever and Bray (1930). The cochlear microphonic reproduces faithfully the waveform of the stimulating auditory signal, and is usually measured by an electrode from the round window niche. The cochlear microphonic has no "threshold" other than the lower limits of the recording apparatus; that is, the cochlear microphonic (CM) is produced to any auditory signal, no matter how slight. Current nomenclature refers to the cochlear microphonic as the "cochlear potential" (CP).

The electrical potential from the auditory nerve is the action potential, noted initially by Derbyshire and Davis (1935). The action potential consists of nerve impulses in the eighth nerve triggered by the CM. The action potential response consists of a well synchronized volley of impulses called N_1, which may be followed by smaller waves known as N_2 and N_3. Although initial clinical attempts to use auditory electrical potentials centered around the cochlear microphonic, the compound action potential response is currently proving most valuable in clinical use.

The compound action potential has a latency of about 2 msec when the cochlea is stimulated by an abrupt sound stimulus. Although the individual action potential in each auditory nerve fiber is a diphasic spike potential, the response of the whole auditory nerve is a compound potential which gives information from the basal turn of the cochlea, and to a lesser extent from the middle turn (Beagley and Fisch, 1981).

Lempert et al. (1947) reported results of ECoG which they conducted at the time of surgery in 11 patients. They stated that the location of the active electrode was very crucial and that contact with the round window yielded the largest magnitude potentials. They commented that good electrode contact with the round window was difficult to achieve because the typical otologic middle ear surgical approach provided only limited access to the round window niche. They concluded that recording the human cochlear potential was not a practical clinical procedure. They substantiated through 3 years of experience that the recording procedure was indeed objective, precise, and easily reproducible. The value of conducting ECoG at the time of surgery, however, when the otologic diagnosis is already determined, was not nearly as useful as if measurements could be made prior to surgery.

After a few dormant years, research with cochlear potentials was started again by Ruben and his associates at Johns Hopkins Hospital. Ruben, during surgery, placed an electrode on the round window of four patients and obtained good responses from two of them (Ruben et al., 1959). Ruben et al. (1960) reported observations on 17 patients who showed good cochlear potentials in response to pure tones, and noted the presence of the eighth nerve action potential in the same recordings with an N_1 latency of 1.2–2.0 msec.

Ruben et al. (1962) reported obtaining cochlear potentials and action potentials from 50 patients including 15 children tested under general anesthesia. The children were grouped as having "serious difficulties with verbal communication," "seriously impaired speech," or "no evidence of hearing." From the 15 children, 8 gave no cochlear or action potentials, 4 gave good cochlear potentials but no action potentials, and the other 3 showed good cochlear and action potentials. Ruben and his associates suggested that these latter three cases may be the first factual validation of central deafness since proof of a functioning cochlea and eighth nerve was evident in light of a picture of severe hearing loss. From this study, the authors concluded that auditory potential measurement is a good technique to teach us more about problems of childhood deafness.

More recently, investigators have been working to find a technique for measuring auditory potentials other than during surgery. The technique utilized in auditory evoked potentials measurement provided the answer in the form of desk computers used to summate successive small responses to repeated, identical acoustic stimuli. In this manner, an "average" response is obtained to many stimulus presentations. The computer signal averages an evoked response from out of extraneous, random background activity.

The use of computer averaging technique was very important to those interested in ECoG. Since this procedure permitted recording of very small voltage responses, it was no longer necessary to place the electrode as close as possible to the organ of Corti. Thus, Yoshie and his colleagues (1967, 1968, 1969) in Japan published several reports concerning parameters of action potentials of the eighth nerve obtained from the external auditory canal; Sohmer and Feinmesser (1967, 1973) in Israel made action potential recordings from the lobe of the ear; Spreng and Keidel (1967) reported in Germany their recordings from the mastoid scalp area; Portmann and Aran (1971), both Frenchmen, have reported several papers with data obtained directly from the promontory, Cullen et al. (1972) recorded action potential responses from an electrode placed against the lateral side of the tympanic membrane. Simmons and Glattke (1975) stated that, in general, electrodes closest to the cochlea provide the clearest recordings, but they also required penetration of the tympanic membrane. Electrodes placed in the ear canal or on the tympanic membrane yielded recordings with greatly reduced amplitudes, and often provided equivocal results with respect to threshold measurements.

Yoshie et al., (1967) described a typical action potential response, recorded through the average response computer, to clicks of moderate intensity, as an initial negative wave, N_1, followed 1 sec later by a smaller negative wave, N_2, and followed occasionally by a still smaller negative wave, N_3 (Fig. 6.19). The latency of the wave N_1, defined as the time between arrival of the click at the eardrum to the peak of N_1, was 2 to 3 msec. The amplitude of the response as measured from the response baseline to the peak of the wave was a function of click intensity and click interval. The baseline for the action potential wave is an idealized line drawn through the tracing of spontaneous activity at the zero response level. The N_1 response also seemed related to the time interval following the previous click.

In 1968, Yoshie reported that changes in the latency of the action potential seemed closely related to the loudness of the clicks. The latency of N_1, in patients with conductive hearing loss was a very obvious clue to the nature of their hearing impairment. Yoshie reported clinic behavioral auditory thresholds and conductive loss thresholds to be in "good agreement" with their action potential records. A sample record showing average auditory nerve action potentials in response to clicks of varying intensities is shown in Figure 6.20.

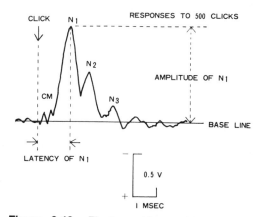

Figure 6.19. Electrocochleographic averaged response as recorded by Yoshie and Ohashi (1969) from an electrode in the wall of the external auditory canal. The stimulus was 500 clicks at 100 dB peak equivalent SPL. This figure illustrates the definition of latency, N_1 amplitude, and the interpolated baseline.

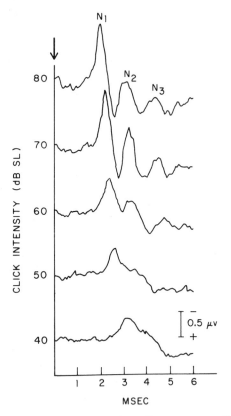

Figure 6.20. Averaged auditory nerve action potentials to 500 clicks at a rate of three per second. Curves were obtained from stimulus presentations of various intensities. Note the increase in amplitude of N_1 as signal intensity increases, and the longer latency of N_1 as the signals approach threshold levels. (Reprinted with permission from N. Yoshie, et al.: *Laryngoscope* 77: 76–85, 1967.)

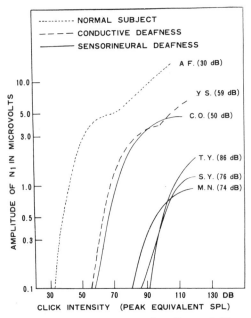

Figure 6.21. Input-output functions of N_1 recorded from the promontory of patients with various types of hearing loss. The dotted curve represents a typical function from a normal-hearing patient; the dashed line was obtained from a conductive loss patient; the four heavy line curves are from patients with sensorineural hearing loss. The numbers in parentheses indicate subjective thresholds for clicks in peak equivalent sound pressure level. (Reprinted with permission from N. Yoshie and T. Ohashi: *Acta Otolaryngologica (Suppl.) 252: 71–87, 1969.*)

Yoshie also examined input-output functions which plotted click intensity against amplitude of the N_1 wave in microvolts. He found that the curve rises rapidly at first from a threshold level of response to an initial hump and then rises again to a second hump which is the maximal level of output (Fig. 6.21). The curve shows an inflection point at which the slope changes in the click intensity region from 70 to 80 dB peak equivalent sound pressure level. Yoshie designated the names low and high intensity portions of the action potential response, or L- and H-curves, respectively.

Clinical application of the ECoG technique has been largely due to the well publicized efforts of Portmann and Aran at the Phono-Audiology ENT Clinic in Bordeaux, France. They have been using the computer-averaging technique since 1967 to record auditory nerve and cochlear microphonic potentials by means of an electrode placed on the promontory through the tympanic membrane (Aran and LeBert, 1968). They report clinical ease of this procedure which is done on adults and children over 8 under local anesthesia. Younger children are tested under general anesthesia, primarily to insure quietness rather than reduction of pain. By placing the active electrode on the promontory, Aran (1971) reports the potential to be approximately 10 times larger than potentials recorded from the external ear canal. Although their measurement technique actually records the sensory response of the cochlea including the cochlear microphonic and summating potential as well as the neural response—the whole nerve action potential, they do not give consideration to the cochlear responses. The cochlear potential is, in fact, eliminated from the recording procedure by a means of reversing the polarity of the stimulating signal and adding it to the picked up cochlear microphonic in the averaging computer. The sum of these two signals in the computer is zero and they essentially cancel each other out of the recording. Meanwhile, the summed action potential is free of CP influence, and quickly presents itself in the recording apparatus.

Critics of the Portmann-Aran technique usually cite their criticism toward the use of the needle electrode of 0.2-mm diameter which is inserted through the tympanic membrane and positioned against the promontory. The apparatus is held in place under tension from a special headband as shown in Figure 6.22. The authors of the procedure state that the healing of the perforation created is almost always very rapid and without complications. They prefer this electrode position because of the stronger auditory system response, and the fact that artifact from the test tone is reduced when evaluating patients with profound hearing loss.

Although ECoG is recognized as an extremely sensitive physiological test of hearing, no standardized clinical approach has yet been established. The technical aspects of ECoG are demanding and interpretation of results requires experience and knowledge of the limitations of the procedure. Most experts agree that ECoG is not a "routine" testing procedure and should be reserved for use with special patients in whom conventional audiometric tests are inconclusive.

Simmons and Glattke (1975) published an excellent review of the current status of ECoG with ample review of the literature for those readers interested in more detail about the technique. A major advantage to the ECoG procedure is that it is able to provide auditory threshold information because the threshold of detection of the action potential (AP) response is within 10 dB of the individual's perceptual threshold for tonal stimuli in the 2000–4000 Hz region. The peak latency of the N_1 component of the AP response is stimulus intensity dependent. In normal hearing subjects, the N_1 peak latency is in the area of 4 msec at threshold, and decreasing to less than 1.5 msec when the stimulus is at 90 dB re threshold (Fig. 6.23).

Beagley and Fisch (1981) report that a wide-band click stimulus threshold with ECoG agrees fairly well with mean behavioral threshold values at 1, 2, 4, and 8k Hz. High frequency tone bursts of 2, 4, 6, and 8k Hz can be used to establish the audiometric configuration for the patient, but reliable threshold information for frequencies of 1000 Hz or lower cannot be established with ECoG. In patients with severe deafness or a nonfunctioning cochlea, no AP will be detected. Spoor and Eggermont (1976) report high correlation coefficients between appropriately filtered clicks and tone burst ECoG threshold data and behavioral audiograms on 100 subjects. They indicate that ECoG is valuable when you need specific hearing threshold information from a patient, not just an estimate of hearing level.

The single most concern in ECoG with children is the need to use anesthesia in an operating room under direction of an anesthesiologist (Simmons et al., 1978). It is necessary to have a healthy child to undergo anesthesia for a purely diagnostic (not treatment) procedure. Simmons and Glattke (1975) state that the ECoG is the most powerful electrophysiologic index of cochlear integrity—when a response is present there is at least some residual hearing at the end-organ, and when there is no response one can be reasonably certain that no residual hearing exists. With transtympanic recording (through the tympanic

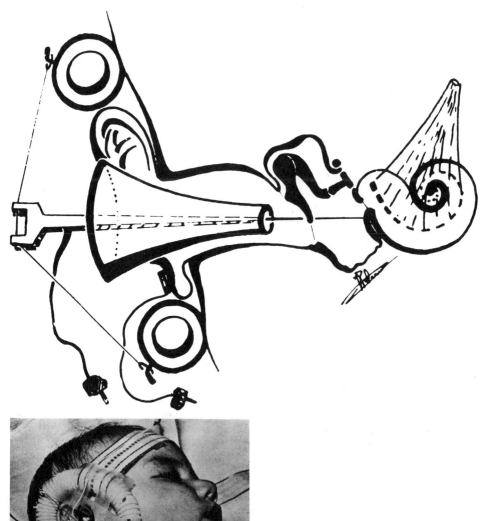

Figure 6.22. The Portmann-Aran technique for positioning the electrocochleographic active needle electrode against the promontory, through the tympanic membrane. (Reprinted with permission from M. Portmann and J. M. Aran: *Acta Otolaryngologica 71:* 253–261, 1971.)

membrane with the needle electrode positioned on the otic capsule) the large promontory responses require relatively few samples to obtain useful data, an entire input-output function for click stimuli can be generated very quickly. In fact, Simmons and Glattke (1975) report that their usual procedures, with measures obtained for both ears with suitable replications, requires less than 1 hour from introduction of anesthesia to final plotting of data.

The facts are not yet all in regarding the best technique to use in ECoG measurements. It seems sure, however, based on evidence accumulated thus far, that ECoG does have strong clinical implication. Its international development will undoubtedly ensure that this new technique is destined to survive and undergo further refinements.

Electrophysiologic Audiometry

Skinner and Glattke (1977) present an

excellent state-of-the-art article on electro-physiologic response audiometry (Table 6.5). They categorize evoked responses which occur within a latency range of 1 to 5 msec as originating from the cochlea and auditory nerve. Responses in the 4–8-msec latency range have the brainstem as their origin. Responses with latencies from about 8–50 msec presumably arise from the upper brain stem and primary projection areas. Slow wave responses from 50 to 300 msec originate as a secondary discharge from the primary cortical projection areas and surrounding secondary and association areas.

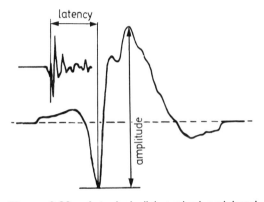

Figure 6.23. A typical click-evoked peripheral response from the promontory of the cochlea by Aran. Note the differences in waveforms, latency, and amplitude measures from the Yoshie procedure as shown in Figure 6.19. (Reprinted with permission from J. M. Aran: *Archiv fur Klenishe und Experimentelle Ohren-, Nasen-, und Kehlkopfheilkunde 198:* 128–141, 1971.)

The longest latency potentials, about 300 msec, are slow shifts that appear to arise from the prefrontal and secondary or association areas of the cortex. Skinner and Glattke summarize that the early, or brainstem, potentials will find the widest application since they can be easily and reliably detected in young individuals and are not affected by sedation. The middle latency responses may be of secondary importance, and late potentials are not reliable for use with young children and are markedly affected by sedation. They indicate that ECoG remains the most reliable of all electrophysiological techniques, but should only be considered after behavioral and other electrophysiological tests have proven inconclusive.

Ruben (1963) suggests a scheme whereby the anatomic diagnosis of sensorineural or nonconductive deafness might be made. The widespread use of such diagnostic tests could make the hearing loss description of "sensorineural" archaic—we could describe hearing loss as either "sensory" deafness or "neural" deafness depending on the procedures. Ruben suggests that knowledge of the exact anatomic location of a child's deafness is very important to the overall management of the individual. He adds that research into the prevention and treatment of nonconductive deafness must depend on our ability to diagnose the anatomical location of the disorder.

Table 6.5.
Electrophysiological Response Classifications[a]

Response Latency Classification	Site of Origin	Response Waveform	Response Latency (msec)	Amplitude (μV)
Electrocochleography	Auditory nerve	Fast	1–5	0.1–10
Early	Brainstem	Fast	4–8	0.001–1
Middle	Brainstem/primary cortical projection	Fast	8–50	1.0–3
Late	Primary cortical projection and secondary association areas	Slow	50–300	8.0–20
Very Late	Prefrontal cortex and secondary association areas	Very slow	300 and beyond	20–30

[a] From P. Skinner and T. J. Glattke: *Journal of Speech & Hearing Disorders*, 42: 180, 1977.

Ruben's suggested diagnostic rationale for the use of physiologic tests in anatomic specificity for locus of deafness was published as early as 1963. X-rays of the temporal bone can be used to identify agenesis of the labyrinth. Vestibular tests, such as electronystagmography, can be indicative of the function of the vestibular portion of the labyrinth, as well as the vestibular portion of the eighth nerve and higher pathways. Electrophysiologic responses of the cochlea, via cochlear microphonics, and the auditory portion of the eighth nerve can be evaluated with ECoG. The presence of cochlear potentials would indicate functioning hair cells in the organ of Corti. If the cochlear potential is absent, then there will be no eighth nerve action potential since there is nothing to stimulate the neurons. The presence of both cochlear potentials in light of a deaf patient would lead the clinician to diagnose the disease to higher auditory centers in the central nervous system. As physiologic tests become more commonplace, clinic procedures for the accurate diagnosis of site-of-lesion deafness will become increasingly a more realistic goal.

EVALUATION OF CHILDHOOD DIZZINESS

There is a scant array of literature regarding vestibular evaluation of children with complaints of dizziness and/or vertigo. We exert considerable time and effort to the problem and prevention of hearing loss in children, yet we often ignore concurrent or subsequent vestibular disorders. This neglect could be due to several factors, perhaps the most common being the fact that vertiginous crises in childhood are often attributed to behavior problems. In addition, the types of vertigo found in adults infrequently occur in young children. When vertigo is described by a youngster (in addition to suspicion of a functional disorder) the possibility of epileptic seizures, brain tumor, or brain stem lesion are considered. Hence, the child with vertiginous complaints may be subjected to a series of lengthy, and expensive medical tests.

More attention should be directed to the likelihood of peripheral disturbances in children suffering from vertigo and/or dysequilibrium. Basser (1964) described a syndrome called "benign paroxysmal vertigo of childhood." He reported that it was quite common in children, but differed significantly from benign paroxysmal vertigo found in adults. The distinction rests on the childhood prevalence, and also the pure paroxysmal nature of the attacks, their brevity, recurrence, absence of any prolonged disequilibrium, and the absence of the febrile illness or upper respiratory infection at the onset. Utilizing electronystagmography (ENG) (Fig. 6.24), Basser successfully documented vertiginous complaints from children. He consistently found caloric responses which were significantly reduced or absent. What a relief to the parents of a youngster complaining of "the world spinning around," to be assured by a physician that their child suffered a benign vestibular insult, which although permanent, would eventually cease to be a problem to the child.

The implications of Basser's report are significant. For one, he demonstrated that children can be lucid in their description of symptoms, and that the traditional ENG can be effectively applied to younger chil-

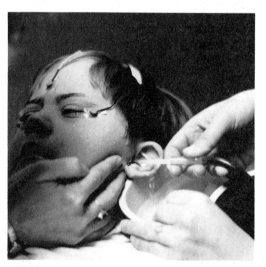

Figure 6.24. Water caloric irrigation with electronystagmography electrodes in place on cooperative youngster.

dren. Most importantly, he brought to light the need to listen more carefully to what vertiginous children are saying; believe their reports, and request a relatively simple and inexpensive evaluation with ENG.

We have a number of youngsters displaying symptoms of vestibular dysfunction, such as ataxia. Within the population of vertiginous children we evaluate are post-meningitis patients, and those with combined renal dysfunction and decreased visual acuity, as in Alport's syndrome. Children displaying visual and vestibular disturbances are of particular concern because of the risk of permanent damage to two of the three systems necessary for maintenance of balance. On occasion we test children who have received long-term and/or high doses of ototoxic drugs which are particularly toxic to the vestibular portion of the inner ear, i.e., gentamicin and streptomycin (Bergstrom and Thompson, 1984).

Despite articles reporting successful application of the ENG procedure with children (Koenigsberger et al., 1970) the consensus still appears to be that ENGs cannot be performed on youngsters under 7 or 8 years of age. It seems likely that this notion arose from clinicians who encountered calibration and tasking problems when attempting to test children with ENG. We also encounter such problems; however, as we modify our audiological testing to suit the needs of the patient, so we do the same with our vestibular testing. We approach the ENG as a play situation, commonly employing various conditioning techniques to help the child adapt and perform adequately.

An ENG should be performed on any child, where strong suspicion exists of vestibular dysfunction. The child who develops bilateral vestibular weakness in infancy or childhood, will often be asymptomatic, and may adapt to the loss in a few days. But, when this child is left in the dark, begins to swim underwater, or grows up to be a deepsea diver, or a construction worker on high buildings—the loss of vestibular function will very quickly and suddenly become apparent. It is our responsibility to recognize and understand the implications of vestibular dysfunction in childhood, and be prepared to undertake appropriate evaluation and/or referral.

A recent excellent overview and discussion of pediatric vestibular evaluation was published by Cyr (1983).

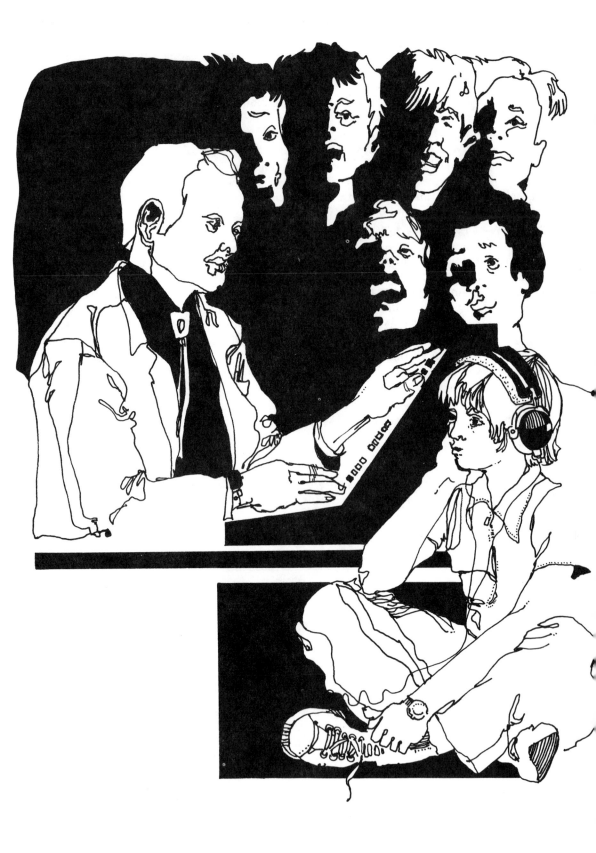

CHAPTER 7

Identification Audiometry with Children

Screening is the process of applying to large numbers of individuals certain rapid, simple measures that will identify those individuals with a high probability of disorders in the function tested. A criterion measurement point is always involved, below or above which the individuals are suspect. Screening is not intended as a diagnostic procedure; it merely surveys large populations of asymptomatic individuals in order to identify those who are suspected of having the disorder and who require more elaborate diagnostic procedures.

Screening for hearing loss in the public schools has been an acceptable practice since 1927. It has been judged in the past to identify successfully the child with a hearing loss that is educationally handicapping (Downs et al., 1965). The literature abounds with descriptions of the progress of audiometric screening dating from the introduction in 1927 of the Western Electric 4-C group speech test (McFarlan, 1927), up to the addition in recent years of tympanometry (Northern, 1980d) as an adjunct to the individual pure tone sweep test, which has been the most acceptable tool for hearing screening in the schools (Darley, 1961).

One also sees reports in the literature concerning a series of attempts that have been made to screen the hearing of 2- to 5-year-olds in as acceptable a way as the hearing of the school child (Downs, 1956; Mencher and McCulloch, 1970). Programs for screening newborns are now firmly recommended but have not yet been implemented universally. It seems that screening of the school-aged child is the only entrenched hearing screening program in the child sphere.

Inasmuch as in this book we are suggesting some innovative approaches to screening methodology at all ages, it might be well to look at the philosophy of screening as viewed, not from the limited view of hearing screening alone but from the vantage point of all the health sciences. A great many public health agencies have taken a long, hard look at the theoretical framework of screening. Discussion of such a framework may help us to reevaluate the entire structure of our previous approaches to hearing screening. From this discussion we will derive a set of goals for screening that lead in turn to some suggested changes in the methodology of screening.

PUBLIC HEALTH ASPECTS OF SCREENING

Screening for disease as early as possible in the child's life is now an accepted public health mandate. It has been recognized that the status of health and the delivery of health care in the United States are at a considerably lower level than that of many other countries of the world. As of 1970, among the nations of the world, the United States ranked 18th in male life expectancy at birth and 13th in infant mortality at birth. The latter is among the commonly accepted indices of the status of health care.

Another accepted indicator of health system functioning is the prevalence of otitis media in a population. The most thorough epidemiologic study of this disease was reported by Eagles et al. (1967) in Pittsburgh. They found 15.2% of the entire school population to have otologic abnormalities in one or both ears, indicative of past or present ear disease. In a 5-year-follow-up study, 1200 of these children—almost 30% of the original population screened—either had otoscopic abnormalities prior to the study or developed them during the 5-year period.

Few reports are available that compare our otitis media statistics with those of other countries, but if one can use perforated eardrums as an index, Hinchcliffe (1972) reported the following:

Finland	7 per 1000
Guam	8 per 1000
Denmark	10 per 1000
USA	20 per 1000
USSR	41 per 1000
Navajo	53 per 1000
India	62 per 1000
Alaskan (Eskimo)	300 per 1000

Audiologic screening for hearing loss has identified similar differences in populations. For example, Fay (1972) found that, among disadvantaged "inner city" children in New York, 19% failed screening tests and were found to have abnormal hearing. Compare this figure with other similarly conducted screening programs of the total school population. Such programs may produce only 2½% abnormal hearing (Doster, 1972), 90% of which is due to medically remediable ear problems. In the National Health Survey (1972) the higher prevalences of hearing losses were found in the lower income group. Another study by Kessner and Kalk (1973) reported that lower educational levels of parents were associated with higher rates of hearing loss.

The effect of a poor environment on intellectual function has been dramatically demonstrated by the studies of Heber and Garber (1970) in Milwaukee. These authors conducted a survey on the IQs of slum-dwelling children, revealing that the children of mothers with IQs below 80 show a progressive decline in mean intelligence as age increases. Furthermore, the survey data showed that the lower the maternal IQ, the lower the child's IQ tended to be. Heber and Garber hypothesized that the mentally retarded mother in the slums creates a social deprivation which predetermines the child's IQ.

Heber and Garber's study is a classic reference for all disciplines. It points the way not only to preventive measures for mental retardation but to possible massive intervention in other areas. What would be the effects on ultimate ear disease if large scale medical treatment were applied to all slum children in infancy? What would be the result if the mothers were taught to apply good aural hygiene to their infants? What effect would good nutrition have on these children? It follows that making something happen in all areas of handicapping conditions is a good thing, devoutly to be sought.

EAR DISEASE IN NATIVE AMERICANS

Otitis media has been one of the most serious health problem among the native American Indian and Eskimo population of North America. Much effort and money has been expended over the past years to gain control over the widespread problems of alcoholism and tuberculosis among American Indians. The success in these health problems, however, brought to light a new health problem—otologic disease and hearing impairment. This fact was cited in the President's Message on Indian Affairs, July 8, 1970, when the four major health problems were listed in order as (1) otitis media, (2) mental health, (3) alcoholism, and (4) maternal and child care.

Health problems are readily evident among native American populations because of their poor home conditions, harsh physical and psychological environment, inadequate water facilities, crowded living conditions, unsanitary waste disposal, inadequate refrigeration, nonexistent insect control, and poor nutrition. With federal financial support great strides in the health care for American Indians and native Alaskans are being made. Cultural barriers, poverty, poor transportation, and lack of education about issues continue to make solutions to health problems more difficult.

Hearing Impairment in Eskimos

As early as 1957 it was reported that the prevalence of active otitis media in Alaskan native children was as high as 17% (Hayman and Kester). In fact, ear disease in Eskimo children is such a common occurrence most Alaskan native parents do not consider otorrhea to be a disease (Maynard, 1969; Maynard et al., 1972). Brody (1964, 1965) reported a study in which 31% of an Eskimo village population had at least one episode of draining ears within the evaluation year, with two thirds of the ear disease group indicating more than one episode of otorrhea. He indicated that ear pathology in Eskimos is established by the age of 2 years, and those children who by age 2 did not have draining ears were unlikely to develop ear pathology.

Several additional studies on Eskimo populations have been published confirming the extraordinary high incidence of middle ear disease. D. Reed et al. (1967) followed 378 Eskimo children during their first 4 years after birth. They reported that the *frequency* of episodes had more influence on the degree of hearing impairment than did the age of onset of the initial otorrhea episode. Ling et al. (1969) examined 525 children and adults in a single village and found active ear disease present in 30.8% of the group. Reed and Dunn (1970) found that 43% of 641 Eskimo children experienced 532 episodes of otitis media, with the highest incidence occurring in children less than 2 years of age. More recently, Kaplan et al. (1973) reported that 38% of a group of Eskimo children had one or more bouts of otorrhea prior to age 1, and 76% of these children commonly ex-

perienced otorrhea when they were subsequently evaluated at 7–10 years of age.

Although impedance screening is reportedly in wide use in Alaska, only a few reports have been published (Harker and Van Wagoner, 1974, 1976). In one study (Van Wagoner and Chun, 1974), more than 700 Southeast Alaskan school-aged children, with 35 of the children under the age of 2 years, were evaluated with pure tone audiometry, otoscopy, and an "abbreviated" impedance technique. Pure tone results could not be obtained on approximately 30% of the group because of their young age; however, impedance results were obtained on all but 1.3% of the group. Some 10% of the children passed the hearing screening but failed the impedance test. It was concluded that ". . . so far as to say in young children, if only one test were available, impedance testing would be preferred."

Ear Disease in American Indians

Review of publications dealing with the incidence of ear disease in various American Indian populations also shows a high percentage of middle ear disorders. Johnson in 1967 reported the incidence of chronic otitis media in the Navajo population to be 12 to 15 times higher than found in Caucasian Americans.

Jaffe (1968) published a widely referenced article concerning the incidence of ear diseases of all types in the Navajo. Aural atresia was found in 58 of 60,000 individuals. Chronic suppurative otitis media was the most common Navajo otologic disease with 4.2% central perforations in 2,000 patients. Jaffe cites inbreeding among the Navajos as a major cause of frequently seen bifid uvula and aural atresias. One hundred years ago there were only 5,000 Navajos, while current Navajo population is estimated at between 125,000 to 150,000.

Other reports have been published on various American Indian tribes (Zonis, 1968, 1970; Gregg et al., 1970; Rossi, 1972; Axelsson and Lewis, 1974; Lewis, 1975;

McCandless, 1975; Johnson and Watrous, 1978).

THEORIES OF HEARING SCREENING

Let us look first at some theories of screening and how they relate to hearing conservation programs. Then we will describe what appear at present to be the most efficacious methods for accomplishing the identification of hearing defects. Two aspects of screening philosophy are relevant to us: (1) the selection of the disorder or disease which should be screened and (2) the evaluation of the screening procedures.

Which Diseases Should Be Screened?

The first question that must be asked is whether a certain disease should be screened. Certain criteria should be applied to the selection of disorders to screen: (Frankenburg, 1976; North, 1976).

Occurrence Frequent Enough or Consequence Serious Enough to Warrant Mass Screening. How prevalent is the disease in the population to be screened? Some balancing of cost with the numbers of children who have the disease must be made. Cunningham (1970) has stated: "From the point of view of a public health program, in order to justify a mass screening program, the condition must be reasonably frequent or if rare it must have serious consequences if not detected." It is estimated that only 1 in 750 children will have some degree of congenital deafness at birth, but, at the age of 2 years, 1 in 3 children will have at least mild hearing losses from ear disease.

In the case of hearing, screening for congenital deafness can be justified on the basis of its severity and resultant disastrous consequences; the screening of the older child can be justified on the basis of numbers alone, as well as on consequences.

The comparison of the yields of various newborn screening programs is shown in Table 7.1 and illustrates the relative status of hearing screening. Not only does hearing screening yield the highest returns among

Table 7.1.
Yield in Screening Tests[a]

Disease Screened	Yield
Phenylketonuria	1 in 15,000 births
Combined immunodeficiency disease	25 in 3 million births
Maple syrup urine disease	1 in 300,000 births
Neonatal hyperthyroidism	1 in 6,000 births
Neonatal hearing screening, high risk register	1 in 750 births

[a] From M. Downs: *Speech, Language and Hearing*, p. 985, edited by N. J. Lass et al. W. B. Saunders, Philadelphia, 1982b, 1983.

these diseases, but it also is more productive of results once the problem is identified. We know that, when phenylketonuria is identified, intervention may not completely alleviate the retardation. And if a child is falsely identified as having phenylketonuria and treated, serious harm can result. Only in maple syrup urine disease and in hearing problems are the results certainly advantageous and the treatment nonharmful if properly applied.

Amenability to Treatment or Prevention That Will Forestall or Change the Expected Outcome. What would be the prognosis for the individual if treatment is instituted, and also if it is not instituted? It perhaps matters little if such a disorder as color blindness is detected early, as no treatment will change it. But the tragic consequences of untreated hearing losses are all too commonly seen: the complete lack of speech or language development at ages when these functions should be well implanted; the deterioration of the parent-child relationship into subtle rejection or bewildered overprotection; and personality deviations of a wide variety, ranging from autistic-like withdrawal to hyperactivity and acting out.

So long as a disease state can be accurately identified, its severity should at the very least be lessened by treatment if we are to regard mandatory screening as a profitable endeavor. The detection and treatment of phenylketonuria may result in the amelioration of the resultant mental retardation, but treatment may be harmful if applied to a child inaccurately designated as symptomatic (Cooper, 1967). Treatment is not always an unmixed blessing.

There is no question that the sequelae of a true hearing loss can be ameliorated if the disorder is given proper treatment. Note, however, the words *true* hearing loss and *proper* treatment, for herein lies the essence of accountability for the audiologist. If a child were falsely labeled as having a hearing loss and were treated with a hearing aid, there is some possibility that noise-induced damage to the ear would result. There perhaps would be little chance of damage, but we cannot evade the possibility.

Availability of Facilities for Diagnosis and Treatment. If a child is identified as being a suspect for a disorder, can he be properly assessed and treated, without too much expenditure of cost and effort? This question largely concerns the state of the art and the number of trained professionals that can be depended upon to produce accurate evaluations and remediation for the child. If 1-year-old Johnny is found in a rural area to have profound deafness, there may not be a facility for his diagnosis and training for hundreds of miles. Or, it can be argued that even in a big city the facilities available may be viewed with a jaundiced eye by critical fellow professionals. When these situations occur—and they doubtless do—can we justify screening for the disorder in that location? The concerned professional must answer YES to that question. Yes, we should screen in rural areas and, when a child is suspect, insist that some agency provide the necessary funds for his travel and follow-up in a larger city center. Yes, we should screen in the poorly staffed Big City, and with a suspect child we should challenge the professionals to attain the requisite skills. Unless we invoke the law of supply and demand, we will never have enough professionals to fill these supremely

urgent needs. The skills are known; they need only to be transmitted to more people.

Cost of Screening Reasonably Commensurate with Benefits to the Individual. Is the screening equipment costly to purchase and to keep up? Do the personnel administering the screening tests require expensive training or high level salaries? We are hard-put to designate any costs as excessive where the health and welfare of many individuals are at stake, but there are sometimes limitations to the funds available in any area. Fortunately, most of the audiometric equipment necessary to screen at any age ranges from $350.00 to $1500.00. Such equipment can continue to be used for long periods of time and for many thousands of tests before any repair or calibration is required. And, as the trend toward nonprofessional aides continues, the cost of screeners continues to decrease.

Cooper et al. (1975) published data regarding efficiency and cost of school screening programs. They reported that the ongoing rate for audiometric screening was about five minutes per student, or 12 students per hour. They also reported data for impedance screening to be about 1.1 min per child or 21 children per hour. Cooper and his associates determined cost of their screening program by establishing an index of cost per accurate referral of failures. To compute the cost per accurate referral, the following formula was developed:

$$\text{Cost/child} = \frac{S}{R} + \frac{C + (M \times L)}{(N \times L)}$$

S = salary of person screening, in dollars per hour
R = screening rate in children per hour
C = cost of equipment in dollars
M = annual maintenance cost of equipment in dollars
L = lifetime of the equipment in years
N = number of children screened per year.

Based on this formula, these authors reported that the cost per child (based on 1000 children) was 43¢ for audiometric screening and 46¢ for impedance screening. The cost per accurate referral was considerably different between the two techniques since audiometry, per se, is not as accurate as impedance measurements in the identification of medical otologic problems. Their cost per accurate referral was $9.62 for audiometric screening, and impedance screening was only $2.77 per 1000 children.

Queen et al. (1981) used the Cooper formula to evaluate their impedance screening program in Kansas City, Missouri. They reported a cost of 0.57¢ per child for impedance screening. Actually they felt this cost may have been overestimated because they did not use supportive personnel to conduct the screening, and they experienced unexpected equipment problems during their screening project.

The cost analysis of screening the infant and preschool population also varies, but in no case would it be considered to be unfeasible when compared with the benefits accrued, even expressed in terms of the manhour economics (see Chapter 1).

A Screening Tool That Validly Differentiates the Disease from Nondisease. Many authors have addressed themselves to the question of the most dependable method for evaluating a screening tool. A discussion of this question follows in the next section. The conclusion is that screening techniques for hearing have reached a higher statistical validity than many of the health screening procedures.

Acceptance by the Public. Once the adequacy of the method has been established, the only remaining problem is to obtain professional and lay acceptance of the procedure. If the procedure is worthy of support, the first requirement is to obtain the approval and endorsement of the medical community. When that has been secured, a program of educating the public can be instituted. Only when widespread acceptance is obtained can the screening program be initiated.

Selection and Evaluation of the Screening Procedure

The success of a screening program depends largely on the effectiveness of the measures used to identify a suspect. The validity of a screening process is poor if it misses many of those who ultimately turn out to have abnormal findings in the function studied. If the process tags as abnormal large numbers of individuals who are actually normal, it is not economical as to time and effort and may cause anxiety to many. It is therefore necessary to set up rigid criteria for the screening procedure in order to select the one which is most feasible.

Reliability. Reliability refers to the reproducibility of the results obtained. Can the procedure be replicated by anyone else who follows the same directions? Several types of reliability may be considered.

Inter-test Reliability. The procedure used must be subjected to repeated tests on the same individual and on different samples of individuals. Does it give the same results when the same individual is tested several times? Does it give comparable results on different groups when the individuals are tested separately? If we test the hearing of a number of school children in the same way three times on three different occasions and obtain significantly different results each time, the instrument used has no test-retest reliability. If we divide our school children into two groups and test each separately, the test results should not vary significantly between groups.

Tester Reliability. The personnel administering the test should be uniformly expert so that two people administering the same test to the same child will obtain similar scores. This requirement is quite different from that of co-positivity and negativity, discussed below, which pits the trained technician against an acknowledged expert. In audiometric screening it means that two testers can screen the same child independently and report similar responses. Brooks (1973) has demonstrated that great discrepancies can exist between two testers' results on the same child.

Function Reliability. All characteristics or functions that are being measured, and their dependent states, should be consistently normal or abnormal, and should not change from moment-to-moment or day-to-day. The presence of the rubella virus in an infant, for example, will not vary over fairly long periods of time, so that the titer test for this virus can be depended upon to measure the real presence or absence of the virus. On the other hand, when one tests the hearing of newborn infants, the state of the infant, on which a response directly depends, can vary from moment-to-moment.

Co-positivity and Co-negativity in Tester and Test. Often a screening test is evaluated by comparing it with a criterion test considered to be, but not known to be infallible. Or a tester may be evaluated by comparing his screening results with those of a presumed expert. Co-positivity is the extent to which the test agrees with the criterion test in identifying positives; co-negativity is the agreement in identifying negatives. We might, for example, compare the efficiency of a criterion test for hearing that uses speech signals, with the efficiency of a fixed intensity pure tone screening test for which accuracy in identifying hearing loss is not known. An expert tester may be selected to conduct the criterion test. Unfortunately, both the criterion speech test and the expert tester may be in error in determining who is abnormal and who is not. On the other hand, however, if the results of the criterion test by an expert have been validated against a standard diagnostic test conducted by a professional, then we must assume they can be utilized in comparing results with those of the screening test. The ideal would be to compare both the screening tests and the speech test results directly with the diagnostic tests by the professional, thus avoiding the intermediate stage.

Sensitivity and Specificity. The validity of an audiometric screening test for hearing is determined first by the agreement between the rating of a child as positive (abnormal) on the screening test and his rating as positive on the diagnostic threshold test, and second by the agreement between the screening test's classification of a child as negative (normal) and

the threshold diagnostic test's designation of him as normal. According to public health terminology (Thorner and Remein, 1967), the accuracy of a screening test in correctly identifying the positive (abnormal) subjects is called *sensitivity*; its accuracy in classifying correctly the negative, or normal, subjects is called *specificity*. Inasmuch as formulations around these terms are in widespread use in the general health areas, we should apply them to our field of screening hearing.

The method of formulating sensitivity and specificity is shown in Table 7.2. Dr. William Frankenburg, co-author of the Denver Developmental Screening Test describes the use of this table:

Perfect agreement between the screening test in the identification of all of the diseased is achieved if a or $(a + b)$ equals $(a + c)$. In such a situation, no diseased subjects would be classified as negative with the screening test, thus c would equal 0. The accuracy of a screening test in correctly identifying all of the diseased subjects is termed sensitivity and is calculated as a percentage by utilizing the formula $a/(a + c) \times 100$. Since it is possible to correctly identify all of the diseased subjects by classifying all of the subjects with positive results as diseased, one must also determine the accuracy of the test in correctly identifying the nondiseased subjects. A perfect agreement between a test and the diagnosis also exists if use of the test makes it possible to classify all non-diseased subjects as negative. To meet this situation, d or $(c + d)$ would have to equal $(b + d)$. Specificity, the

Table 7.2.
Calculation of Sensitivity and Specificity[a]

Screen Test	Diseased	Non-diseased	
Positive	a	b	
Negative	c	d	
	$a + c$	$b + d$	$a + b + c + d$

[a] Sensitivity: Percent of diseased designated positive with screen test $a/(a + c)$.

Specificity: Percent of nondiseased designated negative with screen test $d/(b + d)$.

False positive = b; false negative = c.

Results are random if sensitivity = % positive $a/(a + c) = (a + b)/(a + b + c + d)$.

Results are random if sensitivity + specificity = 100%.

Note: The same computations are made for co-positivity and co-negativity.

second type of test validity, is the agreement between the test in classifying subjects negative and the diagnosis in classifying the same subjects as non-diseased. Specificity is calculated by the formula $d/(b + d) \times 100$. From W. Frankenburg: Evaluation of screening procedures. In *Earlier Recognition of Handicapping Conditions in Childhood,* pp. 45–46, University of California School of Public Health, Berkeley, 1970.)

Relationship between Sensitivity and Specificity. "The relationship between sensitivity and specificity can be represented by two curves, as shown in Figure 7.1. Unfortunately, most biological phenomena have considerable overlap between the nondiseased and diseased subjects. The oversimplified diagram would suggest that designating all subjects to the right of cutting point *A* as abnormal would achieve 100% sensitivity but less than 100% specificity, because the nondiseased subjects with levels between cutting point *A* and cutting point *B* would mistakenly be classified as diseased. Similarly the use of cutting point *B* would result in 100% specificity since the diseased subjects in the area

between the two curves would incorrectly be classified as negative. Thus, when the diseased and nondiseased subjects overlap on a scale it will be impossible to achieve both 100% sensitivity and 100% specificity. Furthermore, the movement of the cutting point to achieve greater sensitivity will invariably result in less specificity; the reverse also holds true. In addition, as the sensitivity is increased there will generally be more overdiagnosis and as the specificity is increased there will be a greater amount of underdiagnosis." (Frankenburg, 1970).

So far as school hearing screening is concerned, the evaluation of the test depends on the selection of the disorder to screen. Melnick et al. (1964) infer that we should screen for evidence of past or present ear disease, and they demonstrate that for this goal the pure tone screening test, and even threshold audiometry, are inadequate. On the other hand, we have assumed that if we set as our goal the identification of educationally handicapping hearing loss, as Downs et al. (1965) suggest, then the pure tone screening test is acceptable. We now

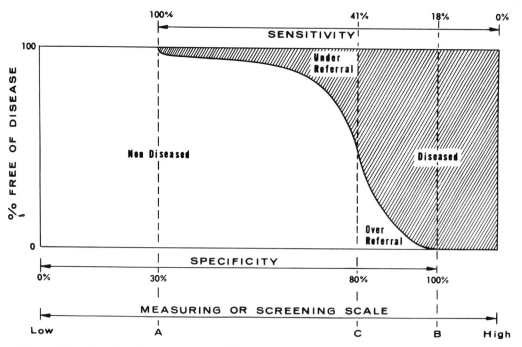

Figure 7.1. Relationship between sensitivity and specificity and overreferral and underreferral.

know that even if the recommended minimal level of 20 dB is used as the screening criterion, it will miss large numbers of children with hearing levels of 15–20 dB—levels that are handicapping to the child's educational progress (see Chapter 1).

An examination of the study by Melnick et al. shows a meticulous survey of pure tone screening, otoscopic examinations, and threshold audiometric tests on 860 school children. It is important to look first at the agreement that was found between the pure tone screening test and the diagnostic threshold pure tone test. Keeping in mind that, when we use a hearing screening test our logical goal is to find a hearing disorder for which a threshold test is diagnostic, Table 7.3 shows the calculated specificity and sensitivity.

The sensitivity of 85% indicates that there is reasonable agreement between the screening test and the threshold test in classifying abnormal hearing, but it means that 21 of 143 children with reduced hearing were not properly identified. Although this is not an ideal situation, it may be satisfactory when one considers cost efficiency factors. This study represents the only one that has compared both threshold and pure tone screening on a large group of children who have also been given otoscopic examinations, and it causes us to examine more closely the routine tests we have so long taken for granted. All that we can say for the screening test is that it has fairly reasonable threshold correspondence with the diagnostic test.

However, when we compare the otoscopic findings in this study with the threshold audiometric tests, a great discrepancy appears, as shown in Table 7.4. It is evident that although the specificity is high for the threshold test, the sensitivity is too low to be acceptable: 90 of 127 otoscopically abnormal children were passed by the threshold test. Such under-referral completely obviates the usefulness of the test if what we are looking for is past or present ear disease.

The obverse of the coin is to treat the threshold audiometric tests as the validation tests—which they well can be considered if we agree that we are looking for hearing loss. When we compare these tests in the study by Melnick et al. against the otoscopic findings, a different picture emerges, as seen in Table 7.5. It is completely valid to do this in order to discover whether otoscopic examinations may miss sensorineural losses, which are significant objectives in any screening program.

These results, of course, approach randomness, indicating that otoscopic examinations in no way identify the important sensorineural losses; 78 children with significant hearing losses were not identified by the otoscopic examinations.

Table 7.4.
Otoscopic Findings[a]

Threshold	Diseased	Non-diseased	Total
Positive	37	78	115
Negative	90	532	622
Total	127	610	737

[a] Sensitivity: 37 ÷ 127 = 29%; specificity: 532 ÷ 610 = 87%.

Table 7.3.
Threshold Hearing Test[a]

Screen Test	Diseased	Non-diseased	Total
Positive	122	13	135
Negative	21	704	725
Total	143	717	860

[a] Sensitivity: 122 ÷ 143 = 85% (overreferrals = 122/13 = 10%).
Specificity: 704 ÷ 717 = 98% (underreferrals = 21/704 = 0.03%).

Table 7.5.
Threshold Tests (as Validation)[a]

Otoscopic (as Screen)	Abnormal	Normal	Total
Positive	37	90	127
Negative	78	532	610
Total	115	622	737

[a] Sensitivity: 37 ÷ 115 = 32%; specificity: 532 ÷ 622 = 86%.

GOALS AND METHODS AT BIRTH

Goals

It is the urgency of securing language input for the infant that makes it mandatory for any congenital hearing loss to be detected at birth whether it is a severe or a mild loss. Even the slight loss due to otitis media has been shown to cause auditory language learning problems if it occurs in the first 2 years of life. So otitis media will be one of the pathologies sought, in addition to the embryologic-related pathologies, the genetic pathologies, and the congenital acquired pathologies. We cannot settle for any lesser goal than detection of hearing loss in the first months of life, nor for any lesser targets than mild as well as severe congenital hearing losses. In their description of a community-based high risk register for hearing loss, Fitch et al. (1982) state that the greater value of such programs may lie in the identification of increased numbers of children with mild-to-moderate conductive losses which are amenable to treatment.

Methods of Screening at Birth

In 1969 a National Committee was formed of representatives from the Academy of Pediatrics, the Academy of Ophthalmology and Otolaryngology and the American Speech-Language-Hearing Association, charged with making recommendations for Newborn Infant Hearing Screening. This Joint Committee first addressed itself to the use of behavioral tests of screening in the nursery, which had been proposed and described by Downs and Sterritt (1964), Downs and Hemenway (1969), and Mencher (1974). Critiques by such careful researchers as Goldstein and Tait (1971) and Ling et al. (1970) were considered, and the Committee issued a statement which did not recommend mass behavioral screening of infants although it urged further research.

The Committee then addressed itself to the possibilities for screening inherent in a high risk register. This means that the record of each infant should be examined to see whether there is any history or physical finding that would give a high probability of hearing loss. Richards and Roberts (1967) reported that a high risk register, to be efficient, should identify a disease that is 14 times more prevalent in the register than in the general population.

The recommendations for a high risk register have been further buttressed by a national Maternal and Child Health Conference that delineated Guidelines for Early Screening (Conference on Hearing Screening Services, 1977). The conference reaffirmed the Joint Committee's program, and made some supplementary suggestions:

1. That audiological follow-up of the high risk infants be made "as soon as possible, but certainly by 7 months"
2. That the mother-child relationship in the first 4 months be safeguarded by education and careful information
3. That informed consent be obtained
4. That information on what to look for in later infancy be given
5. That the development and implementation of adequate identification and diagnostic procedures related to hearing impairments should be undertaken by Public Health Agencies.

Identification and Follow-up in Infant Screening

The effectiveness of any screening program is only as good as the subsequent follow-up program (McFarland et al., 1980). If experienced audiologists are unavailable, or if parents have difficulty gaining access to audiologic assistance, hearing-impaired babies may not receive the necessary follow-up and intervention. The philosophical question remains, who is responsible for follow-up, the parents or the institution? Who should bear the financial burden of further evaluation, the parents or the institution when the baby is called back for additional testing?

Individuals involved in infant screening must also be concerned about the ever-present possibility of progressive sensorineural hearing loss. When high risk babies pass the initial screening test and are later determined to have hearing loss, the question always remains, did the screening test miss this baby or did the hearing loss occur after the hearing screen was applied (Simmons, 1980a)? Simmons argues that genetic delayed-onset hearing losses are probably very rare, and that nearly all, if not all, sensorineural hearing losses in very young children occur before they are discharged from the newborn nursery.

An interesting point can be made by examining reported age of *detection* of hearing loss against age of *confirmation* of hearing loss. Bergstrom (1976) called the situation disgraceful in a referral clinic that hearing loss in a severely to profoundly deaf child is initially suspected, on the average, at age 10 months, detected at age 21 months, and training and amplification first begun at 27 months of age. In 1977, Jones and Simmons published a table showing that the age of suspicion of deafness with 24 infants screened with the Crib-o-gram was approximately 42 days; age of confirmation of hearing loss in these infants was nearly 13 months. Statistics reported in the previous edition of this textbook (1978), based on behavioral infant screening performed at Colorado General Hospital between 1972 and 1976, indicated that the average time of *confirmation* of hearing loss and the beginning of habilitation procedures in these youngsters was 6.5 months. It should be noted that these data all preceded the use of auditory evoked response as a technique to validate hearing loss in infants.

Shah et al. (1978) reviewed 200 questionnaires completed by parents of hearing-impaired youngsters in Toronto. Nearly half of the parents reported that they experienced difficulties and prolonged delays in reaching a firm diagnosis of hearing impairment in their children. Although the mean age of suspicion of hearing loss was 16 months of age, the average additional delay until audiological assessment was completed was 11.5 months, with a range between 0 and 60 months! The parents viewed the chief obstacles as the primary

care physician's unwillingness to accept the parent's opinions; the failure of these physicians to perform simple hearing screening tests; and finally, the reluctance of the physicians to arrange for referral of the child for audiological evaluation. The detection of the child's hearing problem was found to depend on the astuteness and insistence of the parents as well as the alertness of their physicians.

With diligent effort these time lags may be reduced. Data from the University of Colorado Medical Center for the years 1976–1979 show the average suspected age of hearing loss to be 2.1 months, while the age of confirmation of hearing loss was 5 months.

More recently, Simmons (1980b) reviewed the records of 42 babies whose average age of first hearing aid purchase was 22 months. While this statistic alone is not surprising, 83% of these babies were suspects for deafness before they were discharged from the newborn nursery, and 43% of those who were not newborn suspects failed their initial hearing test by 11 months of age.

In his report, Simmons carefully analyzes what happened to these 42 babies since the initial suspicion of deafness and the eventual diagnosis and habilitation. His review of the referral processes and professional judgments is worthwhile reading for all clinicians faced with decision-making responsibilities. His data indicate that the problem is generally not in the audiologist's diagnosis, but in such hearing losses escaping the notice of parents and physicians. Although many of the babies had other medical problems manifested in delayed development of motor skills and moderate-to-severe visual impairments, auditory evoked response testing was conducted in only a few of the babies.

The pattern of delays between the recommendation and the fitting of a hearing aid seemed to be threefold: (1) referral back to the physician for ear examinations and medical clearances, then long, silent intervals without action; (2) babies with multiple physical and developmental problems in which hearing was only part of the total concern of the parents; and (3) parental disbelief or avoidance of the fact that their child had an important hearing loss.

Since the intent of an infant hearing screening program is to identify and habilitate deaf children as early as possible, programs must build in strict time schedules for action following the identification of an infant suspected to have hearing loss. Simmons recommends that any child failing a hearing screen be retested at least once within 2 weeks. A child then suspected of hearing loss should be referred for a formal hearing evaluation, not more than 2 weeks hence, and a final opinion on hearing status should be forthcoming within 6 weeks of the initial hearing screen. A thorough medical examination, impedance audiometry and, if question still exists about the hearing, an auditory brainstem evoked response (ABR) evaluation is a necessity. Even under this rigid time regime, the typical child who is suspect at birth, rescreened at 7 months when behavioral responses are more obvious, will still perhaps require 4 additional months before habilitation is in full swing.

James Jerger of Baylor School of Medicine relates that the clinical audiologist can make two mistakes when counseling parents of an infant suspected to have hearing loss; however, one of the mistakes has considerably more serious consequences than the other mistake. The lesser of the two mistakes is for the audiologist to decide that the infant is deaf—and then determine subsequently that the infant has normal hearing. An embarrassing mistake to be sure, but probably every experienced clinician has fallen prey to this error, but the final outcome of normal hearing is a great relief to all involved with the infant.

The more serious mistake, however, is devastating to the infant in question. In this grave error, the clinician informs the parent that their baby has normal hearing—when in fact the infant has severe-to-profound hearing loss. In this situation, the parent assumes with confidence that the baby hears normally, and by the time the mistake is identified, maximum habilitation may never be achieved.

Armed with knowledge about the potential for these two mistakes in infant hearing assessment, the audiologist must practice extreme care in pronouncing an infant to have normal hearing. When in doubt, it behooves the clinician to assume the infant has a hearing problem until proved otherwise. The audiologist is still the best professional to serve as an advocate for the child, and whose ultimate responsibility is to provide the maximum in support of the infant under evaluation.

PROCEDURES FOR A HIGH RISK REGISTER

WHO Should Conduct Infant Hearing Screening?

Hearing screening is a task for a team of professionals: pediatricians, otolaryngologists, audiologists, nurses, and house staff. Each has his role in the program, but it should be remembered that data collection is a vital part of a project, and therefore the Public Health Agency in the area should be a partner in the activity.

HOW Should Infant Screening Be Done?

INFANT HEARING SCREENING GUIDELINES

In 1972 the Joint Committee on Infant Hearing Screening recommended screening all newborns by means of five criteria to identify infants at risk for hearing impairment and suggested follow-up audiological evaluation of these infants until accurate assessments of hearing could be made. Since the incidence of moderate-to-profound hearing loss in the at risk infant group is 2.5–5.0%, acoustic testing of this group is warranted. Acoustic testing of *all* newborn infants has a high incidence of false-positive and false-negative results and is *not* universally recommended at the present time.

The present Joint Committee represents four professional associations including the Academy of Otolaryngology-Head and Neck, the Academy of Pediatrics, the American Nurses Association, and the American Speech-Language-Hearing Association. The Joint Committee held a meeting in 1982 to propose a new position statement relevant to the current practices of identifying the hearing-impaired infant (birth to one year of age).

I. Identification

The 1982 recommended factors that identify those infants who are AT RISK for having hearing impairment includes the following:

   A. *Risk Criteria*
   1. A family history of childhood hearing impairment.
   2. Congenital perinatal infection (e.g., cytomegalovirus, rubella, herpes, toxoplasmosis, syphilis).
   3. Anatomic malformations involving the head or neck (e.g., dysmorphic appearance, including syndromal and nonsyndromal abnormalities of the pinna).
   4. Birthweight less than 1500 g.
   5. Hyperbilirubinemia at level exceeding indications for exchange transfusion.
   6. Bacterial meningitis, especially *Haemophilus influenzae*.
   7. Severe asphyxia which may include infants with Apgar scores of 0–3 or infants who fail to institute spontaneous respiration by 10 minutes and infants with hypotonia persisting to 2 hours of age.

   B. *Screening.* The hearing of infants who manifest any item on the list of risk criteria should be screened under supervision of an audiologist, preferably prior to 3 months of age, but not later than 6 months after birth. The initial screening should include the observation of behavioral or electrophysiological response to sound. If consistent electrophysiological or behavioral responses are detected at appropriate sound levels, then the screening process will be considered complete except in those cases where there is a possibility of a progressive hearing loss, e.g. delayed onset, degenerative disease, or intrauterine infections. If results of an initial screening of an infant manifesting any risk criteria are equivocal, then the infant should be referred for audiological diagnosis testing.

II. Diagnosis

The Committee recommends that a diagnostic evaluation of an infant under six months of age include:

   A. *General Physical Examination and History Including*
   1. Examination of the head and neck.
   2. Otoscopy or otomicroscopy.
   3. Identification of relevant physical abnormalities.
   4. Laboratory tests such as urinalysis and TORCH (toxoplasmosis, rubella, cytomegalovirus, herpes, syphilis).

   B. *Comprehensive Audiological Evaluation*
   1. Behavioral history.
   2. Behavioral observation audiometry.
   3. Testing of auditory evoked potentials if indicated.

After the age of 6 months the following are also recommended:
   1. Communication skills evaluation.
   2. Acoustic immitance measures.
   3. Selected tests of development.

For infants at any age, the Committee suggests the following when indicated:
   1. Audiograms of parents and siblings.
   2. Thyroid function tests.
   3. Polytomography of middle and inner ears.
   4. Electrocardiograms.
   5. Chromosomal study.

6. Tests for mucopolysaccharidosis.
7. Ophthalmological assessment.
8. Vestibular tests.

III. Management.

The Committee recognizes that habilitation of the hearing-impaired infant may begin while the diagnostic evaluation is in process. The Committee recommends, however, that whenever possible, the diagnostic process should be completed and habilitation begun by the age of 6 months. Services to the hearing-impaired infant under 6 months of age include:

A. Otologic Management
1. Reevaluation.
2. Treatment.

B. Audiologic Management
1. Ongoing audiological assessment.
2. Selection of hearing aid(s).
3. Family counseling.

C. Educational Management
1. Formulation of an individualized educational plan.
2. Information about the implications of hearing impairment.

D. Mental Health Support. Frequently, the hearing-impaired infant may have additional handicapping conditions which require additional services such as physical therapy or neurological evaluation. Parents may need genetic counseling.

After the age of 6 months, the hearing-impaired infant becomes easier to manage in a habilitation plan but s/he will require the services listed above.

IV. Application of High Risk Register

The detailed procedures that are used in identifying the infants in the high risk categories are as follows:

A. Identification Through Query of the Mother. The questions used in the mother's interview are shown in Table 7.6. Although the questions may be easily asked verbally, the form may also be used as a written questionnaire. The mother's answers are recorded on the form by the interviewer, and serve as an important initial sort for the high risk register.

This questionnaire should be given to all new mothers in the hospital at some time after the baby is born. It should be prefaced with an explanation that "We are conducting a survey of all the babies born in this hospital, to see how many families have certain hearing problems. We would appreciate your help in this survey. There is nothing to worry about if you answer yes to any of the questions, so do the best you can with them."

B. Identification Through Visual Observations of the Infant. Cleft Lip or Palate, Including Submucous Cleft. The cleft lip is an immediately observable malformation, but cleft palate—and particularly submucous cleft—will be searched for by a physician. Submucous cleft has been found to be associated with congenital middle ear anomalies, so it is important that the palate be carefully examined.

A bifid uvula always accompanies submucous cleft, but the cleft may be present without this symptom. Palpation of the juncture between the soft and hard palate will reveal a notch in the bony part.

Malformations of the Ears. Abnormal pinnae may be obvious, but they also can be very subtle. Atresia, with partial formation of the pinna, or a small tab of skin where the pinna should be, are easily observed. Often however, the ears are merely low-set, or they may not have complete formation of helix, antihelix, tragus, or antitragus. A small tab of skin may occur in front of the pinna, on the cheek, with an otherwise normal-looking ear. Sometimes these symptoms are accompanied by cranial malformations of the nose, eye orbits, maxillae, or cranial bones, so any oddlooking feature may be a clue (Black et al., 1971a).

C. Identification Through Search of the Medical Records and Physical Examination. Whoever is assigned to examine the mothers' and infants' medical

Table 7.6.
Mother's Interview

MOTHER'S NAME:_____

ROOM NO.:_____

1. Do you know any of the baby's relatives who now have a hearing loss which started before the age of five? Think hard about all of your family and the baby's father's family . . . .

   Yes _____ No _____

   A. In no, proceed to question No. 2.

   B. If yes, ask the following:

      (1) Who were they? (relationship to baby)

         (A)._____ (B)._____ (C)._____

      (2) Do you know what caused the loss? . . . .

         Yes _____ No _____

         (A)._____ (B)._____ (C)._____

      (3) What makes you think the onset of the hearing loss was before age five?

         (A)._____ (B)._____ (C)._____

      (4) Did he/she wear a hearing aid before age five? . . (A) _____ (B) _____ (C) _____

         Does he/she still wear an aid? . . . . (A) _____ (B) _____ (C) _____

      (5) Did he/she attend a special school for the deaf? . (A) _____ (B) _____ (C) _____

         Did the person attend public school? . . . . (A) _____ (B) _____ (C) _____

      (6) Did he/she have a speech problem? . . . . (A) _____ (B) _____ (C) _____

2. During your pregnancy, did you have 3-day measles, German measles, rubella, or a rash with a fever? . . . . Yes_____ No_____

   WHEN: 1st 3 mo._____ Middle 3 mo._____ Last 3 mo._____

3. During your pregnancy, were you around anyone who had 3-day measles, German measles, rubella, or a rash with fever? . . . . Yes_____ No_____

   WHEN: 1st 3 mo._____ Middle 3 mo._____ Last 3 mo._____

4. Do you have any reason to be concerned about your baby's hearing? . . . .

   Yes_____ No_____

   If yes, why?_____

5. What pediatrician or clinic will be caring for your baby when he/she leaves the hospital? _____

   _____

   Approximate location_____

6. Nearest relative or friend: Name:_____

   Address:_____

   Phone:_____

Table 7.7.
Chart Review

	MOTHER'S ROOM NO._____	
	BABY'S NAME:_____	
	BABY'S HOSP. NO.:_____	
	BIRTHDATE:_____ SEX:_____	
	DISCHARGE DATE:_____	
	NURSERY LOCATION: MR. HR. NB	
	CARD PUNCHED: Yes No	

INFANT CHECK LIST

Mother's Name_____ Hosp. No._____ Father's Name_____
Home Address_____ City_____ State_____ Zip_____ Phone No._____
Pediatrician/Follow-up Clinic_____ Location_____
Birth Weight_____ Birth Length_____ Head Circumference_____ Gestation Age_____
Volunteer_____ Chart Review Dates_____ /_____ /_____

HIGH RISK CRITERIA

	YES	NO
1. Birth weight (B/W) less than 1500 g or/over 5000 g.		
2. Apgar 7 or less at 5 minutes. (Severe asphyxia—arterial pH level lower than 7.25, coma, seizures or the need for assisted ventilation.)		
3. Jaundice-hyperbilirubinemia: history of exchange transfusions. B/W: 1000–1250, 1251–1500, 1501–2000, 2001–2500, >2500 Bilirubin Level: 10.0, 13.0, 15.0, 17.0, 18.0		
4. Any of the following conditions: Skeletal and cranial defects _____, skull abnormalities _____, short neck _____, absent clavicles _____, dwarfism _____, malformations of extremities and digits _____, cleft lip _____, cleft palate (overt or submucous) _____, underdeveloped maxillae or mandible _____, external ear abnormalities _____.		
5. Family history of deafness.		
6. Rubella, rubella exposure.		
7. Cytomegalic inclusion disease (CMV), herpes, toxoplasmosis, syphilis, meningitis.		

REMARKS:

records must be well trained in interpreting doctors' abbreviations and terminology (as well as their handwriting). The items to be searched for are shown in Table 7.7.

BEHAVIORAL TESTS

The present authors feel that there is some virtue in using the arousal test in the newborn nursery, but most profitably for the high risk population. The advantage is that those infants with severe to profound deafness will be identified while still in the nursery. The Nova Scotia Conference on Early Identification of Hearing Loss (Mencher, 1976) also recommended that behavioral screening test would be employed, if desired, in the form of the arousal test and only in conjunction with a high risk register.

Arousal Test

The arousal test (Fig. 7.2) technique was standardized at the Winnipeg Conference as follows (Mencher and Gerber, 1981):

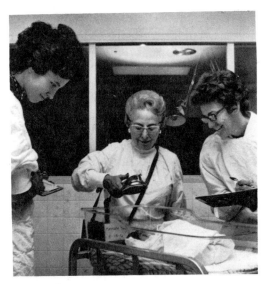

Figure 7.2. Trained volunteers performing the arousal test with sleeping newborns.

A. Instrumentation. It is recommended that a signal of 90 dB (SPL) or less be the criterion level for the test. A high frequency, narrow band signal is preferable. The instrument should be calibrated with a sound level meter so that the intensity at a given distance is known. Some form of calibration check should be available at least once a week.

B. Environment. A study should be made of the noise level of the nursery area, with a sound level meter. If the usual level in the nursery at the time testing will occur is greater than 60 dB, a quieter room should be found. The cribs can then be wheeled into this room one by one, and the babies tested.

C. Pretesting Observation of the Infants' State. The baby should not be tested until he is sleeping quietly. There are varying stages of the depth of sleep in babies this age, and some of the stages may not permit any response at all. The best state of sleep for testing purposes is a light sleep state, and this is the one most commonly seen. To test for this state, flip the eyelid slightly or touch the eyelid lightly with finger or a tongue blade; if there is a quiver of the eyelid, however small, the infant is in a light sleep state. Any other small movement of the body to this stimulus also indicates the light state. This fact should be recorded before testing proceeds.

A deep level of sleep is indicated if there is no movement of the eyelid or any part of the body in response to the flicking of the lash. This state is the second best for testing purposes, but the fact should be noted on the record form.

If the child appears to remain in one of these two stages of sleep, the testing can continue.

D. Presentation of Signal. The loudspeaker of the testing instrument should be placed at the predetermined distance from the infant's ear. The most accessible ear should be tested. A length of string or a stick attached to the loudspeaker can serve as a measuring device.

The signal button should be depressed for a 2-sec signal duration. The infant should be observed for no more than 3 sec following the end of the signal. Any activity after this length of time must be considered random, and cannot be recorded as a response.

E. Criteria for Response. *The only response that can be accepted is an arousal from sleep.* The acceptable criteria for an arousal response are: (1) opening of the eyes; (2) a stirring movement of the whole body, indicating arousal from sleep; and (3) a strong and immediate eye blink, followed by one of the above responses.

After the infant has quieted again, the signal should be presented two more times and the response (or lack of it) should be recorded.

Two credible responses must be seen and agreed upon by the observers before the infant is passed. If only one response out of the initial three trials can be observed to the high frequency signal, a broad band signal (white noise) at 90 dB can be used 3 times to obtain one more response that will confirm the first observed response. If a broad band signal is not available, the narrow band level can be increased to 100 dB.

F. Reporting to the Findings. One member of the team should have the responsibility of making up the list of high risk infants, of referring the critical high risk categories to an otoaudiologic center, and also of referring the positives from the standard high risk screening tests for otoaudiologic evaluation. The information from these lists should be reported to the local public health agency.

Provision should be made to report to the managing physicians the names of the infants who have been placed in the "at risk for deafness" category. Follow-up of these infants can be made by the hospital screening program personnel or by an audiology clinic, or by the public health agency, whichever is appropriate. In any case, the managing physicians of the well-baby clinic to which the child will be taken must be aware of their responsibility in screening the child further for hearing loss or referring to an agency that can do the screening, and then reporting this follow-up to the proper agency.

High Risk Factors for Deafness

The high risk register for deafness should be the basis of any infant hearing screening program. Knowledge of these factors is extremely helpful in eliciting history about children who are discovered to have hearing impairment. A wealth of information is available from studies of various aspects of the high risk register. The clinician should be familiar with this background since an infant with any of these factors in his/her neonatal history has an increased chance of having hearing impairment. Although the factors themselves are easily memorized, audiologists often overlook their significance or do not fully understand the medical implications of each category.

Accordingly, the following discussion presents material on each of the high risk categories. Note that the sequence of the factors is presented in a mnemonic order known as the ABCDs of high risk deafness.

A. Asphyxia. Asphyxia, or anoxia, is a condition in which there is a lack of oxygen and increased carbon dioxide in the blood and tissues. With the introduction of intensive care treatment for very sick babies has come increased skill and technology in resuscitation and mechanical breathing. Short spells without breathing (known as apneic attacks), however, are not uncommon during the neonatal period. Asphyxia may be the single most important factor causing developmental sequelae.

The clinical definition of asphyxia varies somewhat among authors. Scheiner (1980) suggests the use of multiple measures in determining clinically significant asphyxia including the length, degree, frequency and severity of the episodes. The occurrence of asphyxia is commonly related to a number of other medical conditions, so it is difficult to absolutely establish asphyxia as the single cause of a specific case of deafness. MacDonald (1980) points out that a preterm infant is more likely to experience anoxic episodes than a full-term infant. Infants with anoxia may also have a low Apgar score at 1 min and 5 min following birth, low arterial pH level, coma, seizures or the need for resuscitation with oxygen by mask or intubation.

The Apgar method of evaluation has proven most practical as a guide to prognosis and the need for particularly close observation or care in the delivery room and nursery (Apgar, 1953; Apgar and James, 1962). Sixty seconds after the complete birth of the infant, five objective signs including heart rate, respiratory effort, muscle tone, response to catheter in nostril and color are noted, and each is given a score of 0, 1, or 2 as shown in Table 7.8. A total score of 10 indicates an infant in the best possible condition. The Apgar score taken at 1 min is an index of asphyxia and of the need for assisted ventilation. The 5-min score is a more accurate index of likelihood of death or neurologic involvement (Vaughan et al., 1979).

D'Souza et al. (1981) conducted hearing, speech and language studies in 26 children who survived severe perinatal asphyxia. Only 1 child had sensorineural hearing loss, however, nearly one third of their sample had deficits of speech and/or language. Simmons (1980a) implicates anoxia as the single high risk factor that dominates all others in the medical histories of 42 hearing-impaired babies. Although most of these babies had other complications, 73% had anoxic episodes at or shortly after birth.

B. Bacterial Meningitis. Bacterial meningitis develops in approximately 1 of 2500 live births. Neonatal meningitis may develop in utero or following infection at the time of, or subsequent to, delivery. In neonates the infecting bacteria are usually acquired from the mother during delivery. However, bacteria may spread from infant to infant via nursery personnel or contaminated equipment. With the advent of antibiotics, treatment of meningitis is usually successful, although bacterial meningitis is still resonsible for 1–4% of neonatal deaths. Several studies have shown that *Haemophilus influenzae* is the most common bacterial causing childhood meningitis. About 40% of these cases occur during the first year of life. The highest incidence of the disease and the lowest recovery rate are in young infants (Sproles et al., 1969). The clinical manifestations of neonatal meningitis are often subtle and deceptive so that suspicion by the attending physician, coupled with verification by appropriate laboratory studies, provides the only means of diagnosis in newborns (Feigin and Dodge, 1976; Bortolussi and Armstrong, 1978).

The degree of hearing loss associated with meningitis usually ranges from severe-to-profound, but mild-to-moderate hearing loss is also seen. One characteristic of meningitic sensorineural hearing loss in newborns is that some recovery may occur in selected infants following the meningitis episode. In a report of postmeningitis hearing loss in 19 ears, recovery of hearing occurred in 16 ears, with 8 ears showing complete recovery and 8 ears with partial recovery (Rosenhall and Kankkunen, 1980). According to these authors, approximately one fourth of all patients with meningitis hearing loss do recover partially or completely in both ears or only in one ear. Finitzo-Hieber et al. (1981) reports an incidence of 35% sensorineural hearing impairment in 94 infants and children following meningitis. In their study, the highest percent of hearing impairment was associated with *H. influenzae* type meningitis at 55%.

C. Congenital Perinatal Infections. This group of infections is known by the acronym "TORCH" to draw attention to the problem that they are difficult to diagnose because they present with minimal nonspecific symptoms, and yet create devastating developmental complications. The TORCH infections may be acquired by the embryo or fetus during gestation or by the newborn at time of delivery. In the acronym, T stands for toxoplasmosis, R for

Table 7.8.
Apgar Evaluation of the Newborn Infant[a]

Sign	0	1	2
Heart rate	Absent	Below 100	Over 100
Respiratory effort	Absent	Slow, irregular	Good, crying
Muscle tone	Limp	Some flexion of extremities	Active motion
Response to catheter in nostril	No response	Grimace	Cough or sneeze
Color	Blue, pale	Body pink, extremities blue	Completely pink

[a] From V. Vaughan et al.: *Nelson Textbook of Pediatrics*, Ed. 11, p. 393. W. B. Saunders, Philadelphia, 1979.

rubella virus, C for cytomegalovirus, H for herpes simplex viruses and O for other bacterial infections—in the case of hearing impairment we are especially interested in syphilis. The classic paper on the TORCH complex was published by Nahmia in 1974.

TORCH infections are often clinically inapparent, and when the infections are identified, their associated signs and symptoms are nearly indistinguishable. A subclinical infection can result in the same serious defects as one that is clinically apparent. Prognosis for the involved infant is usually grim. Nahmias estimates that 1–5% of all deliveries are infected by one of the TORCH agents, and each year in the United States a minimum of 400 infant deaths results, and at least 2000 additional children are left with significant sequelae.

Nahmias stated that the lack of symptomatology in the pregnant woman makes the diagnosis in TORCH infections very difficult. Even when symptoms are manifest, the diagnosis cannot be confirmed without special laboratory tests. Toxoplasma infections and cytomegalovirus rarely cause a clinically definable syndrome in the pregnant woman; the rash associated with rubella is not specific enough to differentiate it from other entities. In the case of herpes simplex infections, it is not the readily diagnosable cold sores or fever blisters that are of particular concern, but the less discernable genital infections that are often missed at the cervix, the primary site of involvement.

Toxoplasmosis. Congenital toxoplasmosis is typically manifested by chorioretinitis, cerebral calcification, psychomotor retardation, hydrocephalus or microcephaly, and convulsions. Although reports of hearing disorders related to toxoplasmosis are in fact sparse, the congenital infection is so serious that there is no doubt that it may cause hearing loss. Active congenital infection may be fatal in days or weeks, or become inactive with residuals of medical problems in varying degrees and combinations. The full impact of the infection may not become evident until some weeks or

months after its apparent cessation. Apparently, the later in pregnancy the infection occurs, the less severe the clinical symptoms. *Toxoplasma* may be responsible for premature birth, cerebral palsy, blindness and mental retardation (Vaughan et al., 1979).

Toxoplasmosis is acquired in pregnant women as an active disease in 2–7 per 1000, and 30–40% of these women have infected infants (Babson et al., 1980). It is still unclear exactly how the pregnant woman becomes infected, although eating uncooked meat and contact with oocyst-containing feces of cats have been implicated.

Campbell and Clifton (1950) described childhood progressive hearing loss in three of four family members with acquired (not congenital) toxoplasmosis. An infant with toxoplasmosis as a risk factor should be followed for hearing every few months until the age of 1 year or until normal speech development is assured.

Syphilis. Technically speaking, syphilis is a bacterial infection that produces similar manifestations as the viral infections of the TORCH complex, but it can be diagnosed with routine laboratory tests—so it is not usually considered part of the TORCH family. However, we include it so that this infection is not overlooked in the high risk register for deafness.

Early manifestations include nasal discharge (snuffles), rash, anemia, jaundice, and osteochondritis. Later manifestations include saddle nose, saber skin, Hutchinson teeth, mulberry molars, and other dental anomalies. Congenital syphilis may demonstrate a multitude of central nervous system abnormalities including vestibular dysfunction, sensorineural hearing loss, and occasionally aortic valvulitis. Possible accompanying mental retardation depends on severity of neurologic damage.

Auditory impairment may not be present at birth. Onset of hearing loss is generally in early childhood, usually sudden bilaterally symmetrical causing severe to profound impairment. The hearing loss is usually not accompanied by marked vestibular manifestations. Poor hearing function and limited use of hearing aid can be expected due to neural atrophy. The general treatment of congenital syphilis consists of prompt treatment of infant with penicillin. Treatment may be done in utero prior to delivery when an infected mother is identified (Karmody and Schuknecht, 1966).

Rubella. The devastating effects of the rubella epidemic of the 1960s that left 10,000–20,000 children with handicaps is well-known. Although deafness is one of the most common manifestations of rubella with an incidence of 50%, associated problems include heart disease (50%), cataract or glaucoma (40%) and psychomotor/mental retardation (40%) (Cooper, 1969). The present crop of congenital rubella syndrome (CRS) youngsters are now in their late teens, and there appear to be a number of late onset medical disorders including diabetes, endocrine pathology, and central nervous system infections (Harter and Gordon, 1978; Vernon and Hicks, 1980).

With public awareness of the 1960s rubella epidemic, immunization programs developed and the number of congenital rubella cases decreased quickly. As cases of any endemic disease decrease, however, so does public concern, resulting in a reduced number of immunizations. A recent concern is that in some women the vaccine seems to provide immunity to rubella for only 8–12 years (Harris, 1979). Thus, women who were vaccinated during their prepuberty stage may again become susceptible to rubella during their child-bearing years (Vernon and Klein, 1982). Rubella virus is generally acquired by airborne distribution, and enters the maternal respiratory tract (McCracken, 1963).

The gestational age of the embryo or fetus is the critical factor in determining the outcome. Prior to the 8th week of gestation, between 50 and 80% of fetuses exposed to maternal rubella virus become infected; during the 2nd trimester no more than 10–20% of infants become infected; and finally during the 3rd trimester, infection of the fetus is fairly uncommon, 6–10% (Pumper and Yamashiroya, 1975). Live rubella virus, however, may persist for extended periods of time in the newborn infant and serve as a source for spreading the infection to susceptible pregnant women (Vaughan et al., 1979).

Congenital rubella may range from mild, subclinical infection to severe disease. Infants of a mother with known or suspected rubella should be followed carefully throughout childhood since asymptomatic infants may subsequently develop defects later in life. The most commonly delayed manifestation of CRS is progressive sensorineural hearing loss. An excellent monograph has been assembled by Stuckless (1980) on the current status of deafness and rubella.

The hearing loss associated with CRS is severe-to-profound, bilateral, sensorineural with a "cookie-bite" audiometric configuration characterized by the greatest degree of loss in the mid-frequency range, between 500 and 2000 Hz. There seems to be no specific relationship between the time of infection during pregnancy and the degree of hearing loss (Ueda, 1979).

It is often difficult to verify rubella exposure during pregnancy in the postpartum mother, who may have actually had such a mild, subclinical infection that it remained unrecognized. Children with a suspected history of rubella or rubella exposure should be followed with hearing tests until 18–24 months of age, keeping in mind the potential late-onset and progressive nature of rubella hearing loss.

Cytomegalovirus (CMV). Cytomegalovirus is a major cause of prenatal subclinical infections, and the most common of the TORCH complex. Nahmias (1974) estimated that although 20% of pregnant women may have CMV, only 2% of infants are infected at birth, and some 10% of infants are infected by the age of 3 months. Gershon (1981) estimates that 1.2% of infants born in the United States are congenitally infected, but verifies that less than 10% of these infected infants develop severe symptoms.

Cytomegalic inclusion disease is a systemic illness characterized by enlargement of the liver and spleen, jaundice, petechial rash, chorioretinitis, cerebral calcifications, and microcephaly. In contrast to toxoplasmosis and rubella, the visual system is less commonly involved.

Infection of the fetus may be intrauterine, or exposure to the virus as the baby passes through the infected birth canal. There is also strong evidence that CMV may be transmitted transplacentally prenatally or postnatally through infected urine, saliva, breast milk and perhaps feces, tears or through blood transfusions from infected donors (Weller, 1971).

The effects of CMV vary between severe central nervous system destruction to asymptomatic carrying of the virus. In its most severe form, CMV causes global central nervous system infection involving the cerebral cortex, brainstem, cochlear nuclei and cranial nerves as well as the inner ear. Sometimes in the case of asymptomatic CMV an unsuspected hearing loss is present (Davis, 1979).

Some authors feel that fetal risk is related to both the time of infection in utero and to the immune status of the mother (Panjvani and Henshaw, 1981). However, while it is documented that infants with clinically apparent CMV at birth will manifest more significant sequelae, undetected virus has been shown to lead to late-appearing sequelae, namely hearing defects.

Pass and Stasno (1980) reports the incidence of hearing loss to be 30% in symptomatic cases of CMV. Reynolds et al. (1974) reported hearing loss in 9 of 16 patients who had inapparent or subclinical CMV, while Stagno (1977) found hearing defects in 17% of children with subclinical CMV. Hanshaw et al. (1976) verified bilateral hearing loss in 5 of 40 children who had evidence of antibody against CMV, including 3 with profound deafness.

There is no clear-cut pattern in the sensorineural hearing loss attributed to CMV. The hearing loss can range from mild-to-profound and cases of both bilateral and unilateral losses are well documented. There is also evidence of progressive sensorineural hearing loss in the presence of CMV (Pass and Stasno, 1980; Dahl, 1979). Virus excretions may remain active for several years following birth, constituting a contributing factor in the degenerative process. In terms of infant follow-up, it is important to realize that any pattern and degree of hearing loss may occur with CMV. The screening technique of choice with these infants may be auditory evoked potentials since chances of detecting a mild-to-moderate loss is possible. The potential for progressive hearing loss requires follow-up testing within shorter time intervals than when following a child with a nonprogressive risk factor. An audiological evaluation at 3-month intervals would be appropriate for the first year. The fact that asymptomatic virus may later exhibit itself in a hearing loss should alert us to those older children we identify with hearing loss who, as infants, had no positive risk factors.

Herpes Simplex Virus. Herpes simplex virus, commonly referred to as HSV, is rapidly becoming one of the most common sexually transmitted diseases. The most common mode of transmission of HSV to the fetus is during the birth process if the mother is actively infected. HSV is rarely placentally transmitted (Gershon, 1981). However, if HSV is transmitted in this manner it may produce intrauterine malformations.

Herpes simplex virus may cause a severe generalized disease in the neonate with high mortality and devastating sequelae. HSV infects the genital tracts of an estimated 20–25% of the population according to *Medical World News* (1980). HSV infections in the newborn are rarely subclinical or asymptomatic. The majority of cases are thought to be acquired during passage through the birth canal. A cesarean section delivery is indicated for mothers with a known genital infection at the time of delivery. When HSV infection does occur in the neonate, more than 50% are fatal. According to Nahmias and Norrild (1979) only 4% of neonatally infected HSV infants survive without sequelae. Unfortunately, this sexually transmitted infection is apparently on the increase with no cure or effective treatment currently available.

Although specific reports of HSV as a potential cause of hearing loss are not available, histopathologic studies show involvement of the sensory cells of the labyrinth (Ventry et al., 1981). The similarity of HSV to both CMV and toxoplasmosis suggest that careful hearing follow-up of involved infants is appropriate.

D. Defects of the Head and Neck. Anomalies associated with craniofacial and skeletal abnormalities range from the very obvious to slight, subtle defects. Infants at risk for deafness in this category manifest anatomical malformations involving the head, neck, mouth, ears, etc.

Typical indications of a neonate with head and neck defects include babies with craniofacial syndromal abnormalities, malformed, low-set, or aberrant pinna configurations, such as microtia and/or atresia, pre- or postauricular tags and pits, cleft lip and/or palate (including submucous cleft palate), first and/or second arch anomalies including mandibular and maxillary variants and branchial cysts.

It must be remembered that not all infants with such defects will have hearing impairment. The presence of such abnormalities, however, increases the risk of hearing problems in that particular child. These defects, obvious or subtle, will often be noted by the pediatrician or nurse in the medical chart at the time of birth, but unfortunately, seldom is a referral generated to evaluate hearing in the infant.

E. Elevated Bilirubin. Hyperbilirubinemia, or "jaundice," occurs when there is an excess amount of bilirubin in the blood. Rh or ABO incompatability between mother and child may be associated with hyperbilirubinemia, although other physiological problems may also be responsible.

There are two types of bilirubin, conjugated and unconjugated—sometimes referred to as direct and indirect bilirubin. As red blood cells break down, unconjugated bilirubin is routinely released into the plasma serum. This is observed during the healing of a bruise when the surface area under the skin becomes yellow (or jaundiced) due to the presence of unconjugated bilirubin.

The unconjugated bilirubin is bound to plasma albumin and transported to the liver where an enzyme "conjugates" it. That is, the potentially toxic unconjugated bilirubin is joined together with a substance in the body to form a detoxified product. The now "conjugated" bilirubin is normally excreted from the body through the small intestine. When bilirubin cannot be conjugated, it builds up in the serum until it crosses the plasma membrane and is deposited in the brain. Kernicterus is a neurological syndrome resulting from the deposition of unconjugated bilirubin in brain cells causing motor and sensory deficits, mental retardation, or death.

The Joint Committee on Infant Hearing suggests that those infants with a bilirubin level that exceeds indications requiring a blood exchange transfusion are "at risk" for hearing impairment. The Committee on Fetus and Newborn (1982) of the Academy of Pediatrics suggests the serum bilirubin level needed for exchange transfusion is a function of the infants' birth weight (see Table 7.9). The values in this table may be used as a guide in deciding whether to place an infant on the high risk register for deafness or not.

Newborns often have some degree of jaundice following birth because their im-

Table 7.9.
Serum Bilirubin Level for Exchange Transfusion (mg/100 ml)

Birth Weight (g)	Normal Infants	Abnormal Infants
100	10.0	10.0
1001–1250	13.0	10.0
1251–1500	15.0	13.0
1501–2000	17.0	15.0
2001–2500	18.0	17.0
2500	20.0	18.0

mature liver function does not adequately handle the normal breakdown of red blood cells.

The level of bilirubin is not the only deciding factor in determining the need for an exchange transfusion. Consideration is given to seven other factors including perinatal asphyxia, respiratory distress, metabolic acidosis with pH levels less than or equal to 7.25, hypothermia, low serum protein levels, birthweight less than 1500 g, and/or signs of clinical CNS degeneration (Levine, 1979). In his sample of hearing-impaired newborns, Simmons (1980a) cited hyperbilirubinemia as the most common sequela of anoxia causing deafness. Most of his jaundiced babies were also premature, and most of his premature babies had elevated bilirubin levels. Of 8 severely elevated bilirubin babies in the Simmons study, only 2 were uncomplicated by any other factors. Four of the babies developed seizures, cardiac arrests, and evidence of CNS bleeds during or shortly after exchange transfusions. The deafness of these infants may be caused by bilirubin deposition in the cochlear nucleus, or perhaps through intracochlear and intracranial bleeding secondary to hypoxia and/or acidosis.

Hyman (1969) reported multiple abnormalities in 405 infants with hemolytic disease or hyperbilirubinemia. Sensorineural hearing impairment was found in 4.2% of these patients ranging in severity from mild to profound deafness in unilateral and bilateral configurations. Vernon and Klein (1982) suggest that although Rh incompatability was a once major cause of deafness in today's adult deaf population, increased skill in transfusion technology should reduce this factor as a cause of childhood deafness from the current 3–4% to about 1% in the future.

F. Family History. Congenital deafness may be "passed on" or "inherited" from other family members who were deaf or hearing-impaired in childhood. The various patterns of inheritance are described in Chapter 3. Obviously, an infant with a family history of hearing-impaired blood relatives is "at risk" for inheriting that same trait.

Not so simple, however, is the task of eliciting family history from the baby's parents. Unfortunately, family history information is sparse beyond the infant's grandparents. Often, only one parent is available for interview so that little information is available from the "other side" of the family. Information about handicapped relatives is often glossed over by relatives so that considerable uncertainty exists about the true nature, degree, onset or diagnosis of the condition. And finally, the interview technique may bring forth unexpected responses. A parent told us that no deafness existed in their family although a cousin did attend the state deaf school. The parent was quick to add that the cousin was not "deaf"; he "wore a hearing aid and could hear normally." Another parent implicated his uncle, who "was not hearing impaired since childhood . . . but he was totally deaf since birth."

Questions must be phrased carefully to avoid misunderstandings or erroneous responses. We ask, "Do you know any of the baby's relatives who now have a hearing loss which started before the age of 5 years? Please think hard about all of your family and the baby's father's family." If the answer is "yes," we proceed to ask who they were (relationship to the baby). "Do you know what caused the hearing loss? What makes you think the onset of the loss was before the age of five? Did he/she wear a hearing aid before age 5? Does he/she still wear a hearing aid? Did he/she attend a special school for the deaf? Did he/she attend public school? Did (or does) he/she have a speech problem?"

When the family history information is positive, the infant is identified as "at risk" for hearing impairment. It is important to remember the potential progressive nature or possible late onset of hereditary hearing loss. Careful follow-up and thorough parental counseling is advised for these babies "at risk," but who pass the initial hearing screening test.

G. Gram Birthweight Less than 1500.

Infants delivered prior to 37 weeks are considered to have a shortened gestation period and are *premature* or *preterm.* Historically, prematurity was defined by low birthweight. In essence, however, prematurity and low birthweight are usually concomitant, particularly among infants weighing 1500 g or less at birth (about 3 lb), and both factors are associated with increased neonatal morbidity and mortality. It is difficult to separate completely factors associated with prematurity from those associated with low birthweight (Vaughan et al., 1979).

It has been well documented that hearing loss occurs in relatively higher incidence in preterm infants than in full-term babies. The problem of ascertaining the etiology of the hearing loss is difficult because preterm infants often have associated medical complications. Simmons (1980a) states that while it is true that the incidence of prematurity is higher in hearing-loss babies, it is unlikely that prematurity *per se* causes the deafness, but rather neonatal anoxia is the underlying factor. In addition to anoxia, problems associated with the premature infant include hyperbilirubinemia and an increase in bacterial/viral infections. Treatment for infant septemic infection often includes antibiotics, which are themselves potentially ototoxic. Berman et al. (1978) have reported a high incidence of middle ear effusion in low birthweight infants, especially following prolonged intubation.

Davey (1962) found the hearing loss associated with low birthweight infants to be sensorineural with a steep high frequency component. Drillen (1964) tested 433 premature children of school age and found that 17.5% had some hearing deficit. McDonald (1967) found 19 patients with hearing loss out of 1066 infants with birthweights less than 4 lb. Clark and Conroy (1978) studied 204 low birthweight babies and found 5% to have sensorineural hearing loss—each of whom also had elevated bilirubin levels at birth. Abramovich et al. (1979) evaluated the hearing of 111 perinatal care survivors of birthweights of 1500 g or less. They found 10 patients (9%) with sensorineural hearing loss, 1 (1%) with congenital conductive hearing loss, and 21 (19%) with middle ear effusions.

An excellent flow chart of a community based high risk register for hearing loss is shown in Figure 7.3.

Crib-O-Gram

An ingenious automated system for detecting hearing loss in newborns was devised by F. Blair Simmons at the Stanford University School of Medicine in 1974 (Simmons and Russ, 1974; Simmons, 1976; Jones and Simmons, 1977). The technique, known as the Crib-o-gram, uses a motion-sensitive transducer placed under the crib mattress in the intensive care nursery (ICN) or between the crib and frame in the well baby nursery (WBN). The transducer is capable of detecting virtually any motor activity from the infant stronger than an eye blink or facial grimace, including respiration.

The Crib-o-gram is a timed self-cycling system that turns on and shuts off automatically following each complete stimulus presentation and response measurement interval. The current Crib-o-gram is a microprocessor-based unit which performs the test, scores and interprets the results. Preliminary results indicate that the unit can match human scoring in accuracy while decreasing total test time required for each infant (Marcellino, 1979).

The baby's state is monitored automatically by measuring crib movement for 10–15 sec before and 6 sec following each test sound presentation. The test sound presentation is delivered from an earphone placed in the basinette (2000–4000 Hz band pass noise stimulus). The auditory test stimulus is presented 20 or more times over a 7–24-hour period. Responses in the form of baby movement (or lack of responses) are noted by the microprocessor and analyzed until a statistically valid decision can be made by

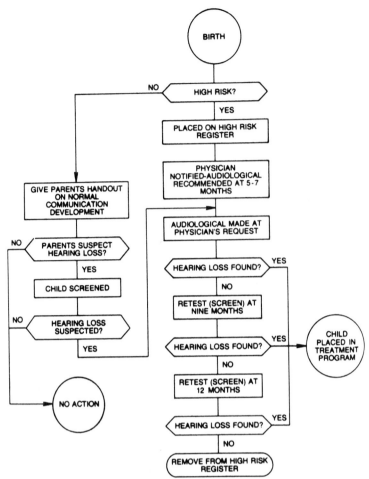

Figure 7.3. Flow chart diagram of a community high risk registry program for deafness. (Reproduced with permission from J. L. Fitch et al.: *Journal of Speech and Hearing Disorders*, 47: 373–375, 1982.)

the unit regarding whether the baby passed or failed the hearing screening. Since a screening test is not a definitive examination, it is possible for an at-risk individual to be missed. Of 42 deaf babies, Simmons considers only two to be screening failures that were identified at a later date (1980a).

The Stanford group has tested more than 12,000 babies with the Crib-o-gram, detecting and establishing firm diagnoses of hearing loss in 42 babies—an incidence of 1:1000 in the well baby nursery (WBN) and 1:52 in the intensive care nursery (ICN) (Simmons, 1980a). The false-positive rate varies around 8% for well babies and 20%

for intensive care graduates (Simmons et al., 1979). McFarland et al. (1980) report sensitivity rates (percentage of hearing-impaired babies detected) and specificity rates (percentage of normal-hearing children who pass the screening test) for the Crib-o-gram. Sensitivity for the WBN was 91% and the ICN was 82%. Specificity for the WBN was 92% and 79% for the ICN. The authors conclude that the poorer specificity in the ICN is likely due to the fact that ICN babies are generally less responsive to all external stimuli due to their poor health and weakened condition.

Simmons (1982) indicates that, for ICN

babies, they must rescreen some 20% of the babies, but the total number is small. They detect one deaf baby out of each 12 rescreened. The screening failure rate is only 0.09%, so if an ICN infant passes the initial screen, the chances of a hearing loss being present are no greater than 0.01%. In the WBN, the screening failure rate is much smaller (8%), and they must rescreen 66 babies per deaf child. The odds on missing a deaf baby in the initial screen are 1:10,000. The incidence of deafness in the WBN is sufficiently small so that mass screening with the Crib-o-gram is impractical.

There is no question that the Crib-o-gram offers considerable promise as an automated newborn hearing screening system. Simmons and his associates continue to up-date their statistics, although they have stated that at least 100,000 infants must be screened and followed to establish firm confidence levels with the technique. The analysis thus far shows that the Crib-o-gram method is a reliable and cost-effective tool for identification of hearing impairment in the newborn nursery.

The Auditory Response Cradle

The auditory response cradle, developed in England as a fully automatic, microprocessor-controlled, newborn screening device has recently been introduced in the United States. The system is comprised of a "cradle" with head and body support which is capable of monitoring four measures of infant behavioral response following auditory stimulation. Trunk and limb movements are monitored by a pressure sensitive mattress; the head jerk component of the startle reflex is monitored by a transducer embedded in the foam of a headrest which is pivoted on low friction bearings to detect head-turn reactions; infant respiratory pattern is sensed by a transducer fitted in a plastic belt which is placed around the upper abdomen of the baby.

A high pass noise of 85 dB SPL (band-width from 2600 to 4500 Hz) is used as the test stimulus and presented through close-coupled ear probes fitted with tips similar to those used for acoustic impedance testing. The auditory stimulus is presented to the infant under test on a number of occasions and resulting motor and respiratory responses detected and stored by the microprocessor. Equal numbers of no-sound "control" trials enable calculation of the probability that the sound responses are genuine and not spontaneous events. When the microprocessor determines that the probability of response exceeds 97%, the baby is considered to have normal-hearing responses and passed. The average test time takes 2–10 min, and consists of between 2 and 10 trial blocks (a trial block is defined as 2 sound and 2 "no-sound" control elements—an element consists of a prestimulus and poststimulus period each lasting at least 5 sec).

Over 2000 babies have been evaluated with the auditory response cradle. To date, infants with severe hearing loss as well as infants with middle ear dysfunction diagnosed as serous otitis media have been identified with this hearing screening technique. Developers of the auditory response cradle report the unit to have exceptionally low false positive errors combined with sensitivity to identify babies with moderate, severe and profound deafness (Bennett, 1979, 1980; Bennett and Lawrence, 1980).

GOALS AND METHODS, BIRTH TO 2 YEARS
Goals

In the period from birth to 24 months, the goals and pathologies are identical with those at birth. We can and should identify even those babies who have mild to moderate hearing losses that might impair their language function. This is the critical age for speech and language development and all efforts should be made to detect even milder impairments. Fortunately, by 4 months the infant begins to show consistent responses to certain sound levels.

There are several techniques available to fit the expanded goals—techniques that can be used in office or well-baby clinics as well as in the audiology laboratory. They consist of orienting (behavioral) tests, impedance audiometry and auditory evoked potentials, and structured questions of the mother.

Methods

Background. Sir Alexander and Lady Ewing (1944), in Manchester, England, first described using noisemakers to obtain orienting responses in infants. Their rather large armamentarium of noises included such things as a toy xylophone, a china cup and metal spoon, tissue paper, a rattle, and voice and unvoiced consonants. The responses they described are those which have withstood the test of time: eye shifts and head turns toward the sound, becoming more definite with increased maturation. Dr. Kevin Murphy (1962), of Reading, England, made detailed observations of the orienting responses and reported refinements. He was able to identify the exact direction of the head and eye movements in relation to chronologic age, thus opening up a valuable line of inquiry.

Procedures

The test of choice for the infant from 2 months to 2 years is production of an orienting response using noisemakers. Before the age of 4 months the response is largely reflexive in nature, and may be difficult to see outside of a sound-treated room. The same criteria should therefore be used between birth and 4 months of age.

In the presence of a lack of response, the tester should repeat the use of a particular stimulus at his discretion until the observer is satisfied that the failure to respond is genuine. Two repetitions should be adequate to establish this fact.

It must be kept in mind that failure of the child to locate the sound does not always indicate that the child did not hear it. The simple fact that he may not be interested in that particular sound can account for this lack of response. For this reason more than one stimulus in a particular range is available for use at the discretion of the tester.

Standards for criteria for failure may be set up by the individual programs. The failure to respond in any way to the sound stimuli is obviously a failed test. Depending on the type of stimuli used, the program may require that the infant respond at least once to one of the lower pitched sounds and once to one of the higher range of sounds (see "Equipment and Environment" below).

The failure to respond does not necessarily mean that the child has a hearing loss, but it does mean that his auditory behavior is not normal. The reason may be a physical or mental impairment. In any case, failure to respond satisfactorily for his age level should mark a child for referral to an audiology and speech center for more detailed testing.

Testing with One Observer. 1. *Equipment and Environment.* A quiet room is required, with little distraction from the outside. The suggested list of equipment is as follows:

a. *Squeeze Toy.* A soft rubber toy should be selected that makes a breathy "whoosh" sound, not a throaty noise. When buying it, compare different ones and find the one that sounds the highest pitches and can be made to sound the softest.

b. *Bell.* A small gold East India import bell produces the highest pitch and also the softest ring. Compare the bells and select the one that is highest and softest. We have measured the output of such bells and found that they produce only frequencies around 4000 Hz when rung slightly, at levels as low as 30 dB SPL. If your bell does not achieve these measurements, try removing the clapper and letting the remaining wire create the sound!

c. *Rattle.* The usual baby rattle is adequate, providing it can be handled to produce a soft rattling sound. One may often find a toy plastic block that has sand-like material in it, that produces a sudden rustling sound. (If you survive the scrutiny of the toy store clerk after making these selections, you are in business as an infant tester.)

One chair is needed, for the mother to sit in with the child on her lap. A colorful toy like a small doll should be available as a distraction, but it should not be too attractive or it will engage the whole attention of the child.

2. *Procedure.* The tester kneels at a 45° angle to the side of the child, with the distracting toy in one hand and the noisemaker well hidden in the other. When the baby's attention is engaged by the toy held in front of him, she makes the sound in the hand held close to the floor, out of the peripheral vision of the child. If an orientation response is seen after one or two presentations, the tester kneels on the other side and uses another noisemaker to test on that side. The tester will learn by experience that for the 0–4-month age level the noisemaker must be produced quite loudly; by 6–9 months, it can be produced more softly; and by 10–12 months it should be made as soft as possible.

The expected response is some sort of head turn toward the sound (see also Chapter 4). An exact description of the head turn and accompanying eye movement should be noted. The expected responses at each age level are as follows (Fig. 7.4):

Age 0–4 months. Eye widening, eye blink (in a very quiet environment), or arousal from sleep as in newborn testing.

Age 4–7 months. By 4 months, a "rudimentary" head turn is seen: a "wobble" of the head even slightly toward the sound.

This response gradually matures until at 6 months the head turn is definite, toward the side of the sound, but only on a plane level with the eyes. He does not fixate the sound source in the lower level where it comes from.

By 7 months there is an inclination to find the sound source on the lower level; the child will look first to the side and then down. He may even be mature enough to find the source directly.

Age 7–9 months. At the beginning of this period he should soon find the sound source on the lower level directly, but if the sound is presented on a level above his head, he will only look toward the side. At the end of this period he may begin to look toward the side and then up, to fixate the higher sound source.

Age 9–13 months. At 9 months, the beginning indirect localization of the higher level will be seen which soon turns to direct localization (Fig. 7.4). We thus see shortly after 1 year of age a direct localization of sounds in any plane.

Age 13–24 months. The same type of orientation prevails for the older child as was seen for the 13-month-old. In other words, the full maturation of the auditory behavior of the child occurs at about 13 months and does not change significantly after that.

Responses Should Also Be Obtained on Selected Developmental and Communication Scales. Here it is recommended that some screening scales be given which identify developmental and communication lags. The Denver Developmental Screening Test (Frankenburg and Dodds, 1967), Bayley Scale (Bayley, 1935), etc., are useful. In addition, a simplified questionnaire for various age levels should be given. The mother can be questioned either by written questionnaire or by oral query, depending upon which suits the needs of the population served. The questionnaire includes information on developmental status and communication abilities in addition to the questions concerning hearing status. It is recommended that this kind of questionnaire be used as a screening device to identify other problems which might benefit from treatment at an early age. The hearing questions are separated from the developmental questions because most of the commonly used developmental milestones are found to be present in otherwise normal deaf babies, and therefore would not identify a hearing loss.

Questions to Ask Mother at the Well-Baby Examination

2 MONTHS

Hearing

1. Have you had any worry about   Yes   No
   your child's hearing?

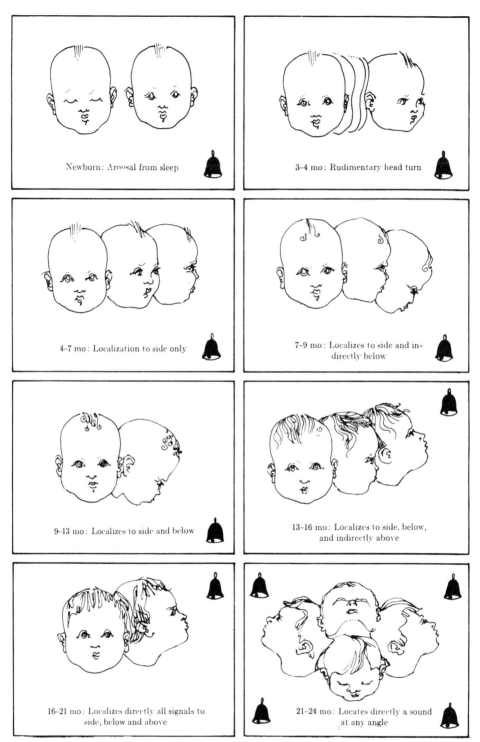

Figure 7.4. Maturation of the auditory response.

2. When he's sleeping in a quiet room, does he move and begin to wake up when there's a loud sound?   Yes   No

Developmental and Communication

3. Does he lift up his head when he's lying on his stomach?   Yes   No
4. Does he smile at you when you smile at him?   Yes   No
5. Does he move both hands together in the same way?   Yes   No
6. Does he look at your face without your making gestures to him?   Yes   No

4 MONTHS

Hearing

1. Have you had any worry about your child's hearing?   Yes   No
2. When he's sleeping in a quiet room, does he move and begin to wake up when there's a loud sound?   Yes   No
3. Does he try to turn his head toward an interesting sound, or when his name is called?   Yes   No

Developmental and Communication

4. Does he lift his head up to 90° and look straight ahead?   Yes   No
5. Does he touch his hands together and play with them?   Yes   No
6. Does he laugh and giggle without being tickled or touched?   Yes   No
7. Does he coo to himself and make noises when he's alone?   Yes   No

6 MONTHS

Hearing

1. Have you had any worry about your child's hearing?   Yes   No
2. When he's sleeping in a quiet room, does he move and begin to wake up when there's a loud sound?   Yes   No
3. Does he turn his head toward an interesting sound or when his name is called?   Yes   No

Developmental and Communication

4. Does he lift up his head and chest with his arms?   Yes   No
5. Does he keep his head steady when sitting?   Yes   No
6. Does he roll over in his crib?   Yes   No
7. Does he reach for objects within his reach and hold them?   Yes   No

8. Does he see small objects like peas or raisins?   Yes   No

8 MONTHS

Hearing

1. Have you had any worry about your child's hearing?   Yes   No
2. When he's sleeping in a quiet room, does he move and begin to wake up when there's a loud sound?   Yes   No
3. Does he turn his head directly toward an interesting sound or when his name is called?   Yes   No
4. Does he enjoy ringing a bell or shaking a rattle?   Yes   No

Developmental and Communication

5. Does he support most of his weight on his legs?   Yes   No
6. Can he sit alone unaided for 5 minutes?   Yes   No
7. Can he sit and look for objects that have fallen out of sight?   Yes   No
8. Can he pick up two objects, one in each hand?   Yes   No
9. Can he transfer an object from one hand to the other?   Yes   No
10. Can he feed himself a cracker?   Yes   No
11. Does he make a number of different sounds and change their pitch?   Yes   No
12. Does he clap his hands in imitation and make noises at the same time?   Yes   No

10 MONTHS

Hearing

1. Have you had any worry about your child's hearing?   Yes   No
2. When he's sleeping in a quiet room, does he move and begin to wake up when there's a loud sound?   Yes   No
3. Does he turn his head directly toward an interesting sound or when his name is called?   Yes   No
4. Does he try to imitate you if you make his own sounds?   Yes   No

Developmental and Communication

5. Does he play peek-a-boo with you?   Yes   No
6. Can he stand for at least 5 seconds, holding onto a crib or chair?   Yes   No
7. Does he try to hold onto a toy when it's pulled away?   Yes   No

8. Is he shy or afraid of strangers?   Yes   No

9. Can he pull himself to standing position alone?   Yes   No

12 MONTHS

Hearing

1. Have you had any worry about your child's hearing?   Yes   No

2. When he's sleeping in a quiet room, does he move and begin to wake up when there's a loud sound?   Yes   No

3. Does he turn his head directly toward an interesting sound or when his name is called?   Yes   No

4. Is he beginning to repeat some of the sounds that you make?   Yes   No

Developmental and Communication

5. Can he pick up a raisin or a pea?   Yes   No

6. Can he get to a sitting position without help?   Yes   No

7. Does he wave bye-bye or pat-a-cake when you tell him to?   Yes   No

8. Can he say "mamma" or "dada"?   Yes   No

Some knowledge of the attributes of the deaf is necessary in order for the questioner to understand why the questions are worded as they are. For example, a deaf child will look around or will wake up when a door slams, when someone stamps a foot on the floor, when a large truck rolls by on the street, or when a loud airplane flies low overhead. Therefore, if the mother states that the child awakens to a loud sound, she must be asked to specify the type of sound that he awakens to.

Another characteristic of the deaf infant is that he is unusually visually alert, and attends to movement in his peripheral vision. Therefore, if the mother reports that he turns around to an interesting sound or when his name is called, the question must be asked if she is sure that the sound is out of his peripheral visual field.

Until the age of 6 months, the deaf infant sounds exactly like the normal infant; he babbles just as much, he increases his vocalizations when the parent appears and coos at him, just as the normal child; and only an expert phonetician could identify the subtle qualitative differences in the babbling sounds that the deaf child makes. Therefore, great care has been taken in the questionnaire not to assume that the baby's vocalizations are any index of his ability to hear.

A very misleading indication is a mother's report that her baby says "mamma" at around the age of 1 year, and that therefore the baby must be hearing at that point. Oddly enough, the mothers of most deaf children make just such a report, and it is universally true that a profoundly deaf infant will appear to be saying "mamma" at around 1 year of age. Actually what he is saying is "amah," which is the most primitive sound that can be made, involving as it does the almost animal-like "ah" vocalization plus the coming together of the lips. It has been postulated that one of the reasons for its development is that in infancy the baby is carried close to the mother, and feels the vibrations or hears low frequencies of his mother's voice, and is thus stimulated to perpetuate the sounds. At any rate, the sounds soon drop off, and nothing remains but the "ah" vocalization in a strident voice.

Auditory Brainstem Evoked Response (ABR) as a Screening Technique in Infants

The application of brainstem evoked response to auditory screening represents a relatively new dimension in the early identification of hearing loss. The rapid development of ABR procedures has resulted in the pursuit of evidence for effective application as a screening technique. Several leading laboratories have evaluated both neonatal normal and high-risk populations with ABR techniques in an attempt to determine the reliability, sensitivity, and accuracy of the procedures. These investigations have lead to controversy over the use of ABR as a newborn hearing screening technique (Fig. 7.5).

Hecox and Galambos (1974) evaluated 35 infants, aged 3 weeks to about 3 years with the ABR technique. They found the

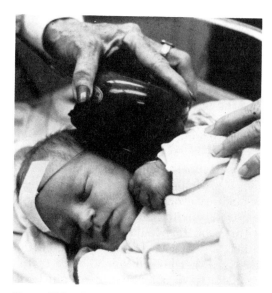

Figure 7.5. Brainstem evoked potential screening being performed on a newborn. (Courtesy of American Telephone Pioneers Infant Hearing Assessment Program.)

latency of wave V to be a function of both click intensity and the age of the subject. The latency at a given signal strength shortens postnatally to reach the adult value (about 6 msec) by 12–18 months of age. At this time, Hecox and Galambos suggested that the reliability and lack of variability of ABR could provide an objective method for assessing hearing in infants.

Schulman-Galambos and Galambos (1979) used ABR as an auditory screening procedure in three groups of newborns. One group consisted of 220 normal-term infants who were within 72 hours of birth and no hearing abnormalities were detected; the second group consisted of 75 intensive care unit newborns in whom 4 were found to have severe sensorineural hearing loss at the time of hospital discharge. The third group consisted of 325 infants, 1 year or older, who had previously been discharged from the ICU. Of these infants, an additional 4 showed sensorineural hearing loss. The authors estimated the incidence of hearing loss in the ICU population to be 1 in 50, and concluded that ABR is a cost-effective screening test.

The application of ABR screening in the neonatal ICU is not without problems. Several investigators have attempted to devise latency norms for premature infants. Weber (1982) conducted two studies, evaluating a total of 400 infants with ABR techniques. The first study established wave V latency norms as well as utilized waves III and V to secure interwave intervals as measures of brainstem maturation. The second study compared the four sets of latency norms to the latencies of an additional group of normal-hearing infants. The results indicated that conceptual age was not as satisfactory for use in ABR latency norms as interwave interval and that wave III may be more appropriate for the measurement of response latency than the more common criterion of wave V latency. The disadvantage is this technique precludes the use of ABR to identify neurological disorders which may extend central conduction time, although traditionally it has not been the intent of ABR hearing screening to also serve as a neurological screening procedure.

A number of investigators have compared ABR between normal and high risk infants in early postnatal life. Salamy et al. (1980) indicate that infants born "at risk" but free of severe auditory defects and major neurological difficulties can be distinguished from healthy (age-matched) controls in terms of the brainstem averaged potential throughout the first post-natal year. Barden and Peltzman (1980) evaluated 61 newborns to study the potential influence of perinatal risk factors for hearing impairment and/or asphyxial brain damage. Their results, although not conclusive, suggest that birth asphyxia and/or low birth weight may be associated with shortened latencies in evoked potential wave forms.

Routine screening of infants from the newborn ICU for auditory impairment with auditory brainstem potentials has been recommended by Marshall et al. (1980) as a clinically feasible and useful procedure. In their study, infants with gestational age of

24–43 weeks and birth weights of 530–2338 g, were classified as pass or fail, depending on the presence or absence of wave V at a latency of 7–11 msec in response to clicks of 60 dB above the normal adult threshold. The failure babies were not correlated with excessive noise exposure or ototoxic medications, but nearly all the babies who failed had intracranial hemorrhage.

Marshall et al. (1980) suggested that the smaller, younger babies failed the ABR screening because of the physiologic immaturity of the small infants and the pathologic severity of the patient's diseases. Starr et al. (1977) reported ABR studies on infants as young as 28 weeks of gestational age and believed that the brainstem response wave complexes could be identified if the stimuli were sufficiently loud. One of the patients in the Marshall study failed the hearing test shortly before clear evidence of a major intracranial hemorrhage became apparent, leading to the intriguing observation that ABR may offer an early technique for detecting significant neurologic dysfunction *before* gross symptoms occur.

Galambos et al. (1982a) conclude that because of the high incidence of hearing loss in infants discharged from the tertiary intensive care nursery, ABR techniques are the most reliable, sensitive, and accurate newborn hearing test available at the present time. In their evaluation of 890 newborns discharged from ICN, 10% suffered from hearing loss in one or both ears, and 2% suffered irreversible bilateral sensorineural hearing losses so severe as to require amplification. When comparing ABR statistics to Crib-o-gram statistics (Galambos et al., 1982b) the authors state, that for every 112 babies correctly identified by ABR, only 64 will be identified by Crib-o-gram.

The argument in disagreement with the statement that ABR is an accurate and cost-effective hearing screening tool for newborns cannot be ignored. Simmons (1982) responded that the identification of hearing loss reported for ABR and for the Crib-o-gram are about the same (1.9 and 2.3%). He questioned the false-positive rate (14%) of ABR testing on infants with abnormal wave V potentials upon discharge from the hospital who, when retested 4–6 months later, were found to have normal auditory acuity. The time-consuming procedures required to complete ABR testing (at least 1 hour) and the necessity for qualified personnel to administer the evaluation may also compromise the cost-effectiveness of auditory evoked potential screening.

Several limitations of ABR evaluations with a neonatal population have been identified by Stockard and Westmoreland (1981). A heightened vulnerability of the neonatal wave potentials to certain technical and subject factors should be of concern. Stimulus intensity, a major source of variability in peak and interpeak latencies, requires nonobjective judgment by the subject to adjust the stimulus intensity to the desired sensation level (SL). This, of course, is impossible to obtain from infants. Uncertainty about the conceptual age versus gestational age of the infant may confuse the interpretation due to the rapid change of maturational levels in auditory transmission time.

Many wave-form criteria of auditory evoked potentials are used to identify a hearing-impaired infant and to distinguish peripheral hearing loss from intracranial pathology (Finitzo-Hieber, 1982): the absolute latency of waves I and V, the latency-intensity function (L-I function), the wave I–V interwave interval (IWI) and the wave V to wave I amplitude ratio. She indicates that accurate infant assessment requires age-specific norms for each of the measurements. These wave forms are first visible in a premature infant at 28–30 weeks *postconception* (or 28–30 weeks gestational age) not postbirth. However, latencies are prolonged and thresholds are elevated when compared to a term newborn. The maturation of the auditory brainstem response is not complete until 12–18 months postterm (term being 38–40 weeks of gestational age). Figure 7.6 illustrates the mat-

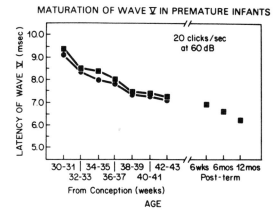

MATURATION OF WAVE V IN PREMATURE INFANTS

20 clicks/sec
at 60 dB

MATURATION OF WAVE I IN PREMATURE INFANTS

20 clicks/sec
at 60 dB

● Despland/Galambos
■ Finitzo-Hieber

Figure 7.6. Maturation of wave V and wave I over time. (Reproduced with permission from T. Finitzo-Hieber: *Seminars in Speech, Language and Hearing*, 3: 76–87, 1982.)

uration of wave V and wave I over time. Note that the critical time is expressed in *postconception* rather than in time *postbirth*.

Finitzo-Hieber (1982) makes the following recommendations in conducting ABR in premature infants: (1) if a premature infant is tested far in advance of discharge, the baby can present with a significant, but transient, impairment which may show partial or complete recovery at the time of discharge. If ABR is to be effective, assessment should take place near discharge time, when the infant is in an open crib and is not less than 37 weeks of gestational age. (2) A single ABR assessment is not sufficient in premature infants. Both improvement and deterioration in auditory func-

tion have been documented on follow-up testing. Therefore, at risk infants should be monitored with ABR every 3 months in the first year of life.

It should then be questioned if ABR monitoring in itself constitutes adequate follow-up for a child. According to Stein et al. (1982), otologic, audiologic, and neurologic examinations, as well as post-discharge ABR, are mandatory before any inferences can be made about hearing loss or neurodevelopmental disorders. The intent of the initial screening procedure will help dictate the appropriate follow-up examinations. A behavioral audiometric evaluation would be necessary to accurately obtain frequency specific information and to determine the existence or extent of a conductive hearing loss.

An extensive review of the literature lead Downs (1982a) to suggest that the legitimacy of ABR testing of infants is at best, uncertain. He stresses the evidence of ABR audiometry's validity, reliability and norms which, thus far, have not met up to the previous high standards imposed upon assessment techniques of our profession. He urges a cautious approach to the application of ABR as a screening procedure. Auditory brainstem response testing, however, is one of the valuable tools available to experienced clinicians for the early identification of infants with auditory disorders.

GOALS AND METHODS, 2–5 YEARS

Goals

The period of 2–5 years gives us real problems in identification. These children are not seen often at well-baby clinics or at doctors' offices. Although Head Start programs are making many children available, there are large numbers who are not seen for health visits unless special efforts are made to reach them. Nursery schools, play schools, and child care centers should be entered for hearing screening programs.

At this age we look primarily for medically remediable hearing losses, on the assumption that the more severely handicapping losses will have been found by 2 years. The chief pathology we are looking for is otitis media—the disease that can result at this age in subtle auditory disorders or permanent middle ear damage. The disorders that should be screened for at this age include middle ear pathologies, viral diseases, and sensorineural hearing loss. The tests that are adequate to identify these disorders are hearing screening, plus acoustic impedance audiometry and/or otoscopic examination.

Methods

Background. Ingenious efforts have been made to develop effective screening methods for the preschool child. The problems arise from the definition of screening as "rapid, simple measurements applied to large numbers of children." Any test that requires a voluntary response from a 2–5-year-old will be neither rapid or simple. The 2–3-year-olds are particularly difficult to test. They can be negativistic, apprehensive, or "eager-beavers"—all attitudes which hardly make for easy testing.

Several solutions have been proposed to implement the screening of preschoolers, but none seem to have solved the 2–3-year-old problems.

The VASC (Verbal-Auditory Screening Test for Children) test culminated efforts to use non-pure tone signals for screening preschoolers (Griffing et al., 1967). In this test, the child is told to point to the picture, on a stand in front of him, that represents the word that is spoken. The stimulus words consist of four randomized lists of the same 125 spondee words, Beginning at a hearing level of 51 dB (re: normal threshold). Each subsequent word is presented at a 4-dB attenuation rate. The last three words reach a level of 15 dB.

The original study reported by Griffing et al. (1967) tested 175 preschool children with the VASC. All the failures were given pure tone tests, as well as every third child who passed. Five of the nine positives were found to have reduced hearing levels; four were normal. Because only one third of the children were given the criterion pure tone threshold test, one cannot apply a sensitivity-selectivity formula to this report.

Procedures

Preschool screening tests are recommended and are listed below in order of their ease of application. The ideal program would utilize both pure tone and acoustic impedance testing. Various studies have shown that impedance will identify from 90 to 95% of all the significant ear pathologies in children. The pure tone screening test may identify 50% of the ear pathologies (Melnick et al., 1964).

1. *Impedance Screening.* See section in this chapter on impedance screening and note recommended guidelines.

2. *Pure Tone Screening Tests*
   a. Play-conditioning procedure for testing the 3- and 4-year-old child (one child with three or four observing).
      (1) Have available a peg board, a ring tower, plain blocks, or other simple toys that are motivating to young children.
      (2) With headphones on your ears, take a block (or peg, etc.) and hold it up to one ear as if listening. Make believe you hear a sound, say "I hear it," and put the block on the table.
      (3) Put the phones on the child's ear and hold his hand with the block up to his ear.
      (4) Sound a 50-dB tone at 1000 Hz and guide his hand to build the block tower. Repeat once or twice and then see if he can do it alone. If he can, go on. . . .
      (5) Set the hearing level to 25 dB and repeat the test. If he responds, go on to the other frequencies (2000–4000 Hz) and repeat the procedure. Praise him for each correct response. After each presentation, place another block in his hand.
      (6) Switch to the opposite ear and

repeat the test starting at 4000 Hz and descending to 2000 and 1000 Hz.

b. Procedure for testing and referrals for the mature 4-year-old and the 5-year-old child are identical to that described for the older child in the next section.

3. *Criterion for Referral.* Failure to respond to 25 dB (ANSI) at any frequency, and/or failure on impedance screening evaluation.

GOALS AND METHODS, 5–18 YEARS

Goals

At school age the primary goal is to keep the child functioning adequately in the classroom. In the past, adequate functioning was considered to be a 25-dB hearing level or better. Now that accumulated evidence, however, has shown that a 15-dB hearing level may be educationally handicapping, the means of securing the educational goals have changed. It is now necessary to identify the milder hearing losses that are caused by middle ear effusions. In the majority of school situations it is impossible to screen at levels lower than 20 dB HL due to the presence of ambient noise.

So for the first time in history the traditional pure tone screening tests must be supplemented by other tests, if educationally handicapping hearing losses are to be identified. The additional test that is proposed is the acoustic impedance test.

Methods

PURE TONE SCREENING TEST

Background. School hearing screening has a long and honorable history. As early as 1924 a group of dedicated otolaryngologists utilized and reported a new instrument for testing the hearing of school children (McFarlan, 1927; Goldstein, 1933). The instrument was developed by Fowler and Fletcher (1926) for the Western Electric Company. The Western Electric 4-A audiometer was a phonograph connected to an assembly of 30 earphones which would simultaneously present well calibrated speech signals to the earphones. In the Western Electric Fading Numbers test, numbers were spoken by both a man's and a woman's voice, starting at 33 dB and ending at 9B (re: normal threshold).

The reason for the change to pure tone testing was that the gross speech signals used in the Western Electric test did not identify children with high frequency losses.

Individual Pure Tone Sweep Test. In 1961 the Conference on Identification Audiometry of the American Speech and Hearing Association issued a monograph providing guidelines for school screening (Darley, 1961). It recommended individual pure tone screening as the most accurate procedure, but stated that group screening tests were less costly and could be used where cost is a factor.

The Conference on Identification Audiometry recommended that four frequencies be tested: 1000, 2000, 4000, and 6000 Hz; 500 Hz was to be omitted because testing environments often produce too high ambient noise levels.

Melnick et al. (1964) conducted a study, which utilized the Conference's recommendations, and found that the use of 6000 Hz as a test frequency produced too many failures. The variable interactions between earphones and children's ear canals at 6000 Hz make this test frequency a poor choice for inclusion in a school screening program. Subsequent to the 1961 conference recommendations, several studies have shown that the use of 500 Hz as a screening frequency is contraindicated to identify middle ear disorders (Eagles et al., 1967; Roberts et al., 1982).

A more recent set of Guidelines for Identification Audiometry was published by the American Speech-Language-Hearing Association in 1975 as an update to the 1961 recommendations. The Guidelines recommend a manually administered, individual, pure tone, air-conduction hearing screening procedure which incorporates the criteria presented below.

The screening test frequencies to be used are 1000, 2000, and 4000 Hz. The screening intensity level should be 20 dB HL (re: ANSI 1969) at 1000 and 2000 Hz and 25 dB HL at 4000 Hz. It is acceptable to screen at 20 dB HL at all three test frequencies, but if the 4000 Hz presentation is not heard, the intensity output should be increased by 5 dB to 25 dB HL. Since most children will hear all three tones at 20 dB HL, the hearing level dial will remain at one setting for the entire screening test. It is important, however, to remember that 25 dB HL is the specified level at 4000 Hz.

Screening Test Failures. Failure of the child to respond at the recommended screening level at any frequency in either ear is to be considered as failure of the screening test. All children who are such "failures" should be rescreened, preferably within the same testing session during which they failed, but definitely within 1 week following the initial screening session. This recommended rescreening, using the same frequencies at the same intensity level, is an essential element for maintaining the efficiency of the hearing screening program.

The children who fail the rescreening should be referred for audiological evaluation by a qualified audiologist. Some persons, particularly younger children, will fail both the screening test and the rescreening test and then yield normal hearing thresholds on the audiologic evaluation. Therefore, a hearing impairment should not be considered identified until after receiving an audiometric evaluation by a qualified audiologist. The following referral priority scheme for audiological evaluation is recommended in the Guidelines for those children who fail the screening and rescreening procedures:

1. Binaural hearing loss in both ears at all frequencies;
2. Binaural hearing loss at 1000 and 2000 Hz only;
3. Binaural hearing loss at 1000 *or* 2000 Hz only;

4. Monaural hearing loss at all frequencies;
5. Monaural hearing loss at 1000 and 2000 Hz;
6. Binaural or monaural hearing loss at 4000 Hz only.

The 1975 Identification Audiometry Guidelines offer several other important suggestions in the procedural operations of a school hearing screening program. Complete audiometer calibration should be conducted at least once every year. In addition, a daily listening check should be performed to ensure that the audiometer is grossly in calibration and that no defects exist in major operational components. Ambient noise levels in the testing room should not exceed 50 dB SPL at 1000 Hz, 58 dB SPL at 2000 Hz, and 76 dB SPL at 4000 Hz as measured with a sound level meter and octave band filters centered on the screening frequencies.

A qualified audiologist should conduct or supervise the identification audiometry program although nonprofessional support personnel may be used for the screening testing after appropriate training. The recommendations for audiologic and medical evaluations should be based on local realities and availability of referral sources.

The paperwork associated with a hearing screening program can be massive. Test forms, calibration data, student records, etc., must be carefully considered and planned prior to the testing sessions. The language used in notices sent to parents and referral physicians about screening or rescreening results should avoid diagnostic conclusions and alarming predictions. Remember that the hearing impairment is not confirmed until the stage of the audiometric evaluation has been completed. The Guidelines recommend personal contact about test results if possible, rather than written notices. Some parents will become overly concerned, others will show little or no concern, and still others would like to cooperate but fear the potential expense that might be involved. If parents believe that their child can "hear," despite the results of the hearing screening, special tact and persuasion will be required to convince them that a problem truly exists. The word "fail" should be avoided in reporting hearing screening results because of its negative connotation. The reporting aspect of the identification audiometry program will require more time and thought than initially is anticipated. Detail concerning the operation of a school hearing screening program has recently been described by Feldman et al. (1981).

Rosenberg and Swogger-Rosenberg (1982) present an interesting discussion and review the status of hearing screening procedures in each state in our country. They have compiled a list, or rather as they describe it, ". . . a chaotic myriad of standards, regulations, guidelines, techniques and recommendations" that they gathered by survey. They noted that most states did have a hearing screening program of some sort, but the extraordinary range of screening techniques and policies is a sad commentary upon our ability to sell a health program in which we believe so strongly.

IMPEDANCE SCREENING

The evaluation of children in hearing screening programs has changed considerably with the use of impedance audiometry. The impedance technique is well suited for use with children since it requires little cooperation, provides objective results, and is quick and easy to administer. However, considerable controversy has arisen about the use of impedance measurements in school screening programs. Brooks (1969, 1973, 1975) has long and often advocated the use of acoustic impedance measurement as a supplement to the standard pure tone hearing screening test in school populations. A large number of studies have been conducted to compare the efficacy of impedance screening in the identification of hearing problems in children. A recent comprehensive review of the status of this topic was published by Brooks in 1980.

The debate about the role of impedance screening was summarized in two points of view by Bess (1980) and Northern (1980b).

Much of the discussion presented below has been taken from these two reports.

The goal of a hearing screening program is to identify those individuals who probably have some hearing problem from those individuals who probably do not have a hearing problem. Children who "fail" the screening tests may or may not have ear problems and are thus "tagged" for additional testing to determine the cause of screening failure. Virtually every state has an active hearing screening program and for nearly 40 years hearing screening has proven to be one of the most acceptable screening procedures in a multitude of health detection programs. Unfortunately, traditional pure tone techniques for screening hearing fail to identify numerous individuals who have mild hearing loss often due to the presence of middle ear disease.

The single "bright light" in the history of auditory screening has been the development of acoustic impedance measurements. It is only natural that the vast numbers of persons responsible for hearing screening programs utilize the best testing techniques to identify children with hearing disorders. The impedance technique is capable of yielding more accurate screening results in the identification of middle ear disease than is possible with otoscopy or pure tone audiometry: a firm fact substantiated in numerous studies.

Professionals active in hearing screening are well aware of the inadequacies of pure tone screening audiometry, and thus welcome the opportunity to supplement their test protocol with impedance screening. The use of impedance in conjunction with pure tone hearing testing increases the overall accuracy of the screening program, reduces the number of children who must be retested prior to referral, and in fact, increases assurance that children who are referred for additional work-up have legitimate otologic problems.

Opponents to the use of impedance in mass screening raise legitimate concern that the technique will identify asymptomatic individuals who have fluctuant otitis media with effusion for which specific treatment may be inadvisable. Although the otitis media with middle ear effusion may resolve spontaneously in many individuals, undetected and untreated middle ear effusions may indeed also create serious otologic complications, speech, language and/or educational problems. Medical complications from otitis media include sensorineural hearing loss, ossicular fixation through adhesions, tympanic membrane perforations and/or retraction pockets, cholesteatoma, ossicular necrosis, mastoiditis, and even meningitis. Although specific treatment may not be in order for every individual with middle ear effusion, certainly accurate identification of such persons is desirable and easily within our technical means.

As shown by Cooper et al. (1975) and Queen et al. (1981) impedance screening is economically the most cost-effective technique for sampling asymptomatic children to identify those individuals who have middle ear problems. Impedance screening is not intended to be a diagnostic procedure; nor is isolated impedance screening advocated without support from audiometry and/or otoscopic examination. Impedance screening will not only identify those individuals who have otitis media with effusion but the technique is also sensitive to all the complications or sequelae of otitis media.

Impedance Validity

Much discussion has been published questioning the validity of impedance screening. Validity is determined by examining the sensitivity and specificity of a screening technique. *Sensitivity* is defined as accuracy in identifying individuals who have the target condition. *Specificity* is the accuracy of the technique in identifying nondiseased individuals. Knowledgeable professionals cannot deny the high sensitivity of impedance screening in correctly identifying individuals with middle ear disease while admitting the low sensitivity of pure tone screening. For example, statistics have shown that pure tone screening missed 259 of 1651 tympanic membrane perforations (17%) and failed to identify 33 of 60 (55%) cholesteatomas. (Northern, 1977a). However, the major criticism of impedance screening relates to its low specificity, or the false identification of individuals who do not have middle ear disease.

Admittedly the monumental number of articles published about impedance screening provides little conclusive data for establishing validity credentials. To determine validity of a screening technique, one screening procedure is used as a criterion measure against which to compare other screening tests. Otoscopy is most often accepted as the criterion test against which to compare screening, in spite of the fact that the accuracy of otoscopy varies tremendously as a function of the individual behind the otoscope (Paradise et al., 1976; Roeser et al., 1977). Otoscopy is so subjective it can be argued that *impedance* should be the criterion procedure because of its objectivity and test-retest reliability. Generally speaking, the use of otoscopy as the criterion produces higher sensitivity agreement since fewer subjects "fail" otoscopy while many subjects may "fail" screening.

Paradise and Smith (1979) analyzed 14 published studies of impedance screening in preschool children and found that only two studies provided ample data from which to calculate validity. In the two cited studies (Paradise et al., 1976; Roeser et al., 1977) impedance sensitivity with otoscopy as the criterion measure was 94% and 97%, while specificity was 42% and 61% respectively. The amount of pathology in the sample population affects the sensitivity rate since it is easy to obtain high agreement between impedance and otoscopy when many normal subjects are examined. The low specificity rates of impedance audiometry are most often due to the use of too rigid failure criteria for peaked negative pressure curves. Adherence to middle ear pressure failure criteria of -200 mm H_2O should do much to alleviate the overreferral, and low specificity problem.

Of course the ultimate validation technique for middle ear effusion is myringotomy. The recent studies reported by Orchik et al. (1978a, 1978b) with impedance and myringotomy in 218 ears has shown that the combined use of tympanometry and acoustic reflex measurement showed a statistically significant correlation with the presence of middle ear fluid. Their studies, as well as the report by Paradise et al. (1976) show the correlation between 'flat" impedance curves and the presence of effusion proven by myringotomy to be 82–90% accurate. This high correlation between 'flat" impedance curves and absent acoustic reflexes speaks highly for referral and medical evaluation of such children.

Additional research of this sort is important if we hope to establish the positive and negative attributes of impedance as a screening test. The importance of the sensitivity-specificity relationship using various combinations of impedance measures in a number of childhood populations cannot be overemphasized. Our goal should be to establish a cutoff which can identify most children with disease but does not result in overreferral. Although abnormal tympanograms appear to be associated with a diseased ear, normal tympanograms do not necessarily imply a nondiseased ear.

In discussing the appropriateness of impedance as a screening tool the aspects of cost and calibration deserve a brief comment. Although estimates have been made of the direct costs of impedance screening (salary, equipment, maintenance, etc), it is difficult to predict the costs of follow-up since we know little about the sensitivity-specificity of this test. A high overreferral rate could well result in unnecessary yet expensive medical management.

Once the presence of middle ear effusion has been identified can it be treated effectively? On this question we have the single most controversial issue as it relates to impedance screening. In part, opposition to mass screening for middle ear disease is based on the knowledge that many effusions are known to resolve spontaneously and that treatment may not be beneficial. As stated by Paradise et al. (1978) "We thus have a disease state—otitis media with effusion—that in most instances may resolve spontaneously; that may have no lasting ill effects; and for which specific treatment may often, if not usually, be inadvisable. Under the circumstances, mass screening programs would stand a good chance of promoting large-scale overreferral and overtreatment, much of the latter inevitably surgical." Such a prospect raises the uncomfortable specter of high indirect costs associated with unnecessary follow-up.

Recognizing that many screening programs were already in operation and that others were soon to be implemented, procedural guidelines and criteria to be used in the screening of preschool and school age children have been developed. A Nashville Task Force (Harford et al., 1978) hoped that the data collected from screening programs already in existence would be obtained in a uniform and systematic manner and that such data could be used to refine future guidelines. Toward this end, the classification scheme shown in Table 7.10 was developed for various screening results. Failure on the initial screening test is determined by an absent acoustic reflex at 1000 Hz (presented at 105 dB HTL in the contralateral mode) or by an abnormal tympanogram. An abnormal tympanogram was defined as one that was either flat or rounded having no discernible peak, or one having a negative pressure equivalent to or greater than -200 mm H_2O. It was recommended that any child who failed the initial screening be retested in four to six weeks. Classification 1 is represented by a pass on the initial screening whereas classifications 2 and 3 are for those children who fail the initial test. As denoted by classification 2, referral is made to an appropriate health care provider if the child fails the retest. A child who passes the retest, as designated by classification 3, is categorized as "at risk" and a close monitoring program is recommended.

An alternative set of screening guidelines was developed by the American Speech and Hearing Association (ASHA, 1978). In these guidelines the need to identify middle ear disease not only was based on medical considerations but also much emphasis was placed on the possible educational, social and psychological sequelae. Although the procedural considerations for both sets of recommendations are remarkably similar, the ASHA guidelines differ from the Nashville report in two significant ways. First, the ASHA guidelines refrain from making any value judgments pertaining to the need for mass screening. That is, they neither recommend nor oppose impedance screening on a routine basis for the detection of middle ear disorders in children. Rather, procedural guidelines are merely outlined for those who wish to implement a screening program. Second, the referral criteria of the ASHA guidelines differ from the Nashville recommendations. The middle ear screening criteria advocated by ASHA are summarized in Table 7.11 and Figure 7.7. Although somewhat more detail is provided, the "pass" and "risk" classifications do not differ significantly from the Nashville schema. The "fail" classification, however, is considerably different in that a failure in the initial screen results in an immediate referral. Recall that the Nash-

Table 7.10.
Nashville Task Force Classifications and Criteria[a]

Classification	Initial Screen	Retest	Subject Outcome
I	Acoustic reflex present and tympanogram normal	Not required	Cleared
II	Acoustic reflex absent and/or tympanogram abnormal	Acoustic reflex absent and/or tympanogram abnormal	Referred
III	Acoustic reflex absent and/or tympanogram abnormal	Acoustic reflex present and tympanogram normal	At risk; recheck at later date

[a] From E. R. Harford et al.: *Impedance Screening for Middle Ear Disease in Children*, p. 6. Grune & Stratton, New York, 1978.

Table 7.11.
ASHA Guidelines and Middle Ear Screening Criteria[a]

Classification	Screening Pass/Fail Criteria Results of Initial Screen	Disposition
1. Pass	Middle ear pressure normal or mildly positive/negative and acoustic reflex (AR) present	Cleared; no return
2. At risk	Middle ear pressure abnormal (and acoustic reflex present) or Acoustic reflex absent (and middle ear pressure normal or mildly positive/negative)	Retest in 3–5 weeks (a) If tympanometry and AR fall into Classification 1: PASS; (b) If tympanometery or AR remain in Classification 2: Fail and refer
3. Fail	Middle ear pressure abnormal and Acoustic reflex absent	Refer

[a] ASHA Subcommittee on Impedance Measurement Guidelines for Acoustic Immitance Screening of Middle-ear Function. *Asha, 20:* 550–555, 1978.

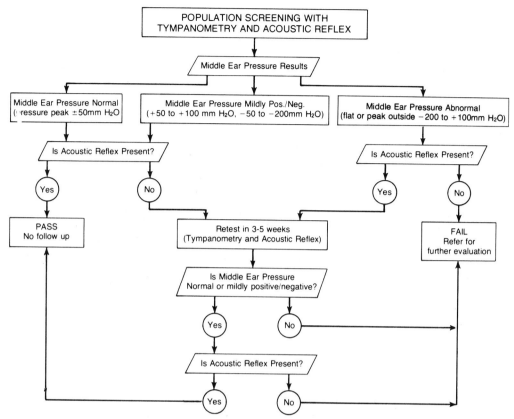

Figure 7.7. Flow chart depicting guidelines for impedance screening interpretation and pass-monitor-fail criteria. (Reproduced with permission from *Asha, 21:* 287, 1979.)

ville conference recommended a retest in 4–6 weeks following a fail on the initial screen.

The current state of affairs in impedance screening programs is that we now have two significant sets of guidelines for those school clinicians who wish to include impedance measurements as part of the hearing screening program. There is still an urgent need, however, for carefully planned and rigorously controlled scientific screening projects to clarify further the benefits and limitations of impedance screening. Further, there is need to gather additional data on the natural history, medical management and educational complications of middle ear effusions.

Lucker (1980) reported results of a screening project in which the ASHA guidelines were followed and pass/fail criteria were applied after a single test session. A

pilot project so conducted yielded a large number of failures, many of whom were not found to have middle ear disorders when examined by their physicians within 2 weeks from the date of referral. Lucker was able to reduce the number of failures in the impedance screening program by altering the ASHA guideline pass/fail critera by retesting all the children in the "fail" catergory one to two weeks following the initial screening prior to referral.

Queen et al. (1981) reported results of an impedance screening project conducted in the Kansas City, Missouri, Public School District involving nearly 20,000 elementary students. Although they attempted to utilize the ASHA guidelines, they soon found need to delete the acoustic reflex from the test procedure except in "borderline" cases, i.e., -200 mm H_2O middle ear pressure. They also combined the ASHA recommended AT RISK and FAIL categories into a simple REFERRAL category for retesting at a later date. They report that their initial retest rate was 17%, compared to a 25% rate reported by Lucker (1980). They finally identified 6.2% of their total elementary population for further audiologic evaluation.

AUDITORY SCREENING OF THE MENTALLY RETARDED

Standards for institutions serving the mentally retarded as set forth by the Accreditation Council for Facilities for the Mentally Retarded (1971) provide operational guidelines for audiology services. In reference to audiometric screening, the standards state that all new residents, children under 10 at annual intervals, other residents at regular intervals, and any resident referred shall be screened. In addition, many facilities provide outpatient evaluation and services which include audiometric screening. As a result audiologists in such facilities are finding themselves faced with great numbers of retarded, of all ages and functioning levels, for audiometric screening.

Comprehensive audiologic assessment implies pure tone thresholds, speech audiometry, and any other significant diagnostic information obtainable. However, when large numbers of mentally retarded are involved, the need for a more efficient method of screening becomes evident. A variety of conditioning techniques, evoked response audiometry, special diagnostic procedures, as well as other auditory assessment techniques, have been suggested; although these may be reliable clinical tools, the technical problems of applying them to rapid mass screening have not been resolved. Subjective approaches which employ behavioral observation alone give limited information and no indication of cause of hearing loss.

We have developed a screening procedure for the retarded based on behavioral observation as a function of mental age (Downs, 1970) and acoustic impedance audiometry

(Lamb and Norris, 1970; Northern, 1971a, 1978c, 1980d). Our screening technique is designed for use with the severely and profoundly retarded and other patients who would be classified as difficult to test. It is not proposed as a substitute for pure tone screening when pure tone results are obtainable within the limitations of a screening program. Rather, it is designed for use when traditional clinical assessment techniques are not applicable.

The subject is seated or held in the sound suite facing one speaker. Initially the stimulus is presented through the opposite speaker so that if the subject localizes he must make an overt lateralization, which is very obvious, to seek the sound from the speaker furthest away from him. If he localizes, as soon as his head is turned toward the speaker, the examiner quickly switches the signal to the other side. Speech is primarily used as the sound stimulus, but a variety of other stimuli can be employed. It is sometimes necessary to change the stimuli during testing to pure tones, warble tones, white noise, or complex noise.

Observations are made by an audiologist and, if possible, trained observers. Response categories include (1) responses which indicate awareness such as eye opening, quieting, assuming a listening attitude, smiling, laughing, cessation of activity; (2) localization responses which are the overt learned responses that take the place of generalized body movements as the child matures; (3) startle responses which are the involuntary reflexive responses that are expected 65 to 85 dB above threshold and include eyeblink, orientation reflex, tonic neck reflex, Moro reflex; and (4) no response.

Step 1

An ascending approach should be employed in an attempt to obtain response from the subject at levels of 45 dB HL or better. Awareness, or preferably localization by 45 dB HL constitutes passing the observational portion of the screening.

Step 2

If no response is obtained by 45 dB, ascend in 10-dB steps in an attempt to elicit a response. It is necessary to vary the time between presentations in an attempt to catch the subject off guard. If the subject shows awareness or localizes by 65 dB HL and a startle can be elicited, it may be concluded that he either has grossly normal hearing or a mild-to-moderate hearing loss.

Step 3

Even when a subject shows awareness and/or localization at levels below 45 dB, an attempt is made to elicit a startle. If no startle is obtainable the subject fails screening and probably has a hearing loss. Even as the examiner attempts to elicit a startle at high intensity levels, it is important to continue to watch for awareness and/or localization responses. Responses at these levels will provide inferences about auditory sensitivity.

Step 4

The final step in the screening procedure is impedance audiometry. Tympanograms and acoustic reflexes, if possible, are obtained bilaterally. The objective measurements obtained with the impedance audiometer not only rule out or establish conductive problems but serve as an objective means of examining the more difficult-to-test students.

Operant conditioning techniques may also be used as screening methods for the mentally retarded. In general, however, they involve a threshold search and are therefore described in Chapter 5 under clinical testing.

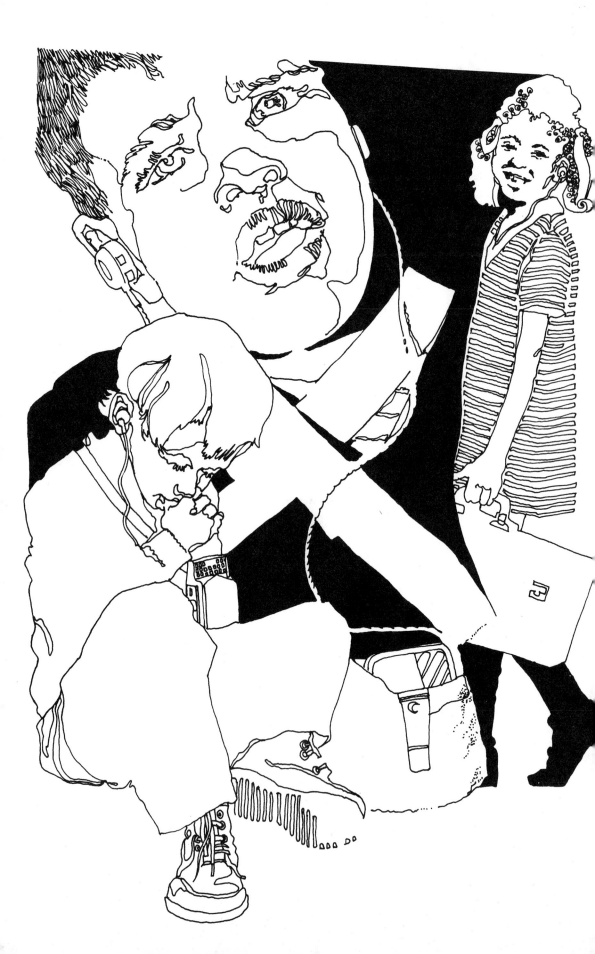

CHAPTER 8

Amplification for Hearing-Impaired Children

There is little doubt that the single most important invention to help the hearing-handicapped child is the electronic hearing aid. There is an old adage, ". . . as we hear, so shall we speak," and it is this very close relationship between hearing, speech, and language that is so important to the deaf child. Several electronic gadgets have been invented to help the deaf child learn to speak, including voice pitch indicators, speech timing equipment, vowel indicators, voice/nonvoice meters, speech spectrum displays, visible speech machines, etc. None of these inventions, however, is more fundamental to the deaf child's education, and his ability to learn speech, than properly fitted hearing aids.

The task of selecting hearing aids for a child is not to be taken lightly. Selection of hearing aids for the hearing-impaired or deaf child must not be undertaken by the inexperienced clinician or the nonprofessionally trained individual. The procedure involved in the process of selecting hearing aids for a child involves many people including the otolaryngologist, the pediatrician, the audiologist/dispenser, the speech pathologist, the teacher of the deaf, as well as other auxiliary professionals such as the public health or school nurse and the social worker. These individuals must work together closely, in a coordinated effort, to ensure that the hearing-impaired child obtains maximal benefit from amplification.

The audiologist is clearly the individual to coordinate and guide the hearing aid selection procedure. The audiologist, because of his extensive training, is able to identify the nature and degree of the child's hearing loss—which may in itself be an extremely difficult task. The audiologist ensures that proper medical clearance is obtained prior to the hearing aid selection procedure. He is able to evaluate the performance of various hearing aids on the child and, through the use of an electroacoustic hearing aid test chamber, make an earmold impression, select and dispense the hearing aids to obtain the best amplification available for the patient's hearing loss. As part of this entire process, the audiologist must counsel the parents about the new hearing aids, their care and use; he must arrange for therapy for the child and special training if necessary. And finally, he is able to devote the necessary time to follow-up the progress of the patient, and maintain an ever vigilant eye to be sure the hearing aids are in top operating condition. The audiologist must be careful not to use the hearing aids as a device to test a youngster's hearing, as it is no substitute for an accurate, knowledgeable hearing assessment. Do not confuse the problem by mixing the audiometric evaluation with the hearing aid evaluation.

Clinical hearing aid evaluations with children should include ample consideration for therapy. Many hours are involved in the preselection hearing aid workup for the hearing-impaired child. Nearly as much time may then be necessary to select the proper hearing aid and earmold. Additional telephone calls and letters may be necessary to appropriate agencies to obtain financial assistance for the purchase of the aid. Electroacoustic analysis of the hearing aids is important to confirm proper fitting. But the time consumed by these procedures is only fleeting seconds when compared to the long-term therapy and follow-up programs that the child will need through the remainder of the school years.

Tremendous technologic advances in the hearing aid have been made over the past three decades. Only a few years ago, hearing aids were heavy, cumbersome units with large, unsightly battery requirements. The electronic hearing aid became a reality in the 1930s; the vacuum tube became part of the system in the 1940s; transistors permitted the hearing aid to be a much smaller unit in the 1950s. Today, tiny "solid state" electronic devices have reduced the instrument and its power source to a practical size and weight—with satisfactory cosmetic appeal to most consumers. Recent developments in the microphone component of the hearing aid have extended both ends of the frequency reproduction range. Microphones are now available that are truly directional—amplifying only sounds that are immediately in front of the hearing aid and at the same time attenuating sounds emitted from the sides or back of the listener.

Hearing aid technology has improved considerably over the past decade, and today's instruments are infinitely better than the hearing aids of even 5 years ago. Critics complain that we should not be satisfied with today's hearing aid, and that technologic advances must still be pursued.

The operation of the hearing aid has been likened to a miniature hi-fi set designed as a group of tiny components, which picks up sound wave vibrations from the air and converts them into electrical signals. Actually, modern hearing aids are much more than just ultraminiature electroacoustic amplifiers. They are sophisticated, personal signal processing systems, comprising not only the hearing instrument itself, but also a technically elaborate acoustic coupling system which plays a significant role in processing and modification of the acoustic signal, as well as conducting the signal to the tympanic membrane (Ely, 1981). Although the major amplification, signal limiting, and complex controlling functions are achieved within the hearing aid itself, spectral shaping takes place not only in the hearing aid but also in the acoustic coupling system which includes the earmold, earhook and tubing (Fig. 8.1). Readers interested in more information about hearing aids are referred to Pollack (1980), or Hodgson and Skinner (1981). A large number of textbooks concerning all aspects of hearing aids are now available to the interested reader. Recommended textbooks include Studebaker and Bess (1982), Libby (1980), and Bess et al. (1981).

Few studies have reported on the status of hearing aids worn by children. Persons working with children who use hearing aids are familiar with the "maple syrup syndrome," in which the hearing aid catches all sorts of debris and quits working. Gaeth and Lounsbury (1966) interviewed 134 hard of hearing elementary school children and their parents as part of a longitudinal evaluation program. Electroacoustic measurements showed that only 16% of the children were wearing hearing aids that could be considered adequate, and only 50% of the children were obtaining adequate hearing from the aids.

Zink (1972) reported results from a 2-year longitudinal electroacoustic hearing aid program of analysis of aids worn by children. He warns that, just because a child wears his hearing aid faithfully, the assumption cannot be made that the aid is functioning adequately. In the evaluation of 92 hearing aids in use by children, only 55% were found to be acceptable. Zink recommends that each amplification unit in regular use receive regular longitudinal electroacoustic analysis. Often, a child's difficulty in adjusting to amplification or his reluctance for continued hearing aid use may be traced to poor function of the hearing aid (Zink and Alpiner, 1968). Potts and Greenwood (1983) described a daily hearing aid monitoring program the results of

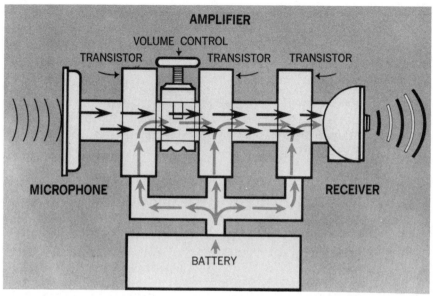

Figure 8.1. The components of a modern hearing aid. (Reproduced with permission from E. Corliss: Facts about Hearing and Hearing Aids. A Consumer's Guide from the National Bureau of Standards, U.S. Dept. of Commerce. Washington, D.C., U.S. Govt. Printing Office, 1971.)

which created a significant decrease in the incidence of hearing aid malfunction in their school. The program was based on a detailed visual-auditory inspection (Table 8.1) and routine electroacoustic analysis. These authors commented that the increased emphasis on hearing aid performance appeared to promote other improvements in the child's utilization of amplification.

The regulations of the recent Education for All Handicapped Children Act of 1975 (P.L. 94-142) state that each public agency shall ensure that hearing aids worn by hearing-impaired students in school are functioning properly (*Federal Register*, August 23, 1977, 121a.303). Positive hearing aid maintenance programs can be conducted within educational settings (Hanners and Sitton, 1974). Bendet (1980) reports a successful public school hearing aid maintenance program carried out by the teachers of the hearing-impaired students.

FDA regulations were put into effect in August 1977 for the protection of potential hearing aid consumers. These regulations include the following rules related to hearing aids for children:

1. Before purchase of a hearing aid, an individual with a hearing loss must have a medical evaluation of the hearing loss by a physician (preferably a physician specializing in diseases of the ear) within 6 months preceding the sale of the aid.

2. Adult patients, under carefully defined circumstances, can sign a waiver of the medical clearance requirements. However, there is no waiver option for persons under 18 years of age. The physician who examines the child must provide a written statement that the patient's hearing loss has been medically evaluated.

3. In addition to seeing a physician for a medical evaluation, a child with a hearing loss should be directed to an audiologist for evaluation and rehabilitation since hearing loss may cause problems in language development and the educational and social growth of a child.

HEARING AIDS

The basic principle is to provide as much useful amplification as possible, taking best advantage of whatever residual hearing exists. Innovative experimenters have attempted to transform certain acoustic fea-

Table 8.1.
Total Looking/Listening Check for Hearing Aids[a]

Remove aid from child, noting "as worn" volume setting.

Component	Looking	Listening (use sounds /a/ /u/ /i/ /ʃ/ /s/)
Earmold	Opening clear? Cracks, rough areas?	
Battery	Read voltage (replace at 1.1 or below)—Compartment clean?	
Case	Cracks? Separating?	Press case gently—Interruption in amplification?
Microphone	Clean? Visible damage?	
Dials	Clean? Easily rotated?	Rotate—Reasonable gain variation? Static?
Switches	Clean? Easy to move?	Turn on and off—Static?
Cord (body aid)	Cracked? Frayed? Connection plugs clean?	Run fingers down cord—Interruption in amplification? Connections tight?
Tubing (ear level aid)	Cracks? Good connection to mold and aid? Moisture? Debris?	Cover opening of earmold and turn to maximum gain—Feedback?
Receiver (body aid)	Cracks? Firmly attached to earmold snap ring?	Distortion? Static? Reduced gain? Substitute spare receiver and recheck.
Oscillator (bone aid)	Cracks? Plug clean? Attached well to band?	Listen with oscillator on mastoid, ears plugged to block air-conducted sound.
Variable Controls	Proper SSPL, frequency response, gain setting?	5 speech sounds clearly amplified? Gain sounds normal for this aid?
Distortion		Clear quality?
Feedback	Recheck receiver snap, tubing, earmold.	Turn to maximum gain to check—External feedback? Internal?

Replace aid and check fit of the earmold to the child's ear.

[a] From P. Potts and J. Greenwood: Hearing aid monitoring. *Language, Speech and Hearing Services in Schools, 14:*163, 1983.

tures into other sensory modalities such as vibrotactile or visual stimuli, or to change the physical acoustic properties of the signal into other auditory characteristics. There appears to be agreement that a more efficient and widespread means of providing maximal benefits of amplification among hearing-impaired children may help alleviate some of the present burdens of deafness (Levitt and Nye, 1971).

Basic to the concept of hearing aid recommendations is a realistic understanding of what the aid can do for the patient. No hearing aid will enable a hard of hearing youngster to perform normally in *all* situations. The primary reason for recommending the use of personal amplification is to enable the child to communicate better with a hearing aid than without it. Such improvement may be possible in only a few select conditions for a child, but he will ultimately learn, with good teaching, to utilize the aid to its maximal benefit. In the words of Mark Ross (1969), "merely because one can 'get along' without a hearing aid is *not* an adequate reason to discourage its use."

Curran (1982) described four basic factors for successful hearing aid fittings that may be applied to children: (1) He identified the importance of the case history and basic hearing evaluation to confirm the patient's hearing status and qualify his/her candidacy for amplification. (2) The method for selection of the hearing aid is often a function of the experience of the audiologist. Although no specific method provides exact, precise information regarding the correct amount of gain, output or frequency response, final selection may be influenced by ergonomic characteristics as described by Rubin (1980) such as needs of the child, cosmetic considerations, manipulation of trimmer controls, availability of options, and of course, cost. (3) The third important factor recommended by Curran is to use instruments which have wide range adjustable trimmers such as a 90-dB saturation sound pressure level (SSPL 90) reduction control, a low-cut tone control of at least 15 dB at 500 Hz, a gain trimmer, a high frequency roll-off trimmer and threshold of compression adjustments. Curran correctly points out that this factor is especially valuable in children's fittings because of the questionable hearing threshold measurements and the fact that the patient's listening skills will change over time after the hearing aids are fitted. (4) The fourth factor is by far the most important, modifications to the hearing aid coupling system. The coupling system, including the earmold, tubing, earhook, etc., are all under direct control of the dispenser of the hearing aid. Small, almost imperceptible changes in the physical dimensions of the earmold, and associated "plumbing" system, can produce significant auditory changes in the response of the hearing aid system.

Young children have not developed a "listening strategy" and it is important to reemphasize that the hearing aid evaluation in children is a continuing process. Other factors to be considered require the best possible amplified signal with good quality and clear sound. This *must* be checked electroacoustically by the audiologist-dispenser for *every* hearing aid on *every* child at *every* clinic visit. Townsend and

Olsen (1982) reported that only 69% of new hearing aid instruments they evaluated met the manufacturer's specifications, which stresses the importance of electroacoustic analysis in the clinic setting. Townsend and Wavrek (1983) surveyed 333 clinics who ranked various electroacoustic analyses in the order of importance to be (1) high frequency full-on gain, (2) maximum SSPL 90, (3) high frequency-average SSPL 90, (4) total harmonic distortion, and (5) frequency response curve.

Other important factors to be considered in children's hearing aids include the need for flexibility to fit a variety of educational amplification input options, a good tele-coil that has good frequency response with external inputs and allows for both microphone and tele-coil function simultaneously. Common wisdom requires that a child's hearing aid be exceedingly durable, and of course consideration should be given to a protection plan for extended warranty, loss, or damage.

Today's audiologist-dispenser must be especially cognizant of the methods of hearing aid response modification technology. Ely (1981) points out that, within the hearing aid, level and spectral modifications can be implemented to produce a uniform effect over the entire spectrum or to selectively effect frequency ranges of the overall spectrum. Modifications to the hearing aid response can be influenced by consideration of a number of factors including the microphone location, frequency response adjustments, the earhook and tubing length, diameter, configuration and filter characteristics, the earmold shape and size, the seal or openness of the earmold (which can strongly influence low frequency amplification), and the ear canal space between the tip of the earmold and the tympanic membrane. The clinical side of the evaluation reminds us that, even when the above considerations have been accurately worked out for maximum benefit in amplification, changes in the impedance of the tympanic membrane and middle ear due to pathology may render the "best fitting" somewhat less than desired. All of these factors must be second nature to the audiologist-dispenser who works with hearing-impaired children (Curran, 1982).

The Earmold

The earmold itself is an essential feature of the hearing aid system. It provides support for the aid, directs the amplified sound into the ear canal, and prevents acoustic feedback if fitted properly. If the earmold does not fit properly, it will cause feedback in the form of whistles and squeals, or produce local irritation and soreness.

Ross (1972) points out that the earmold is an integral part of the electroacoustic events that begin with the hearing aid and end with the patient's ear canal. Northern and Hattler (1970) have shown that variations in earmolds can alter the electroacoustic characteristics of the hearing aid as shown in Figure 8.2. Accordingly, it is important to evaluate a hearing aid with the

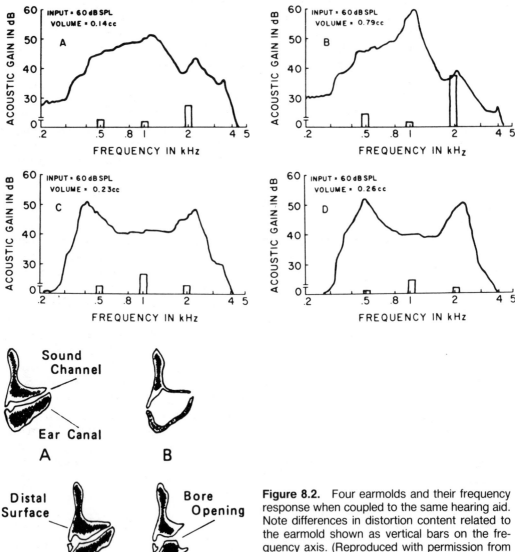

Figure 8.2. Four earmolds and their frequency response when coupled to the same hearing aid. Note differences in distortion content related to the earmold shown as vertical bars on the frequency axis. (Reproduced with permission from J. L. Northern and K. W. Hattler: *Journal of Speech and Hearing Research, 13:*162–172, 1970.)

earmold which is to be used with it. This may mean two visits with the child, one to take the earmold impression, and an additional session after the permanent custom earmold has been fabricated. It is particularly difficult to conduct hearing aid evaluations with children using stock earmolds, since they often do not fit well in the child's ear canal and most certainly do not represent how the hearing aid will perform and sound to the child when he has his own earmold. The pinna continues to grow in size in children until about 9 years of age. Thus, earmolds may have to be remade every 3–6 months in the child's early years, or once a year after age 5, to ensure adequate fit.

The earmold can be crafted in many ways to enhance the hearing aid, with open vents, various tubing, filters, etc. The material of the earmold is relatively nonsignificant, as long as a good tight fit of the mold is achieved in the ear canal. The most important factor about the earmold is that acoustic feedback must be prevented if the hearing aid is to be used for maximum benefit. This may require special attention on behalf of the audiologist-dispenser and several remakes of the earmold in children with difficult-to-seal ear canals. Fifield et al. (1980) describe a new ear impression technique to prevent acoustic feedback with high powered hearing aids, while Ross and Cirmo (1980) describe reducing feedback in a postauricular aid by implanting the receiver in the earmold.

Jerger and Thelin (1968) noted that one of the most important electroacoustic characteristics of a hearing aid is the absence of peaks and valleys to produce a relatively smooth frequency response curve. They explored a number of electroacoustic variables and found that an index of irregularity of frequency response was the best predictor of aided performance. Through developments in subminiature transducers and electronics, the physical performance of hearing aids has been vastly improved, and problems previously associated with the earmold and acoustic coupling are now

sufficiently understood so that a smooth frequency response of the hearing aid, as perceived by the user, can be individually tailored in a highly predictable manner (Killion, 1982).

The development of transducers with wide band capabilities by Knowles Electronics in the early 1970s, and the suggestion by Knowles that the "stepped diameter" approach to the conventional acoustic coupling system could be extended to the earmold to improve the high frequency response of the aid has had tremendous impact on the fidelity of amplification.

Libby (1982) improved on Killion's earmold designs and eliminated problems which made use of innovative earmold construction to utilize venting, predictable damping elements and acoustic horn effects. Killion (1976) noted that venting is effective below 1000 Hz, damping is a useful technique to influence the frequency range from 1000 to 3000 Hz, and the acoustic horn effects above 3000 Hz can be accomplished by changes in the diameter and length of the tubing. He pointed out that construction of the earmold becomes increasingly important in preserving the high frequency response of the hearing aid. To meet these needs, a one-piece tapered, internally stepped bore horn, known as the "Libby horn," is shown in Figures 8.3 and 8.4. The Libby horn is an extremely important aspect of hearing aid fittings and can be used effectively to conserve high frequency components of amplified sound which are so important to hearing-impaired children in the learning of speech and auditory discrimination. The Libby horn can be used with occluded or nonoccluded earmolds, tube fittings, or contralateral routing of signals (CROS)-type hearing aid fittings.

Patients with high frequency hearing loss consistently demonstrate significant speech discrimination improvement with "open" earmolds when compared with responses using "standard" earmolds (Dodds and Harford, 1968; Hodgson and Murdock, 1970; McDonald and Studebaker, 1970;

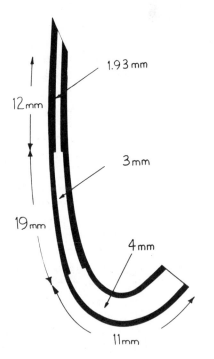

Figure 8.3. The Libby horn. One piece tapered internal stepped bore with Killion 8CR configuration. (Reproduced with permission of Libby and Associated Hearing Instruments, Inc.)

Frank and Karlovich, 1973). Unlike the standard earmold, the open earmold does not occlude the ear canal, but serves merely to hold, in the canal, the tube which carries the acoustic signal from the hearing aid. The open earmold provides the listener with a mixture of the amplified sound and the natural sounds from the listener's surroundings. The open earmold is commonly used in CROS fittings but can also be used ipsilaterally with certain precautions.

Frequency response measured in real ear canals with a probe tube microphone reveals that energy in the low frequency range—below 1000 Hz—is considerably reduced when an open earmold is placed in the ear canal, but is increased when a standard earmold is used (Lybarger, 1972). This phenomenon suggests that the open earmold prevents overamplification of the low frequencies for which persons with high frequency hearing loss often have essentially normal hearing sensitivity. This low frequency attenuation may eliminate upward spread of masking phenomenon.

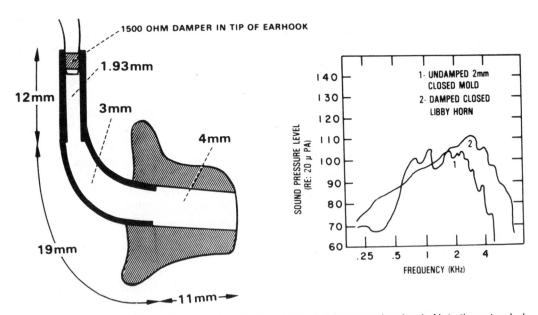

Figure 8.4. An acoustic modifier earmold with Libby horn and dampened earhook. Note the extended high frequency spectrum. (Reproduced with permission from E. R. Libby: *Hearing Instruments*, 32:10, 1981.)

Since the low frequency sounds are attenuated with an open earmold, the hearing aid effectively becomes a mild and high frequency emphasis instrument. The system provides amplification in the range of the listener's greatest hearing loss, while allowing the listener to hear and process the natural acoustic cues in the environment (phase, time, localization, low frequency information, etc.) which are known to improve discrimination in hearing impaired individuals (Johnson, 1975).

McCandless and Miller (1972) have observed that the utilization of open molds results in a reduction of low frequency energy at the tympanic membrane, which in effect reduces the patient's total sound pressure level exposure significantly—by as much as 20 dB at some frequencies. This reduction in overall SPL exposure may reduce the likelihood of induced temporary hearing loss from cochlear overload.

The primary limitation of the open earmold is the risk of acoustic feedback. This is particularly true when the open earmold is used ipsilaterally. Courtois and Berland (1972) examined parameters of ipsilateral fitting with open earmolds while using post auricular hearing aids. Their findings were that: (1) the narrower the ear canal, the less risk of acoustic feedback; (2) hearing aids with high frequency emphasis are more likely to create feedback than instruments with wider frequency response; and (3) gain levels of 30 and 40 dB can be achieved without inducing feedback.

Classification of Hearing Aids

Hearing aids may be classified in several ways. One system of classification is based on the place where the hearing aid is actually worn—body-type hearing aids or ear level hearing aids. The on-the-body model of hearing aids has a relatively large microphone, amplifier, and power supply enclosed in a case which is attached to the clothing, placed in a pocket, or carried in a harness around the chest. An external receiver attaches directly to the earmold and is driven by power supplied through a thin flexible wire from the instrument case. Body-type hearing aids usually provide greater gain and power output than ear level instruments. Since the microphone and receiver are separated by considerable distance, the probability of acoustic feedback (or squeal) from amplified sound that leaks out around the earmold and "feeds back" into the microphone of the hearing aid is reduced. Acoustic feedback is usually caused by an ill-fitting earmold.

Body-type hearing aids are now less often recommended for children because of current improvements in ear level hearing aids. In spite of their size, bulk, and cord, body aids can be firmly carried by young children in garment type carrier harnesses. The body aid is more durable and less likely to be broken than ear level instruments. The external controls are easier to adjust, although this often creates problems with children who play with the aids or inadvertently turn the hearing aid volume down or shut it off. Body aids may be too often recommended for children and not enough consideration given to ear level instruments.

Ear Level Hearing Aids. Ear level instruments include behind-the-ear models, eyeglass models, or all-in-the-ear aids. The all-in-the-ear instruments fit directly into the ear canal. They have no external wires or tubes and are very lightweight. They are generally used with patients of all degrees of hearing loss, from mild to severe. The all-in-the-ear instrument may be used with children and adults.

The behind-the-ear model hearing aid has all its components housed in one curved case which fits neatly behind the pinna and rests against the mastoid surface. A short plastic tube connects the earmold to the hearing aid case. Ear level hearing aids are generally not as powerful as body-type aids and deliver up to 70 dB full-on gain and 125–130 dB saturation sound pressure level. Since the microphone and receiver are in the same case, and in very close proximity to the earmold, increased opportunity exists for acoustic feedback.

Ear level hearing aids have been the most popular type of amplification instrument since the early 1960s. The reasons for the success and popularity of the ear level hearing aid are many. This type of aid is less conspicuous than the body hearing aid; it does not amplify clothing noise since it is worn on the head; and most important, from the audiologist's point of view, hearing reception is at a more natural position on the head. Our success with the behind-the-ear hearing aid with children has been very good and we tend to recommend this type of aid whenever possible. We have fit ear level instruments on youngsters as young as 2 years of age with little problem.

The eyeglass-type of hearing aid was quite popular when it first appeared on the commercial market in the late 1950s. The eyeglass unit is essentially the same aid as the behind-the-ear type except that the plastic case that encloses the components is part of the eyeglass temple piece. These units have become less popular in recent years, and we seldom recommend eyeglass aids for children. The major problem is that when repairs are necessary on either the eyeglass set or the hearing aid, both units are lost to the user while service is performed.

As children grow older they become more concerned about the cosmetic appearance of their hearing aid. As they reach those trying "teen" years, they often find excuses for not wearing their body-type hearing aid. Many of these patients can use powerful ear level instruments, and we are always happy to make this recommendation when possible. Better to underfit the patient with a hearing aid that will be willingly used, than to force the use of an unwanted hearing aid that will not be worn.

Monaural-Binaural Hearing Aids. Monaural hearing aid systems are those which provide amplification for one ear only. A binaural hearing aid system consists of two complete hearing aids including microphones, amplifiers, and receivers—one complete system for each ear. Some manufacturers house both systems in one case with two separate cords and receivers plugged into the sides of the unit. Generally, binaural fittings are accomplished with two separate hearing aid units of the same make and model.

A long controversy has existed among professionals concerning the benefits of the binaural hearing aid system over the monaural system. Obviously, the binaural system is twice as expensive as the monaural systems. However, hearing-impaired adults often state the binaural system increases the directional sense, helps separate wanted sounds from annoying background noise, and is well worth the additional expense.

Children are unable to make judgments regarding monaural versus binaural hearing aid use, and the decision falls to someone else. The clinical evaluation procedure is typically hardpressed to show superior performance with binaural hearing aids over a monaural hearing aid, and this single fact has stoked the monaural-binaural controversy for years. Initial studies that were published produced contradictory results (Jerger and Dirks, 1961) with no clear-cut evidence that binaural fittings were indeed superior to monaural aids. Clinicians and the hearing aid industry quickly lined up on opposite sides over the monaural-binaural issue.

Common sense, however, as well as patient preferences (Haskins and Hardy, 1960; Kodman, 1961; Dirks and Carhart, 1962), supports the view that two ears are better than one. Research reported by many investigators including Koenig (1950), Carhart (1958, 1965), Belzile and Markle (1959), and Harris (1965) matched binaural hearing aid performance, often through the delivery of speech discrimination test materials in simultaneous competing noise signals, substantiating the superiority of binaural listening. According to Hirsh (1971) the principal advantage afforded by binaural listening is the improvement of discrimination in noise due to the ability to localize the sound source. Ear level binaural aids are especially advantageous since the microphones are at the level of the head, separated by the head, resulting in improved time-intensity parameters of the wanted signal.

In the fitting of hearing aids for children, audiologists now recommend a hearing aid for each ear. Binaural hearing aids usually improve the user's ability to localize the directionality of a sound. Another factor in favor of binaural aids for children is that the critical listening situation is often in a noisy classroom with poor acoustic properties, so that the child's head movements will naturally favor the desired signal.

The easiest candidates for binaural hearing aids are those children with bilateral, symmetrical hearing loss. Ross (1969) advocates the use of binaural aids in children with severe hearing losses, based on his experience that children fitted with two aids seem to make better progress than those fitted with just one hearing aid. The clinical and experimental evidence of binaural fittings with children support Ross' viewpoint (Bender and Wig, 1962; Fisher, 1964; Ramaiya, 1971). A survey of over 1000 cases treated with binaural hearing aids in Scandinavia reported by Jordan et al. (1967) led to a conclusion that binaural hearing aids should be the standard treatment in every case of binaural hearing loss.

The CROS Hearing Aid. In 1965 a new concept in hearing aid fittings was reported by Harford and Barry of Northwestern University. They fitted 20 subjects with severe unilateral hearing loss with a special instrument that utilized a microphone on the side of the head with the bad ear, and transmitted sound electrically as picked-up by this microphone to the good ear through an open-type earmold. They named this special instrument CROS, or contralateral routing of signals. This simple procedure opened up many new applications of amplification for hearing-impaired persons.

The basic premise of this amplification system is to improve hearing by eliminating

the "head shadow effect." This arrangement, of placing the microphone beside the patient's poorer ear and feeding the amplified sound to the better ear, prevents the head from blocking sounds, directed to the bad side, from reaching the better ear. The most common arrangement for this apparatus is in an eyeglass frame as shown in Figure 8.5. Some patients, who do not wear glasses, use a wire or a thin plastic tube draped around the back of their head, often under their hair, to connect the microphone to their good ear, or use an FM wireless set. In some designs, the sound is directed into the better ear by only a plastic tube without an earmold. The open-type earpiece is an essential part of the CROS system, since the good ear when left unoccluded allows normal reception of sound directed to the better ear.

While the CROS-type hearing aid is undoubtedly a great help to persons with unilateral hearing loss, it quickly turned out that this type of hearing aid would be very useful to the large group of people who have bilaterally symmetrical high frequency hearing loss. These persons may have normal hearing up to 1000 Hz, but then show significant hearing loss for the higher test

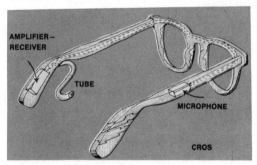

Figure 8.5. The CROS hearing aid with the microphone located on one side and the amplifier-receiver on the opposite side. This hearing aid system picks up sound on the "bad" ear side, transmits it electrically, and amplifies the signal to the "good" ear. (Reproduced with permission from E. Corliss: Facts about Hearing and Hearing Aids. A Consumer's Guide from the National Bureau of Standards, U.S. Dept. of Commerce. Washington, D.C., U.S. Govt. Printing Office, 1971.)

frequencies. In the past, these persons were often told that a hearing aid would not benefit them because, although it would amplify the high frequency sounds that they were missing, the aid would also amplify the low frequency sounds too much to be useful to them. It has been long recognized that these persons do have difficulties in hearing. Fletcher (1929) wrote that elimination of frequencies in communication above 1500 Hz reduces only 10% of the energy available, but reduces discrimination ability by 35%.

The use of an open-type earmold, or the use of a tube without an earmold enhances speech discrimination for persons with high frequency hearing loss (Dodds and Harford, 1968, 1970; Green, 1969; Hodgson and Murdock, 1970). Lybarger (1968) explained that the success of the open canal fitting is due to a reduction in gain and maximal power output so that even very loud sounds in the low frequency spectrum do not produce discomfort to the patient.

The success of the CROS aid was immediate. Some 10 versions of the CROS principle have now been incorporated into various designs and applications, including localization for blind persons with unilateral hearing loss (Rintelmann et al., 1970). The most common variant of the CROS aid is termed the BICROS system (Fig. 8.6). The BICROS consists of two microphones—one above each ear—which send electrical signals to a single amplifier. The output from the amplifier goes to a single receiver which delivers sound to the better ear through a conventional earmold.

CROS instruments were specifically not recommended for children by Harford and Barry (1965) and Harford and Dodds (1966) since they believed unilateral hearing loss children could not appreciate the benefits from CROS fittings. Matkin and Thomas (1972) verified that children do benefit from CROS hearing aids. They report the need for careful consideration of CROS aids in youngsters with unilateral hearing loss only, or new hearing aid users in their teenage years. Children with bilat-

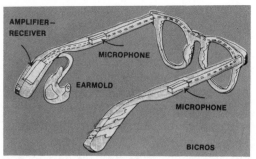

Figure 8.6. The BICROS hearing aid. This amplification system is a variation of the CROS aid consisting of two microphones which deliver sound to a single amplifier and to one ear. (Reprinted with permission from E. Corliss: Facts about Hearing and Hearing Aids. A Consumer's Guide from the National Bureau of Standards, U.S. Dept. of Commerce. Washington, D.C., U.S. Govt. Printing Office, 1971.)

eral high frequency hearing impairments do very well with CROS fittings.

In our experience, the CROS fitting can be beneficial to children when their motivation to hear is good, and the interest of their parents in the handicapping condition is evident. Our successful fittings of CROS instruments are enhanced if the youngster already wears glasses. The dispenser hearing aid is a most important ingredient in the CROS aid for children, and the clinician must work closely with him. Rental trials with CROS aids may be of benefit to allow the parent an opportunity to judge how much use the youngster obtains from the aid. CROS fittings can be so rewarding that the clinician must be cautious to not overfit hearing-impaired persons with this system.

Extended Frequency Hearing Aids. Conventional hearing aids attempt to provide optimal amplification for the speech frequency range between 200 and 5000 Hz. For years, however, attempts have been made to produce amplification systems which can provide supplemental speech cues for the profoundly hearing-impaired. The frequency response of the hearing aid has been under consideration by several researchers.

In recent years, special amplification systems have been developed to enable the deaf with residual hearing in the low frequencies to use amplification. These special hearing aids provide greater low frequency acoustic stimulation than does the conventional hearing aid. Initial evaluation of these amplification systems by their proponents were reported to be favorable, but later studies have produced conflicting results.

One system extends the lower frequency limit of amplification with a special wide range microphone, in several research projects. Ling (1964), as well as Briskey and Sinclair (1966), reported that the use of low frequency hearing aids increases the awareness of deaf children and improves their voice and speech patterns.

A second low frequency emphasis system developed by a Swedish engineer, Bertil Johansson (1961, 1966) is the transposer hearing aid. The aid was designed to transpose or change high frequency information as present in the spectra of phonemes [s] and [ʃ] into low frequency energy. It was felt that since many persons with profound sensorineural hearing loss have residual hearing in the low frequencies only (below 1.5 kHz), this transposed information could be processed as cues for high frequency phonemes.

Early studies on performance with the transposer hearing aid involved hearing-impaired children and normal-hearing adults having simulated losses. The studies produced conflicting results. Wedenberg (1971) and Johansson (1966) showed significant improvement in speech discrimination for nonsense syllables and monosyllabic words, using the transposer hearing aid.

Ling and Druz (1967), Ling (1968), and Ling and Maretic (1971) conducted several studies using Johansson's transposer as well as other transposing devices with hearing-impaired children. They found that while significant improvement in discrimination of monosyllabic words was evident for the transposed mode of amplification, this improvement was also noted for conventional amplification. Their conclusion

was that intensified training rather than transposition accounted for the improvement. Ling (in Levitt and Nye, 1970) indicated that his result from several years work on extended low frequency aids has not been very encouraging and that he was clearly doubtful about the value of frequency transposition.

More recently Berlin (1982) described a new form of hearing loss in which hearing is poor in the standard audiometric ranges but nearly normal at frequencies between 8,000 and 15,000 Hz. In his report, Berlin described the development of an upward-shifting translating hearing aid which has a frequency response extending well beyond 10,000 Hz. Candidates for this special translating hearing aid are difficult to diagnose. They typically have unusually good speech and sensitivity to environmental sounds in the presence of poor speech perception, severe pure tone hearing losses with unusually good speech-detection thresholds. Their audiograms suggest severe-to-profound deafness, poor speech understanding, and good speech production. Many of these patients reject standard hearing aids and often function well without them.

PRINCIPLES OF HEARING AID FITTING FOR CHILDREN

The selection of a hearing aid for a child is the exclusive responsibility of the audiologist. It challenges the ultimate skills of even the most experienced person. One of the requisite experiences in fitting very young children is practice with the fitting of current models on adults. Even a little on-going exposure to the way current hearing aid models perform on various adults with hearing losses is helpful. Extrapolation can then be made from the adult who is easily testable to the child who is not easily testable!

When the child has both receptive and expressive speech and language sufficient for speech reception testing, the selection of an aid is fairly simple. It is the nonverbal child who poses the greatest problem—

either the infant and very young hearing-impaired child or the older, profoundly deaf nonverbal child. No specific rules can be formulated to detect the hearing aid selection, but a few general principles can be proposed, plus the always present exceptions that accompany them.

Hearing Aid Fitting Rationale

Weber developed a rationale and procedure for selecting hearing aids for children when objective audiological information is limited (Weber and Northern, 1980). He was especially concerned about the common procedure of audiologists to select a specific hearing aid for a nonverbal, non-cooperative child based on aided awareness thresholds measured with speech, narrow band noise, and/or pure tone signals. Inevitably, he believes, the aid of choice is the instrument which yields an awareness threshold closest to audiometric zero. Weber states that although this technique will establish the "effective gain" of various hearing aids, the procedure may fail to identify the instrument most effective for providing maximum speech discrimination ability.

Hearing Aid Power. Hearing aids should not be selected because of their power output alone—known as the saturated sound pressure level (SSPL 90). The hearing aid with the greatest power output is not always the appropriate hearing aid for the patient with the most severe hearing loss. The potential danger of creating additional hearing loss with powerful hearing aids is discussed in detail elsewhere in this chapter and must be given some consideration in the selection of power for a hearing aid being fitted on a child.

The Colorado Department of Health makes the following recommendations in regard to maximum power when selecting hearing aids for children:

1. The maximum speech sound pressure level for a child should not exceed 110 dB SPL—except for patients with a conductive component to the hearing loss. The degree of conductive loss should determine the power selection in excess of 115 dB SPL;

2. All hearing aids fitted on children with a SSPL greater than 105 dB should have compression amplification circuits;

3. Patients should be instructed to schedule regular periods of "down time" or "off time" every day to reduce cochlear fatigue.

Hearing Aid Gain. A number of methods are currently used to determine the appropriate gain of a hearing aid. Each of the methods suffers some disadvantages:

1. Loudness Discomfort Level. This technique is based on the premise that the gain selected should limit the SPL at the patient's ear to a level not to exceed the patient's loudness discomfort level for speech. This method predicts only the upper limit of the hearing aid, and is not particularly helpful in selection of a gain level appropriate for normal daily use.

2. SRT Method. One of the most common techniques for selecting gain requirement is the selection of a hearing aid capable of producing gain that approximates the person's hearing loss for speech (SRT). That is, a person with an unaided SRT of 60 dB (HL) would be fit with a hearing aid producing 60 dB of gain, which theoretically would provide the person with an aided SRT of zero dB HL. Clinical evidence supporting this concept is lacking; in fact, this method, when applied to a patient with a recruiting ear, can be highly undesirable.

3. Use-Gain Method. McCandless (1976) measured the use-gain selected by 200 hearing aid users who were instructed to adjust the gain to a comfortable loudness level setting with conversational speech level input. He found that the use-gain approximated about 50% of the amount of hearing loss. According to the formula, a person with a 60-dB HL pure tone average in the speech frequencies will require a gain level of 30 dB. This method may prove to be helpful in determining gain requirements for patients with mild to moderate hearing loss. However, the presence of a recruitment factor with a more serious sensorineural hearing loss may provide an inappropriate estimate of gain need.

4. *Acoustic Reflex Method.* With this suggested procedure, the patient is fitted with a hearing aid to one ear with an impedance meter probe tip placed in the contralateral ear. Using constant input of average environmental sounds or conversational speech, the gain control of the hearing aid is slowly raised until the acoustic reflex is barely observed in the contralateral ear. A gain setting is accomplished by adjusting the controls just below this level which will be safely under the patient's loudness discomfort level (McCandless and Miller, 1972; Olson and Hipskind, 1973; Snow and McCandless, 1976). This method enjoys several advantages. This technique appears to determine gain level which provides maximum intelligibility for speech (Rappaport and Tait, 1976). The method also provides information from which SSPL of the hearing aid can be determined. This technique allows the audiologist to select appropriate gain level for the pediatric patient from whom limited subjective information may be available. Unfortunately, the acoustic reflex is often absent as cochlear hearing loss becomes more severe, usually beyond 75 dB HL (Northern, 1984a).

5. *Most Comfortable Loudness Level Method* The most comfortable loudness (MCL) level method allows the subject to set the hearing aid to a gain setting that is comfortably loud while listening to speech at conversational levels. Studies have indicated that individuals who are experienced users of hearing aids consistently tend to adjust the gain of their instrument to a level at which discrimination for speech is maximum (Markle and Zaner, 1966; Rappaport and Tait, 1976). Of course, this method requires the patient to be able to manipulate the hearing aid gain control to make a determination of what level is comfortably loud, which may be a task perhaps beyond the skills of most pediatric patients.

Irrespective of the method selected for determining gain requirements, the patient's *dynamic range* of hearing must always be considered. The intensity range of hearing between the threshold of sensitivity and the loudness discomfort level (LDL) has been defined as the dynamic range of hearing. It has long been known that a restricted dynamic range tends to occur in patients with sensorineural hearing loss. Rubin and Ventry (1975) reported that the dynamic range was so restricted that mean MCLs were only 10 dB greater than speech detection threshold (SDT) for speech in 20 profoundly deaf students enrolled in Lexington School for the Deaf. The range between speech detection thresholds and speech most comfortable loudness levels in individuals with sensorineural hearing loss may become less as the hearing loss increases (Danaher and Pickett, 1972).

Investigators exploring the loudness discomfort level for normal hearing subjects and subjects with hearing loss from cochlear lesions have found that there is agreement between these studies to indicate that an ear suffering from cochlear lesions and in normal ears, the loudness discomfort level for pure tone speech frequencies, running discourse, and bands of noise with frequency spectrum common to normal modern hearing aids, can be expected to be found at levels falling between approximately 95 and 110 dB (SPL). The upper limit of the intensity function appears to be constant, while the threshold of hearing is the sole variable.

Data from the above studies suggest that persons with uncomplicated cochlear lesions should utilize gain levels which would raise conventional conversational speech (approximately 70 dB SPL) to a level not to exceed about 110 dB SPL, or a gain level no greater than about 40 dB irrespective of the magnitude of the hearing loss.

Based on the above considerations the Colorado Department of Health recommends the following procedures to determine hearing aid gain for children:

a. The acoustic reflex response method with conventional speech input is the method of choice in nonverbal children for determining hearing aid gain.

The most comfortable loudness method should be used whenever possible, or when acoustic reflexes are not present

b. The following procedure is suggested for children who are inexperienced hearing aid wearers and for whom no acoustic reflexes are demonstrable:

(1) Assumption will arbitrarily be made that the patient's loudness discomfort level will be 105 dB SPL;

(2) Speech awareness level will be obtained and converted to SPL;

(3) Midpoint between 105 dB SPL and speech awareness level should be calculated and increased by 5 dB. Hearing aids should be selected which will provide this desired SPL with conventional speech input;

(4) The hearing aids can then be tested in a hearing aid test box. The hearing aid gain control is adjusted to achieve the desired SPL (as in 3 above), with a 70 dB SPL speech spectrum noise input. The hearing aid gain control is marked at this setting to enable the gain level to be maintained when the aid is worn by the child;

(5) The child should be entered in an auditory training program where therapists can help select the most comfortable level.

Frequency Response of Hearing Aids. Early in the history of hearing aid fitting a controversy arose between the "selective" frequency response proponents and those preferring a "flat," more uniform response curve. The controversy soon became rather one-sided, with the selective fitting proponents enjoying the recognition and acceptance of the majority. The selective method was based upon the patient's audiogram and provided amplification only where most needed. Amplification was restricted to the frequency areas in which the user still had residual hearing to be reached. However, in 1946 reports of the Harvard Study began to question the advantage of selective fitting. The Harvard group conclusions were very emphatic that selective fitting was of no value, and that a uniform response would almost invariably yield as good, if not better, speech discrimination response. "For every subject the best performance could be obtained by using either the flat response system or the high pass 6 dB per octave tilt." Studies by Watson (1944) and Davis et al. (1946) concluded that the most important frequencies for understanding speech fall between 300 and 3000 Hz, and that frequencies beyond these two extremes were less important. As a direct result of these studies, hearing aids were designed with this limited frequency response characteristic, and the model has prevailed until recently.

A variety of tests have been devised to measure intelligibility for speech through hearing aids. Tests consisting of consonant-vowel combinations in nonsense syllables, monosyllabic words, multiple syllable words, phrases, pediatric "synthetic" sentences, sentences, and running discourse have been devised to be presented in quiet, through filters which restrict the frequency response, and presented with a background of broad band noise or competing running discourse.

Generally, speech discrimination is least difficult in quiet than in the presence of noise or conflicting running discourse. Speech discrimination becomes progressively less difficult from nonsense syllables, to words, to sentences, to running discourse. Words presented in isolation are more difficult to discriminate than the same words presented in phrases or sentences. Success in discrimination of nonsense syllables to running discourse is known to be frequency related. For instance, in normal hearing subjects, recognition of consonants in nonsense syllables is about 90% when all frequencies above 1000 Hz are passed, whereas speech that contains only frequencies below 1000 Hz is only 27% intelligible. Monosyllabic words (such as the CID W-22 Word List) are about 40% intelligible when frequencies above 1000 Hz are filtered out, while about 80% of continuous discourse is intelligible under the same filter conditions (Giolas and Epstein, 1963).

There has been a reevaluation of the position of the importance of low frequency hearing aid amplification. Ling (1964) showed that amplification with flat frequency response extending to 100 Hz resulted in higher intelligibility than the frequency response of conventional aids. Jerger and Thelin (1968) presented synthetic sentences through commercial hearing aids to subjects with normal hearing and with sensorineural hearing loss. They found a high correlation between speech intelligibility and frequency spectrum below 1000 Hz. The wider the spectrum below 1000 Hz—passing more low frequency energy—the greater the intelligibility.

Although the primary energy for consonants and monosyllabic words is found in the high frequencies, Rosenthal et al. (1975) examined the extent to which cues for consonant reception are contained in the lower frequency range. A split-band technique was used in which the gain in intelligibility was measured when low frequency band was added to high frequency band. The studies concluded that when low bands (as low as 55–110 Hz) are presented simultaneously with a high band (1100–2200 Hz), discrimination for consonants is improved significantly in normal hearing subjects.

However, the relative intensity level of the low frequency band with the high frequency band is critical. Bilger and Hirsh (1956), Martin and Pickett (1970), Danaher and Pickett (1975), Franklin (1975), clearly demonstrated that when a low frequency sound is presented at high intensity levels, a type of masking is produced which reduces the subject's ability to detect sounds in the higher frequency regions. This effect is termed "upward spread of masking" and occurs in normal hearing subjects and most subjects with sensorineural loss. When amplified with a low frequency emphasis aid,

moderate levels of environmental noise may be sufficiently intense to produce spread of masking, making speech intelligibility frustratingly difficult for the hearing-impaired listener.

The audiologist's task, then, is to discover an acoustic system that will provide the patient with all of the acoustic cues necessary to achieve maximum use of his/her residual hearing for daily—real world—communication, while minimizing the degradation of signal through "upward spread of masking" in most (preferably all) listening situations. This task is of course confounded when the patient is very young, nonverbal or noncooperative!

The hearing aid system selected for a very young child should be determined by the patient's audiometric configuration which may be estimated as awareness threshold levels using speech, narrow band noise, and/or pure tone signals. The system can be finer tuned as the child matures to a level when reliable information may be forthcoming. We suggest the following considerations:

1. A child demonstrating an audiometric configuration of normal/near normal hearing levels extending upward through 500 Hz, with high frequency hearing loss bilaterally should be tested in the binaural state using open earmolds coupled with high frequency emphasis hearing aids ipsilaterally. If acoustic feedback prevails, hearing aids with broader frequency response patterns can be utilized;

2. A child demonstrating bilateral profound hearing loss with a "corner audiogram" of hearing levels measurable only at 125, 250, and/or 500 Hz at high intensity levels should be tested in the binaural state, with hearing aids producing low frequency energy extending downward to at least 100 Hz (and preferably lower). The standard earmold should be utilized.

In our experience successful results have been obtained from hearing aids on 15-dB average losses, and unsuccessful fittings have been made on 25-dB average losses in children. In this borderline area all that can be said is that hearing aids should be considered for a child, and sometimes tried out, before a decision is made. Successful fittings at 15 dB have often been made in the child, dull-normal in intelligence, who needs every bit of hearing he can get in the educational situation. Young children with recurrent otitis media and resulting hearing losses of 15–25 dB are also good candidates for hearing aid trial. The unsuccessful fittings at 25 dB have been in the child whose intelligence on superior listening strategies allow him to function well without an aid. Occasionally behavior problems preclude successful fittings at this level.

When considering an aid for slight losses in the 15–25-dB range, consultation should be requested with the teacher, parents, and managing physician. If a trial of an aid is attempted, reports should be requested from everyone dealing with the child. Only in this way can a meaningful decision be made.

There are special cases in which a hearing aid may be recommended even when normal hearing prevails at a given time. These are the children whom we call "recalcitrant otitis media" cases, and there is a series of over 50 of them in our files. They originally present, at 6 months to 6 years, with serous otitis media and hearing losses of 30–40 dB. Myringotomies are performed, and the hearing returns to normal. However, in a short time there is a recurrence of ear disease, the tubes may be extruded, and the hearing drops again. Myringotomies are performed again, and after a period of normal hearing the children present with 20–30-dB hearing losses. These episodes may be repeated four, five, six, or seven times and the hearing will be normal only for short periods. Over a space of 1–3 years, it can be seen that as much as two thirds of the time the children are functioning with below normal hearing levels of 15–30 dB.

In such recalcitrant cases, consultation with the otolaryngologists managing the cases has produced the decision that hearing aids should be obtained for the children.

The aids will be used at such times as the hearing is reduced, and parents and teachers are counseled as to the indications of when the aids should be used. No child should be without adequate hearing for any period during his formative and educational years. Eventually the tendency to ear disease may be outgrown, and normal hearing will be present. In the meantime, the child is protected against periods of inadequate hearing.

The kind of hearing loss also makes a difference in the judgments of whether to fit with a hearing aid. Strangely enough, the conductive hearing loss may be in greater need of an aid having greater gain and output than the sensorineural loss. The reason is that at above threshold levels the loudness sensation in a conductive loss is less than in the sensorineural loss. The latter is most generally accompanied by recruitment, giving a louder sensation at above threshold hearing levels. It is also more difficult to keep a hearing aid on a child with mild sensorineural loss than on one with a mild conductive loss. Many times the child with 25–30-dB average sloping sensorineural loss will actually function better without an aid. In such cases, trials with aids over a period of time will have to reveal how this particular child functions. Arbitrariness in recommending aids is to be avoided when dealing with such cases. The otolaryngologist, the parents, and the teachers should be a part of all decisions that are made.

The Hearing Aid

Wherever possible an ear level type is the aid of choice for a child. We have placed the cut-off point at 3 years, arbitrarily, but the exceptions will be numerous. For some very active children of 3 or 4, the parents may not be able to maintain an ear level aid. The behavior levels of other older children may not permit such an easily accessible aid. On the other hand, a quietly behaved 2½-year-old may be given consideration for an ear level aid. Parents should be warned that a great many such aids end up either flushed down a toilet or chewed up by the family dog or thrown out of a window or used as a pacifier. The parents can make the decision whether they can handle the problems of the ear level aid. They will then assume the responsibility of seeing that it is cared for, and protected against loss.

Bone conduction aids have been advised for those children who have atretic canals, microtia, or recurrent ear disease. There is no objection to a child's wearing bone conduction aids at any age. We have placed them on infants 1 month old, who have stenotic canals or microtia, with excellent results. No obvious misshaping of the head has occurred, but special padding should be applied to the end clip and sometimes to the entire headband. Soft felt material or Styrofoam can be used to pad the band. The transmitter can be placed in back, if the baby lies on his stomach, or in front when he lies on his back.

The only provision to make in placing a bone conduction aid on children is that it be understood that this type will not be worn permanently. Experience with older people who have always worn bone conduction aids is that when a decrease in the sensorineural hearing renders the bone conduction reception inefficient, it is very difficult for them to change to air conduction. It is like learning a new language and they neither like it nor do well with it. Although it is impossible to speculate on what the chances are of a decrease in sensorineural hearing, at some point a decision should be made to change to air conduction aids where possible. It should be done with a child before the time that a change will be strongly resisted.

The cut-off point for ear level aids has been placed at 75-dB hearing loss. This point is an arbitrary one, and may vary with individual needs. The level may also become higher with new developments of tightly fitting earmolds and new hearing aid design. The ideal would be for all hearing-impaired children and adults to wear ear level aids, regardless of degree of loss.

Hearing aid manufacturers are actively researching these new designs, and may soon meet this challenge. Also, with the new trend toward lower SSPL in hearing aids for even severe losses, the 75-dB cut-off should not be considered a fixed rule.

Another exception to the 75-dB loss criterion is for the adolescent child. At the age of 12 or 13, the child who has worn a body aid all his life will suddenly become self-conscious about it and begin to reject wearing it. The young boy suddenly feels that the obvious cord and receiver of the aid draw attention to him as a handicapped person. It impugns his masculinity. The young girl whose breasts are developing finds it difficult to wear two body aids inconspicuously, and even one hearing aid is bulky. She also wants to wear swimming suits in the summer, and dislikes the attention that is drawn to the aids. These are normal, legitimate complaints that should be given careful consideration. The old adage, "the best hearing aid is the one that is worn," should be remembered. If it can be shown that an ear level aid gives performance reasonably close to that of the body aid, it should be recommended. Often the youngster will make his own decision after a trial of the head-worn aid; some have admitted that their hearing reception is not as good, and have gladly gone back to the body aid. Others have taken to the ear level aid eagerly and well. As in all other factors, the individual's special needs must be evaluated.

Which Ear to Fit?

It has been our philosophy that, whenever possible, two separate hearing aids should be fitted on a child. The observations made by teachers, families, and the children themselves over many years have convinced us that in general it is a sound approach. The criterion for binaural fittings has been the presence of identical or fairly similar losses in each ear. Real advantage has been demonstrated through fitting a moderate loss in one ear with a moderate hearing aid and a severe loss on the other ear with a more powerful aid. In such cases it is only when the child is old enough to give speech responses that we attempt it.

The selection of which ear to amplify when a monaural fitting is decided upon rests on several factors. The general principle is to fit the ear which will give the child the better hearing. But the degree and kind of loss in each ear sometimes figure largely in the decision. In the case of conductive losses in both ears, 25 dB in one and 35 dB in the other, equal performance can be expected. Therefore, the worse ear would be fitted, leaving the better ear to hear what it is able to. In such cases one might obtain a 5–10 dB aided speech threshold in the better ear and a 10–15 dB aided threshold in the worse. Even with the measurable improvement in thresholds with the aided better ear, the worse ear should be fitted.

When asymmetric mild and moderate sensorineural losses are present, it is possible that the worse ear will tolerate the aid more easily than the better ear. However, care should be taken in making the decision, as a well designed high frequency emphasis aid may give optimal discrimination in the better ear. It is obvious that each case of problem fittings must be decided on its own merits.

Dichotic Listening

Dichotic listening is achieved when different auditory signals arrive simultaneously at the listener's two ears. In dichotic listening research, more words are recognized by the right ear than the left ear. The right ear also recognizes consonant-vowel nonsense syllables significantly better than the left ear (Dirks, 1964; Nagafuchi, 1970; Shankweiler and Studdert-Kennedy, 1970). Rosenthal et al. (1975) and Franklin (1975) demonstrated that consonant discrimination is improved when the signal is passed through low frequency bands combined with a high frequency band. When presented in the dichotic state, speech discrimination may be improved, irrespective of the audiometric configuration of the person's hearing loss. The Colorado State Department of Health recommends that all patients with binaural sensorineural loss be tested in the dichotic state with an aid in the right ear set for high frequency amplification and an aid in the left ear set for a low frequency emphasis.

HEARING AIDS AND ACOUSTIC IMMITTANCE MEASUREMENTS

Although acoustic immittance (impedance) measurements have long been recommended for routine inclusion in every hearing evaluation, only in the past few years have clinicians recognized the potential contribution of acoustic impedance measurements to hearing aid selection, fitting and management. Madell (1976) stated that acoustic impedance testing should precede *every* hearing aid evaluation session. Thorough discussions of impedance measurements and their utilization in hearing aid clinical practice may be found in materials published by Northern (1978a) and McCandless and Keith (1980).

Rubin (1976) cited the importance of impedance measurements with deaf children because of the high incidence of middle ear pathology. She reported that, in 1 year, 50% of the hearing-impaired toddlers and babies in the Lexington Infant Center had cases of middle ear effusion, and that each of the children was given ongoing impedance testing during each session of the hearing aid evaluation to be aware of possible hearing changes. She indicated further that the audiologist must be certain that a child's middle ears function normally when "real ear" hearing aid measurements are used to evaluate specific hearing aids.

Ear Canal Volume and Hearing Aids

The use of the acoustic impedance meter to measure ear canal volume between probe tip cuff and the tympanic membrane has special significance for hearing aid selection and utilization. This procedure is known as the physical volume test (PVT) and is described in Chapter 6. The electroacoustic impedance meter relies on the physical principle that the intensity of a sound measured in a closed cavity is a direct function of the size of the cavity. Thus, a signal of given intensity introduced into a large cavity and a small cavity successively will produce two different sound pressure levels (SPL), and a higher sound pressure level will be measured in the smaller cavity.

The average enclosed ear canal cavity volume will be between 1.0 and 1.4 cc for an adult, and 0.8–1.0 cc for a child. In infants, the physical volume may be 0.5 cc. These same ear canal volumes exist when the ear canal is tightly sealed with a non-vented, occluding earmold.

Clinicians are aware, of course, that hearing aid specifications are reported in dB relative to a hard-walled 2.0-cc coupler. Hearing aid response curves are altered as a function of the type of earmold coupling and ear canal resonance. Less appreciated, however, is that the hearing aid specifications relative to a 2.0-cc cavity are altered significantly when the hearing aid is coupled tightly to an ear canal that is less than 2.0 cc in volume. In fact, each time the cavity volume is reduced by one-half, sound pressure is increased by 6 dB. It can be expected that hearing aid sound pressures measured in a 2.0-cc cavity will be delivered to an adult 1.0-cc ear canal with 6 dB more intensity than that shown on the standard hearing aid frequency response curve (Cole, 1975). Small children with ear canal volumes of approximately 0.5 cc may actually receive 12 dB more amplification than that shown on the hearing aid technical specification sheet. That is, an instrument with an SSPL 90 of 130 dB, as measured in a 2.0-cc coupler, becomes capable of delivering 142 dB SPL when coupled to an ear having a 0.5-cc space between the tip of the earmold and the eardrum (Fig. 8.7).

Jirsa and Norris (1978) examined changes in hearing aid performance characteristics resulting from a reduction in

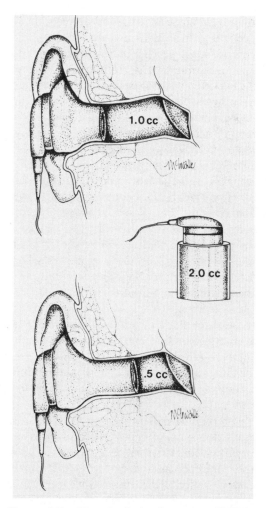

Figure 8.7. The physical volume test (PVT) is an important consideration in hearing aid fittings. Hearing aid specifications are obtained from a 2.0-cc cavity. When the hearing aid is fitted to ear canals of smaller volumes, the sound energy is increased 6 dB in a 1.0-cc ear canal, and 12 dB in an ear canal of only 0.5 cc.

coupler volume from 2.0 cc to 1.0 cc and 0.5 cc, in an effort to determine the differences that might exist between cavity size and SPL. Results showed the expected inverse relationship between cavity size and SPL. That is, as volume was reduced, the SPL developed inside the cavity increased. In addition, Jirsa and Norris examined the relationship between threshold improvement and acoustic gain, aided and unaided speech reception thresholds, and ear canal volume, in eight hearing-impaired children. Acoustic gain as measured via the threshold improvement procedure was compared to that measured in the standard 2.0-cc and the experimental 1.0-cc and 0.5-cc couplers. Results showed that functional threshold improvement always exceeded the 2.0-cc coupler acoustic gain measure. Conversely, when gain was determined in a coupler approximating the volume of the child's real ear canal, the relationship between real ear (functional) and coupler gain measures was considerably closer. The results reported by these investigators again suggest that it is important to consider the increase in SPL that will occur in real ears when determining appropriate acoustic gain and maximum power output (SSPL 90) requirements from electroacoustic data. Failure to account for these differences may result in overamplification and cause the child either to reject the aid, or reduce the hearing aid gain to allow for a more comfortable listening level (Schwartz and Larson, 1977).

Common complaints from hearing aid users relate to loudness discomfort from amplification. Gaeth and Lounsbury (1966) and McCandless and Miller (1972) noted that virtually all hearing aid wearers turn their aids to levels lower than clinicians deem appropriate. A recent national survey indicated that more than one half of former hearing aid users stopped wearing their aids, or use their aids only part time, because of excessive loudness. Bragg (1977) reported that the most common problem in hearing aid fitting is "overamplification." Clinicians who select hearing aids based on 2.0-cc coupler measurements must be aware, therefore, that overamplification may result from coupling an aid and a full earmold to an ear having a volume of less than 2.0 cc. According to Sachs and Burkhard (1972) the 2.0-cc coupler underestimates aided SPL relative to the human ear canal by as much as 15 dB in the higher frequencies. The acoustic immittance meter can provide important information if the PVT is conducted to establish ear canal volume prior to selection of the hearing aid.

HEARING AID SELECTION PROCEDURES

In the words of Mark Ross, ". . . for most hearing-impaired children, the early and appropriate selection and use of amplification is the single most important habilitative tool available to us." In his excellent material on hearing aid selection for preverbal hearing-impaired children, Ross emphasizes the need for hearing aid preselection procedures including analysis of the electroacoustic characteristics of various aids, and examining features of the hearing aids to eliminate consideration of those aids which are not appropriate to provide the child with maximum auditory information consistent with his hearing loss. His key word in the hearing aid selection is "flexibility" since initial information concerning the child's residual hearing may be limited, and since the audiologist-dispenser has some control over the response of the hearing aid itself through earmold and tube considerations, the selected aid must have adjustable output and frequency response systems (Ross and Tomassetti, 1980).

Dr. Ross summarizes his thoughts about hearing aid fittings in children by stating that the goal for most children is properly used and adjusted binaural hearing aids, preferably at ear level. He views the hearing aid selection on the basis that all initial electroacoustic recommendations are tentative and may need to be altered in time, and that foremost, it must be remembered that children's hearing aid selection and fitting must be considered an ongoing process that is part of a complete habilitation program. Matkin (1981) writes that the focus of routine audiologic monitoring of amplification must include the child's auditory status and the function of the hearing aids, but also the function of the auditory training system (in school) and the parent's participation in the habilitation program.

The Preverbal Child, Birth to 2- or 3-Year-Olds

The initial choice of those hearing aid brands from which to select an aid for the preverbal child should be made on the basis of principles that will include dealer criteria:

Service. Is the dispenser who sells the particular brand of hearing aid known to be reliable, to be available at all times, and to handle children well and to be licensed if required? Is he willing, if requested, to make some sort of trial/rental arrangement? In case of damage or malfunction of the aid, will he offer a temporary loaner aid as a substitute while the repairs are made? Are warranties adequate, or does he have some type of insurance program? Does he offer a reasonable time payment plan? Is he able to make an adequate earmold, and if it is not adequate at first, will he remake it at no extra cost? Does he communicate well with you, offering his ideas freely and listening to yours? An experienced hearing aid dispenser with whom one has a relationship of mutual confidence can be of great assistance in offering suggestions as to the improvement of the fitting or ways of making the wearing of it mechanically better. Any audiologist who refuses to enlist a responsible dispenser's suggestions and advice is missing one of the most valuable adjunct guides he can obtain. No audiologist knows everything that is to be known about the performance and wearing variations of a given aid.

Appropriateness for Children. Is the hearing aid known to be sturdy and long lasting? Are heavy duty cords available? Does the transmitter minimize clothing noise, in the case of a body-worn aid? Is the aid able to be worn so that food and liquids will not spill into the microphone? Are the controls sturdy and not easily breakable? (Wheel controls are better than levers.) Are the prong inserts at both ends of the cord strong? Is the size the most convenient that can be selected for loss?

Pretested Approval. If a public or private agency is purchasing the aid for the child, is the aid on their approved list of pretested models? After a few general brands have been selected, the aids within these brands which furnish the approximate gain, power output, and frequency response for a specific kind of loss can be chosen for further consideration.

A further narrowing down of the list is made by specific application of the dynamic range principle described previously. To do this, fair approximations of threshold levels and tolerance limits should be known. Attempts should be made to observe tolerance limits under earphones. If possible, an audiometer with higher outputs than the standard levels should be used, up to 120 and 130 dB. An infant may cry or start when his maximal tolerance level is reached. Using this level in relation to the threshold levels obtained by observations or objective techniques, the desired gain and maximal power output may be estimated.

The list at this point will be narrowed down to three or four aids. Now, subjective observations will begin. Wearing each aid, the child should be given various levels of gross speech through a loudspeaker. Thresholds of awareness should be obtained, plus observations of reactions to louder levels. The instruments which produce evident discomfort at low speech levels can be eliminated. "Reasonable" levels can be estimated in relation to the degree of hearing loss. An approximation of what should be expected is as follows:

Degree of Loss	Reasonable Level of Awareness
100 dB HL+	45–55 dB HL
75–100 dB HL average	35–50 dB HL
50–75 dB HL	20–35 dB HL
25–50 dB HL	10–25 dB HL

A greater gain can be tolerated by the child with a conductive or mixed loss than by one with a sensorineural loss. For example, a child with a conductive loss of 60 dB HL average can easily tolerate a gain that brings his awareness level to 20 dB HL or even less. But a sensorineural loss of that degree will not allow the child to tolerate receiving such thresholds; 25–30 dB HL may be the best that can be expected for him. It is simply not realistic to expect normal or near-normal thresholds of awareness on children. They will not wear an aid giving those levels, despite all our ambitions to bring them to normal levels.

To make a final evaluation, acoustic reflex tests may now be given with the choice hearing aids as described by Snow and McCandless (1976). The aid with the best dynamic range should be chosen.

The Nonverbal Child, 2 or 3–16-Year-Olds

The child 2 or 3 years and older who can be play-conditioned or taught hand-raising responses to sounds can be given a satisfactory hearing aid evaluation. The principle of such an evaluation is to compare the unaided audiogram and the speech awareness levels with similar measures using

hearing aids. The initial choice of which hearing aids to try may be made on the basis of the principles listed in Table 8.2.

On the basis of those principles and criteria, no more than three aids need be selected for trial on a young child; more might exceed the attention limits of a child for a testing session. In fact, it may be necessary to schedule more than one testing session for the 2-, 3-, or 4-year-old. His tolerance for testing has a limited time span and it is fruitless to try to extend it. Some bright 2- or 2½-year-olds are able to learn play-conditioning techniques for speech or pure tones and sustain their interest for very short periods of time. A 2-year-old may surprise you by learning simply play-conditioning long enough to give a speech awareness level or a threshold at one frequency during short periods of time. Two or three frequencies are sufficient to place the loss: 500 and 2000 Hz, or 500, 1000, and 2000 Hz. This is the major frequency range of hearing aid amplification.

Given a threshold audiogram, plus observed tolerance limits obtained from observation or acoustic reflexes, the following is a suggested procedure for hearing aid selection.

Table 8.2.
Synopsis of Standard Hearing Aid Specifications

Saturation sound pressure level	Curve (minimum range recorded 200–5000 Hz)
Saturation sound pressure level (maximum)	dB (+ 0 dB tolerance)
High frequency—average saturation sound pressure level 90	dB (average of 1000, 1600, 2500 Hz outputs) ± 4 dB tolerance
Full-on gain	Curve (60 dB input, 50 dB for automatic gain control aids)
High frequency—average full-on gain	dB (average of 1000, 1600, 2500 Hz gain) ± 5 dB tolerance
Reference test position	17 dB below high frequency saturation sound pressure level 90. Input 60 dB
Reference test position automatic gain control aids	Maximum gain; input 50 dB
Reference test gain	dB (average of 1000, 1600, 2500 Hz at reference test position)
Frequency response at reference test position	Curve (input 60 dB, 200 to 5000 Hz)
	Low band (below 2000 Hz + 4 dB tolerance)
	High band (above 2000 Hz + 6 dB tolerance)
ANSI frequency range	Hz (average of 1000, 1600, 2500 Hz minus 20 dB)
Total Harmonic Distortion 500, 800, and 1600 Hz	(Reference test position, input 70 dB, at each frequency)

On each hearing aid selected for trial, obtain the five measures listed below. (The approximate volume setting can be estimated from the hearing aid analysis charts in relation to the mid-point of the dynamic range.)

1. Using gross speech, obtain a speech awareness level through play-conditioning techniques or hand-raising. The simple word "now" is as good a speech signal as any.

2. Using warbled pure tones, obtain an aided free field audiogram on each aid. Use intermediate frequencies in addition to the standard frequencies (750, 1500, 3000 Hz) if possible.

3. Test the tolerance limits of the aid on the child by raising the speech level gradually until the child evinces discomfort.

4. Evaluate the aids first on the basis of the best speech awareness in relation to tolerance levels. The measure of highest tolerance limits should be given precedence over the lowest speech awareness levels. An aid giving a 15- or 20-dB HL speech awareness level but producing tolerance limits at 65 dB should be eliminated in favor of one with a 25–30-dB HL awareness level with a tolerance limit of 75 or 80 dB HL.

5. The next evaluation of aids should be made on the basis of the aided pure tone thresholds. The threshold at 2000 Hz is the most critical, and the aid showing the best threshold there should be given preference. The contour of the audiogram should be fairly even, without high peaks at any frequencies.

This procedure should allow a selection of one or two acceptable aids which can be recommended. If there is any question, a trial of the finally selected aids can be suggested. During the trials, observations of the child's performance with each aid can be made by parents, teachers, or clinicians. From these observations the ultimate selection can be made.

The Verbal Child, 3–16 Years

When receptive language is present in the child, some gross discrimination testing can be accomplished with hearing aids; when in addition there is expressive language present, finer discrimination tests are applicable, with varying degrees of sophistication.

A minimum of three and a maximum of five should be selected for trial. In the descriptions of testing at various age levels which follow, there will be overlapping in the ages at which children can perform the tests. The variable factors are the degree of hearing loss, the level of language skills, and the intellectual function of the child. A mentally retarded child of 9, for example, may have to be handled like a 3-year-old. Previous audiometric testing should have determined the level of testing that can be used on each child.

Age 3–5 Years. It will be unusual for a hearing-handicapped child of this age to attend long enough for detailed discrimination tests. He will require motivational techniques, even for speech reception testing. Therefore, toys or pictures of objects should be used to sustain interest in the test. The steps that can be followed are:

1. Set the gain of each aid in accordance with a recommended procedure. An aid should never be tested at full volume, as some distortion may occur at high levels.

2. Obtain a speech reception threshold using the toys suggested in Chapter 5, or the picture tests described. Work as fast as possible, foregoing the standard three-out-of-six-words criterion for threshold. Select as threshold the last word repeated on a descending threshold starting at 40 dB and proceeding rapidly downward in 5-dB steps. Express pleasure or clap your hands at each response. Record the level.

3. Starting at 40 dB, sweep upward in 5-dB steps, giving a "buh-buh" at each step. Observe carefully the first sign of discomfort the child shows. He may wince, or put his hand to his ear, or grimace, or even remove the receiver. Record this level.

4. Use as criteria for selection the combination of the best SRT and highest tolerance level, giving more weight to the tolerance level. No aid with a tolerance level

much under 65 dB should be chosen, nor an aid with an SRT higher than 30 dB. These general criteria can be set because the child of this age who has receptive language probably has a mild to moderate hearing loss. He should be expected to hear speech comfortably loud at 40 dB HL with an aid. He need not be expected to have a 10- or 15-dB HL threshold, unless it can be obtained with a high tolerance level. This last condition often obtains in cases of conductive loss, but rarely is found in sensorineural losses.

Age 6–10 Years. The cooperative child at this age can be given more sophisticated speech reception tests. Always determine which of the children's spondee words he is familiar with, if he will at least try to repeat the discrimination words. These steps can be followed:

1. Set each aid at an appropriate gain level between one-half and two-thirds volume.

2. Obtain a speech reception test using 8 to 10 children's spondees, giving them to him first in the sound room. Start at 40 dB HL and descend in 5-dB steps, giving one word at each level. Bracket the threshold level with no more than three words around threshold. Keep the child's interest by smiling with pleasure at each response, and praising him when he is through.

3. Give a half-list of PB-K words at 40 dB HL maintaining his attention with praise. The 40-dB level is selected because the goal for the child should be to hear normal conversational speech level. Some people prefer to use 45 dB as the criterion for normal speech level, and the choice of either is an arbitrary one. Verbal children of this age most likely have moderate to moderately severe losses at worst, and should be expected to understand normal conversational speech with an aid. His responses may not be clear enough on any words to be correct, but you should set up a mental criterion of what he is probably hearing correctly, even if he cannot pronounce it correctly. A consistent criterion will produce meaningful results. Another

useful criterion is the latency of his responses. One aid may provide the child with a signal that permits immediate response; another aid may produce hesitation on each word. This observation should be noted.

4. Starting at 40 dB HL, ascend in 5-dB steps, giving a spondee at each level. Watch for the first sign of discomfort. If he has sufficient understanding, he can be instructed to tell you when it becomes too loud. In this case, make three presentations of the ascending levels, and record the average level of the three discomfort responses.

5. Use as criterion for final selection of the aid, the combination of the best discrimination score, the best SRT, and the highest tolerance level. Speech discrimination is given the greatest weight, tolerance level follows closely, and SRT is of the least importance.

Age 10–16 Years. Depending on the language level and capacity of the child, standard or slightly modified adult techniques can be used at this age range. The six steps are:

1. Turn each aid to a MCL gain setting. Speaking normally at a distance of 3 or 4 feet, ask him, "Do you like it this loud?" ... "Is it better this loud?" Often he will indicate a quite definite preference for one volume setting, if he understands.

2. Obtain an SRT with 12 or 15 spondees that have been previously presented to him. Standard speech reception threshold technique can be used, but should be shortened in the case of poor attention span.

3. Give a one-half list of PB words at 40 dB HL or of PB-K words if it appears indicated. In the case of poor articulation, again set up mental criteria of what you will accept as correct. Consistency is the essence in these judgments. Knowledge of the kinds of logical substitutions that are commonly made by hearing-impaired children will help decide on the criteria. The judgments must be made rapidly, and comprise another skill in the art of audiology.

4. Instruct the child to tell you when your voice becomes "too loud" for him, and

give spondees in 5-dB ascending steps from 40 dB HL. Repeat three times and take the average of the response levels.

5. Use as criteria for the final selection the best discrimination score, the highest tolerance level, and the best SRT, in that level of importance. At this age the child may voice a preference for one aid over the other. If it is not the aid that performed the best, determine on what basis he made his choice. If it is on size, shape, or color, try to point out better features of the aid that performed best. Assure him that he will hear the best with the selected aid. Letting him listen again with both aids may persuade him. Rarely, an extremely obstinate child will refuse the aid selected. In this case it is well not to make an issue of it. One should always keep in mind the audiologist's adage: "The best hearing aid is the one that is worn." Occasional compromise is better than a permanently uncooperative hearing aid user.

CAN HEARING AIDS DAMAGE HEARING?

Clinicians often worry that powerful hearing aids fitted to children may cause additional hearing damage due to overamplification. In fact many case studies have been published over the years showing that the use of a hearing aid can indeed cause temporary and permanent threshold shift resulting in further hearing loss (Holmgren, 1940; Harford and Markle, 1955; Truex, 1957; Sataloff, 1962; Roberts, 1970).

Kasten and Braulin (1970) presented a case study in which they could create deterioration in patient's hearing through the use of a hearing aid. Their patient was a 10-year-old girl with bilateral, moderate sensorineural hearing loss. She wore a body-type hearing aid satisfactorily in one ear for 14 months and then began to complain that the aid was not helping as much as it did previously. An audiometric evaluation showed marked worsening of the hearing in the aided ear and no change in the hearing of the unaided ear. Kasten and

Braunlin alternated the hearing aid between ears and were able to show temporary deterioration in the aided ear, regardless of which ear wore the hearing aid. The aid in question had an average gain of 39 dB and average saturation sound pressure level of 120 dB. They recommended a less powerful hearing aid of 30-dB gain and 100-dB saturation sound pressure level. When a less powerful hearing aid was fitted to the patient, and worn alternately between ears, evaluations verified that the temporary deterioration of hearing was no longer present.

Two patients exhibiting temporary increases in sensorineural hearing loss following hearing aid use were reported by Heffernan and Simons (1979). The use of different hearing aids with decreased power output did not cause temporary threshold shifts. Based on their experiences Heffernan and Simons offer specific follow-up routine to include: (1) check of performance with the new hearing aid within 30 days of purchase, (2) electroacoustic analysis of the new aid within 30 days of purchase, (3) monthly appointments thereafter to monitor hearing thresholds until the hearing levels have stabilized for at least 3 months of continual hearing aid use, (4) reevaluation at least every 3 months for the next calendar year, and (5) annual otologic and audiologic evaluations as long as the aid is worn.

Heffernan and Simons also suggest that initial introduction of amplification should always be on a monaural basis. If subsequent testing for at least 3 months reveals that no hearing change has occurred with the new hearing aid, then the recommendation for the second hearing aid can be immediately implemented. The second hearing aid, however, must be monitored in the same maneuver as the first.

Rojskjaer (1960) reported an evaluation of 390 cases of all types of hearing loss treated with hearing aids for 5 years or more. He found 9 cases with additional hearing loss in the aided ear. No cases were noted where hearing deteriorated in nonaided ears. Naunton (1957) reviewed charts of 120 patients selected from a population of 1480 cases. He compared thresholds from the nonaided ear with the aided ear of these patients, and concluded that changes in hearing due to hearing aid use are statistically and clinically nonsignificant. On the contrary, in a similar study by Kinney (1961) with 178 patients, sufficient numbers of unilateral traumatic hearing losses were attributed to amplification that he recommended that aids fitted to children with sensorineural deafness be limited to less than 40 dB of gain. Kinney also recommended frequent audiologic follow-up visits for children who wear hearing aids.

Macrae and Farrant (1965) evaluated changes in the aided and unaided ears of 87 children and concluded that (a) individuals with sensorineural hearing loss should be fitted with limited maximal power output hearing aids, (b) frequent audiologic follow-up of aided children should be required, (c) children should alternate use of the aid in each ear whenever practical, and (d) users should be cautioned about wearing hearing aids in high ambient noise environments. Macrae (1968a, 1968b) found substantial temporary threshold shift in the aided ears of children with sensorineural deafness following use of powerful hearing aids. He measured the hearing levels of four children from a school for the deaf on Friday afternoon after the youngsters had worn their hearing aids all week. He then kept the aids, and deprived the children of amplification for 66 hours, until the following Monday morning. Hearing levels in all four children showed improvement on Monday morning which again deteriorated after 4 hours of hearing aid use.

Jerger and Lewis (1975) described an incident of progressive hearing loss in a young patient attributed to excessive sound pressure from a high power hearing aid. These authors suggest caution in fitting high power hearing aids binaurally in children, and propose alternating a single hearing aid between ears every other day to afford each ear 24 hours of rest between exposures.

Reilly et al. (1981) examined the effects of hearing aid use on progressive hearing loss of children. Careful examination of the role of amplification and the time period of progressive hearing loss, "probably" implicated the hearing aid in 11% of the patients, and "questionably" implicated the hearing aid in an additional 20% of the cases. These authors warn that it is unwise to conclude that hearing aid use is the cause of hearing deterioration without considering all other plausible factors.

Details of several experimental investigations regarding the use of amplification and its effect on residual hearing have been summarized by Ross and Lerman (1967) and Rintelmann and Bess (1977). Humes and Bess (1981) published a tutorial on the potential deterioration in hearing due to hearing aid use based on studies of temporary threshold shift induced by overamplification.

The evidence for powerful hearing aids causing threshold changes in the aided ear certainly seems, to us, to confirm this unfortunate circumstance as a real possibility to be considered by clinicians. It is our hope that the attention of additional researchers and hearing aid manufacturers will be drawn to this problem. Further developments will hopefully assist in identifying children, in advance, who might suffer trauma from hearing aid use. There is much we still do not know about some basic psychophysical facts related to hearing loss and hearing aid use. Danaher and Pickett (1972) noted in subjects with profound hearing loss that their most comfortable hearing level may actually be 125 dB SPL, with a loudness discomfort level of 128 dB SPL. Many patients with profound hearing loss have no loudness discomfort at any level, while other patients, with seemingly similar hearing loss, have loudness tolerance problems so severe that they cannot tolerate any type of amplification.

Markides (1976) studied the effects of hearing aid amplification in four groups of children ($N = 100$) as a function of hearing aid output and frequency response. Each group of children was tested every 6 months for a 3-year period. Although his reported mean results showed insignificant group differences, analysis of individual children showed that seven of the subjects showed 10–15-dB deterioration in aided ears at 4000 Hz.

Darbyshire (1976) and Titche et al. (1977) examined large groups of children with hearing aids for signs of possible effects of amplification on auditory sensitivity. The conclusion that hearing aids have no damaging effects on the hearing sensitivity of children was reported in each study.

A comprehensive review of the literature by Mills (1975) provides the most logical conclusions available. In general, he states, "the results of all studies indicate that habitual use of a hearing aid is not associated with additional deterioration of hearing in a large majority of persons tested. In some subjects, however, decreases in auditory sensitivity are observed." However, Mills questions whether the additional hearing losses are due to genetic or to disease-related factors, or whether they are due to the chronic temporary threshold shifts of 5–20 dB reported on many hard of hearing adults who use powerful hearing aids. Chronic threshold shifts of 5–20 dB may be a small cost for the many benefits of a hearing aid, states Mills.

We wholeheartedly support the recommendations of Ross and Lerman (1967) to alleviate, or lessen, the possibility of inadvertent traumatic hearing loss related to overamplification.

1. Additional hearing loss is most likely related to use of extremely high levels of maximal power output which exceed 130 dB SSPL; hearing aid recommendations for children with sensorineural hearing loss should include only hearing aids with less than 130 dB SSPL.

2. Although we recognize that traumatic hearing loss may be related to hearing aid use, the incidence seems quite small, and our concern is by no means to be interpreted as contraindicatory to amplification. In fact, we believe that denying a child a hearing aid during the critical language

years may only be saving his hearing for no good purpose. If the aid is fitted too late, it will not help anyway.

3. Frequent follow-up audiometric and hearing aid evaluation is an absolute must for all children with sensorineural hearing loss who wear hearing aids. We reevaluate our aided children twice a year.

A PRIMER FOR PARENTS OF A HEARING-AIDED CHIILD[1]

A number of excellent materials are now available to help parents deal with their aided hearing-impaired infants and children. We especially recommend the Parent-Infant Communication curriculum developed by Sitnick et al. (1978) and the programmed Orientation to Hearing Aids produced at the National Technical Institute for the Deaf in Rochester, New York, by Ganger et al. (1980). The material reproduced below is given to parents at the time their youngster is fitted with the initial hearing aid to help them with possible immediate problems that may occur.

Let's Start with the Hearing Aid

Your audiologist has fitted your child with the best hearing aid available. It may be one aid or two—one for each ear. Whichever it is, trust the audiologist's judgment that it is the best fitting for your child.

Think of the hearing aid as you would a pair of glasses. Both are something that a child must learn to wear during all his waking hours. He will put the aid on in the morning just as he puts on his clothes.

It may take a little time for your child to get used to wearing the aid. It is not easy to suddenly hear a lot of loud noise after having lived in a quiet world. That is why a special program of gradually getting him used to the aid is being outlined for you. Some children can get used to the aid very quickly; others take more time—and much patience.

---

[1] Much of this material is taken from pamphlets prepared by M. Downs and D. Pollack between 1951 and 1961 at the University of Colorado Medical Center.

Decide right now that you are not going to be embarrassed or apologetic about the aid. If adults or other children show interest in the aid, make a point of explaining that some people cannot see very well and wear glasses which help them to see more clearly; your child cannot hear well, and must wear a hearing aid. If he cannot talk, explain that, because he can hear more clearly, he will learn to talk. Parents have noticed that other children like to hold the receiver to their ears and listen—they may call it a little "radio" and they feel the hard of hearing child is very fortunate to possess something they do not have.

Another thing you must be clear about is what you should expect from the aid. Even at best it will take some time before the sounds that are heard through the aid become meaningful. It takes a newborn baby a full year of just listening to speech before he, himself, can produce even one word. If your child has not heard speech before, he will be like a newborn baby in relation to learning what sounds mean. It may take him more than a year or it may take him less to develop the understanding of what speech means.

The Home Program

Usually children will become accustomed to wearing aids if you follow the very simple kind of program outlined in this section. The next section discusses problems which may arise.

The First Week. *Short Periods Only.* For 10 min if you can retain his interest, increasing gradually to 30 min per period.

1. Wear the aid in a quiet room at home, preferably occupied by only two or three people. Do not take the new aid when you visit friends or are in a movie theatre.

2. Set the aid at a low volume, saying "Hello———, isn't this fun," etc., gradually increasing the volume until your child shows a slight awareness of your voice.

3. During the first week you might put the aid on while he is eating, so that he has a pleasant association with it.

4. Turn off the aid and remove the ear insert *before* the child becomes tired or restless. Do not show any impatience or anxiety if the child rejects the aid—you can always try again later. If the aid is persistently rejected, seek expert advice from an audiologist.

Prepare activities for these periods so that they are really enjoyable: You might read stories; make a scrapbook together, cutting out pictures and talking about them; model clay (but don't build blocks: it's too noisy!); play games like Picture Lotto or dressing paper dolls; draw or crayon, talking quietly about the colors, etc.; look out of the window—talk about the things you can see; or follow any activities that are being given by his therapist: color matching, nursery rhymes, etc.

The Second Week. *Two or Three Periods a Day for Approximately 1 Hour per Period.* Continue with the games and activities enjoyed before and add phonograph records, television, or musical programs on the radio. Adjust the volume and teach your child to adjust the volume of the aid—if the music is soft, the child will increase the volume until he can hear it, and vice versa. Very young children will enjoy watching you sing, dance, march, etc., to music or will tolerate rhythmic activities to music, such as Looby Lou, Mulbery Bush, etc. They do not usually enjoy just sitting and listening to music for some time.

Add Sounds Around the House. Using low volume, introduce your child to the sounds made by the telephone, vacuum cleaner, water running, clock, etc. Exaggerate, with a pleasant expression, your own reactions to these sounds.

If your child is receiving *speech training,* use the aid for the exercises, etc., to be practiced at home, whenever this is specifically recommended.

Go outdoors and take a walk (after turning the volume fairly low); listen carefully and identify all the sounds you hear—children's voices, dogs barking, horns blowing, etc., always drawing your child's attention to them and indicating who or what made these sounds. If your child will not wear his aid for any length of time, postpone this until later.

The Third Week and Later. Now is the time to encourage the idea that wearing the aid is as necessary as wearing shoes! Put it on when your child is dressing and try leaving it on for 2 or 3 hours at a time—that is, *if your child has already made a successful adjustment to the aid.*

Your child may now start to wear his instrument for a longer time, wherever he goes, so that he will eventually be in a hearing world all day. Arrange for these experiences; turning the volume fairly low, go outdoors and take a walk if you have not tried this before; go to the movies, sitting 8–15 rows from the front, as close to center as possible; play outdoors (if the play is not too boisterous or noisy), gardening, sandbox, swings, etc.; go to the zoo, the band in the park, etc.

Children with moderate losses often enjoy games at this time in which they have to depend on hearing. For example, cover your face and ask your child to point to certain toys or perform certain actions. (Color the dog black, make your doll dance, ring the bell, etc.) You, and your child, may be surprised how much he is now hearing and understanding. Very young children enjoy sound discrimination games: indicating whether you blew a horn or rang a bell, knocked on the door, etc.

Children with a hearing impairment have great difficulty in locating sound, and will enjoy games to overcome this. For example, they close their eyes and point to the corner of the room in which you ring a bell or call their names.

Problems in Hearing Aid Use

If you are having trouble keeping the hearing aid on your child, it may help to know that other parents have had the same troubles. Here are some of the problems and complaints others have had, with suggestions as to what to do about them (Downs, 1966, 1971).

Complaint: THE RECEIVER AND EARMOLD WON'T STAY IN THE EAR—THEY KEEP COMING OUT.

Remedy: In the case of a very young infant, the whole outer ear and ear canal may be too small to allow both the earmold and the receiver in it. To remedy this, the audiologist may recommend that the receiver be attached to a short tube leading to the earmold. The receiver can then be positioned just behind the ear flap, and the tube strengthened with wire so it will hold its conformity to the ear. This is a compromise that should only be used when necessary.

After a year or 18 months of age, the ear should be large enough to hold both the receiver and the earmold. If they still keep falling out, ask to have another earmold made, preferably of soft plastic material. Experiment several times if necessary to see if a perfect fit can be obtained. Remember that whenever you have an earmold fitted, you should demonstrate to your child what is going to happen: Take a large doll, lay it on its side, and put a piece of clay or cotton into the doll's ear. Show the child that this is what will happen to him. Lay him on his side and put cotton in his ears very gently. Praise him for lying still. A little preparation now saves a lot of screaming later.

Sometimes the cord keeps getting in the way of small hands, and the receiver is accidentally pulled out. Try placing the aid on the back instead of the front, and anchor the cord on the back of the shirt collar with a safety pin. Slip the cord through the safety pin, rather than piercing it.

If the earmold still keeps coming out, you may have to devise a knitted band for him to wear on his head to hold the receiver in place. Or, in the case of a girl, a ribbon or a little bonnet can be used.

Complaint: JOHNNY CONTINUALLY PULLS THE RECEIVER OUT OF HIS EAR, SO THE EARMOLD MUST BE HURTING HIM, OR THE AID MUST BOTHER HIM, OR PERHAPS HE DOESN'T NEED AN AID AND IT DOESN'T DO HIM ANY GOOD.

Remedy: You have probably let Johnny get the upper hand, Mother. But just to be sure, check the aid carefully.

1. If there is some real irritation from the earmold that is hurting him, there is a way to find out: make an appointment with your ear doctor, and put the earmold in Johnny's ear for an hour before you see the doctor. He will then examine the outer ear and ear canal for evidence of irritation. If there is, the mold can be remade with special attention to the spot that is irritating, or the "high spot" on the mold can be ground off and repolished.

2. If the aid is "bothering him," the audiologist can tell by doing tolerance tests at different volume settings of the aid. If certain levels of sound cause Johnny to blink, or to jerk, or to cry, then the audiologist will make the proper adjustment in the aid.

3. If you feel Johnny "doesn't really need the aid," you should ask the audiologist to make another evaluation. He will show you the levels at which Johnny hears, and where he doesn't hear. Often, after a child has worn an aid for a while and has learned to identify sounds in his environment, he will respond to some sounds even when he is not wearing the aid. He is responding to "reduced cues"—that is, once he is aware of the importance of sounds, he will attend to some that are loud enough just to reach his threshold. He may be hearing only a part of a sound, very faintly, but he now pays attention to it. This does not mean that his hearing has improved or has become normal, much as we would like that to happen. It is very exciting to know that he is making use of every bit of residual hearing he has, and it is a good sign for his future functioning with the aid.

If you continue to have trouble keeping Johnny from taking off the hearing aid, you can work toward training him never to touch the receiver or to take it off. The following program may take 3 or 4 days of your time, but it will succeed in convincing Johnny that you mean business.

First Week. The first thing in the morning, show the child the earmold and aid, and set them near the clock. Point out that at 9:00 you will put the aid on for 5 min, and then you will take it off. He need not understand the time concept, but he will get the idea that you know what you're going to do and that you intend to do it consistently. When 9:00 comes show him the time and put the earmold in without turning the aid on. If he does not object to the mold, play quietly and lovingly with him for 5 min, and then remove it. If he protests actively, hold his arms and legs, placing him sidewise on your lap so his feet can't kick you. Do not let him take the mold out. After 5 min, remove the aid and put it back near the clock. Point out the next time of application.

Apply the aid in this way four times a day, showing him what you are going to do, and *do it*. He must learn that you are in control of the situation, not he. By the end of the fifth or sixth day of this routine he will tolerate wearing the mold, you may be sure.

When he has tolerated the mold, at the next session turn the aid on to one-fourth volume and talk quietly into it, "Hello, isn't this nice? How's Johnny?" Then put it into his pocket or harness, and leave it on for 5 min. Play with a favorite game or toy during that time. If necessary, again hold down his arms and legs, avoiding flying feet!

Second Week. Apply the hearing aid as above four times a day for 15 min, turning the volume to one-third position. (Place a small piece of adhesive tape over the volume wheel to hold it at that position.) Play quietly or read for the first 5 min, then take him around the house to investigate various noises. Point out the door bell and listen to it ring; show him the vacuum cleaner, the refrigerator, the washer, and listen for their noises. Each time, point to your ears and say "I hear it—its a BIG sound" (or a little one)—and demonstrate big and little with your hands.

Third Week. Apply the hearing aid as above four times a day for 30 min, turning the volume a little above one-third. After 5 min of quiet play with him, go about your household tasks, placing him near you in a crib, playpen, or on the floor. As you work, call his attention to all the sounds you make in your work: banging pans together while washing dishes—"Listen, Johnny, what a BIG sound;" clinking glasses together—"What a LITTLE sound;" shaking out towels from the laundry—"What a funny noise." Whenever a dog barks, a truck goes by, or someone knocks at the door, call his attention to it and imitate the sound.

Fourth Week. Apply the hearing aid as above four times a day for 45 min, turning the hearing aid almost to the prescribed level.

Fifth Week. Apply the hearing aid as above four times a day for 1 hour, turning it to the level that has been prescribed, e.g., one-half, two-thirds, three-fourths volume. it is a good idea to put a dab of nail polish on the wheel at a point that will tell you where the prescribed level is. As long as necessary, place a strip of adhesive over the wheel so the child cannot turn it.

If the aid squeals, or feeds back when the volume is placed at the desired level, try some Vaseline around the canal piece. If this doesn't prevent feedback, go immediately to have a new earmold fitted. Never allow the feedback to dictate where the volume control is set, even though it may be necessary to have new earmolds made every 3 or 6 months.

Sixth Week and Thereafter. Increase the time of wearing the aid gradually until by the second month he is wearing it all day long with the following exceptions: (1) three 10-min rest periods a day (turn the aid off; you needn't take the mold out); (2) rough play outdoors; and (3) nap time.

There may, of course, be other problems which you, as a parent, will have to overcome. Consult with your audiologist whenever you need help in solving a problem situation; chances are it is not the first time he has heard the problem. More than likely, he will have some helpful suggestions for a remedy.

AMPLIFICATION IN THE CLASSROOM

One of the most important aspects of amplification is its use in the school or educational setting. Important technological advancements have occurred in the past few years which makes amplification in the classroom an essential component in the education of hearing-impaired children. Excellent reviews of the current status of classroom amplification have been written by Freeman et al. (1980), Bess and Gravel (1981), Boothroyd (1981), Bess and McConnell (1981), Sinclair and Freeman (1981), and Bess and Logan (1983).

The acoustic environment in which hearing-impaired students do their learning typically has high noise levels and poor acoustic reverberation conditions. Olsen (1981) and Finitzo-Hieber (1982) have shown that classroom acoustics are an important consideration which can be deleterious to the hearing-impaired student. To be sure, certain architectural improvements can be made in school rooms to help reduce unwanted noise and limit reverberation, but in these days of mainstreaming it is unlikely that all school classrooms can be modified to meet the needs of the hearing-impaired student. Sanders (1965) reported the mean noise values of normal school occupied classrooms to be as high as 69 dB.

The personal hearing aid is, of course, the most common means of providing school room amplification. The major drawback to the personal unit is its dependence on close distance to the speaker to achieve a high signal-to-noise effect. Unfortunately, this is difficult to control in the typical classroom, and as the teacher moves away from the child wearing a personal hearing aid, the increase in distance contributes quickly to the demise of signal amplification for the hearing-impaired child. When faced with a weak sound signal, the hearing aid user must turn up the gain of the unit, which also increases the background noise creating unavoidable masking effects (Kothman, 1981).

These problems have led to the development of radio frequency transmission units (FM) with wireless microphones. The wireless microphone is worn by the teacher which strengthens and stabilizes the reception of the speaker's voice while simultaneously minimizing the effect of background sounds (Powers, 1980). External receivers may be coupled to the personal earmolds worn by the hearing-impaired child. The student receivers can be adjusted to make them adaptable to a wide range of individual needs.

Even more recently a number of newer techniques permit the "dovetailing" of the personal hearing aid to the FM system (Bess and Gravel, 1981; Bess and Logan, 1983). The coupling of the FM system to the personal hearing aid can be accomplished by several techniques including electrical, induction or acoustical. The advantages to an FM radio transmission through a wireless microphone attached close to the mouth of the speaker, sending high fidelity signals to the personal hearing aid of the hearing-impaired child (who may be as far as 200 meters (650 feet) away) are obvious. The personal hearing aid has been carefully selected by the audiologist to the individual needs of the patient, and the FM system works to reduce loss of signal due to distance and minimize environmental noise.

The application of the FM-personal hearing aid system are much broader than just school room use. These systems are practical for at home use, learning sports activities, driver's education, and large group theater or auditorium activities. The FM system is no longer a "special instrument" consideration, but an important part of every hearing-impaired child's daily life. Audiologists, physicians and educators must become more aware of the application of educational amplification systems.

IMPLANTABLE AUDITORY PROSTHESES

For several years surgical centers in this country and abroad have been experimenting with the implantation of electrodes into the cochlea in order to stimulate the hearing nerves and obtain some hearing where none was before. A number of adults and children have received implants at this time.

Some centers have begun placing implants in children, and there is impetus toward implanting younger and younger children. Because audiologists may be managing children who are being considered for implants Downs (1981) reviewed the implant program and developed a stance toward it.

Many patients throughout the country have been implanted and are being studied both for auditory skills and for equipment design. The original design incorporated a single electrode introduced into the cochlea, usually the basal turn of the scala tympani. More recently multiple electrodes are being investigated with a promise of improvement in results. Revisions of the implants have been deemed necessary every 2 years or more.

Bilger's (1977) extensive psychoacoustic evaluation of implanted adult patients specified the nature of the auditory discriminations possible with the prostheses. The typical implant patient could hear the speech frequencies most sensitively. For narrow bands at 250 and 500 Hz subjects could discriminate intensity differences as well as normal subjects, but at 2000 Hz none could achieve adequate intensity discrimination. Adequate pitch perception was present only for frequencies below 250 Hz.

Subjects were able to discriminate differences in signal duration, temporal patterning (rhythm), and spectrum (tone vs. narrow band). Many subjects could discriminate among pairs of speechlike sounds, but did not appreciate them as speechlike. Subjects could identify two-syllable words when they knew exactly which words of a small set would be presented. They also identified common environmental sounds when they knew which sounds were likely to be heard.

Ratings of speech intelligibility showed that the quality of most of the subject's speech was enhanced when the prosthesis was activated.

The audiologists' position toward implants should be one of caution tinged with respect for the scientific progress that is being made. Where children are concerned there are far more caveats than with adults. What follows is a proposed list of criteria that may be useful to those who are managing the education of young children who may be considered for surgical implants.

According to Downs (1981) a child who falls into any of the categories below should not be a candidate for an implant:

1. A child who can receive results with a hearing aid that are equivalent to the results that implants have been shown to produce. A hearing aid rehabilitation program utilizing all the techniques that are used for post-implant patients is thus mandatory.

2. A child whose parent cannot invest the time in the rehabilitation process that is requisite to a good outcome. Number of siblings, psychological stability, and socioeconomic factors should be considered.

3. A child whose parents could not tolerate the necessity for periodic revisions of the implants, currently approximately every 2 years. Financial as well as psychological factors should be considered.

4. A child who has only one ear that is acceptable for an implant. One ear should be available for implant 20 or 30 years hence, when more effective techniques may have been developed.

5. A child who is not able to respond reliably to the psychophysical measures that might be necessary to achieve alignment of the coils used in the equipment.

6. A child who is at risk for recurrent of otitis media including:
   a. Close family members with recurrent otitis.
   b. History of otitis media with first bout under 1 year of age.
   c. Bacterial meningitis caused by otitis media.
   d. Upper respiratory allergies.
   e. Cleft palate.
   f. Down's syndrome.
   g. Prematurity.
   h. Native American heritage.
   i. Any child under 8 years of age with an uncertain history of otitis media.

A comprehensive review of the status of cochlear implants at the House Rehabilitation Center has been published by Berlinger and House (1981).

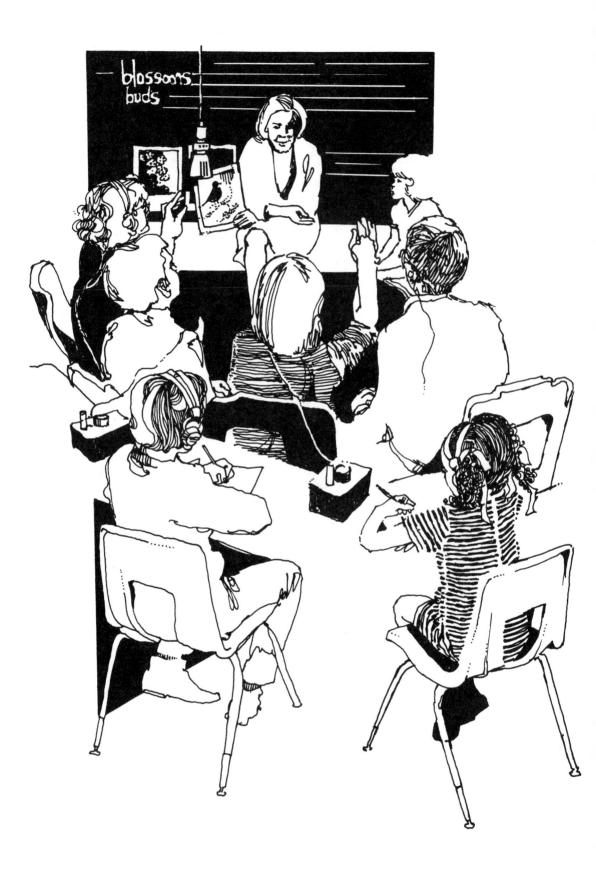

CHAPTER 9

Education for Hearing-Impaired Children

AUDIOLOGY AND EDUCATION OF THE HEARING-IMPAIRED CHILD

One of the first issues to be clarified in this chapter is that of terminology and definition. Our definition of "hearing-impaired" children includes all those children with hearing loss who are handicapped to such an extent that some form of special education is required. Obviously, this broad definition includes these we traditionally define as "deaf." The Conference of Executives of American Schools for the Deaf defines "the deaf" as having a hearing loss of 70 dB HL or greater in their better ear, while the "hard-of-hearing" student has a loss of 35–69 dB HL in the better hearing ear. Amon (1981) defines "deaf" as a hearing impairment so severe that a child experiences difficulty in processing linguistic information through hearing, with or without amplification. Although it is easy to speak in general terms about the education of deaf and/or hard-of-hearing students, the point must be made that these groups are by no means homogeneous, and there is no single educational "method," "system" or "approach" that is uniformly applicable to all members of each group.

Of all the information published throughout the years in previous editions of this textbook, this chapter, "Education for Hearing-Impaired Children," elicits more controversial commentary from our colleagues than any other chapter. But such is the nature of this topic, and it is unlikely that the information presented below will satisfy all readers. Our goal is to acquaint speech-language-hearing students with the single most important aspect of management of the child with hearing impairment—achieving the maximum potential of the child through education.

The audiologist is often hard put to maintain the distinction between himself as an expert and himself as an advocate. When he expresses an objective judgment within the field of his expertise, he is on safe ground; but when he advocates a chosen position on questions of general policy not directly related to his expertise, he must recognize his tenuous position.

In this book we have described objective measures that have been fairly adequately standardized, and we have also outlined subjective assessments that lend themselves to some measurable degree of judgment. Here we are under a fair amount of control. However, in the field of directing hearing-impaired children into educational channels, the audiologist becomes an advocate of a cause. Most audiologists do not have complete familiarity with all training methods and what they can do, nor do they have an understanding of all the variables that will affect the child's functioning in a given training method. In order to rectify these inadequacies, we point out that the audiologist, in addition to his own empirical testing, must seek the judgments of various physicians, educators, psychologists, sociologists, and others. With these people he must evolve a decision concerning the direction of management of the child—one that is flexible enough to change with the further accumulation of information. When the audiologic clinician makes such a judgment, he has become an informed advocate utilizing the information gathered from many disciplines which, however far from the ideal, is still the best anyone can know for the child.

It is our philosophy that the audiologist can become an "advocate without a cause" in the field of educational management for the child. He should not be biased in the direction of any training method or philosophy. He should consider only what will best ensure the child's maximal ultimate development. In this book we try to give the audiologist the tools with which he can arrive at a working construct concerning the direction of management for a child.

But, in another sense, the audiologist can espouse advocacy for principle or cause alone. This is in the sense of fighting for the child's right to be given a chance to show what he can do, despite contrary evidence. We would be something less than human if we failed to let hope play a part in judgments of multiple handicapped children. We also would be less than human if we failed to glow with satisfaction when a child who was scheduled for institutionalizing becomes trainable with hearing aids and hearing therapy, upon our insistence—or when an infant who was thought to be incapable of developing useful auditory perceptions becomes in every way a hearing person with adequate speech and language abilities.

Among the fundamental rights that we as surrogates for children should demand from society is a child's right to achieve his maximal potential communication abilities. Even if a child be deaf, or blind, or crippled in any way, we should demand of society that special provision be made to help him override the disability and become as "normal" as his limitations will allow. The world-famous child psychologist, A. L. Gesell, said in a 1956 publication, "The . . . aim should not be to convert the deaf child into a somewhat fictitious version of a nor-

mal hearing child, but into a well-adjusted nonhearing child who is completely managing the limitations of his sensory deficit." An excellent description of the current state of affairs in the field of education of hearing-impaired learners was written by Ferguson et al. (1982).

GOALS OF EDUCATION FOR THE DEAF

Adequate Language Skills

Language deprivation is the most serious of all deprivations, for it robs us of a measure of our own human-ness. Whether caused by sensory deprivation, by experiential deprivation, or by central disordering, in some degree it keeps one from the complete fulfillment of one's powers.

Language is the desideratum that we most wish for the hearing impaired. For too long we have been misled into placing oral speech as the primary goal for all of these children, never realizing that the enrichment of their lives may be sacrificed for the ability to mouth words. What words?—And in what relationships? If one is not able to think in highly complex language symbols, does it matter whether he is able to vocalize any of them? And, most important, how can he verbalize adequately unless he has an adequate symbol system to utilize?

The premise of our proposal for the management of the hearing-impaired child rests upon language as the primary goal to be sought for the child. Whatever route will lead the way through his neurologic labyrinth to reach language understanding, that route must be taken. We must be ruthless in discarding methods and methodologies, entrenched techniques, and individual philosophies. We hold no brief for any established method or educational technique— nor any not yet established. Any, or all, should be selected for use when the need warrants. What is important is that an approach be selected on the basis of what is best for the child, not for the institution. For too long the child has been forced to be tailor-made to the program; we must now tailor-make a program for each individual child's needs. The primary goal is always to tap the innate language skills by whatever means possible. Secondarily only will we aim for intelligible oral expression of that language—a skill that itself depends upon the acquisition of a high degree of language competence.

Not only speech, but reading and writing skills are also dependent upon language skills. One forgets that the sequence of development of language skills is first, listening; second, speaking; third, reading; and fourth, writing (Mackintosh, 1964). A foundation of competence in the input of language (listening) is requisite to the expressive skills of speaking and writing. Likewise, a firm basis of language input is requisite to capability in reading, which is the secondary receptive input skill. These facts are basic to the organization of a therapeutic and educational program for a hearing-impaired child.

It is the deficiency in language skills which is the spectre that haunts the clinician who sees a generation of hearing-impaired children grow to adulthood. Fully half of all the children in our clinical experience with severe to profound losses who were started at a very early age in an auditory-oral program did not develop language commensurate with their potential intellectual level. Their language levels are typified by the results of a recent demographic survey conducted by Gallaudet College (Reis, 1973a). This study reported the results of standard achievement tests in 19,000 deaf and hard-of-hearing children in the United States. Both oral and manual educational techniques were represented. One of the most significant test results indicates that the highest average score in paragraph meanings, which represents language comprehension, was obtained by the 19-year-olds and was equivalent to normal fourth grade level!

Preschool oral programs have not seemed to be successful in raising the level of language, lipreading, and reading skills. Vernon and Koh (1970) reported well-controlled studies demonstrating that, by age 9, no differences existed between deaf children who had had oral preschool programs and those who had not had such training.

Such studies do not refute the hypothesis that early language training can raise the level of language of the deaf; they do demonstrate that oral training at the preschool level is not effective for many children. What does seem to be effective is exposure to manual language patterns at a young age. A large number of studies show that the deaf children of deaf parents have a significantly higher level of language than all other deaf children, that they have equivalent speech development, that they achieve academically at a higher level, and that they tend to be better adjusted than all other deaf children (Vernon and Koh, 1970; Quigley and Frisina, 1961; Meadow, 1968b; Stuckless and Birch, 1966). The plethora of reports confirming these facts can hardly be controverted by even the most zealous auditory-oral advocates.

Sound Mental Health

The most effective learning takes place in the context of warm, nurturant relationships within the family. This is particularly important for the very young child during his critical years for language development. Whatever type of program a child is receiving, his parents should be given close emotional support and guidance in their management of the child's problems. The results should be the development of the child's self-confidence, high self-esteem, and the ability to relate well to people in the environment.

The warm relationship between parents and child can be fostered by helpful, supportive communications from physician and educational personnel. The initial phase of reporting the child's deafness to the parents is crucial to the parents' attitude toward the problem. Time should be allowed for them to air their feelings and their sorrow over having an "imperfect" child. Grief must be expressed if acceptance of the handicap is to come. These natural feelings should be shared with empathy and understanding. The physician and the audiologist can create the kind of atmosphere out of which nurturant attitudes can grow.

Together with the physician and audiologist the parents can choose an educational program for their child which will allow the continuation of a good parent nurturing. As Schlesinger (1973) pointed out: "Early parent-child communication is a traumatic issue between hearing parents and their deaf children. Although the hearing parents talk to and in front of the child, they can only guess at his level of understanding." Frustration results, both for parents and child. Thus it is important that an educational program be chosen which minimizes this frustration. It should be noted that such problems are not present in the relationships of deaf parents to their deaf children. Denton et al. (1974) stated: "Deaf parents, as they communicate to and in front of the child, can test the child's understanding more easily. The child ... can learn the symbols, the signs the parents use, and learn to understand and reproduce them more easily."

Whatever program is chosen, the goal should be to foster the kind of communication that allows good "mothering" and "fathering." The goal of sound mental health is essential to any achievement that can be desired for the deaf child.

Intelligible Speech

It is no accident that speech skills take only third place in the hierarchy of goals for the hearing impaired. Intelligible speech without good language skills is an exercise in futility; intelligible speech is an emotionally disordered mind in a useless function. Only after the two previous goals have been assured do we ask for the development of understandable speech. Articulate speech is greatly to be desired, but a program producing excellence only in this skill and not in language or emotional stability cannot be highly rated.

Easy Communication with Peers

Too often an evaluation is made on the basis of how a child communicates with his teachers and his parents. But his real need is to communicate well with his peers, with whom he must spend the rest of his life. Unless he is able to understand and be understood by his peer group on their own level and according to their standards, it does not matter how well he can be understood in the structured milieu of his home or school. Watch the child whose teacher has said: "He's doing so well—see how clearly he repeats these words."

How does he get along with his peers—can they understand him and communicate with him, within the needs of their play? The real world of normal hearing is a harsh one for the hearing-impaired child, and not many achieve the easy, normal communication with their normal hearing peers that is our goal for them.

The point is not to force a child into a peer relationship where he cannot compete or be accepted, but to choose a peer community where he can communicate easily, without stress or censure. Eventually this child may find a spouse to share his life. Can he find one from the peer group in which he has been placed? Unless there is easy communication together it is difficult to find a compatible partner.

Easy communication can be secured in milieus other than the one we consider the most desirable—the normal hearing world. For example, in the manual-deaf community all peer communication is easy, for all are alike. This kind of milieu need not be considered a last resort, but rather a means of securing a highly satisfactory goal for a hearing-handicapped child.

These four goals do not limit the range of objectives that one might have for the deaf and hard-of-hearing child. However, any other goals that we might enumerate—high employability, job satisfaction, enrichment of life—all depend upon how well these basic four are secured. All follow from these fundamental aims.

THE EDUCATIONAL CONTROVERSY

Certainly there is a need for a variety of experts in the field of deafness. The difficulty comes from the fact that few "experts" have the important ingredient of objectiveness when it comes to evaluating the field of deaf education. The professional groups who know most about this area are the teachers themselves or program administrators. Yet these people are limited in number and isolated from new parents of a deaf child.

The new "educational audiologist" may prove to be the appropriate intermediary trained in deafness education and management with special emphasis in audiological aspects of hearing-impaired children. These individuals, albeit few in number at this time, are a great asset to the interdisciplinary team because of their background and experience in diagnostic evaluation and habilitation of hearing-impaired children. With technological knowledge and educational management competencies, the education audiologist can provide a solid bridge between the basic science areas and the social sciences of education and psychology (Ross, 1982). Bess and McConnell (1981) produced an excellent textbook based on this concept which brings together audiology, education and the hearing-impaired child.

The major area of controversy boils down to differences of opinion between those who advocate oral and manual approaches to deaf education. Current terminology divides deaf education into auditory/verbal and visual/oral methods. The real problem here may be the inability of advocates of "methods" to take a positive "child-centered" approach rather than protecting their own self-interests and avoiding exposing their own biases. According to Moffatt (1972), proponents of both views agree that, when severe hearing loss exists, learning to talk with your hands is easier than learning to speak aloud. The supporters of the oral system feel that the child who uses the manual system will ultimately be forced into a "deaf society" because of his limited communication abilities (Rupp, 1971). Proponents of the manual system feel that deaf children learn more easily when taught primarily through the "visual" mode, and thus develop a wider base of knowledge for future use.

According to Luterman (1976) the auditory/verbal approach presupposes that lipreading or visual awareness of the face need not be taught; rather, the impaired auditory modality must be trained while allowing the child to use visual information as he needs it. This approach differs from the multisensory (visual/oral) system in which no formal work is attempted in lipreading; nor is the child's attention deliberately directed toward the speaker's face. While all agree that auditory training is an important part of the auditory/verbal and the visual/oral program, the visual/oral proponents view auditory training as a supplement to vision.

This controversy is so appealing to the public that daily newspaper editorials often contain letters regarding deaf education, and lay magazines become jousting grounds for opposing educational factions. *Harper's Magazine* some years back published an essay (Kenny, 1962) advocating reconsideration of the common lipreading system in deaf education and proposing use of the sign language in more schools. A few months later, the Editors of *Harper's* indicated that they had received "a flood of mail" within 3 weeks of the article from 22 states and Europe! Opinion reflected in the letters was reportedly evenly split for and against the Kenny point of view, but the fact that so many took sufficient interest to express an opinion shows the tremendous overlay of emotional concern.

The Education for All Handicapped Children Act of 1975 (Public Law 94-142)

The passage of the Education for All Handicapped Children Act of 1975 (otherwise known as Public Law 94-142) represents a landmark in federal recognition of their responsibility to provide funding for the costs of special education that will ensure a basic minimum level of program quality for handicapped children and their parents. The law assures the right of all children to be educated in the school districts in which they live.

The basic purposes of the law are to ensure that every handicapped child in the country will be able to receive a free, appropriate public education. The education is to be free—at no charge to the child or parents, appropriately designed to fit the special needs of the child and public—that is, the state education department has the legal responsibility to provide appropriate educational services under public auspices at public expense. The basic goals of this legislation broadens the options available to educate deaf students, recognizes the diverse needs of individual children, and supports the need for early identification and diagnosis.

The specific provisions of the law include (1) a free, appropriate public education for all handicapped children; (2) the identifiction, location, and evaluation of all handicapped children; (3) the preparation and implementation of an individualized education plan (IEP) for each involved child; (4) assurance of education in the least restrictive environment; (5) procedural safeguards for parents—"due process"; (6) maintenance of rights for children placed by the state in private schools; (7) in-service training; and (8) related services (including some health-related services). Although the 1970s will be remembered for this encompassing law, the economic conditions of the 1980s may create serious challenges for the enactment and fulfillment of the law's provisions. The "education of all handicapped children" is a multibillion dollar per year undertaking for which most of the funding has been allocated to the state and local communities (Palfrey, 1980).

Davila and Brill (1976) published an editorial supporting the concept of Public Law 94-142. They point out, however, that the law itself is not a panacea, nor will it automatically improve services and education for deaf students. The small numbers of the deaf require grouping deaf children with other deaf children in day programs or residential school settings. The law is not an automatic decree that "the least restrictive environment" and maximal integration are synonymous. Considering the ultimate objective of producing well-educated, socially adjusted and responsible adults, the "least restrictive environment" is not necessarily the one that is closest to home or has the maximum integration in schools.

In many ways, the law has been enacted before answers are ready concerning meeting the educational mandates. Many questions still exist regarding identification, evaluation and education of hearing-impaired and deaf children. One of the major tenets, which has received mixed reviews, relates to the placement of children in the "least restrictive environment." Although "mainstreamed children" have experienced some of the obvious benefits of association with age-similar peers, they have also experienced isolation and rejection within the classroom.

A number of interesting statistics were published in the Annual Survey of Hearing Impaired Children and Youth (Karchmer and Trybuss, 1977) regarding a national survey to determine how many and what kind of hearing-impaired children were involved in mainstreaming programs. Within the limitations of their survey, of the nearly 50,000 children samples, nearly 20% were participating in mainstreaming programs. As one might expect, 62% of these children had mild or moderate hearing loss, and were likely to be *post*lingually deaf. In contrast, the prelingual, severe-to-profoundly deaf children were usually in full-time special education programs. Bess and McConnel (1981) summarize the factors associated with a higher degree of success in mainstream programs to include the onset of hearing loss after oral language has been established, middle or upper income family background, and an ability to speak intelligibly.

Conway (1979) points out that mainstreaming is indeed becoming a reality for a high percentage of hearing-impaired students. Success in mainstreaming, however, is dependent upon careful selection of appropriate students. Thompson and Thompson (1981) warn that educators must be wary of getting caught up in a group movement that may not reflect the needs of an individual child, and in fact, may actually be detrimental to the achievement of that child's goals. They state that decisions about school placement should necessarily be made on the basis of the individual child's needs *and* on the basis of the availability of continued professional support by qualified persons after the placement has been made.

Excellent discussions of the implications of Public Law 94-142 for hearing-impaired and deaf children have been published by Bess and McConnell (1981) and Amon (1981). Amon points out that, in the past, it could be assumed that if a school hired certified teachers of the hearing-handicapped, and provided room, materials and equipment for the hearing-handicapped children, that the school's educational and legal mandate had been fulfilled. But, she continues, *no one system, method or program can meet all the needs of hearing-handicapped children.*

The United States Supreme Court reached its first decision involving the Education for All Handicapped Children Act in 1982. Although in this specific suit, the Rowley case, the Court found that a young deaf student did not require a sign language interpreter in school, it affirmed the right of all handicapped children to receive personalized instruction and the supportive services they need to benefit from their IEP. In addition, the Court upheld the basics of the law that parents are to share in the planning and development of their child's IEP, and if the parents are not satisfied, they can appeal through the due process of law. The Court determined that Ann Rowley, the deaf daughter of deaf parents, was doing well in school with other supportive services, and that the state was meeting the mandate of the Public Law by "... providing personalized instruction with sufficient supportive services to permit the child to benefit educationally from that instruction." The Court was not unanimous in its decision, and it is likely that additional legislational challenges in the future will be presented to test Public Law 94-142.

CURRENT STATUS OF EDUCATION OF THE DEAF

The Babbidge report (1965) produced by a national committee sponsored by the Department of Health, Education, and Welfare stated that "the American people have no reason to be satisfied with their limited success in educating deaf children and preparing them for full participation in our society." The Babbidge report cites the underlying cause of this poor result as a failure to launch an aggressive assault on the basic problems of language learning by the deaf, and lack of progress in the development of improved systematic and adequate programs for educating the deaf at all grade and age levels. Since the initial contributions of early deaf educators such as Abbé de L'Epée, Thomas Hopkins Gallaudet, and Alexander Graham Bell, education of the deaf is sometimes exactly where it was 150 years ago. However, innovations in medical technology, sophistication in psychology and linguistics, and improvements in personal and classroom amplification systems should stimulate the educational establishment to improve the educational level and skills of the deaf and hearing-impaired students.

McClure (1973) blames the "ostrich syndrome" demonstrated by certain deaf educators as one of the reasons for failure in deaf education progress. The "ostrich syndrome" is manifested by (1) an inability to accept change, (2) an inability to recognize the educational implications of modern research on deafness, (3) a tendency to do little research and to castigate investigators who depart from the traditional approaches, and (4) an overwhelming desire to bury their heads in the sand hoping that current trends will disappear or that contradictory research will suddenly appear to maintain the status quo. For example, many schools for the deaf and special classrooms for the hearing impaired are still not treated acoustically in a manner to benefit the children with hearing problems. Although most programs employ "audition" of some sort in teaching, a large gap exists between the research based facts about classroom acoustics and the application of these principles in the classroom.

Where are today's deaf students? Each year the April issue of *The American Annals of the Deaf* is devoted to a directory of information concerning all deaf education programs in the United States.The 1982 Directory issue indicated that nearly 44,000 deaf children were enrolled in 485 schools and special education classes. Approximately, 16,200 of these pupils were located in only 66 public and private *residential* schools. The 650 day classes and day school programs, public and private, accounted for 26,784 deaf students. An additional 633 students were listed in 26 multihandicapped or specific handicap facilities.

An interesting fact of note in these figures is that numerous deaf students attend residential-type programs. Traditionally, residential schools are aligned with manual education while private, day school programs are oral in nature. Such dichotomy, however, is currently not so specific. Additional statistics from the 1982 Directory issue indicate that one-third of these residential school students attend as day pupils. Thus, some 32,000 pupils can be categorized as day students, while only some 11,000 can truly be considered residential or "live-in" students.

All educators would agree that the most vital aspect of any child's intellectual development is language. Upon the child's successful handling of language skills

hinges his progress in school and in life. His ability to communicate his thoughts, wants, and needs to others, and in turn his understanding of thoughts and feelings of others, depend on crucial language skills. It is not by chance that these skills have been immortalized as the first two of the three R's.

The deaf child's problems have been clearly summarized by Louis Fant (1963) of the Department of Education at Gallaudet College and we are indebted to him for the following discussion. He believes that hearing plays a vital role in language development to build concepts and clarify them. The deaf child lacks this valuable input channel and accordingly throughout life has trouble developing and clarifying concepts. The entire process is slowed down and becomes laborious.

Language and concept developments, according to a scheme developed by Fant, clearly proceed hand-in-hand with communication. For the hearing child, the early states of communication are primarily via speech and hearing, and may be categorized into five components:

1. Reception: Sensory data are fed into the brain via the senses.

2. Symbols: Words, signs, gestures which are used in *Reception*.

3. Encoding: Meaningful arrangement of symbols.

4. Transmission: Meaningful sending of encoded material to someone else.

5. Decoding: The receiver's mind now utilizes the message and extracts meaning from it.

Fant states that for smooth, free-flowing communication, all five components must be operating efficiently. There must be a sufficient number of symbols to represent the message (vocabulary).There must be sufficient skill to encode the symbols (grammar). There must be sufficient mechanisms for transmission such as speech and writing. The process of decoding involves understanding vocabulary and grammar which form the very basis of the most important factor, the substance or content of the message itself. Incomplete communication and frustration result from a breakdown anywhere along the line.

So the educator of the deaf faces the problem with every deaf child. The deaf child is stuck at the very first element of the communication process. His mind is deprived of the rich sensory data supplied normally through the auditory mechanism. He often has a meager supply of symbols to use for labeling, categorizing, and storing. New symbols are difficult to come by. The deaf child functions on the concrete level of mental operations and, thus, abstract operations are most difficult for him because they are performed with words—the very commodity of which he never has enough. Abstract operations demand precise encoding and decoding and mastery of "word" concepts. Deaf children seldom attain sufficient language skills to master abstract operations even after arduous effort.

And finally, Fant points out that the usual process of trial and error learning—or teaching for that matter—is seriously hampered for the deaf child. The deaf child cannot hear his errors of vocabulary or grammar. Attempts to correct the deaf child's errors are chancy undertakings. Because of the often indistinct transmissions (speech), the listener cannot be certain that the child made an error in his use of words or grammar or whether the listener just did not understand his speech. Suppose the listener thinks an error was indeed committed; imagine his task in trying to correct the error. Or suppose an error was committed, but the listener is unsure and, because of the problems in trying to correct the error situation, is content to deduce an answer and let the error go. Thus, the child's error is reinforced and will surely be perpetuated.

One is never really sure what the hearing-impaired child is thinking because of difficulties in communication. Consider this example relayed to us by a teacher of the deaf. In her classroom of hard of hearing preschoolers, when some object would drop accidentally on the floor with a loud noise, the concept was conveyed to the children by the teacher who quickly held her hands over her ears and showed exaggerated facial expression of disdain. The children could see the situation cleary and quickly followed example with similar behavior each time an object was dropped. A few days later following this lesson, a pencil was dropped on a soft carpet accidentally. As expected, the preschoolers clapped their hands over their ears and made exaggerated faces! To what were they reacting? Surely not "noise" as the teacher thought she was teaching a few days previously. And so every concept must be carefully considered by the deaf educator from the eyes and mind of the hearing-impaired child.

Today the problems of teaching the deaf are further complicated by the fact that a greater proportion of our deaf young people were born deaf, or were deafened before the acquisition of language than was the case 25 years ago. In fact, today, with medical achievements creating more control over the various etiologies of deafness, the communication dilemma is even more of a problem, for there are fewer adventitiously deaf children who might have some language acquisition prior to their deafness, entering our deaf education programs. Today's hearing-impaired child is usually congenitally deaf, and exhibits many more difficulties and frustration in meeting language needs and speech skills than his predecessor who may have lost his hearing after the critical language age of 2 years. Further, many of today's deaf children, if born 20 years ago, might not have lived to enter school. Today they live, often exhibiting multiple handicaps and creating very special problems for the educator of the deaf to solve. Northcott (1981) indicates that 91% of all hearing-impaired children have two normal hearing parents, 6% have one normal hearing parent, while 3% have two deaf parents.

Kohl (1966) expressed a different view concerning the problem of education for deaf youngsters. He noted that the deaf child, who most of the time has two hearing parents, experiences rejection through dislike, pity, and misunderstanding from the hearing world as soon as his deafness is discovered. It is thus not surprising that the deaf children of deaf parents seem to be much happier and better adjusted than deaf children who have hearing parents. Kohl believed that most deaf children thus have social problems which complicate their language disability. Accordingly, the frustrated deaf child is noted to show outbursts of anger and rage which accompany him throughtout his school years. In schools for the hearing-impaired run by hearing teachers, the deaf children may develop strong emotional ties and loyalties to each other which prepare them to enter an exclusive and excluded community of the deaf as adults (Northern et al., 1971). An excellent review of the psychosocial problems of deaf children and their families was published by Malkin et al. (1976).

McClure (1973) believes the problem is not so much the development of better teachers and of greater skills, although these are desirable, as to put into effect that which we already know. The deaf child learns primarily through vision, so we must make the imperceptible become perceptible. When we instill in deaf children the desire to communicate and provide the necessary language skills to do so, teaching speech will become a far easier task.

Ling (1975) reviewed the numerous advances made during the past few years. He cites progress in new approaches to language acquisition; new emphasis on early detection, diagnosis, and treatment during infancy; the more systematic use of improved hearing aids; development of a variety of educational services leading to placement within regular schools; and new subject teaching techniques, as positive signs in the area of education of deaf children. Ling feels, however, that we continue to have a severe shortage of qualified personnel working with hearing-handicapped children who can utilize these progressive advances in their teaching programs.

THE METHODOLOGIES

Many claims have been made for success of education of the deaf. Most of the claims, however, are from teachers of the deaf who have a personal belief in their own teaching techniques. Most claims, furthermore, are mere testimonials supported by a demonstration from one or two deaf children who have performed exceedingly well under the advocated, or advertised, method. Closer scrutiny seldom turns up any objective scientific evidence to support the proposed case. Few new systems withstand the test of time. In this section we will limit our discussion to the oral, manual, and total communications philosophies of deaf education and a few of the most significant variations of these three major categories. Although virtually volumes of material have been written on the methodologies in education of the deaf, we can provide only a basic, and necessarily shallow, synopsis in these pages.

The Aural/Verbal Method

Essentially three methods of oral education for deaf children are in use in the United States today. The traditional approach is to use them in the order described below. If the first method does not seem to do the job, then the second approach is attempted, and finally the third method is utilized. All three oral methods have the commonality that they essentially depend on training lipreading and audition and wholly exclude the use of any natural signs or gestures. The greatest appeal of the oral methodology is to hearing parents of deaf children, since the main aim of the system is to make the deaf youngster a part of the hearing society through good speech and lipreading.

Silverman and Lane (1970) report that 85% of children enrolled in schools for the deaf are instructed by the oral method, at least in their early years. The fundamental assumption of the oralists is that every deaf child should be given an opportunity to communicate by speech. They prefer that children taught by the oral method not be mixed with manually communicating children, even in living dormitories, because these oral "speaking" children must adjust to the child who cannot talk, and thus valuable practice in oral communication is lost. Advocates of this method indicate that an employer is more inclined to hire a deaf person to whom he can give oral instructions over an equally capable deaf person to whom he must communicate in gestures and writing. Proponents of this approach feel that orally trained children do very well in life and that training in speech and lipreading permits an earlier adjustment to a world in which speech is the chief means of communication.

According to McConnell and Liff (1975) children who become good listeners also use vision as necessary to become good lipreaders. Since the two events do not happen simultaneously, it is necessary to establish the acoustic channel as the primary input channel if all possible. The use of the visual channel then seems to come naturally as needed. Conversely, if the visual channel is established first as the main source of the child's perceptions and information, the use of hearing does not come naturally, but only laboriously and slowly and with much intensive training.

The first and primary oral method may be termed *pure oralism* or *auditory stimulation*. It developed in America at the Clarke School for the Deaf during the late 19th century. All sign language is discouraged, and the child is exposed to sounds and spoken language at every opportunity. He is fitted with hearing aids and every excuse for auditory stimulation is utilized. In theory, the deaf youngster is to "hear" everything that a youngster with normal hearing might be exposed to, only the auditory stimulation must be conducted with more deliberate action and intensity than usual circumstances might dictate. The method starts with visual attention to lipreading and includes isolated sound elements, sound combinations, words, and fi-

nally, speech. Much of the work is done at home, and if a nearby preschool for the hearing handicapped is not available, a home-study course is offered by the John Tracy Clinic in Los Angeles.

When auditory stimulation alone or lipreading is not sufficient to initiate satisfactory speech and language development, the second oral method known as the *multisensory/syllable unit method* is called into use. It is essentially the same as the pure oral procedure with lipreading, except that reading and writing of orthographic forms of English are included. Sight and touch are utilized as well as sound. This system is probably the most widely used oral method.

Everything in the deaf child's environment is labeled and his attention is drawn to the relation between the written form and the object, as well as the relation between the written form and the spoken word. The teacher may use the motokinesthetic approach to learning speech, where the child mimics speech production by feeling the teacher's face and reproducing the same breathing and vibration effects.

The third oral method is called the *language association-element method* or *"natural language" method*. It was proposed and developed by the long time principal of the Lexington School for the Deaf in New York City, Mildred Groht, who felt that the deaf child should learn to speak through activity (Groht, 1958; Hart, 1964). This type of program is developed around activities, and teachers continually talk to the deaf children and encourage them to ask questions with speech. Activities are supplemented with specialized instruction in lipreading and speech.

At times it is difficult to separate these aural/verbal education approaches and some electric programs choose to utilize the best from all three methods. It would seem that the children who do best in such programs are those with good residual hearing and good listening skills.

Opponents of the aural/verbal methods cite several objections to the approach. In general, their complaints are against lip-reading itself, and the fact that the oral method depends too heavily on lipreading as the primary mode of reception. Lipreading is too ambiguous because (a) many sounds and words look alike on the lips (homophenous words such as mat, pan and bat); (b) too many sounds are not visible because they are made in the back of the throat such as k, g, ng; and (c) too many people do not speak clearly and distinctly and speaking styles vary tremendously.

Opponents state that lipreading is an art mastered by very few—regardless of the motivation or training involved. Those who have the talent may do very well and serve as demonstration students. The opponents claim the majority of orally trained deaf pupils never master lipreading. It depends on acute vision, good lighting, and exposure of the lips and is extremely limited by distance between speakers. Lipreading is useless in dimly lit environments, within groups of talkers, or for speaker-audience formats.

Lipreading provides an inadequate means for the deaf child to monitor his own language. What is more frustrating than two aural/verbal deaf pupils, both encumbered by language disabilities and speech articulation errors, attempting to lip read each other? The intense concentration required for lipreading may place too much emotional stress on the child's personality and may produce inordinate anxieties.

Arguments against the oral multisensory approaches have been summarized by Stewart et al. (1964). They state that children cannot effectively handle several simultaneous sensory stimuli at the same time. They cite previous reports that use of a combined multisensory system may actually reduce the efficiency of performance, and that success in such methods demands that all sensory systems operate in a normal manner and that one sensory input system is not always the same as other sensory input systems in deaf children.

A well-recognized variant of the oral method is the so-called "unisensory" or "aural approach" to education of the deaf (Pollack, 1970; Rupp, 1971). Rupp cites the features of an auditory emphasis program as (a) audition is the most suitable perceptual modality by which a child learns speech and language, (b) it develops the impaired hearing modality to its fullest by focusing attention on audition, (c) the unisensory approach has applicability to the very young child, and (d) normalcy of environmental contacts at all levels is necessary for success of the method. The unisensory approach is dependent on very early identification, early parental guidance, early amplification, and total exposure to normal language stimulation.

The unisensory approach to deaf education has numerous advocates, and is practiced throughout the United States. Pollack (1971) states that much is to be gained from a unisensory, or acoupedic, approach for a child whose major deficit is congenital hearing loss. She feels that the youngster becomes more fully responsive to his environment, has a more natural voice quality with fluent speech, learns language more easily and naturally, and becomes a better lipreader. The stated goal of the acoupedic approach is the successful integration of children with hearing impairment into a hearing world. Pollack (1982) recently published a most informative "how to" article dealing with early amplification and auditory/verbal training of hearing-impaired infants.

Temporal bone studies from children with profound deafness have been reported with total absence of the cochlear structures or eighth nerve tissue. Any sort of hearing in such a child is absolutely impossible. Amplification can provide no benefit except possible tactual cues. Such a child is not a good candidate for the auditory/verbal method (Fig. 9.1).

Eric Greenway, the well known British educator of the deaf, has indicted oralism:

... for almost a century we have witnessed the great oral experiment ... In theory it is ideal

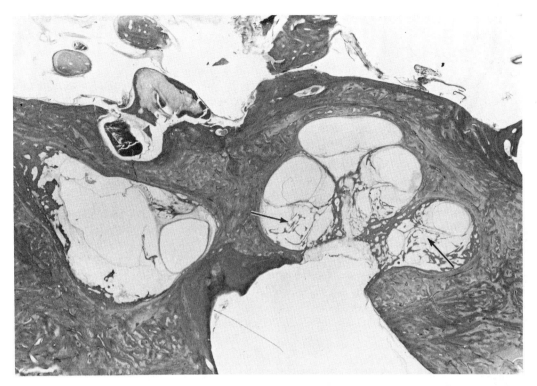

Figure 9.1. Midmodiolar section from the temporal bone of a patient whose deafness was caused by meningitis. Note the partial ossification that has taken place in the scala vestibuli portion of the cochlea (*arrows*), and the lack of eighth nerve fibers and spiral ganglia. This patient had no measurable hearing. The absence of essential sensory and neural structures makes amplification with a hearing aid useless. (Courtesy of I. Sando, M.D., University of Colorado Medical Center.)

and there are essential virtues in its principles. In many respects it has been a courageous attempt to bring the deaf into the world of the hearing by simulation of the normal means of communication. But an honest appraisal of the results shows plainly that it has not met with the overall success that teachers hope for or that the deaf themselves desire and demand . . . It cannot be denied that there have been some outstanding successes with an exclusive oral system, but for the majority it fails because it is unable to provide the fullest and most congenial means of communication. (From E. B. Greenway: The communication needs of the deaf child. In *Report of the Proceedings of the International Congress on the Education of the Deaf*, pp. 433–439. Washington, D.C., Gallaudet College, 1964.)

Luterman (1976) evaluated language skills in 49 hearing-impaired children. Of these, 27 had received visual/oral treatment and 22 received auditory/verbal treatment. Illinois Test of Psycholinguistic

Abilities and Northwestern Syntax Screening Test (NSST) testing showed no difference between the two groups, despite a 2-year advantage for the visually/orally trained children. Thirty-six percent of the auditory/verbal group were totally integrated as compared to less than 10% of those with the visual/oral approach. These results suggest an educational advantage in the auditory/approach compared to the more traditional visual/oral approach.

However, a classic study initiated at the University of Minnesota in 1969 and terminated in 1975 suggests other conclusions (Weiss et al., 1975). The children in seven well-known programs for the deaf and hard of hearing were studied intensively during these years. The programs provided a diverse representation of approaches to deaf education, ranging from auditory/verbal to visual/oral. One of the findings regarding children who were integrated into mainstream education was that these children had had better hearing acuity and superior articulation prior to integration. It seemed conclusively evident that children do not speak better because of integration, but are integrated because they speak better.

Other measures in the 6-year Minnesota study compared relative communication efficiency between modes of training. Children were found to receive communication most efficiently when stimuli were presented simultaneously through speech and signs. Next were simultaneous speech and fingerspelling, followed by speechreading and sound. The least efficient means was sound alone. In the area of expressive speech, the better articulation scores were made by the better hearing students. The type of training seemed not to affect articulation scores; rather, skill in articulation related purely to the emphasis on auditory training and articulation given by a program.

The Visual/Oral Methods

It is said by many, including the vast majority of deaf adults, that the sign language is the common, natural language of the deaf. The signs have concrete meanings. Words can be spelled on the fingers to connect the signs into sentences. According to Ridgeway (1969), "... the sign language with deaf children is part mime; it is beautiful to watch, highly expressive and receptive."

Education of the deaf has not always been dominated by the oral methods. Some 100 years earlier than the advent of the oral method, L'Abbé de L'Epée, a French priest, undertook the education of two deaf sisters in the year 1750. Fingerspelling had been used earlier to teach language to the deaf in France, but to it L'Epée added a "natural language of gestures." He established a school to teach the deaf in Paris in 1860, and was later succeeded by his equally famous pupil, L'Abbé Sicard.

In 1815 an American named Thomas Hopkins Gallaudet, a minister from Hart-

ford, Connecticut, met a young deaf neighbor girl, Alice Cogswell. Gallaudet was deeply taken by Alice's plight of mutism and the fact that she had no place to go to school. He sought support from families of other deaf children and ultimately went to Europe to study methods of teaching the deaf. He visited London and was refused access to Watson's Asylum, where secret and expensive educational methods were jealously guarded. However, he met L'Abbé Sicard and was invited to Paris to learn L'Epée's system of sign language. From this warm welcome in France, he returned to America with a young deaf teacher, Laurent Clerc, and established the first school for the deaf in the United States in 1817, the American School for the Deaf in Hartford. The school was replicated throughout the United States, and L'Epée's sign language was fused with the natural gestures used in America and became the basis for our present day sign language (Stokoe, 1960).

Years later, Thomas Hopkins Gallaudet, enjoying the success of establishing schools for the deaf across the United States was still not satisfied. As an old man he passed his vision of visions onto his son, Edward Miner Gallaudet, and his dream was realized with the establishment of Gallaudet College in 1864, the world's first college for the deaf, in Washington, D.C. The last decade has seen the establishment of the National Technical Institute for the Deaf associated with Rochester Institute of Technology in New York as a second college program for the deaf—more than 100 years following the dedication of Gallaudet College.

The language of signs has been subjected to systematic analysis by several investigators including Stokoe (1960), Tervoort (1964), and Bornstein (1973, 1978, 1979). Their conclusion is that sign language is an independent language that is neither a translation of oral language nor a poor imitation of it. Natural gestures and fingerspelling depend on situational understanding; when a sign has a tendency to become repeated and understood by more than one person the sign is "formalized" and no longer a natural gesture. The manual alphabet and samples of sign language from David Watson's fine book *Talk with Your Hands* (1964), are shown in Figures 9.2 and 9.3.

Louie Fant, one of the finest interpreters for the deaf in the United States, and author of the book, *Say It with Hands* (1964), points out the importance of facial expression as one communicates with the sign language. The face, in fact, carries most of the meaning and many of the subtleties needed to enrich the communication. The limitations of sign language are also recognized and acknowledged by the experts. It is limited in scope and expressive power when compared to oral language. The sign language is bound to the concrete, and limited in expression of abstractions, metaphor, irony, and humor.

The standardization of American Sign Language, or "Ameslan," has been enhanced by two important developments: the valuable contribution of Stokoe's *Dictionary of American Sign Language* and second, the establishment of a National Registry of Interpreters for the Deaf (RID), with three levels of certification according to interpreting skill based on standardized tests administered by expert hearing and deaf interpreters.

The argument of the manualists is a relative one. They define the role of an educational program as that of providing an education to the deaf child which is equitable to the education of a hearing child. The manualist questions the implementation of speech and lipreading into the curriculum to the diminution of the three R's. He differentiates between language skills and speech/lipreading and submits that language skills are paramount to speech both educationally and socially.

Garretson (1963), a respected deaf educator and long time advocate of the use of fingerspelling and signs in spite of the fact that he was brought up in the oral tradition, cites the following factors as assets for the manual method:

1. Denying a child the right to use his hands along with speech and lipreading creates anxiety and emotional stress on the pupil.

2. With the use of fingerspelling, signs, and speech, there is no doubt as to what is being communicated.

3. Signs on the hands are considerably larger and clearer than lip movements.

4. Fingerspelling and signs do not discriminate against anyone and all have equal opportunity to participate and learn from classroom activities.

Garretson concluded that during the last 75 years of education of the deaf, signs and fingerspelling had never been made compulsory for the student, while speech- and lipreading are usually taught in special sessions in schools for the deaf. The fact that the manual system has persisted among deaf adults, and is the preferred method of communication by the majority of the deaf, speak for the value of the manual system.

Mention should be made of two early variants of the manual system known as the combined method and the simultaneous method. The combined method utilizes speech, speechreading, hearing aids, and fingerspelling. The simultaneous method is essentially the same as the combined method with the addition of the language of signs.

One of the major drawbacks to Ameslan is that its syntax is not conducive to the development of acceptable English. With the Ameslan system it is difficult to express pronouns; verb tense is indicated by context; signs follow each other according to convenience and not necessarily accepted English order; and what is acceptable for communication is the *general concept*, not the *specific intent*. Proponents of the oral methods use this syntax problem as a major objection to manualism.

The Rochester Method

The New York state deaf residential school staff questioned the educational validity of signed English. They noted that deaf children, who had been taught in the oral method during elementary school years and then introduced to Ameslan still were

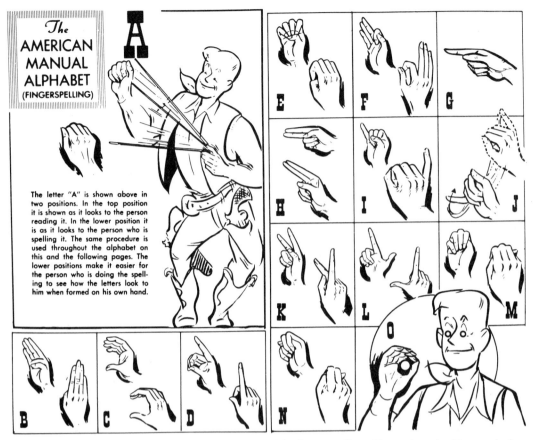

Figure 9.2. The American manual alphabet used in fingerspelling. (Reproduced with permission from D. O. Watson: *Talk with Your Hands*. Winneconne, Wis., 1964, © 1963.)

not acquiring educationally acceptable English. There arose subsequently the Rochester method which is the simultaneous use of speech and fingerspelling—a sort of "writing in air" technique superimposed on normal speech (Scouten, 1964). This technique is also known as "visible speech" because the teacher is able to face the class and synchronize what is said and shown on the lips with a more visible form of English as spelled on the hands.

The more visible approach of the Rochester method is the best supplement to an otherwise oral method because it is a pure, visible, English medium. It represents a multisensory visible oral-plus approach to language development. This method is said to continuously emphasize the traditional oral approach, supplemented by simultaneous and very visible fingerspelling.

Total Communication

Comparatively recently, in terms of deaf education tradition, a philosophy termed total communication has arisen. The proponents of total communication recognized the educational advantages of visible speech, yet they also noted certain difficulties. The manual dexterity of the preschool child limits his ability to fingerspell quickly, and his limited attention span makes it difficult to attend intensely on "flying fingers and fleeting flexible faces" for an all day instruction session.

The Conference of Executives of American Schools for the Deaf agreed upon a definition of total communication: total communication is a philosophy requiring the incorporation of appropriate aural, manual, and oral modes of communication

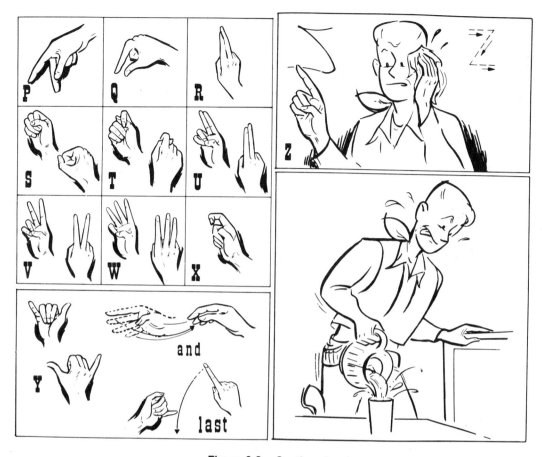

Figure 9.2—*Continued*

in order to ensure effective communication with and among hearing-impaired persons (Brill, 1976).

Total communication, as it is stressed by its advocates, is a *philosophy* and not simply another method for teaching deaf children. The basic premise is to use every and all means to communicate with deaf children from infancy to school age. No particular method or system is to be omitted or stressed. The student is exposed to natural gestures, Ameslan, fingerspelling, facial expression, body English, all accompanied simultaneously with speech heard through hearing aids. The idea is to use any means that works to convey vocabulary, language, and idea concepts between the deaf child and everyone to whom he is exposed. The important concept is to provide an easy, free, two-way communication means be-

tween the deaf child and his family, teacher, and schoolmates. In some environments and educational facilities, total communication is practiced continually with all pupils throughout their school years.

The concept of total communication appealed very quickly to the manually oriented observers, since it really involves little in terms of compromise on their part.

Opponents of total communication complain that if a teacher of the deaf really favors one method over another, the teacher will unwittingly move the students in the direction of that approach under the guise of teaching total communication. Some educators believe that it is not possible to evaluate the effectiveness of any one approach while using all the approaches at the same time. These arguments, however, seem to miss the main

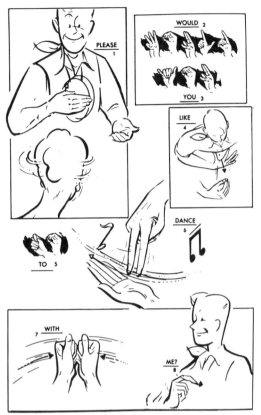

Figure 9.3. Signs and fingerspelling used in the sentence, "Please, would you like to dance with me?" (Reproduced with permission from D. O. Watson: *Talk with Your Hands*. Winneconne, Wis., 1964, © 1963.)

concept of total communication which says that it is paramount to communicate without regard for which "method" is really doing it. The total communication approach has been criticized because it is too much of a shotgun approach to education of the deaf. Critics argue that the overstimulation of the deaf child is actually detrimental to communication.

For years, the approach to deaf education was to start all children in an oral-type program for their early years of school. At some point in time, second or third grade or age 7 or 8, the child would be evaluated with regard to his educational progress and the oral method. If he was doing well, he would be continued in an orally oriented program. If he was not doing well he would

be transferred into a manually oriented class. For most children, this timing of selecting their educational method so long after the critical years of language and speech development makes education prognosis very poor. Total communication in the early years seems to be an important new concept in behalf of the deaf child, and should add years of head start toward his formal education. The concept of total communication has caught on and spread quickly in the United States. The progress, thus far, is encouraging and the change in attitude from stressing a particular "method" to overall concern for the deaf child's needs to be immersed in two-way communication, may turn out to be the most significant change in deaf education for over 100 years.

The dynamic change in methods of educating deaf children is dramatically brought to light in a survey reported by Jordan et al. (1976). Responses to questionnaires were received from 43% of 796 programs. Of the 343 programs, 302 indicated that they had changed from the oral/aural method. Some 333 programs reported that they changed their educational methods to total communication.

Deafness Management Quotient (DMQ)

Downs (1974) proposed a Deafness Management Quotient (DMQ) formula to predict whether a hearing-impaired child could be successful in an oral educational program or whether he required the supplementary visual information of a total communication program. The proposed formula consists of weighted scales which take into account many aspects of the child and his environment. Table 9.1 shows the DMQ, weighted on a 100-point scale, with a suggested score of 81 or better to qualify for an auditory/verbal program.

Luterman and Chasin (1981) applied the DMQ to 31 severely hearing-impaired children who had attended a preschool nursery program and were now 6–13 years of age. They reported that those children with high

Table 9.1.
Suggested Scale for Deafness Management Quotient (DMQ)—Total: 100 Points

Residual hearing: 30 points possible
    0 = no true hearing
    10 = 250–500 < 100 dB   Add 10 points for conductive ele-
    20 = 250–500–1000 < 100 dB   ment to hearing loss
    30 = 2000 < 100 dB

Central intactness: 30 points possible
    0 = diagnosis of brain damage
    10 = known history of events conducive to birth defects
    20 = perceptual dysfunction
    30 = intact central processing

Intellectual factors: 20 points possible
    0 = MR < 85 IQ
    10 = average   85–100 IQ
    20 = above average: >100 IQ

Family constellation: 10 points possible
    0 = no support
    10 = completely supportive and understanding

Socioeconomic: 10 points possible
    0 = substandard
    10 = competely adequate

Auditory program leading to oral: 81–100 points

Total communicative program: 0–80 points

DMQs were found to be in mainstreamed classes while those children with low DMQs were indeed in total communication programs. The children with high DMQ scores were deemed superior in their use of hearing, language and speech, and were more oral. Luterman and Chasin stated that the DMQ is a viable sorting device for distinguishing auditory/verbal children from those requiring total communication. They suggested the addition of a measure of the child's use and acceptance of amplification as being more important than the pure tone average.

CURRENT SIGN SYSTEMS

During the past few years, several manual sign systems have been developed as improvements to Ameslan since their design is such that they represent English. It is too early to judge the merits or impact of these new sign systems on the deaf consumer and user, but their presence is certainly creating attention and controversy. The new systems are described here to orient readers to the basic philosophies, approaches, nomenclature, and differences, since these approaches have been developed to overcome apparent inadequacies of the American Sign Language or Ameslan. Excellent materials regarding these current sign systems have been published by Bornstein (1973, 1978, 1979). The new systems have as their premise that Ameslan, with linguistically generated variations, can be the visual equivalent of spoken English. Furthermore, they share the idea that if this type of system is introduced to the deaf child at a very early age, the language skills, total experiences, mental health, and communicative abilities will be improved over our traditional approaches.

The new sign systems discussed below have several principles in common as described by Cokely and Gawlik (1973). The basic premise is that deaf children need a visual symbol system to develop their language competency to its fullest potential. They assume that the more syntactically correct the symbols, the more it will aid in development of language in the deaf child. Apparently, all argue that although the American Sign Language is an adequate communication tool, its syntax is such that it is not necessarily related to the grammatical structure of English. And finally, with exception of "cued speech," each believes that a visual symbol system can be developed to incorporate basic Ameslan signs with modifications that encourage the use of meaning through context that is consistent with the form of spoken English.

The new sign systems are in a state of flux and transition. Incongruities and contradictions may be seen within the systems. To judge the systems today would be imprudent and unfair, and decisions, as of yet with few data, must be based on personal intuition. The advent of the systems reflects dissatisfaction with the American Sign Language as a basic languge instructional tool. Final judgment must be reserved until the results can be examined objectively.

Cued Speech

Cued speech is a method of communication developed by R. Orin Cornett for the hard-of-hearing in which 8 hand configurations and 4 hand placements are used to supplement the visible manifestations of natural speech. Cued speech was hailed in 1967 as a possible answer to the oralism versus manualism controversy. The 12 cues described above are used around the chin, cheek, and neck, drawing attention to the speaker's face and lips. The cued speech system provides a visable phonetic analog of speech in the form of lip movements supplemented by hand cues with both vowel and consonant cues (Cornett, 1967, 1975).

According to Cornett (1975) most users of the auditory-only and multisensory approaches do not introduce the written language until there is sufficient foundation in the basic oral skills to permit mutually supportive use of oral communication and written language. He feels that cued speech offers specific advantages for supportive use in oral programs. The greatest advantage of cued speech is that it facilitates the acquisition of the vocabulary and the syllabic-phonemic-rhythmic patterns of the spoken language without interrupting the natural process of communication to interpolate the written form.

Cornett argues that another advantage to cued speech is that it meets the objections of total communication and other manual-language advocates, that early communication through exclusively oral methods is insufficient to meet the psychosocial needs of the child. Cued speech forces the use of information on the lips by the hearing-impaired child without subjecting him to the confusion of lipreading. And, finally, Cornett states that cued speech is self-limiting in that the child with speech does not use cues to hearing persons, and that he ignores the cues he does not need.

Actually, the cues are not intelligible without proper mouth motions. Because "cueing" is completely dependent upon spoken language and lipreading, it satisfies the oralist's demand that emphasis be placed on learning to communicate with those who do not know sign language (Miles, 1967). It reportedly takes about 30 hours for a hearing person to achieve fairly fluent use of cued speech, but critics of the system complain that the cued speech system is too complex for easy learning. Cued speech has been under widespread evaluation in several institutions, but results of data gathering are inconclusive at this time.

Seeing Essential English (SEE₁)

This sign system, originated by David Anthony in 1962, and developed in Southern California, uses modifications of Ameslan to resemble English. SEE₁ is intended for use by all age groups, and now has as its basis an impressive two-volume manual which includes an introduction to the system, how it is used, grammar and syntax guidelines, and over 5000 vocabulary entries (Anthony et al., 1971). The SEE₁ system has the largest vocabulary of any of the new systems.

SEE₁ signs represent word forms or word parts such as roots, prefixes, or suffixes. The signs are used in combinations to form any desired word. To reflect English syntax, SEE₁ emphasizes complete English word order. Verb tense is clearly indicated and irregular verb forms have signed representation. In general terms, English words are represented by the traditional American sign word plus a suffix and/or prefix. English compound words are often made up of elements different from the single sign element often used in Ameslan. As a result, SEE₁ words often do not closely resemble the original source sign in Ameslan. SEE₁ is similar enough to Ameslan that American Sign Language users can almost read it in context, but may not be able to identify specific SEE₁ signs without previous exposure or explanation.

Signing Exact English (SEE₂)

This sign system was developed in 1972 by a group of former members of the Seeing Essential English group, headed by Dr. Gerilee Gustasan. It is perhaps unfortunate that the new group did not select another name for their system that did not mimic Anthony's SEE system. Cokely and Gawlik (1973) use the notations, SEE₁ and SEE₂ to differentiate the two systems. According to Bornstein (1973), the reasons leading to the development of Signing Exact English is that SEE₁ utilized too many signs that were too distant from Ameslan, was too radical in its use of the root word, and too complex for the needs of parents and teachers. Accordingly, SEE₂ uses signs which represent words rather than roots, as well as basic affixes as needed. Signing Exact English has a vocabulary of some 2800 words published in booklet form.

Signing Exact English is also intended to be used by young children. It is readily apparent, then, that a situation can develop whereby parents and children who interact with persons trained in another system will use different signs for the same word. According to calculations reported in Bornstein (1973), 61% of the SEE₂ vocabulary is based on traditional Ameslan signs, 18% modified Ameslan signs, and 21% entirely new signs. When SEE₂ signs were compared with SEE₁ signs, some 80% of the traditional sign group were identical in both systems. Bornstein concludes that difficulties created by these sign word differences are relatively minor.

The Verbo-tonal Method

In about 1952, Professor Petar Guberina from the University of Zagreb, Yugoslavia, began developing a method to improve foreign language teaching through emphasis on the spoken rhythm of the language to be learned. He later applied his theory and methods to teaching deaf children and adults—still with emphasis on the rhythm of spoken language and on speech perception and production as an interacting loop system.

According to Craig and Craig (1972), the verbo-tonal approach is characterized by (a) emphasis on low frequencies (below 500 Hz) and on vibratory clues in perception of spoken language patterns; (b) matching of special amplification devices known as SUVAG to the deaf person's optimum "field of hearing"; (c) use of body movements to assist both in production and perception of speech; (d) emphasis on acoustic memory for language patterns aided by body movements and by articulatory movements from the production of speech; (e) providing speech and language work in active "play" type situations, so that much longer periods of concentrated work on spoken language are possible; and (f) emphasis on language in meaningful context of "situations."

Guberina's concept is based on his theory that the low frequencies of spoken language do not mask the high spoken frequencies. He believes that amplifications of auditory clues, below 500 Hz, to include rhythmic patterns and the sound fundamentals, can actually help the deaf person to perceive the higher speech frequencies. In an additional effort to reach the low frequency residual hearing of profoundly deaf children, the verbo-tonal approach includes the use of vibrators, or bone oscillators, to provide vibratory cues in the perception of language rhythms and sound patterns. Body movements are an important part of the technique and lipreading is taught only incidentally. In the United States the verbo-tonal technique has been under development by Carl Asp and his associates at the University of Tennessee since 1967.

The goal of verbo-tonal therapy is to help hearing-impaired children develop good oral communication skills which will allow them to freely interact with normal-hearing people. A review of a number of studies of international verbo-tonal programs summarized by Guberina and Asp (1981) concludes that these programs have been "extremely successful in integrating the deaf children who begin therapy at 2 or 3 years of age . . . and that these children can continue in therapy beyond the first grade suggest that the children who are integrated are not the exception—they are the rule."

Signed English (Siglish)

This system uses 2500 words to aid the language development of the preschool child. Some 1700 of these signs can be represented by existing Ameslan signs. Siglish was developed by Bornstein and his associates at Gallaudet College (Kannapell et al., 1969). Signed English substitutes American Sign Language words for English words without changing the English syntax structure. Signed English is intended to be an educational tool to facilitate the learning of English, and not a substitute for American Sign Language.

Bornstein et al. (1980) and Bornstein and Saulnier (1981) report results of an initial evaluation of Signed English. They studied 20 hearing-impaired children over a 4-year period. During this period of time, the childrens' receptive vocabulary grew at a rate

43% of that manifested by normal-hearing children. The vocabulary level of these children at age 8 was similar to that reported for comparable hearing-impaired children at age 11 taught by other methods. Although no syntax development was noted until after the first year of the program, syntax then developed at a steady, and seemingly, accelerating rate in subsequent years.

Complex English words are represented by natural Ameslan words in whatever form they exist. The authors of this technique indicate in Bornstein (1973) that they are not convinced that an altered form of the sign word actually facilitates learning of the English word form.

Signed English incorporates some 14 sign markers used after the sign word to denote plurals, verb tense, possessive forms, gerunds, etc. In an interesting project, a number of children's classic stories such as "Goldilocks and the Three Bears" and "Little Red Riding Hood" (Bornstein et al., 1972) have been illustrated in color, with line drawings of sign words in Signed English form. Signed English has the unofficial endorsement of the National Association of the Deaf, and is used in many state residential schools for the deaf as well as at Gallaudet College.

MAINSTREAMING

Mainstreaming is one of the single most important issues in education of deaf children to appear in the last few decades. By formal definition, mainstreaming is "an educational programming option for handicapped youth which provides support to the handicapped student(s) and his teacher(s) while he pursues all or a majority of his education within a regular school program with nonhandicapped students." In short, mainstreaming is the current term for the practice that used to be known as "integration" of the hearing-impaired student into regular classrooms with hearing children. Mainstreaming is a procedure which is already well established in the United States and is the crest of a fast-moving wave in education circles. The real push for mainstreaming has been the stimulation provided by the "least restrictive" portion of the new federal law known as the Education for All Handicapped Children Act of 1975. Excellent materials on mainstreaming hearing-impaired youngsters have been published by Northcott (1979) and Hoversten and Fornby (1981).

The organization of educational programs for hearing-impaired students is undergoing considerable change in many states. The change is from serving only a few students, mainly in residential schools, toward serving many deaf students in local community programs with a system that provides a variety of educational opportunities to the hearing-handicapped child and his parents (Macklin, 1976). Northcott (1973) clearly stated, however, that partial or full-time integration for hearing-impaired students into regular classes is not a realistic goal for every child; nor is the policy of self-containment from kindergarten through grade 12 suitable for all hearing-impaired children. A recent survey reported by Craig et al. (1976) indicates that integrated programs are offered by 30% of residential schools, 65% of day schools and 73% of day classes. In this survey of 440 responding programs, some 7,500 deaf students, out of a possible number of 17,000 total deaf students in all schools responding to the questionnaire, are currently integrated with hearing students for some part of their instructional day.

As with every major issue in education of the deaf, controversy rages over the pros and cons of mainstreaming. Vernon and Prickett (1976) report that we have some 25 years of experience with integration of hearing-impaired students to provide us with much historical precident on *how not to* mainstream.

Bricker (1978) suggests that integration is a means of eliminating the deleterious effects of segregation and the stigma often attached to the "handicapped" student. Normal children are thus exposed to the handicapped child with positive and en-lightened responses toward the integrated person. Of course, it is also possible that a negative response to the integrated child, or handicapping condition, is also possible, with devastating results to the integrated child.

Birch (1976) indicates that mainstreaming deaf children is to be done only after thorough preparation, with sensitivity to the needs of all parties, and with careful monitoring and support. He states that degree and onset of hearing loss are not the primary factors in selecting children for mainstreaming. Regular classroom teachers are very accepting of hearing-impaired pupils, and are willing to design programs for complete or partial mainstreaming depending on the child's capabilities, requirements, and the school's resources. Birch concludes that the philosophy of mainstreaming has deep, strong roots. Mainstreaming has been tried for years, and its success is the reason for its continued survival and growth.

One of the key factors in successful mainstreaming is the guarantee that hearing-impaired students will not be "dumped and forgotten" into the regular classroom. This proviso is covered by the requirement in Public Law 94-142 for all handicapped children to receive personalized instruction and supportive services they need to benefit from an individualized educational plan, known as the IEP. The IEP is confirmation for hearing-impaired children that a more objective and scientific educational decision-making process will be followed. Withrow (1981) feels that with the use of IEPs, educators can no longer rely on biases and preconceived ideas of what is "best" for the hearing-impaired child.

The most outstanding description of a successful program of mainstreaming is known as the Holcomb Plan—which is a model plan being implemented in Newark, Delaware (Holcomb and Corbett, 1975). Total communication is used in every deaf school whenever possible. The deaf child is put into a class with hearing children only when a tutor-interpreter is available to translate everything said in the classroom into sign language and fingerspelling. The tutor-interpreter is a trained teacher of the deaf so that the teacher aide function is utilized constantly to help the hearing-impaired student. The tutor helps the deaf child to keep up with the rest of the class and grasp fully what is going on at all times. Acceptance of such a program in the regular school is enhanced by teaching all normal hearing students and classroom teachers elements of sign language and fingerspelling.

Special consideration must be given when hearing aids are worn by the hearing-impaired child mainstreamed into the regular classroom without regard for the acoustic characteristics of the normal school room. Poor signal-to-noise ratios produce detrimental effects on speech discrimination and understanding by the hearing-impaired student using amplification aids. A recent study of this problem in the Detroit metropolitan area indicated that hearing-impaired children with malfunctioning hearing aids studying in regular classrooms suffered a high scholastic failure rate (Robinson and Sterling, 1980). Mussen (1981) has prepared an excellent chapter to aid speech-language clinicians and teachers with one or more hearing-impaired children in their regular classrooms in special techniques to enhance listening and auditory training skills of the handicapped youngsters.

A thought-provoking essay questioning the quality of a mainstreamed education for prelingually deaf children was written recently by Brill (1975), a veteran of 25 years as the Superintendent of the California School for the Deaf in Riverside. He worries that we are in an era of simplistic solutions to complex programs. Until a few years ago many deaf children were postlingually deafened as a result of some childhood illness. However, today's deaf children are mostly *prelingually* deaf and present different educational problems.

Brill points out that the deaf child learns best when he is in a small class composed of children who are about the same age and educational level. It is likely that a limited geographical area will contain only a small number of deaf children of about the same age and educational level. Mainstreaming philosophy requiring the right to an education in the least restrictive or most typical school setting possible has held first, that every child is generally best placed in a regular classroom; secondly, that he is best placed in a special class by being provided special supportive services while still in his local school; and that only as a last resort should he be separated physically from all of the so-called typical children in his educational placement.

Brill concludes that the claimed integration of deaf children in a special class with the hearing children in a school is most frequently a token integration. The typical deaf child with a tremendous communication handicap is not best placed in a regular classroom. The teacher in the regular classroom does not have the competencies to meet the child's special needs. The prelingually deaf child is almost never appropriately placed in a regular classroom. The policy of placing the child with less severe hearing loss in integrated programs while the profoundly deaf child attends a specialized deaf school eliminates destructive conclusions or comparisons of academic or social achievements.

In view of the current social climate, mainstreaming is here to stay. In the midst of the wide appeal of the mainstreaming approach, there obviously exist grave concerns about the misplacement of deaf children. Ferguson et al. (1982) cautions that care must be excercised so that professionals and parents do not perceive mainstreaming as "the only way to go." These respected educators of the deaf feel that special schools, including residential schools, should remain a part of our educational system for hearing-handicapped children. Ling (1975) likens the deaf education controversy to cyclic sunspot activity. It has flared up on numerous occasions in the past and abates only when the protagonists realize that there is no one method or mixture of methods that can possibly meet all the needs of hearing-impaired children and their parents.

DEAFNESS AND VISUAL ACUITY

The concern for visual acuity in deaf children cannot be overemphasized. Given the importance of good vision to persons with hearing loss, the *American Annals of the Deaf* devoted a recent issue detailing the relationship between deafness and vision (Johnson and Caccamise, 1981). It was recommended that (a) an indepth ophthalmological examination be done routinely for every child with hearing loss, (b) reassessment of visual and auditory function be conducted periodically for all persons with severe-to-profound hearing losses, and (c) information be provided for hearing-impaired persons, parents and professionals concerning the importance of visual assessment and visual hygiene for persons with hearing loss.

Clinicians should be well acquainted with the symptoms of *retinitis pigmentosa* which are not uncommon in deaf individuals. Retinitis pigmentosa is generally characterized by an initial loss of night vision followed by loss of peripheral field vision. These symptoms are usually initially noted during the teenage years.

Retinitis pigmentosa is defined as a disorder associated with a group of diseases which are frequently hereditary, marked by progressive loss of retinal response (as elicited by the electroretinogram), retinal atrophy, attenuation of the retinal vessels, and clumping of the pigment, with contraction of the field of vision. Retinitis pigmentosa may be transmitted as a dominant, recessive, or X-linked trait.

The combination of retinitis pigmentosa and deafness is known as Usher's syndrome. Vernon (1969, 1976) noted that Usher's syndrome is currently the leading cause of deaf-blindness. The incidence of Usher's syndrome among the congenitally deaf is approximately 3–6%, while its occurrence in the general population is 3 per 100,000. The concern for identification of Usher's syndrome in the congenitally deaf child is very important, because the child will need extensive special education, counseling, social-emotional support and vocational consideration. Although most hearing loss associated with retinitis pigmentosa is severe-to-profound in degree, some moderate sensorineural hearing loss patients have been reported. The hearing loss may also be progressive, and may start at the same time as the visual degeneration.

Hicks and Hicks (1981) presented a five-stage program for dealing with deaf youngsters with symptoms of retinitis pigmentosa. Stage I is an *awareness period* between the ages of 6 and 12 years and consists of a comprehensive diagnosis and explanation of the disease to the child and parents. Stage II involves *general counseling*, including genetic counseling, educational and career planning. Stage III is the *general planning and community resource identification* stage during which the child is established with an appropriate resource agency which can assume primary responsibility for case management. By this period, the deaf patient has probably suffered considerable loss of vision. Stage IV consists of the *specific planning and adjustment counseling* stage, and deals with the middle adult years and stresses. And finally, Stage V, the *adjustment* stage, deals with the later adult years when the Usher's syndrome has rendered the deaf client a complete loss of usable vision. This is an extremely important article to acquaint the uninitiated with the real severity of this problem.

PARENT TRAINING

For perhaps too many years, attention of professionals has been devoted solely to the hard-of-hearing or deaf child, and little consideration has been given to the parents. We believe that the parents of the deaf child may be the key to one of the most significant factors in the deaf youngster's development. And fortunately, during the past few years, parent-oriented habilitation programs for children with hearing impairment have emerged. The importance of families of hearing-impaired children and the role they play in the development of the handicapped child is the subject of a monograph, well worth reading, prepared by Murphy (1979).

Horton (1975) summarized the objectives of parent training programs into five categories:

1. To teach parents to optimize the auditory environment for their child;

2. To teach parents how to talk with their child;

3. To teach parents strategies of behavior management;

4. To familiarize parents with the principles, stages and sequence of normal development, including language development, and apply this frame to reference in stimulating their child;

5. To supply affective support to aid parents in coping with their feelings about their child, and to reduce the stresses that a handicapped child places on the integrity of the family.

The major emphasis of parent training include emotional support for the parents by helping them recognize, realize, accept, and understand the implications of their child's hearing problem. This increased awareness should help reduce anxiety and worry often expressed by parents of handicapped children. Education for the parents is important so that they might fully understand the nature of their child's hearing loss with realistic ramifications of the educational future for their youngster. The parent is taught to understand child growth and development as well as the need for communication skills, social contact, and emotional expression. A clear reference source such as Caplan's *The First Twelve Months of Life* (1973) is especially valuable to parents. Parents must be involved in the choice of the communication system the family wishes to use with the hearing-handicapped child. The choice between communication systems is secondary to the desirability of the parents being in agreement, enthusiastic, and committed to the system

of their choice. Professionals can provide guidance, exposure, and background to the parents, but the final choice, should be made with full cooperation and agreement with the parents. Imposing the use of signs on parents who lack confidence in their ability to interact with the child is a common cause of failure. If the parents choose to use signs, the entire family must develop fluency with this means of communication.

Another project in parent training is to teach the parents how to utilize and adapt daily activities of the home as experiential teaching events for the preschool child. Hopefully, the result is a stimulating home environment for the hearing-impaired child, where auditory, speech, and language development is a daily, ongoing, and natural activity for the youngster. Some programs have a model home completely furnished and operational with kitchen, bathroom, bedroom, playroom, etc. The home is stocked with typical utensils and furnishings. Parents spend time with the parent-training supervisor to learn how to develop a repertoire of experiences and activities to stimulate interaction with their children. Video tape is used extensively to observe parent-child interaction with immediate feedback to the parents in order to increase their abilities with their children.

A number of practical publications are now available to help the professional deal with parents of hearing-impaired children, including Stewart (1978), Stream and Stream (1978), Luterman (1979), and Mitchell (1981). A good study course for parents is now available as a two-part guide—*Talk To Me* (Alpiner et al., 1977).

Major cities and most large clinic programs have parent-centered projects underway, and it would appear that the deaf child will be the ultimate beneficiary of support and education aimed at his parents during the initial stages of discovery of the hearing loss. Meadow and Trybus (1979), in a review of emotional problems of the deaf, report three family variables of importance to a deaf child's mental health: (a) degree of parental overprotectiveness, (b) development of unrealistic expectations for the child's progress, and (c) effectiveness of parent-child communication.

An important study which examined the attitudes and stress of hearing families with a profoundly deaf preschool child was recently published by Greenberg (1980). The author studied 28 families that were equally divided into those using oral and simultaneous communication, and then further divided these groups into subdivisions based on communicative ability (high vs. low). Mothers completed questionnaires and interviews on stress concerns, parent attitudes, and their child's developmental level. Results showed few differences between simultaneous and oral families. However, comparison of the four subgroups indicated that those with high competence simultaneous communication skills had more positive attitude and less stress than highly competent oral communication families. Simultaneous communication children received a higher estimated social age than the oral communication children. It is interesting to note that deaf children have often been characterized as low in social maturity and self-concept, impulsive, immature and egocentric. Studies such as that conducted by Greenberg would suggest the need for additional research on key variables in the deaf childs' life, such as the family, which undoubtedly have significant impact.

IN SUMMARY

Dr. Julia Davis (1981) of the University of Iowa recently discussed utilization of audition in the education of the hearing-impaired child. She describes the population of hearing-impaired children as "vastly heterogeneous," and correctly points out that the best use of the residual hearing in each child will require different procedures and emphasis. In summary, as Davis states, "...we really must stop arguing over whether children use the auditory system *alone* or in conjunction with visual or tactual information during educational endeavors. If the energy spent in futile attempts to convince each other of the supremacy of one educational method over another had been spent in devising ways to maximize reception through *all* modalities, including hearing, it is unlikely that the educational achievement levels of hearing-impaired children would be as low as they are today."

CONCLUSION

The field of preventive medicine gives us an analog: it has been said that "medicine is unique among the sciences in that it strives incessantly to defeat the object of its own invention." This object, of course, is disease—and there is a parallel in audiology. Since our beginnings in the mid-forties, we have measured, described, researched, cataloged, analyzed, and synthesized the entity of hearing loss exhaustively—and now, having defined it, we must busy ourselves with preventing the devastation of its effects on children. In such terms preventive audiology becomes a viable endeavor—a discipline devoted to preventing the effects of ear disease on the individual who suffers from it. Such prevention can only be accomplished by early detection of the condition and by proper provision for remedial therapy and education.

We must be patient and await fresh methods and occasions for research. We must be ready, too, to abandon a path which we have followed for a time, if it seems to be leading to no good end.

Sigmund Freud (1948)
Beyond the Pleasure Principle

We have measured, described, researched, cataloged, analyzed, and synthesized the entity of hearing loss. Now we must busy ourselves with the prevention of its devastating effects on children.

Jerry L. Northern
Marion P. Downs

Appendix of Hearing Disorders

A synopsis of various syndromes associated with congenital deafness is presented in this appendix of hearing disorders. The material is a summary of information we feel is pertinent to the clinician. The information is by no means intended to be exhaustive or even complete; our intent is to provide a concise, clear, and informative reference regarding special patients who have an inordinately high risk for impairment of their hearing. We recognize that children with symptoms that are variants from our generalized information about each disorder will be seen, and that readers will immediately wish to revise our summary. So be it; our intent is to provide only an orientation, or a guide, to clinicians who might come into contact with children who demonstrate these disorders and to instill a desire to learn more about the disease.

General References

Some students may wish to consult more general reference sources for detailed accounts of syndromes included in this section of the book, or to pursue information on syndromes not included in this Appendix. Such general references cover much more than individual articles, and may touch on many aspects of the disorders not covered in our necessarily scant summaries. Accordingly, such a list is given below which we have found immeasurably useful in our review of birth defects associated with hearing loss.

Bergsma D (ed): *Birth Defects Compendium*, ed 2. New York: Alan R. Liss, 1979.

Bess F: *Childhood Deafness: Causation, Assessment and Management*. New York: Grune & Stratton, 1977.

Black FO, Bergstrom I, Downs M, et al: *Congenital Deafness. A New Approach to Early Detection Through a High Risk Register*. Boulder, Colo.: University of Colorado Associated Press, 1971.

Ford FR: *Diseases of the Nervous System in Infancy, Childhood and Adolescence*, ed. 5. Springfield, Ill.: Charles C Thomas, 1966.

Fraser GR: *The Causes of Profound Deafness in Childhood*. Baltimore: Johns Hopkins University Press, 1976.

Gellis SS, Feingold M: *Atlas of Mental Retardation Syndromes*. Washington, D.C.: U.S. Dept. of HEW, 1968.

Gorlin RJ, Pindborg JJ: *Syndromes of Head and Neck*. New York: McGraw-Hill, 1964.

Hemenway WG, Bergstrom L: Symposium on congenital deafness. *Otolaryngol Clin North Am. 4:* 1971.

Jablonski S: *Illustrated Dictionary of Eponymic Syndromes and Diseases*. Philadelphia: W. B. Saunders, 1969.

Jaffe B (ed): *Hearing Loss in Children*. Baltimore: University Park Press, 1977.

Konigsmark BW, Gorlin RJ: *Genetic and Metabolic Deafness*. Philadelphia: W. B. Saunders, 1976.

Lindsay JR: Profound childhood deafness. *Ann Otol Rhinol Laryngol* (suppl 5) 82: 1973.

Siegel-Sadewitz V, Shprintzen R: The relationship of communication disorders to syndrome identification. *J Speech Hear Disord* 47:338, 1982.

Smith DW: *Recognizable Patterns of Human Malformation*. Philadelphia: W. B. Saunders, 1970.

Warkany J: *Congenital Malformations*. Chicago: Year Book, 1971.

Absence of the Tibia

(Robert's Syndrome)

Skeletal disorder; recessive trait; characterized by congenital absence of one or both tibias (lower legs) and shortened, malformed fibulas, and severe, congenital sensorineural hearing loss (Pashayan et al., 1971).

Achondroplasia

(Chondrodystrophia Fetalis)

A congenital skeletal anomaly characterized by slow growth of cartilage, retarded endochondrial ossification, and almost normal periosteal bone formation (Fig. A.1). As a result those affected are very short in stature with disproportionately short limbs, large heads with prominent foreheads, depressed nasal bridge, and "button" nose. Mentality is usually normal but retardation may appear secondary to hydrocephalus and increased cranial presssure. Deafness may be present. Respiratory, pulmonary, and other complications increase with age. Diagnosis may be suspected by clinical examination, but is confirmed by radiographic evaluation.

This is a hereditary dominant disorder; however, over 80% of cases are due to fresh mutation, both parents being normal. Incidence increases with increasing parental age.

Both conductive and/or sensorineural loss may be present. Middle ear anomalies include fusion of ossicles to surrounding bony structures as well as dense thick trabec-

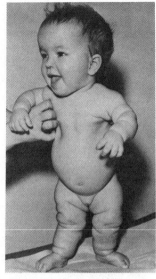

Figure A.1. Achondroplasia. (Reproduced with permission from T. H. Shepard and B. Graham: The congenitally malformed: achondroplastic dwarfism: diagnosis and management, *Northwest Medicine*, *66:* 451–456, 1967).

ulae without islands of cartilage in the endochondrial and periosteal bone. Associated anomalies of the inner ear include deformed cochlea and thickened intercochlear partitions. Incidence of serous otitis high.

General treatment consists of genetic counseling and surgical treatment as indicated (Cohen, 1967; Langer et al., 1967; Langer, 1968).

Acoustic Neuroma

(See Von Recklinghausen's Neurofibromatosis)

Acrocephalosyndactyly

(See Apert's Syndrome)

Albers-Schönberg Disease of Osteopetrosis

(Chalk Bone Disease; Ivory Bone Diseases; Marble Bone Disease)

Craniofacial and skeletal disorder; recessive form associated with deafness. Brittle, but paradoxically sclerotic thickened bones. Head may be somewhat enlarged; retarded growth in one third of cases. Visual loss noted in about 80% of cases which may lead to blindness. Mental retardation in 20% of cases, facial palsy, unilateral or bilateral in 10%. Little detailed audiometric data available, but 25–50% of patients are reported to have moderate, progressive sensorineural or conductive hearing loss (Johnston et al., 1968; Jones and Mulcahy, 1968; Myers and Stool, 1969).

Albinism with Blue Irides

(Oculocutaneous Albinism)

Integumentary and pigmentary disorder; dominant; scalp hair white, fine, and silky, sometimes with patches of pigmentation. Fair skin. Possible heterochromia of iris. Severe sensorineural congenital deafness (Tietz, 1963; Reed et al., 1967).

Alport's Syndrome

(Hereditary Nephritis with Nerve Deafness)

Renal disorder associated with deafness and ocular

anomalies. Characteristics include autosomal dominant inheritance with men more severely affected than women, progressive nephritis with uremia, ocular lens abnormalities such as cataracts, and progressive sensorineural hearing loss. Hearing loss occurs in 40–60% of cases; ocular defects in 15%. Hearing impairment is typically mild to severe, high frequency, usually bilaterally symmetrical, and may occur alone or in combination with the renal disease. Hearing loss is more frequent and tends to be more severe in men. Age of onset of hearing impairment is in preadolescence (Bergstrom et al., 1973; Rintelmann, 1976; Johnsson and Arenberg, 1981).

Amyloidosis, Nephritis, and Urticaria

(Muckle-Wells Syndrome)

Dominant. Onset in teens of recurrent uritcaria (vascular reaction of skin with elevated patches and itching) with malaise and chills with onset of recurrent limb and joint pain. Amyloidosis (starchy-like substance in the blood) precedes nephropathy and renal failure. Progression of hearing loss parallels progression of renal failure resulting in severe hearing impairment by third or fourth decade of life. Endocrine and metabolic disorder with progressive sensorineural hearing loss of late onset.

Apert's Syndrome

(Acrocephalosyndactyly)

Skeletal and associated skull malformations which include craniofacial dysostosis, syndactyly, brachiocephaly, hypertelorism, bilateral proptosis, saddle nose, high arched palate, ankylosis of joints, and spinal bifida and mental retardation (Figs. A.2 and A.3). Syndactyly (fusion of fingers and toes) is complete on both hands and feet. Hearing loss

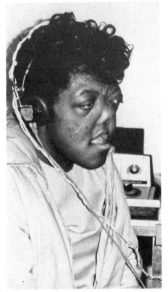

Figure A.2. Apert's syndrome.

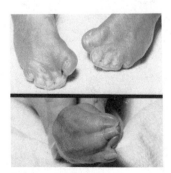

Figure A.3. Apert's syndrome.

common. Characteristic "tower skull," with flat forehead.

Most reported cases appear sporadic. When reproduction is possible, the disorder is apparently of autosomal dominant transmission. There also appears to be a high mutation rate related to increasing parent age. Manifestation present at birth. Risk of occurrence is 1 in 160,000.

Audiometric findings usually show flat conductive loss. However, a sensorineural component is suspected in some cases. Surgical explorations have revealed congenital stapedial footplate fixation, abnormal patency of cochlear aqueduct, and enlarged internal auditory meati. Impedance audiometry shows manifestations of conductive hearing loss with low compliance and absent acoustic reflexes (Bergstrom et al., 1972; Lindsay et al., 1975).

Atopic Dermatitis

Recessive. Congenital moderate nonprogressive sensorineural hearing loss which may not be detected until school years. About age 10, affected persons develop lichenified, skin eruptions especially on forearms, hands, elbows, and trunk and arms. Very rare. Integumentary and pigmentary disorder with congenital sensorineural hearing loss (Konigsmark et al., 1968, 1970).

Brevicollis

(See Klippel-Feil Syndrome)

Cardioauditory Syndrome

(See Jervell and Lange-Nielsen Syndrome)

Cerebral Palsy

Recessive or sporadic trait; 1 out of 330 babies is born with cerebral palsy. Paralysis due to a lesion of the brain, usually suffered at birth, and characterized by uncontrollable motor spasms. Cerebral palsy involves paralysis, weakness, incoordination, or other abnormality of motor function due to pathology of the motor control centers of the brain. Damage to the brain may occur during embryonic, fetal, or early infantile life. Essentially nonprogressive, clinical symptoms of the disorder include spasticity (40%), athetosis (40%), ataxia (10%), or combinations of these basic motor dysfunctions. Mental deficiency and convulsive disorders are common. Feeding problems, retarded growth, eye difficulties such as strabismus and nystagmus, developmental delay, orthopedic problems, communication disorders, and educational problems often are evidenced in varying degrees. Damage to the brain may occur during embryonic, fetal, or early infantile life and may result from an antecedent disorder such as trauma, metabolic disorder of infection, destructive intercranial cerebral processes, and/or developmental defects of the brain. Location of the lesion may be in cerebral cortex, basal ganglia, or other sites in the pyramidal system or extrapyramidal system; coexistent involvement in both systems is observed. Less frequently, cerebellar damage may be evident. Patients may have mild to moderate sensorineural

hearing loss, typically more severe in high frequencies.

Cervico-oculoacoustic Dysplasia

(See Klippel-Feil Syndrome)

Cleft Palate and/or Lip

High incidence of recurrent middle ear effusion episodes. Approximately 35–50% of cleft palate babies have associated anomalies (Fig. A.4). See Chapter 3, pages 62–63 for additional information (Bzoch, 1979).

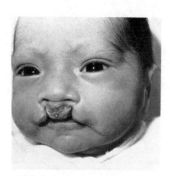

Figure A.4. Bilateral cleft palate and lip.

Cleidocranial Dysostosis

(Cleidocranial Dysplasia, Osteodental Dysplasia)

A general disorder of skeleton due to retarded ossification of membranous and cartilaginous precursors of bone characterized by congenital absence of clavicles, softness of skull, and irregular ossification of bones (Fig. A.5). In addition, shortness of stature, narrow drooping shoulders, widely spaced eyes, irregular

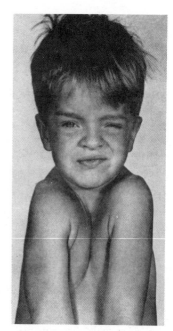

Figure A.5. Cleidocranial dysostosis. (Reproduced with permission from I. S. Jaffee: Congenital shoulder-neck-auditory anomalies, *Laryngoscope, 58:* 2119–2139, 1968.)

or absent teeth, and high arched palate or submucous cleft have been noted. Concentric narrowing of external auditory canals. Mental development is usually normal. Chromosome analyses show normal karyotypes. Autosomal dominant with high percentage and wide variability in expression. About one third of the cases appear to be sporadic. Occasional progressive deafness is reported. May be conductive or sensorineural due to retarded bone ossification.

Cockayne's Syndrome

Recessive, Dwarfism, mental retardation, retinal atrophy, and motor disturbances. Progressive disorder. Appearance normal at birth. Growth and development normal through first year. During second year growth falls below normal range and mental-motor development becomes abnormal. Minimal diagnostic characteristics include dwarfism, retinal degeneration, microcephaly, cataracts, neurologic impairment including progressive mental retardation, sun-sensitive skin, thickening of the skull bones, disproportionately long extremities with large hands and feet, eye disorder, and progressive sensorineural hearing loss of later onset, usually of moderate-to-severe degree. Prognosis is poor with severe blindness and deafness. Hearing aid is possible; however, mental retardation precludes much success (MacDonald et al., 1960; Riggs and Seibert, 1972).

Craniofacial Dysostosis

(See Crouzon's Syndrome)

Crouzon's Syndrome

(Craniofacial Dysostosis)

Abnormally shaped head characterized by a central prominence in the frontal region, a peculiar nose resembling a beak, and marked bilateral exophthalmos caused by premature closure of cranial sutures (Fig. A.6). Shape of the skull depends on which sutures are involved. Mentality may be low but usually is not unless there is brain damage secondary to increased intracranial pressure. Bifid uvula and cleft palate may be present. Autosomal dominant

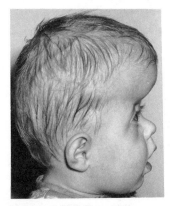

Figure A.6. Crouzon's syndrome.

with variable expression. Approximately one fourth of reported cases arise as fresh mutations. Detected at birth or during first year. Ears may be low set. About one third of cases have nonprogressive conductive hearing impairment. May have mixed type deafness. Middle ear manifestations include deformed stapes with bony fusion of promontory, ankylosis of malleus to outer wall of the epitympanum, distortion and narrowing of middle ear space, and absence of the tympanic membrane, and perhaps bilateral atresia. Stenosis or atresia of external canal common. Early surgical intervention is usually recommended to prevent damage to the brain and eyes. Genetic counseling is recommended (Dodge et al., 1959; Vulliamy and Normandale, 1966; Baldwin, 1968).

Cryptophthalmus

Eye disorder. Recessive. Adherent eyelids which hide the eyes, often accompanied by external ear malformations. In its most severe form, unilateral or more often bilateral extension of skin of the

forehead completely covers eye or eyes to the cheeks. In less severe form, the upper or lower eyelid may be absent. Syndactyly of fingers and/or toes may be present. Laryngeal atresia has been reported. Cleft lip/palate is not uncommon. Hearing loss is of mixed type, with atresia of external auditory canals (Fraser, 1962; Ide and Wollschlaeger, 1969).

Cytomegalovirus Disease (CMV)

Intrauterine viral infection causing growth retardation and numerous associated defects. See Chapters 3 and 7 for additional information.

Diastrophic Dwarfism

Craniofacial disorder. Recessive trait. Marked shortness of stature, characteristic hand deformity with short fingers, and severe bilateral clubfoot. The auricles show cystic swellings in infancy which later develop into cauliflower-like deformities which may calcify. There is 25% incidence of cleft palate. Congenital sensorineural hearing loss (Langer, 1965).

Down's Syndrome

(Trisomy 21 Syndrome; Mongolism)

Syndrome (fig. A.7) is the result of a chromosomal abnormality, either as a 21 trisomy, translocation trisomy (Fig. A.8, *A* and *B*) or as mosaicism. High incidence of occurrence—1 in 770 live births. Clinical findings include a list

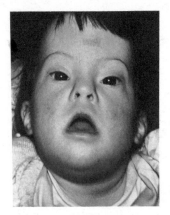

Figure A.7. Down's syndrome.

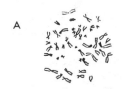

DOWN'S SYNDROME

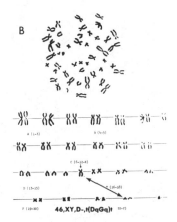

Figure A.8A. Karyotype of Down's Syndrome (note extra 21st chromosome). (Courtesy of A. Robinson, M.D., Cytogenetics Laboratory, University of Colorado Medical Center, Denver.)

of 50 features with varying penetrance. Mental retardation is almost universal. Characteristic personality that is warm, friendly, and affectionate. Common diagnostic features include flattened facial features, oblique palpebral fissures, flat occiput, short limbs, short broad hands, short fingers (especially the fifth finger), depressed nasal bridge, congenital hearing defects, absent moro reflex in infancy, mouth breathing,

Figure A.8B. Karyotype of Down's Syndrome (note translocation). (Courtesy of A. Robinson, M.D., Cytogenetics Laboratory, University of Colorado Medical Center, Denver.)

dental abnormalities, and mental retardation. Ear symptoms in Down's syndrome include small pinnae, narrow external ear canals, abnormal ear configuration and a strong tendency for repeated bouts of otitis media. Incidence of hearing loss is very high with implications of sensorineural, conductive and mixed hearing problems. Anomalies of middle ear ossicles have been reported. Risk of occurrence increases with age of mother: 1 in 1,200 at age 25, but increasing to 1 in 100 for a 40-year-old. See Chapter 3 for additional information.

Duane's Syndrome

(Cervico-oculoacoustic Dysplasia)

Eye disorder. Recessive. Congenital paralysis of the sixth cranial nerve (abducens palsy) with retracted bulb and severe congenital sensori-

neural and/or conductive deafness. Striking appearance because head seems to sit directly on trunk. The abducers paralysis prevents external rotation of eyes, may be unilateral or bilateral; occasional cleft palate. Various ear anomalies have been described including perauricular tags, malformation, atresia or absence of external ear canal, abnormal ossicles, etc. Congenital and nonprogressive (Singh et al., 1969; Cross and Pfaffenbach, 1972; Kirkham, 1969; Stark and Borton, 1973).

Dyschondrosteosis

(See Madelung's Deformity)

Ectodermal Dysplasia

(Ectrodactyly, Ectodermal Dysplasia, and Cleft Palate; EEC Syndrome, Lobster-Claw Syndrome)

Integumentary and pigmentary disorder sometimes accompanied by congenital progressive sensorineural and/or conductive hearing loss. Depressed vestibular function. Abnormality of middle and inner ears has been described. Syndrome seems to have dominant transmission with poor penetrance and variable expressivity. Peculiar lobster-claw deformity of hands and feet, nasolacrimal obstruction and cleft lip-palate. Microcephaly and/or mental retardation present in about 20% of cases (Preus and Fraser, 1973; Robinson et al., 1973; Pashayan et al., 1974).

Engelmann's Syndrome

(Craniodiaphyseal Dysplasia, Diaphyseal Dysplasia)

Skeletal disorder; dominant and/or recessive transmission. Radiologically, this syndrome is characterized by bilateral fusiform enlargement of the diaphyses of the long bones. Skull base may be sclerotic. Deafness is universal and may appear as progressive sensorineural mixed, or conductive in nature (Nelson and Scott, 1969; Sparkes and Graham, 1972).

Fanconi Anemia Syndrome

(Infantile and/or Adolescent Renal Tubular Acidosis)

A syndrome of many causes, some of which are inherited, yet often unidentified. Exposure to toxic agents directly precedes most acquired cases. The clinical manifestations are dependent upon the causes of the syndrome. All aspects of the disorder reflect impaired renal tubular transport. Growth retardation common. In the infantile form, high frequency sensorineural deafness was noted in infancy; in adolescent form, slowly progressive sensorineural deafness noted during teen years (McDonough, 1970; Walker, 1971).

Fehr's Corneal Dystrophy

(Harboyan Syndrome)

Eye disorder. Recessive. Age of detectability is usually between 5 and 9 years. Congenital corneal dystrophy with slow progression leading to blindness at age 40. Progressive sensorineural deafness of delayed onset (Maumenee, 1960; Harboyan et al., 1971).

Friedrich's Ataxia

Nervous system disorder. Recessive. Progressive spinocerebellar ataxia appearing between the ages of 7 and 18 years. Nystagmus, optic atrophy, oculomotor paralysis, retinitis pigmentosa, cataracts, cardiac complications and organic psychological problems. Progressive sensorineural deafness of late onset which may be mild or severe, possibly progressive, symmetrical or asymmetrical with better hearing in the mid-frequencies (Sylvester, 1958, 1972; Shanon et al., 1981).

Goiter, Stippled Epiphysis, and High Protein-Bound Iodine (PBI)

Endocrine-metabolic disorder. Congenital metabolic defect associated with thyroid overactivity, congenital profound sensorineural deafness, birdlike facies, pigeon breast, and winged scapulae. Goiter appears in early infancy. Congenital sensorineural hearing loss (Refetoff et al., 1967).

Goldenhar's Syndrome

(Oculoauriculovertebral Dysplasia)

Eye, oral, musculoskeletal anomalies (Fig. A.9). Eye ab-

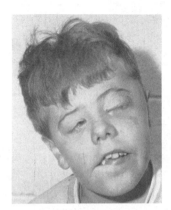

Figure A.9. Goldenhar's syndrome.

normalities include cleft or upper lid, epibulbar dermoids, extraocular muscle defects, and antimongoloid obliquity. Auricular abnormalities include auricular appendices, unilateral posteriorly placed ear, unilateral microtia, atresia of external auditory meatus (40%), and blind-ended fistulas. Oral abnormalities include unilateral facial hypoplasia of ramus and condyle, high arched palate, and open bite. Musculoskeletal abnormalities such as hemivertebrae and clubfoot. Congenital heart disease. Mental retardation not common. Etiology unknown, but may not be hereditary. Most cases are sporadic. Possibly secondary to vascular abnormality during embryologic development of first and second arches. Conductive hearing loss present in 40–50% of reported cases due to atresia of external auditory canals (Sugar, 1966; Berkman and Feingold, 1968).

Hallgren's Syndrome

Eye disorder. Recessive. Congenital sensorineural

hearing loss. Retinitis pigmentosa, progressive ataxia, and mental retardation in 25% of cases. Some patients show later psychosis; 90% have profound deafness (Hallgren, 1959).

Hand-Hearing Syndrome

(Hand Muscle Wasting and Sensorineural Deafness)

Dominant inheritance. Patients manifest familial congenital bilateral or unilateral sensorineural hearing loss of varying degrees. A congenital hand abnormality is seen in both normal hearing and deaf patients (Fig. A.10). Congenital contractures of the digits and wasting of finger muscles. No pain and no other deficits (Stewart and Bergstrom, 1971.)

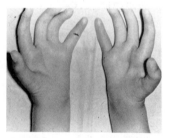

Figure A.10. Hand-hearing syndrome.

Hemifacial Microsomia

Craniofacial disorder with unknown etiology. Abnormalities are unilateral and include ear aplasia and hypoplasia with various pinna malformations. Preauricular tags are present in nearly all cases. External ear canals may be absent or present with the open-

ing covered with skin. Other characteristics include eye abnormalities, lower palpebral fissure in the affected side, microphthalmia, cysts, iris, and choroid colobomas and strabismus, hypoplastic facial muscles, malocclusion (90%), hypoplasia of the maxilla and mandible (95%). May have unilateral conductive hearing loss.

Hereditary Hyperphosphatasia

(See Paget's Disease)

Herrmann's Syndrome

(Photomyelonus, Diabetes Mellitus, Nephropathy, and Sensorineural Deafness)

Nervous system disorder; dominant inheritance. Photomyoclonic and grand mal epilepsy. Later course of syndrome includes personality changes leading to severe dementia, slurring of speech progressive hemiparesis, and mild ataxia, renal disease, and diabetes. Age of detectability is 3rd or 4th decade. Progressive sensorineural hearing loss of late origin (Herrmann et al., 1964).

Hurler Syndrome- Hunter Syndrome

(Mucopolysaccharidosis I and II)

Hurler's is felt to be autosomal recessive, and Hunter's is x-linked recessive (Fig. A.11 and A.12). Although the two disorders are clinically identical, Hunter's is generally

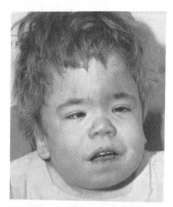

Figure A.11. Hurler's-Hunter's syndrome.

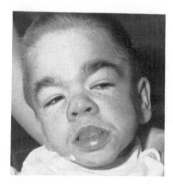

Figure A.12. Hurler's-Hunter's syndrome.

less severe and affects only males. Hurler's can affect both sexes. In contrast to patients with Hurler syndrome, patients with Hunter syndrome usually do not show gross evidence of corneal clouding. Patients have normal appearance at birth but during early months of life onset of progressive abnormal traits. Often described as an "inborn error of metabolism." Diagnostic features include growth failure, marked mental retardation, progressive coarsening of facial features, chronic nasal discharge, joint stiffness, and biochemical evidence of intracellular storage and acid mucopolysaccharides. Death usually occurs before 10 years of age in patients with Hurler syndrome, while patients with Hunter syndrome in mild form may survive until adulthood, or those with severe type may die before puberty. Auditory symptoms have not been satisfactorily described according to Konigsmark and Gorlin (1976). They describe most Hurler syndrome patients to have some degree of progressive deafness. Hunter syndrome has been accompanied by deafness in about half the cases; although the loss is usually not severe and most likely mixed sensorineural and conductive in nature. Otolaryngologic manifestations include upper and lower respiratory infections, narrow nasal passages, hypertrophied adenoids, mucopurulent rhinorrhea, and noisy breathing. Affected individuals are prone to eustachian tube dysfunction and middle ear effusions (Kelemen, 1966; Leroy and Crocker, 1966; Hayes et al., 1980).

Hydrocephalus

A condition characterized by abnormal accumulation of fluid in and around the brain (Fig. A.13). May be congenital or acquired; typically detected at birth or within first 3 months of life. Mental retardation if not treated. Risk of occurrence is 1 in 2000. Accompanied by enlargement of the head, prominence of the brain, mental deterioration, and convulsions. With successful shunt treatment 80% of children reach 5 years of age and 80% of survivors are normal or educable. No data available regarding hearing impairment (Shulman, 1973).

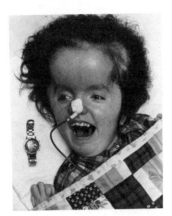

Figure   A.13. Hydrocephalus.

Hyperprolinemia I and II

A biochemical phenotype. No proven association with clinical disease, although identified frequently in pedigrees containing renal disease or convulsive disorders. Recessive disorder. Metabolic problem. Hearing loss has been described as sensorineural in some individuals affected with Type I disease (Schafer et al., 1962).

Hyperuricemia

Endocrine-metabolic problem. Dominant transmission with variable expressivity. Slowly progressive ataxia beginning in second decade. Renal insufficiency. Cardiopathy, myopathy and gout have been noted in some patients. Progressive sensorineural hearing loss of late onset usually high frequency in nature; may progress to total hearing loss with vestibular abnormalities (Rosenberg et al., 1970).

Jervell and Lange-Nielsen Syndrome

(Cardioauditory Syndrome, Surdocardiac Syndrome)

Cardiovascular disorder affects 0.3% of congenitally deaf persons. Autosomal recessive trait. Consanguinity is common. Profound congenital bilateral sensorineural deafness accompanied by electrocardiographic abnormalities, fainting attacks, and, occasionally, sudden unexplained death in childhood. Death usually occurs between 3 and 14 years of age in over half the cases of cardiac problems. Hearing loss is usually symmetrical. Often erroneously diagnosed as a seizure disorder and thus improperly treated (Jervell and Lange-Nielsen, 1957; Friedmann et al., 1966; Wahl and Dick, 1980).

Keratopachyderma and Digital Constrictions

Integumentary disorder, dominant trait. Hyperkeratosis involving the palms, soles, knees and elbows. Ring-like furrows developing on fingers and toes. Mild to severe congenital sensorineural deafness, mainly for frequencies above 4000 Hz, which may be slowly progressive. May include renal disease (Bitici, 1975).

Klippel-Feil Syndrome

(Wildervanck's Syndrome; Brevicollis; Cervico-oculoacoustic Dysplasia)

Craniofacial disorder (Fig. A.14) of debatable etiology

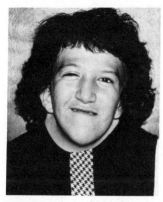

Figure A.14. Klippel-Feil syndrome with right facial paralysis.

probably due to faulty mesodermal differentiation at about the 2nd month of gestation. Involves fusion of some or all cervical vertebrae and is characterized by a short neck with limited mobility which gives the impression that the head sits on the shoulders. Diagnostic criteria include involvement of ear, eye and neck. Other malformations may occur such as clubfoot and cleft palate. Associated neurologic disturbances. Debatable etiology. If familial, autosomal dominance with poor penetrance and variable expression. Faulty segmentation of mesodermal somites in utero, defects in maternal intestinal tract, and environmental factors have been suggested. Summary of syndrome characteristics includes multifactorial inheritance, fusion of cervical vertebrae, abducens nerve palsy, occasional cleft palate, torticollis, severe sensorineural or conductive hearing loss. May range from mild conductive to profound sensorineural. Temporal bone and roentgenogram findings include narrow to absent external auditory meatus and/or

middle ear space, deformed ossicles, narrow oval window niche, underdevelopment of cochlea and vestibular structures (ENGs abnormal), absence of semicircular canals, absence of eighth cranial nerve. Central nervous system involvement is also frequently described and may contribute to audiologic findings. This syndrome is much more common in females (McLay and Maran, 1969; Singh et al., 1969; Stark and Borton, 1973; Windle-Taylor et al., 1981).

Knuckle Pads and Leukonychia

Dominant. Callous-like thickening over dorsal aspects of interphalangeal joints of fingers and toes first observed in infancy and early childhood. Progressive whitening of finger and toenails (leukonychia). Integumentary-pigmentary) disorder; congenital sensorineural or conductive hearing loss. Hearing loss usually noted in infancy or early childhood. Cochlear involvement, of mixed mild-to-moderate degree (Bart and Pumphrey, 1967).

Laurence-Moon-Biedl-Bardet Syndromes

Eye disorder with progressive sensorineural hearing loss of recessive inheritance. Patients with the Laurence-Moon syndrome have retinitis pigmentosa, mental retardation, hypogenitalism and spastic paraplegia. Patients with Biedl-Bardet syndrome show obesity and retinitis pig-

mentosa in association with polydactyly, hypogonadism and mental retardation (Weinstein et al., 1969; Konigsmark and Gorlin, 1976).

Leri-Weill Disease

(See Madelung's Deformity)

Lobster Claw Syndrome

(See Ectodermal Dysplasia)

Long Arm 18 Deletion Syndrome

Abnormalities include mental retardation, microcephaly, short stature, hearing impairment with malformations of auricles and external auditory canals, retinal changes, facial peculiarities, and a high count of whorls on the fingers (Fig. A.15). Congenital heart disease, horseshoe kidney, cryptorchidism, spinal defects, and

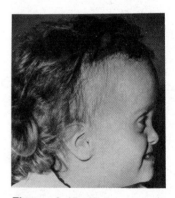

Figure A.15. Long arm 18 deletion syndrome. (Reproduced with permisson from D. Bergsma: *Birth Defects Compendium*, ed. 2, National Foundation-March of Dimes. New York: Alan Liss, 1979.)

PARTIAL DELETION OF 18 LONG ARM

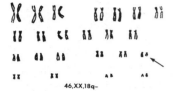

46,XX,18q-

Figure A.16. Karyotype of partial deletion of long arm of 18th chromosome. (Courtesy of A. Robinson, M.D., Cytogenetics Laboratory, University of Colorado Medical Center, Denver.)

foot abnormalities have also been described. Genetic imbalance syndrome involving partial deletion of the long arm of the 18th chromosome (Fig. A.16). If translocation is responsible for deletion, transmission to children is possible. Conductive hearing loss associated with external and middle ear anomalies most frequently reported. Temporal bone study has shown collapsed Reissner's membrane in all turns of the cochlea; rolled and retracted tectorial membrane, hypoplastic cochlear aqueduct (Smith, 1962; Kos et al., 1966; Sando et al., 1969; Bergstrom et al., 1974).

Madelung's Deformity

(Dyschondrosteosis; Leri-Weill Disease)

Craniofacial-skeletal disorder. Dominant. Characterized by deformity of the distal radius and ulna bones and mild dwarfism. Congenital bilateral conductive loss with abnormal ossicles and narrow external auditory canals (Nassif and Harboyan, 1970).

Malformed Low-Set Ears Syndrome

Craniofacial disorder with unilateral or bilateral, mild to severe, conductive hearing loss associated with malformed low-set ears (usually bilateral). Conductive loss usually worse in the most affected external ear. May be accompanied by mental retardation in 50% of cases (Mengel et al., 1969).

Marfan's Syndrome

Craniofacial-skeletal disorder of dominant inheritance. Characteristic symptoms include arachnodactyly, scoliosis, joint hypermobility, dislocated lenses and cardiac anomalies. Deafness associated with Marfan's syndrome is rare (Konigsmark and Gorlin, 1976).

Measles

A highly contagious viral infection involving the respiratory tract. The skin becomes covered with red papules that appear behind the ears and on the face before spreading rapidly down the trunk and onto the arms and legs. Measles may be complicated by bacterial pneumonia, otitis media, and by a demyelinating encephalitis. According to Bergstrom (1977) measles may cause hearing loss due to invasion of the inner ear via the blood stream or central nervous system or through purulent labyrinthitis secondary to suppurative otitis media.

Meningitis

Infection of inflammation of the meningeal membrane surrounding the brain and spinal cord. May be a complication of otitis media. Etiology is varied and may be due to bacteria, virus, or fungi. Symptoms include stiff neck, headache, high fever, nausea, vomiting, and sometimes coma. Approximately 40% of children with deafness due to meningitis have at least one other major handicapping condition. Recovery of auditory function following meningitic deafness has been documented in numerous reports. Fairly common cause of sudden, severe-to-profound sensorineural deafness (8–16%) usually bilateral, but occasionally unilateral. See Chapter 3 for more information (Vernon, 1967b; Roeser et al., 1975; Keane et al., 1979; Finitzo-Hieber et al., 1981).

Möbius Syndrome

(Facial Dysplagia)

Dominant. Craniofacial nervous system disorder (Fig. A.17). Bilateral congenital fa-

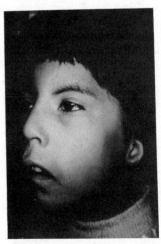

Figure A.17. Möbius syndrome.

cial paralysis, due to paralysis of cranial nerves VI and VII, severe but incomplete, with varying degrees of ophthalmoplegia, external ear malformations, micrognathia. Hands, feet, or digits may be missing; tongue paralysis and mental retardation may be present. Middle ear anomalies may be associated, as well as aberrant facial nerve. Congenital sensorineural and/or conductive hearing loss (Kahane, 1979).

Mohr Syndrome

(Oral-Facial-Digital II; OFD II)

Deformities of face, mouth and fingers transmitted as recessive trait. Characterized by cleft lip and lobulated tongue, broad nasal root, hypoplasia of the mandible, poly and syndactyly. Oral deformities may cause speech problems conductive hearing loss associated with malformed ossicles (Rimoin and Edgerton 1967).

Mongolism

(See Down's Syndrome)

Muckle-Wells Syndrome

(See Amyloidosis, Nephritis, and Urticaria)

Multiple Lentigines Syndrome

(Leopard Syndrome)

Integumentary-pigmentary disorder. Dominant trait. Freckly, dark brown, small spots concentrated on the neck and upper trunk. The term LEOPARD syndrome is an acronym derived from *len*tigines, *e*lectrocardiographic defects, *o*cular hypertelorism, *p*ulmonary stenosis, *a*bnormalities of genitalia, *r*etardation of growth, and sensorineural *d*eafness in 15% of cases. Hearing loss is usually detected in childhood (Gorlin et al., 1969; Voron et al., 1976).

Mucopolysaccharidosis

(See Hurler Syndrome-Hunter Syndrome)

Mumps

A contagious viral disease occurring mainly in children. It is acquired by aspiration with the heaviest inoculation of virus being in the salivary and parotid glands. The incubation period is 18–22 days, with fever and painful inflammation of the involved glands. Symptoms are most pronounced during the first 2 days and subside slowly over the next 4 or 5 days. Classic symptoms involve fever, headache, anorexia, malaise, earache, and enlargement of parotids. Relatively common cause of sudden, total unilateral sensorineural hearing loss. Hearing loss is nearly always permanent. Bilateral total deafness has been reported, but only in rare instances. Exact incidence of hearing loss is difficult to ascertain due to undetected, or undiagnosed, unilateral cases. Deafness may be approximately 5% (Fowler, 1960; Vuori et al., 1962).

Muscular Dystrophy

Recessive, or x-linked. Muscle wasting of various types classified by transmission mode, age of onset, damaged muscle set, rate of disease development, associated problems. *Pseudohypertrophic* muscular dystrophy usually begins prior to age 5 years and affects most body muscles including cardiac and pulmonary systems. *Facioscapulohumeral* type affects face, shoulder, and upper arm muscles; slowly progressive with age of onset at 13–14 years. *Limb-girdle* initially affects muscles of hips and shoulders. *Myotonic* muscular dystrophy associated with diabetes mellitus and cataracts, usually of late onset at age 30 to 40 or older. Severe infantile muscular dystrophy noted to be accompanied by sloping, sensorineural hearing loss of mild to moderate degree. Risk of occurrence is 1 in 100,000; childhood form is usually noted during initial 3 years of life. Extremely rare in females (Black et al., 1971a).

Myoclonic Epilepsy

Dominant nervous system disorder with variable expressivity. Seizure disorder characterized by myoclonic movements which include jerking motions involving head, trunk and limbs. Slowly progressive ataxia. No mental retardation. Progressive sensorineural hearing loss of late onset (May and White, 1968).

Myopia and Congenital Deafness

Recessive transmission. Patients demonstrate a combination of symptoms including myopia, congenital moderate to severe, nonprogressive sensorineural hearing loss and low intelligence in some cases (Eldridge et al., 1968).

Neprhrosis, Urinary Tract Malformations

Sex-linked or recessive transmission. Renal disorder with congenital conductive hearing impairment. Characterized by renal anomalies, nephrosis, digital anomalies, bifurcation of uvula. Congenital moderate-to-severe conductive type hearing impairment (Winter et al., 1968).

Norrie's Syndrome

(Oculoacousticocerebral Degeneration)

X-linked recessive with progressive eye degeneration leading to total blindness. Approximately one-third are severely mental retarded, one-third are mildly retarded, and one-third of normal intelligence. Auditory impairment is progressive of late onset, usually bilaterally symmetric sensorineural hearing loss in one-third of cases (Holmes, 1971).

Oculoacousticocerebral Degeneration

(See Norrie's Syndrome)

Onychondystrophy

Recessive integumentary disorder characterized by rudimentary fingernails and toenails, triphalangeal thumbs with congenital severe sensorineural hearing loss (Goodman et al., 1969).

Optic Atrophy and Diabetes Mellitus

Autosomal recessive with onset in childhood of progressive visual impairment. Diabetes mellitus onset prior to second decade, with childhood progressive sensorineural hearing loss (Stevens and Macfayden, 1972).

Optic Atrophy and Polyneuropathy

Recessive or x-linked transmission. Symptoms include progressive visual loss with bilateral and symmetric optic atrophy beginning in second decade leading to rapid deterioration of vision. Polyneuropathy from childhood. Progressive severe sensorineural deafness in childhood that tends to affect high frequencies. Risk of occurrence is 1 in 100,000 or less (Iwashita et al., 1970).

Opticochleodentate Degeneration

Eye and nervous system disorder. Recessive trait. This fairly rare syndrome is characterized by progressive visual and sensorineural hearing loss, as well as progressive spastic quadriplegia. Vision is normal until about 1 year of age with total blindness at about age 3 years. Microcephaly, mental deterioraton, and speech problems may be evident, with death in later childhood (Konigsmark and Gorlin, 1976).

Osteogenesis Imperfecta

(Van Der Hoeve's Disease)

High percentage of infant death, multiple fractures may be present at birth, weak joints, blue sclera, thin and translucent skin, yellowish-brown and easily broken teeth, deafness. Deformities such as kyphoscoliosis and pectus excavation (Fig. A.18), internal hydrocephalus, nerve root compression, cardiovascular lesions, and thin atrophic skin may also occur. Also known as "brittle bone" disease. Etiology is hereditary autosomal dominant, present at birth. Majority of severe cases are sporadic and because of clinical variability, detection may range from birth through adulthood. Of reported cases, 60% have conductive hearing loss reportedly due to otosclerotic changes, the footplate of the stapes, and the posterior semicircular canal. Temporal bone findings show diminished or immature bone formation in otic capsule and ossicles. Degeneration of stapes crura so no contact is possible between crura and footplate. Sensorineural hearing loss has also been demonstrated in high frequencies. Genetic counseling, magnesium ther-

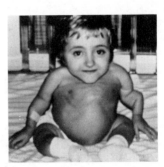

Figure A.18. Osteogenesis imperfecta.

apy, orthopedic correction. Rate of occurrence is about 2–5 per 100,000 births. Otologic surgery is usually successful. Estimates of hearing loss range between 26% and 60% of cases (Hall and Rohrt, 1968; Bretlau et al., 1970; Quisling et al., 1979; Riedner et al., 1980).

Osteopetrosis

(See Albers-Schönberg Disease)

Otopalatodigital Syndrome (OPD)

Sex-linked recessive craniofacial-skeletal disorder. Features include cleft palate, stubby clubbed fingers and toes, wide-spaced nasal bridge giving pugilistic facies, low set and small ears, winged scapulae, downward obliquity of the eyes, and down-turned mouth. Mild mental retardation and congenital conductive-type hearing loss due to ossicular abnormalities (Buran and Duvall, 1967).

Paget's Disease (Juvenile)

(Hereditary Hyperphosphatasia)

Recessive skeletal disorder. Juvenile form is characterized by progressive skeletal deformities that become apparent during the second or third year of life. May result in sporadic cranial nerve involvement. Progressive enlargement of head and long bones. Occasional progressive mixed-type hearing disorder due to

continued new bone formation at the skull base (Thompson et al., 1969).

Pendred's Syndrome

(Goiter and Profound Deafness)

Recessive endocrine-metabolic disorder. The goiter is usually apparent by age 8 years, but may be noted at birth in some cases. Auditory manifestations are variable but usually demonstrate a moderate to profound sensorineural hearing loss. Hearing loss is usually detected in first 2 years of life, and almost always symmetrical. Risk of occurrence is about 1 in 14,500. Fairly common disorder related to profound deafness (Batsakis and Nishiyama, 1962; Fraser, 1965; Illum et al., 1972).

Piebaldness

Divided into three integumentary-pigmentary syndromes by Konigsmark and Gorlin (1976). (a) Recessive piebaldness and profound congenital sensorineural deafness. Head, hair, upper chest, and both arms showed substantial depigmentation. Normal vision with blue irides. (b) X-linked pigmentary abnormalities and congenital sensorineural deafness. Similar pigmentary skin changes as seen in (a) above. Profound deafness. (c) Dominant piebald trent, ataxis and sensorineural hearing loss. About 80% have ataxia and mental retardation, and 60% have progressive sensorineural deafness (Woolf et al., 1965).

Pierre Robin Syndrome

(Cleft Palate, Micrognatha, and Glossoptosis)

Dominant, craniofacial-skeletal disorder. Oral findings include cleft palate, smallness of jaw and chin, downward displacement or retraction of the tongue. Ears may be low set. About 20% of cases associated with mental retardation. Congenital amputations, hip dislocation, sternal anomalies, spina bifida, hydrocephaly and microcephaly have been reported. A variety of cardiac anomalies have been reported. Congenital conductive and/or sensorineural hearing loss. A 10-year follow-up study of 55 cases showed high incidence of speech-language-hearing problems. Risk of occurrence is 1 in 30,000 (Williams et al., 1981).

Pili Torti

Recessive integumentary disorder. Dry, brittle, flat, twisted hair of scalp, eyebrows and eyelashes accompanied by moderate to severe bilateral severe sensorineural hearing loss (Singh et al., 1973).

Preauricular Abnormalities

Includes preauricular pits, preauricular tags (Fig. A.19), and branchial fistulas which may be multiple, and usually bilateral. Dominant craniofacial disorder often accompanied by conductive hearing loss, or profound sensori-

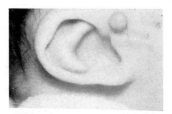

Figure A.19. Preauricular abnormalities.

neural hearing loss, and sometimes external ear canal atresia. Preauricular tag and/or pits usually require no treatment except for cosmetic surgery or excision if draining (McLaurin et al., 1966; Melnick et al., 1976).

Pyle's Disease

(Craniometaphysical Dysplasia)

Recessive form of craniofacial-skeletal disorder. Expressivity is somewhat variable; facial features include hypertelorism, broad nasal ridge, enlarge paranasal area and cranial sclerosis. Nystagmus is common. Progressive sensorineural and/or conductive hearing loss (Miller et al., 1969; Gladney and Monteleore, 1970).

Refsum's Syndrome

Recessive eye disorder. Onset in second decade with visual loss, night blindness due to retinitis pigmentosa, progressive ataxia, muscle wasting, obesity, ichthyosis, and polyneuritis. Major clinical symptoms include triad of retinitis pigmentosa, peripheral neuropathy and cerebellar ataxia. May be related to enzymatic defect. Sensorineural

progressive hearing loss (50%) with one side often worse than the other (Fryer et al., 1971; Nance, 1973).

Renal-Genital Syndrome

Recessive disorder. Renal anomalies and internal genital malformations. Malformation of middle ear with low set auricles and stenotic external canals. Moderate to severe conductive hearing loss (Winter et al., 1968; Turner, 1970).

Renal Tubular Acidosis

(Fanconi Anemia Syndrome)

Richards-Rundle Syndrome

(Ataxia-Hypogonadism Syndrome)

Recessive trait. Nervous system disorder. Includes ataxia, muscle wasting in early childhood. Progressive severe mental retardation, absent deep tendon reflexes with failure to develop secondary sexual characteristics. Early onset of progressive, severe, sensorineural hearing loss; horizontal nystagmus (Richards and Rundle, 1959).

Rubella, Congenital

Rubella embryopathy is today the most important prenatally acquired cause of profound childhood deafness. Infants with congenital rubella virus infections have a variety of defects of varying severity

depending on the embryonic stage during which the infection occurred. Hearing impairment can result from fetal rubella not only during the first trimester of pregnancy, but also in the second and even third trimester (Bordly et al., 1968). Several million persons were affected by the widespread rubella epidemic in the United States during 1963 to 1965.

Diagnostic features include transient neonatal manifestations of low birth weight, hepatosplenomegaly, purpura, bulging anterior suture, corneal clouding and jaundice. Anemia, pneumonia, meningitis, encephalitis may develop. Major associated problems include hearing loss (50%), heart disease (50%), cataract or glaucoma (40%), and psychomotor and mental retardation (40%) (Cooper et al., 1969). A major feature of the rubella embryopathy is a characteristic "salt and pepper" retinal pigmentation, noted in rubella children without cataracts, which does not interfere with visual acuity. Dental abnormalities, microcephaly, and behavioral problems are common in congenital rubella children.

Rubella deafness is commonly sensorineural in nature, often severe to profound in degree. Although sometimes complicated by a conductive component, the typical configuration in rubella deafness tends to be flat or gradually sloping downward from low to high frequencies. Evidence of central auditory deafness due to central nervous system lesion has been reported. Variation in audiometric configuration is common.

The pathology of rubella deafness includes a variety of inner ear abnormalities, middle ear and external ear anomalies. General treatment includes special education considerations as necessary, with possible surgery for cataracts when indicated. Early amplification and auditory training is mandatory when significant hearing loss is determined. See Chapter 8 for additional information (Stuckless, 1980).

Saddle Nose and Myopia

(Marshall Syndrome)

Dominant transmission. Characterized by severe myopia, saddle-nose defect, congenital and/or juvenile cataracts, and congenital progressive sensorineural hearing loss of moderate degree (Ruppert et al., 1970; Zellweger et al., 1974).

Sensory Radicular Neuropathy

Dominant trait, nervous system disorder. Onset in late teens or early adulthood of lightning pains that involve the distal extremities with painless ulcerations of feet. Progressive moderate to severe sensorineural hearing loss (Mandell and Smith, 1960; Stanley et al., 1975).

Symphalangism

Dominant skeletal disorder. Stiff fingers and toes due to bony ankylosis of the proximal interphalangeal joints.

Congenital conductive hearing loss due to stapes fixation (Spoendlin, 1974).

Syphilis, Congenital

Infectious disease, contracted from infected mother to unborn fetus. Sensorineural hearing impairment of slow progressive nature. Pattern of deafness shows variation dependent upon time of onset and rapidity of progression. Youngster may initially show normal hearing. Typically associated with other sensory defects. See Chapter 3, page 80 for additional information (Kerr et al., 1973).

Treacher Collins Syndrome

(Mandibular Dysostosis, First Arch Syndrome)

Major diagnostic features include facial bone abnormalities of structures formed from the first branchial arch including downward sloping palpebral fissures, depressed cheek bones, deformed pinna, receding chin, and large fish-like mouth with frequent dental abnormalties (Fig. A.20). Atresia of auditory canal, defects of auditory canal and ossicles, and cleft palate are common. Mental deficiency reported in about 5% of cases.

Treacher Collins is a genetic defect leading to multiple congenital anomalies. Autosomal dominant with incomplete penetrance and variable expression. More than half of cases reported are fresh mutations.

The external ears may be

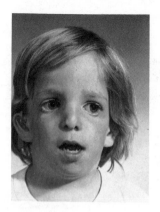

Figure A.20. Treacher Collins syndrome.

small, displaced, or simply nubbins. Atresia of external auditory canal is common. The middle ear is often poorly developed, the tympanic ossicles being absent or deformed. Hypoplasia of the horizontal semicircular canal of the cochlea has been observed, as have branching of nerve to horizontal canal cristae bilaterally and abnormalities of bony and membranous vestibular labyrinth. Deafness generally complete conductive, but may be sensorineural.

General treatment includes genetic counseling, surgical repair of ear anomalies, hearing aid if recommended, orthodontic treatment, and speech therapy if indicated (Herberts, 1962; Fernandez and Ronis, 1964; Frazen et al., 1967; Sando et al., 1968; Lindsay, 1971a, 1971b).

Trisomy 13–15

Major diagnostic features include chromosomal aberration resulting in minimal characteristics of microphthalmia, cleft lip and palate, and polydactyly. A host of other abnormalities may be present including mental retardation; deafness; broad nose hypotelorism; microcephaly; heart and/or skin defects; retroflexed thumbs; "rockerbottom" feet; seizures; renal, abdominal, and genitalia abnormalities. Those affected frequently suffer with feeding problems, failure to thrive, jitteryness, apneic spells, hypotonia, and jaundice. Meiotic nondisjunction appears to be the cause of the extra chromosome in 13–15 group (Fig A.21). Trisomy 13 syndrome with 47 chromosomes frequently associated with increased maternal age. External ears are low set in 80%; malformed ears in 80%; cleft lip/palate in 50–80%. Middle ear findings have included deformed stapes, distorted incudostapedial joint posteriorly, and absence of stapedial muscle and tendon. Inner ear abnormalties have included distorted and shortened cochlea, shortened endolymphatic valve, abnormal branch of nerve to posterior semicircular canal crista from posterior cranial fossa, degeneration of organ of Corti, tectorial membrane, stria vascularis, and saccule. Other studies have been normal. Genetic counseling, other

as may be indicated. Prognosis is poor; 95% die by 3 years (Cohen, 1966; Maniglia et al., 1970; Black et al., 1971b; Scherz et al., 1972).

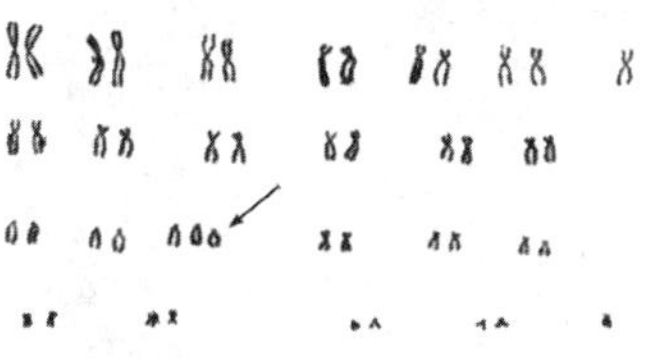

Trisomy 18

Due to chromosomal aberration, features present at birth include being underweight with an undernourished appearance, possible limpness at first soon becoming hypertonic. Microcephaly with triangular shape due to occipital prominence and receding chin. Skin is loose. Flexion of hand with overlapping of index finger over third, "rocker-bottom" feet, short sternum, small pelvis, and agenesis of bones of the extremities. Congenital heart disease, renal abnormalities, cleft lip and palate, deformed ears may also be present. Mental retardation usually profound.

Due to nondisjunction of one chromosome in 17–18 group (Fig. A.22). Advanced maternal age is common. Possibility of recurrence in same family is rare unless translocation is present.

Audiometric testing shows failure to respond to sound. Middle ear anomalies include malformed stapes, deformed

incus and malleus, exposed stapedial muscle in the middle ear cavity, absence of stapedial tendon, absence of pyramidal eminence, a split tensor tympanic muscle in separate bony canals, abnormal course of the facial and chorda tympani nerves, and underdevelopment of facial nerve.

Other anomalies reported include atresia of external canals, decreased spiral ganglion cells, anomalies of cochlea, absence of utriculoendolymphatic valve, and absence of semicircular canals and cristae. Genetic counseling, other treatment is indicated. By 1 year 90% die (Smith, 1962; Kos et al., 1966; Keleman et al., 1968; Sando et al., 1969; Chrysostomidou et al., 1971).

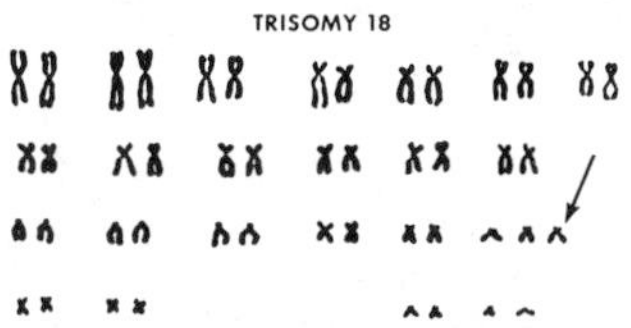

Trisomy 21

(See Down's Syndrome)

Turner's Syndrome

(Gonadal Dysgenesis)

Chromosome defect, not inherited. Low hairline, webbing of neck, widely spaced nipples, shieldlike chest, webbing of digits. Chromosomal abnormality recognizable at birth by webbing or loose folds of skin of short neck, swelling of dorsa of hands and feet, deep creases on thickened palms and soles, hypertelorism, epicanthic folds, ptosis of upper lids, elongated "gothic" ears, high arched palate, micrognathia, pinpoint nipples, and enlarged clitoris. Fingernails are hypoplastic and appear small. Later manifestations include shortness of stature ocular manifestations,

Figure A.21. Trisomy 13–15 (D₁) karyotype. (Courtesy of A. Robinson, M.D., Cytogenetics Laboratory, University of Colorado Medical Center, Denver.)

TRISOMY 18

47,XX,18+

Figure A.22. Trisomy 18 karyotype. (Courtesy of A. Robinson, M.D., Cytogenetics Laboratory, University of Colorado Medical Center, Denver.)

hearing impairment, impairment of taste, congenital cardiovascular disease, anomalies of kidneys, and sexual infantilism. It occurs only in females. Mentality may be normal. Mild sensorineural and conductive hearing loss has been reported. Anderson et al. (1969) reported audiometric findings from 79 patients with Turner's syndrome. Of the 79 patients, 64% had sensorineural hearing loss with a bilaterally symmetrical dip in the mid-frequency range. An additional 22% showed a conductive or mixed hearing loss. Conductive hearing loss has been attributed to frequent middle ear infections in infancy and early childhood, but congenital hearing loss has also been observed (Stratton, 1965; Anderson et al., 1971).

Usher's Syndrome

Recessive, genetic condition including congenital deafness and progressive loss of vision leading to eventual blindness. The hearing loss is bilateral, moderate to severe, sensorineural. Patient initially notices difficulty seeing at night during early teens or twenties; narrowing of visual field (tunnel vision); retinitis pigmentosa. May have additional disorders such as mental retardation, vertigo, psychosis, loss of smell, abnormal EEGs, and epilepsy. Prevalence among profoundly deaf children has been estimated between 3 and 10%. Early diagnosis is important for provision of appropriate rehabilitation endeavors, genetic counseling, screening of relatives. Can vary greatly in age of onset, severity, and speed of progression.

Vestibular response to ca-

loric testing are generally abnormal; 90% of 177 patients (Hallgren, 1959) had severe bilateral congenital deafness, whereas 10% had moderate (30 to 70 dB) sensorineural hearing loss, more marked in higher frequencies. In many cases, the deafness is so profound that hearing aid use is not successful; no treatment for retinitis pigmentosa. Most patients are forced to retire by age 30 or 40, because of vision problems and associated disabilities (Kloepfer et al., 1966; McLeod et al., 1971; Hicks and Hicks, 1981).

Van Buchem's Syndrome

(Hyperstosis Corticalis Generalisata)

Recessive craniofacial-skeletal disorder. Generalized osteosclerotic overgrowth of the skeleton. Paralysis of cranial nerve VII and sensorineural deafness are frequent. Onset during puberty demonstrated by narrowing of skull foramina causing cranial nerve paresis with visual and mixed-type hearing loss. Lion-like facial expression with square jaw (Fosmoe et al., 1968).

Van Der Hoeve's Disease

(See Osteogenesis Imperfecta)

Von Recklinghausen's Neurofibromatosis

Usually a slowly progressive disease of autosomal dominant inheritance characterized by café-au-lait spots associated with cutaneous tu-

mors. The tumors may occur in nodules along a peripheral nerve occasionally producing motor or sensory disturbances. Virtually every part of the central nervous system may be affected by the disease process. Cranial nerve signs may be the result of a glioma or neuroma. Optic nerve and acoustic neuromas, particularly in children, are the most frequent cranial nerve tumors. Slow to rapid progression of sensorineural hearing loss; prevalance is about 1 in 3000. Congenital skeletal problems may also be associated with this disease. Malignant degeneration of the CNS tumors may ultimately cause death. Treatment is genetic counseling and surgery (Nager, 1964; Hitselberger and Hughes, 1968; Young et al., 1970).

Waardenburg's Syndrome

Genetic hearing loss with integumentary system characteristics; inherited as autosomal dominant characteristic with variable penetrance. Major diagnostic features include white forelock (20%)

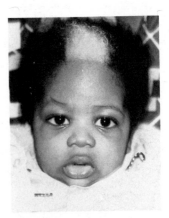

Figure A.23. Waardenburg's syndrome.

(Fig. A.23); lateral displacement of medial canthi (95–99%); iris bicolor or heterochromia (45%); prominence of root of nose; hyperplasia of medial portion of eyebrows (50%). Other findings include thin nose with flaring alae nasae, "cupid bow" configuration of lips, prominent mandible, and occasional cleft palate (5%). All characteristics are not found in each patient. Mental retardation is not typical.

Congenital mild-to-severe sensorineural hearing loss is present in 50% of patients, and may be unilateral, bilateral and/or progressive. Hearing impairment may be evidenced primarily in low and middle frequencies, but profound deafness may also be present. Histopathologic findings include absence of organ of Corti and atrophy of spiral ganglion (Marcus, 1968; Marcus and Valvasori, 1970; Pantke and Cohen, 1971).

Wildervanck's Syndrome

(Otofaciocervical Dysmorphia)

Multifactorial inheritance. Depressed nasal root, protruding narrow nose, narrow elongated face, flattened maxilla and zygoma, prominent ears, preauricular fistulas, poorly developed neck muscles. Facial asymmetry combines the Klippel-Feil characteristics with retraction of the eyeball, sixth nerve paralysis, and total deafness. Integumentary and pigmentary disorder: congenital sensorineural hearing loss. Female preponderance, 1:10.

References

Abahazi DA, Greenberg HJ: Clinical acoustic reflex threshold measurement in infants. *J Speech Hear Dis* 62:514–519, 1977.

Abbs JH, Sussman HM: Neurological feature detectors and speech perception: A discussion of theatrical implications. *J Speech Hear Res* 14:23–36, 1971.

Abramovich S, Gregory S, Slemick M, et al: Hearing loss in very low birthweight infants treated with neonatal intensive care. *Arch Dis Child* 54:421, 1979.

Accreditation Council for Facilities for the Mentally Retarded: Standards for Residential Facilities for the Mentally Retarded. Chicago. Joint Commission on Accreditation of Hospitals, 1971.

Ades HW: Central auditory mechanisms. In Fields J, Magoun HW, Hall VE: *Handbook of Physiology, Vol. 1.* Washington, D.C.: American Physiological Society, 1959.

Ahram DM, Nation JE: Preschool language disorders and subsequent language and academic difficulties. *J Commun Disord* 13;159–170, 1980.

Alberti PWRM, Kristensen R: The clinical application of impedance audiometry. *Laryngoscope* 80:735–746, 1970.

Alpiner JG, Amon C, Gibson J, et al: *Talk to Me.* Baltimore: Williams & Wilkins, 1977.

Altmann F: Histologic picture of inherited nerve deafness in man and animals. *Arch Otolaryngol* 51:852–890, 1950.

American Academy of Otolaryngology Committee on Hearing and Equilibrium and the American Council of Otolaryngology Committee on the Medical Aspects of Noise: Guide for the evaluation of hearing handicap. *JAMA* 251:19, 2055–2059, 1979.

American Academy of Pediatrics, Committee on Children with Handicaps: The physician and the deaf child. *Pediatrics* 51:1100, 1973.

American Academy of Pediatrics, Committee on Environmental Hazards: Noise pollution: neonatal aspects. *Pediatrics* 54:476, 1974.

American Academy of Pediatrics, Joint Committee on Infant Hearing: Position Statement 1982. *Pediatrics* 70:496–497, 1982.

American National Standards Institute, *Specifications for Audiometers.* ANSI S36-1969. New York: American National Standards Institute, 1969.

American National Standards Institute/Acoustical Society of America: Specification of Hearing Aid Characteristics, S3.22-1976. New York: American National Standards Institute, 1976.

American Speech-Language-Hearing Association Guidelines for Acoustic Immittance Screening of Middle-Ear Function. *Asha* 21:283–288, 1979.

American Speech-Language-Hearing Association, Joint Committee on Infant Hearing Position Statement. *Asha* 24:1017, 1982.

American Speech and Hearing Association Guidelines for Identification Audiometry. *Asha* 17:94–99, 1975.

American Speech and Hearing Association Guidelines for Manual Pure-Tone Threshold Audiometry. *Asha* 29:297–301, 1978.

American Speech and Hearing Association Task Force: The definition of a hearing handicap. *Asha* 23:293–297, 1981.

Amon C: Meeting state and federal guidelines. In Roeser R, Downs M: *Auditory Disorders in School Children.* New York: Thieme-Stratton, 1981, ch 2.

Anderson H, Barr B: Congenital pseudo-mixed deafness. *Laryngoscope* 77:1825–1839, 1967.

Anderson, H, Filipsson R, Fluur E, et al: Hearing impairment in Turner's syndrome. *Acta Otolaryngol (Suppl)* 247:1–26, 1969.

Anderson H, Lindsten J, Wedenberg E: Hearing defects in males with sex chromosome anomalies. *Acta Otolaryngol (Stockh)* 72:55–58, 1971.

Anderson MS, Bentinck BR: Intracranial schwannoma in a child. *Cancer* 29:231–234, 1972.

Aniansson G: Methods for assessing high frequency hearing loss in everyday listening situations. *Acta Otolaryngol* 320 (suppl), 1974.

Anson BJ: *An Atlas of Human Anatomy,* ed 2. Philadelphia: W. B. Saunders, 1963.

Anson BJ: Developmental anatomy of the ear. In Paparella MM, Shumrick DA: *Otolaryngology, Vol. I. Basic Sciences and Related Disciplines.* Philadelphia: W. B. Saunders, 1973.

Anson BJ, Donaldson JA: *The Surgical Anatomy of the Temporal Bone and Ear.* Philadelphia: W. B. Saunders, 1967.

Anthony DA, et al: *Seeing Essential English.* Univ. Northern Colo., Greeley, 1971.

Apgar V: A proposal for a new method of evaluation of the newborn infant. *Anesth Analg* 32:260, 1953.

Apgar V, James L: Further observations on the newborn scoring system. *Am J Dis Child* 104:419, 1962.

Aran JM: The electrocochleogram: recent results in children and in some pathological cases. *Arch Klin Exp Ohren Nasen Kehlkopfheilkd* 198:128–141, 1971.

Aran JM, LeBert G: Les réponses nerveuses cochleaires chez l'homme: Image du fonctionnement de l'oreille et nouveau test d'audiométrie objective. *Rev Laryngoscope (Bordeaux)* 89:361, 1968.

Arciszewski RA: The effects of visual perception training on the perception ability and reading achievement of first grade students. *Dissertation Abstracts* 29(12A), 4174, 1969.

Arenberg IR: Meniere's disease. *Otol Clin North Am* 8:2, 1980.

Arey LB: *Developmental Anatomy*. Philadelphia: W. B. Saunders, 1940.

Armitage SE, Baldwin BA, Vince MA: The fetal sound environment of sheep. *Science* 208:1173–1174, 1980.

Arnst D, Katz J (eds): *Central Auditory Assessment: The SSW Test, Development & Clinical Use*. San Diego: College Hill Press, 1982.

Aslin R, Pisoni D, Jusczyk P: Auditory development and speech perception in infancy. In Haith M, Campos J: *Infancy and the Biology of Development* (Vol. II of Carmichael's Manual of Child Psychology, ed 4, PH Mussen (ser ed).) New York: John Wiley & Sons, 1983.

Atkinson M, Canter G: Variables influencing phonemic discrimination performance in normal and learning disabled children. *J Speech Hear Disord* 44:543–556, 1979.

Axelsson A, Fagerberg SE: Auditory function in diabetics. *Acta Otolaryngol* 66:49–64, 1968.

Axelsson A, Lewis C: Aspects of delivery of ear, nose and throat care to Montana Indians. *Health Care and the Poor* 89:6, 551–557, 1974.

Babbidge HS: Education of the Deaf. A Report to the Secretary of Health, Education, and Welfare by his Advisory Committee on the Education of the Deaf. U.S. Govt. Printing Office, 1965, 0-765-119.

Babson SG: *Diagnosis and Management of the Fetus and Neonate at Risk*, ed 4. St. Louis: C. V. Mosby, 1980.

Baker B, Northern J: Medical conditions of the external ears. *Maico Audiological Library Series* 14:(No. 7), 1976.

Baldwir JI: Dysostosis craniofacialis of Crouzon. *Laryngoscope* 78:1660–1675, 1968.

Balkany TJ: Otologic aspects of Down's syndrome. *Semin Speech Lang Hear* 1:39, 1980.

Balkany TJ, Berman SA, Simmons MA, et al: Middle ear effusion in neonates. *Laryngoscope* 88:398–405, 1978.

Balkany TJ, Mischke RE, Downs MP, et al: Ossicular abnormalities in Down's syndrome. *Otolaryngol Head Neck Surg* 87:372, 1979.

Ballenger JJ: *Diseases of the Nose, Throat and Ear*, ed. 12. Philadelphia: Lea & Febiger, 1977.

Ballentine HT, White JC: Brain abscess: influence of antibiotics on therapy and mortality. *N Engl J Med* 248:14–19, 1953.

BAM World Markets, Inc., Box 10701 (Dept. BHK), University Park Station, Denver, Colorado 80210.

Barber HO: Head injury: Audiological and vestibular findings. *Ann Otol Rhinol Laryngol* 78:239–252, 1969.

Barden T, Peltzman P: Newborn brain stem auditory evoked responses and perinatal clinical events. *Am J Obstet Gynecol* 136:912–917, 1980.

Barr DF: *Auditory Perceptual Disorders*, ed 2. Springfield, Ill.: Charles C Thomas, 1976.

Bart RS, Pumphrey RE: Knuckle pads, leukonychia and deafness; a dominantly inherited syndrome. *N Engl J Med* 276:202–207, 1967.

Bartoshuk AK: Response decrement with repeated elicitation of human neonatal cardiac acceleration to sound. *J Comp Physiol Psychol* 55:9–13, 1962a.

Bartoshuk AK: Human neonatal cardiac acceleration to sound; Habituation and dishabituation. *Percept Mot Skills* 15:15–27, 1962b.

Bartoshuk AK: Human neonatal cardiac responses to sound: a power function. *Psychon Sci* 1:151–152, 1964.

Basic Education Rights for the Hearing Impaired: The National Advisory Committee on Education of the Deaf, Office of Ed., Dept. of HEW, 1973, Publication No. (OE) 73-24001.

Basser LS: Benign paroxysmal vertigo of childhood: a variety of vestibular neuronitis. *Brain* 87:141–152, 1964.

Batsakis JG, Nishiyama RH: Deafness with sporadic goiter: Pendred's syndrome. *Arch Otolaryngol* 76:401–406, 1962.

Bax M: The intimate relationship of health, development and behavior in the young child. In Brown CC: *Infants at Risk: Pediatric Round-Table 5*, New Brunswick, N.J.: Johnson & Johnson, 1981, pp 106–113.

Bayley N: The development of motor abilities during the first three years. *Monogr Soc Res Child Dev* 1:1–25, 1935.

Beagley HA, Fisch L: Bio-electric potentials available for electric response audiometry: Indications and contra-indications. In Beagley HA: *Audiology and Audiological Medicine*. Oxford: Oxford University Press, 1981, ch 31, vol 2.

Beal DR: Prevention of otitis media in the Alaskan native. In, Glorig A, Gerwin K: *Otitis Media*. Springfield, Ill.: Charles C Thomas, 1972, pp 156–162.

Beck HL: Counseling parents of retarded children. *Children* 6:225–230, 1959.

Belzile M, Markle DM: A clinical comparison of monaural and binaural hearing aids worn by patients with conductive or perceptive deafness. *Laryngoscope* 69:1317–1323, 1959.

Bench J, Collyer D, Mentz L, et al: Studies in behavioral audiometry. III. Six-month-old infants. *Audiology* 15:384–394, 1977.

Bench RJ: Sound transmission to the human foetus through the maternal abdominal wall. *J Genet Psychol* 113:85–87, 1968.

Bench RJ: Infant audiometry. *Sound* 4:72–74, 1971.

Bench RJ, Boscak N: Some applications of signal detection theory to paedo-audiology. *Sound* 4:3, 1970.

Bender R, Wig E: Binaural hearing aids for hearing impaired children in elementary schools. *Volta Rev* 64:537–542, 1962.

Bendet R: A public school hearing aid maintenance program. *Volta Rev* 82:149, 1980.

Bennett FC, Ruuske SH, Sherman R: Middle ear function in learning disabled children. Paper presented at the Child Development Section of the American Academy of Pediatrics, San Francisco, 1979.

Bennett M, Ward PH, Tait CA: Otologic-audiologic study of cleft palate children. *Laryngoscope* 78:1011–1019, 1968.

Bennett MJ: Trials with the auditory response cradle; I. Neonatal responses to auditory stimuli. *Br J Audiol* 13:125, 1979.

Bennett MJ: Trials with the auditory cradle; III. Head turns and startles as auditory responses in the neonate. *Br J Audiol* 14:122, 1980.

Bennett MJ, Lawrence RJ: Trials with the auditory response cradle; II. The neonatal respiratory response to an auditory stimulus. *Br J Audiol* 14:1, 1980.

Beratis S, Rubin M, Miller RT, et al: Developmental aspects of an infant with transient moderate to severe hearing impairment. *Pediatrics* 63:153–155, 1979.

Bergsma D (ed): *Birth Defects: Compendium*, ed 2, The National Foundation—March of Dimes. New York: Alan R. Liss, 1979.

Bergstrom L: Viruses that deafen. In Bess FH: *Childhood Deafness: Causation, Assessment, & Management.* New York: Grune & Stratton, 1977, chap 4, pp 53–68.

Bergstrom L: Medical problems and their management. In Roeser R, Downs M: *Auditory Disorders in School Children.* New York: Thieme-Stratton, 1981, ch 6.

Bergstrom L: Congenital deafness. In Northern JL: *Hearing Disorders*, ed 2. Boston: Little, Brown, 1984.

Bergstrom L: The routine reevaluation of the congenitally deaf child. Paper presented at the Colorado Otology-Audiology Workshop, Aspen, Colo., 1981.

Bergstrom L, Hemenway WG: Otologic problems in submucous cleft palate. *South Med J* 64:1172–1177, 1971.

Bergstrom L, Thompson P: Ototoxicity. In Northern JL: *Hearing Disorders*, ed 2. Boston: Little, Brown, 1984, ch 10.

Bergstrom L, Hemenway WG, Downs MP: A high risk registry to find congenital deafness. *Otolaryngol Clin North Am* 4:369–399, 1971.

Bergstrom L, Neblett LM, Hemenway WG: Otologic manifestations of acrocephalosyndactyly. *Arch Otolaryngol* 96:117–123, 1972.

Bergstrom L, Jenkins P, Sando I, English GM: Hearing loss in renal disease: clinical and pathological studies. *Ann Otol Rhinol Laryngol* 82:555–577, 1973.

Bergstrom L, Stewart J, Kenyon B: External auditory atresia and the deletion chromosome. *Laryngoscope* 84:1905–1917, 1974.

Berkman MD, Feingold M: Oculoauriculovertebral dysplasia (Goldenhar's syndrome). *Oral Surg* 25:408, 1968.

Berko J, Brown R: Psycholinguistic research methods. In Mussen PH: *Handbook of Research Methods in Child Development.* New York: John Wiley & Sons, 1960, p 531.

Berlin CI: Ultra-audiometric hearing in the hearing impaired and use of upward-shifting translating hearing aids. *Volta Rev* 84:352–363, 1982.

Berlin CI, Catlin FI: Manual of Standard Pure Tone Threshold Procedure, Programmed Instruction: Tactics for Obtaining Valid Pure Tone Clinical Thresholds. Johns Hopkins Med. Institutions, 1965.

Berlin CI, Loew SS: Temporal and dichotic factors in central auditory testing. In Katz J: *Handbook of Clinical Audiology.* Baltimore: Williams & Wilkins, 1972, p 280.

Berlin CI, Lowe-Bell SS, Janetta PJ, et al: Central auditory deficits after temporal lobectomy. *Arch Otolaryngol* 96:4–10, 1972.

Berlin CI, Lowe-Bell SS, Cullen JK, et al: Dichotic speech perception: An interpretation of right-ear advantage and temporal offset effects. *J Acoust Soc Am* 53:699–709, 1973.

Berliner K, House W: Cochlear implants: an overview and bibliography. *Am J Otol* 2:277–282, 1981.

Berlow SJ, Caldarell DD, Matz GJ, et al: Bacterial meningitis in sensorineural loss: a prospective investigation. *Laryngoscope* 90:1445–1452, 1980.

Berman SA, Balkany TJ, Simmons MA: Otitis media in the neonatal intensive care unit. *Pediatrics* 62:198–202, 1978.

Berry J: Parents of the handicapped as consumers: Some thoughts for physicians. *Clin Pediatr* 20:363, 1981.

Bess FH: Impedance screening for children: a need for more research. *Ann Otol Rhinol Laryngol* 89(Suppl 68):228, 1980.

Bess FH: Children with unilateral hearing loss. *J Acad Rehabil Audiol* 15:131–144, 1982.

Bess FH, Gravel J: Recent trends in educational amplification. *Hear Instruments* 32:24, 1981.

Bess FH, Logan S: Amplification in the educational setting. In Jerger J (ed): *Pediatric Audiology.* San Diego, Calif.: College-Hill Press, 1984.

Bess FH, McConnell F: *Audiology, Education, and the Hearing Impaired Child.* St. Louis: C. V. Mosby, 1981.

Bess FH, Powell RL: Hearing hazard from model airplanes. *Clin Pediatr* 11:621–624, 1972.

Bess FH, Lewis HD, Cieliczka DJ: Acoustic impedance measurements in cleft-palate children. *J Speech Hear Disord* 40:13–24, 1975.

Bess FH, Schwartz DM, Redfield NP: Audiometric, impedance and otoscopic findings in children with cleft palates. *Arch Otolaryngol* 102:465–469, 1976.

Bess FH, Peek B, Chapman J: Further observations on noise levels in infant incubators. *Pediatrics* 63:100, 1979.

Bess FH, Freeman B, Sinclair JS. (eds): *Amplification in Education.* Washington, D.C.: A. G. Bell, 1981.

Bess JC: Ear canal collapse. *Arch Otolaryngol* 93:408–412, 1971.

Bilger R (Ed): Evaluation of subjects presently fitted with implanted auditory prostheses. *Ann Otol Rhinol Laryngol* 86(Suppl 38):(3, Pt. 2), 1977.

Bilger RC, Hirsh JJ: Masking of tones by bands of noise. *J Acoust Soc Am* 28:623–630, 1956.

Billings BI, Lowry LD: Tympanometry, impedance and aural reflex testing in a cleft palate population. *Cleft Palate J* 11:21–27, 1974.

Birch JW: Mainstream education for hearing-impaired pupils: Issues and interviews. *Am Ann Deaf* 121:69–71, 1976.

Bitici OC: Familial hereditary progressive sensorineural hearing loss with keratosis and plantaris. *J Laryngol Otol* 89:1143–1146, 1975.

Bjorkesten G: Unilateral acoustic tumors in children. *Acta Psychiatr Scand* 32:1–5, 1957.

Black FO, Bergstrom L, Downs MP, et al: *Congenital Deafness: A New Approach to Early Detection Through a High Risk Register.* Boulder, Colo.: Colorado Associated University Press, 1971.

Black FO, Sando I, Wagner JA, et al: Middle and inner ear abnormalities, 13–15 (D_1) trisomy. *Arch Otolaryngol* 93:615–619, 1971b.

Blager FB: The effect of otitis media on speech and language development. *Semin Speech Lang Hear* 3:313, 1982.

Bland RD: Otitis media in the first six weeks of life: diagnosis, bacteriology and management. *Pediatrics* 49:187–197, 1972.

Blennow G, Svenningsen N, Almquist B: Noise levels

in infant incubators (adverse effects?). *Pediatrics* 53:29, 1974.

Bloom L, Lahey M: *Language Development and Language Disorders.* New York: John Wiley & Sons, 1978.

Bluestone CD: Relative value of tonsil and adenoid surgery in preventing otitis media. In Wiet RJ, Coulthard SW: *Otitis Media: Proceedings of the Second National Conference on Otitis Media,* Columbus, Ohio: Ross Laboratories, 1979, pp 73–78.

Bluestone CD: Article in *Washington Post,* May 27, 1981.

Bluestone CD, Shurin PA: Middle ear disease in children: Pathogenesis, diagnosis and management. *Pediatr Clin North Am* 21:379–400, 1974.

Bluestone CD, Beery QC, Paradise J: Audiometry and tympanometry in relation to middle ear effusions in children. *Laryngoscope* 83:594–604, 1973.

Bocca E, Calearo C: Central hearing processes. In Jerger J: *Modern Developments in Audiology.* New York: Academic Press, 1963, pp 337–370.

Boothroyd A: Group hearing aids. In Bess F, Freeman B, Sinclair J: *Amplification in Education.* Washington, D.C.: A. G. Bell, 1981.

Boothroyd A: *Hearing Impairments in Young Children.* Englewood Cliffs, N.J.: Prentice-Hall, 1982.

Bordley JE, Brookhouser PE, Hardy J, et al: Prenatal rubella. *Acta Otolaryngol (Stockh)* 66:1, 1968.

Borg F, Moller AR: The effect of ethylalcohol and pentobarbital sodium on the acoustic reflex in man. *Acta Otolaryngol* 64:415, 1968.

Bornstein H: A description of some current sign systems designed to represent English. *Am Ann Deaf* 188:454–463, 1973.

Bornstein H: Signed English: a manual approach to English language development. *J Speech Hear Disord* 3:330–343, 1974.

Bornstein H: Sign language in the education of the deaf. In Schlesinger I, Namir L: *Sign Language of the Deaf: Psychological, Linguistics and Social Perspectives.* New York: Academic Press, 1978, pp 333–359.

Bornstein H: Systems of Sign. In Bradford L, Hardy W: *Hearing and Hearing Impairment.* New York: Academic Press, 1979, pp 331–361.

Bornstein H, Saulnier K: Signed English: a brief follow-up to the first evaluation. *Am Ann Deaf* 124:69–72, 1981.

Bornstein H, Kannapell BM, Saulnier KI, et al: Signed English Basic Pre-School Dictionary; Little Red Riding Hood, Goldilocks and the Three Bears, etc. Washington, D.C.: Gallaudet College Press, 1972.

Bornstein H, Saulnier K, Hamilton L: Signed English: a first evaluation. *Am Ann Deaf* 125:467, 1980.

Borton T, Smith CR: Heart rate response audiometry: bases, clinical techniques, and limitations. *Ear Hearing* 1:121, 1980.

Borus J: Acoustic impedance measurements with hard of hearing mentally retarded children. *J Ment Defic Res* 16:196–202, 1972.

Bower T: Competent newborns. In Levin R: *Child Alive.* Garden City, N.Y., Anchor Press/Doubleday, 1975.

Bower TGR: Repetitive processes in child development. *Sci Am* 235:38–47, 1976.

Boyd SF: Hearing loss: Its educationally measurable effects on achievement. M.S. thesis, Department of Speech Education, Southern Illinois University, Carbondale, 1974.

Brackbill Y, Downs MP: Cited in Brackbill and Fitzgerald's "Development of the sensory analyzers during infancy." In Lipsitt LP, Reese H: *Advances in Child Development and Behavior.* New York: Academic Press, 1969, pp 4, 173–208.

Brackbill Y, Fitzgerald HE: Development of the sensory analyzers during infancy. In Lipsitt LP, Reese H: *Advances in Child Development and Behavior.* New York: Academic Press, 1969, pp 4, 173–208.

Brackbill Y, Adams G, Crowell DH, et al: Arousal level in neonates and preschool children under continuous auditory simulation. *J Exp Child Psychol* 4:178–188, 1966.

Brackman DE: Electric response audiometry in a clinical practice. *Laryngoscope* 87 (Suppl 5):1–33, 1977.

Bragg V: Toward a more objective hearing aid fitting procedure. *Hear Instruments* 28:6–9, 1977.

Brandes PJ, Ehinger DM: The effects of early middle ear pathology on auditory perception and academic achievement. *J Speech Hear Disord* 46;301–307, 1981.

Bransford J, Nitsch K: Coming to understand things we could previously understand. In Kavanagh J, Strange W, *Speech and Language in the Laboratory, School and Clinic.* Cambridge, Mass: MIT Press, 1978.

Bredbereg G: Cellular pattern and nerve supply of the human organ of Corti. *Acta Otolaryngol Suppl* 236, 1968.

Bretlau P, Jorgensen MB, Johansen H: Osteogenesis imperfecta. Light and electronmicroscopic studies of the stapes. *Acta Otolaryngol (Stockh)* 69:172–184, 1970.

Bricker D, Bricker W: A programmed approach to operant audiometry for low-functioning children. *J Speech Hear Disord* 34:312–320, 1969.

Bricker DD: A rationale for the integration of handicapped and nonhandicapped preschool children. In Guralnich MJ: *Early Intervention and the Integration of Handicapped and Nonhandicapped Children.* Baltimore: University Park Press, 1978.

Bridger WH: Sensory discrimination and habituation in the human neonate. *Am J Psychiatry* 117:991–996, 1961.

Brill RG: Mainstreaming: format or quality. *Am Ann Deaf* 120:377–381, 1975.

Brill RG: Definition of total communication. *Am Ann Deaf* 121:358, 1976.

Briskey RJ, Sinclair J: The importance of low frequency amplification in deaf children. *Audecibel* (Winter) 7–20, 1966.

Brody JA: Notes on the Epidemiology of draining ears and hearing loss in Alaska with comments on future studies and control measures. *Alaska Med* 6;1, 1964.

Brody JA, Overfield T, McAlister R: Draining ears and deafness among Eskimos. *Arch Otolaryngol* 81:29–33, 1965.

Brooks D: An objective method of detecting fluid in the middle ear. *Int Audiol* 7:280–286, 1968.

Brooks D: The use of the electro-acoustic impedance bridge in the assessment of middle ear function. *Int Audiol* 8:563–569, 1969.

Brooks D: Electroacoustic impedance bridge studies on normal ears of children. *J Speech Hear Res*

14:247–253, 1971.

Brooks DN: Hearing screening: A comparative study of an impedance method and pure tone screening. *Scand Audiol* 2:67–76, 1973.

Brooks DN: Middle ear effusion in children with severe hearing loss. *Impedance Newsletters* (American Electromedics, New York) 4:6–7, 1975.

Brooks DN: Impedance in screening. In Jerger J, Northern JL: *Clinical Impedance Audiometry.* Acton, Mass.: American Electromedics Corp., 1980.

Brooks DN, Wooley H, Kanjilal GC: Hearing loss and middle ear disorders in patient's with Down's syndrome (mongolism). *J Ment Defic Res* 16:21–29, 1972.

Bross M, Harper D, Sicz G: Visual effects of auditory deprivation: common intermodal and intramodal factors. *Science* 207:667–668, 1980.

Brown JB, Fryer MP, Morgan LR: Problems in reconstruction of the auricle. *Plast Reconstr Surg* 43:597–604, 1969.

Brown KS: The genetics of childhood deafness. In McConnell F, Ward PH: *Deafness in Childhood.* Nashville, Tenn.: Vanderbilt University Press, 1967, pp 177–202.

Brown KS, Chung CS: Genetic studies of deafness at the Clarke School for the Deaf, Northampton, Mass. In Report of the Proceedings of the International Congress on Education of the Deaf. Washington, D.C., U.S. Govt. Printing Office, 1964.

Brown RM Jr, Haigler C, Cooper K: The biomodal perception of speech in infancy. *Science* 218:1138–1141, 1982.

Bruner JS: *Processes of Cognitive Growth: Infancy.* Worcester: Clark University Press, 1968.

Buran DJ, Duvall AJ: The oto-palato-digital (OPD) syndrome. *Arch Otolaryngol* 85:394–399, 1967.

Bryan EM, Nicholson E: Congenital syphilis. *Clin Pediatr* 20:81–87, 1981.

Burgener GW, Mouw JT: Minimal hearing loss effect on academic/intellectual performance of children. *Hear Instruments* 33:7–17, 1982.

Butterfield EC: An extended version of modification of sucking with auditory feedback. Working Paper 43, Bureau of Child Research Laboratory, Children's Rehab. Unit, University of Kansas Medical Center, 1968.

Butterfield G: A note on the use of cardiac rate in the audiometric appraisal of retarded children. *J Speech Hear Disord* 27:378–379, 1962.

Byrne D, Tonisson W: Selecting the gain of hearing aids for persons with sensorineural hearing impairments. *Scand Audiol* 5:51–59, 1976.

Bzoch KR (ed): *Communicative Disorders Related to Cleft Lip and Palate*, ed 2. Boston: Little, Brown, 1979.

Cameron J, Livson N, Bayley N: Infant vocalizations and their relationship to mature intelligence. *Science* 157:331–333, 1967.

Campbell AMG, Clifton F: Adult toxoplasmosis in one family. *Brain* 73:281–290, 1950.

Caplar F (ed): *The First Twelve Months of Life: Your Baby's Growth Month by Month.* New York: Grosset & Dunlap, 1973.

Carhart R: Speech reception in relation to pattern of pure tone loss. *J Speech Disord* 11:97–108, 1946.

Carhart R: The usefulness of the binaural hearing aid. *J Speech Hear Disord* 23:41–51, 1958.

Carhart R: Monaural and binaural discrimination against competing sentences. *Int Audiol* 4:5–10, 1965.

Carhart R, Jerger J: Preferred method for clinical determination of pure tone thresholds. *J Speech Hear Disord* 24:330–345, 1959.

Carter CO: *An ABC of Medical Genetics.* Boston: Little, Brown, 1969.

Cass R, Kaplan P: Middle ear disease and learning problems: A school system's approach to early detection. *J Sch Health* 49:557–560, 1979.

Cazder CB: Suggestions from studies of early language acquisition. In Language in Early Childhood Education. National Association for the Education of Young Children, Washington, D.C., 1972.

Chiappa KH, Ropper AH: Evoked potentials in clinical medicine, Part I. *N Engl J Med* 306:19, 1140–1150, 1982; Part II, 306:20, 1205–1211, 1982.

Chomsky N: *Aspects of the Theory of Syntax.* Cambridge, Mass.: MIT Press, 1966.

Chow K: Numerical estimates of the auditory central nervous system of the rhesus monkey. *J Comp Neurol* 95:159, 1951.

Chrysostomidou DM, Caslaris E, Alexion D, et al: Trisomy 18 in Greece. *Acta Paediatr Scand* 60:591–593, 1971.

Clark AD, Richards CJ: Auditory discrimination among economically disadvantaged and nondisadvantaged preschool children. *Except Child* 33:259–262, 1966.

Clark B, Conry R: Hearing impairment in children with low birthweight. *J Aud Res* 18:4, 1978.

Clopton BM, Winfield JA: Effect of early exposure to patterned sound on unit activity in rat inferior colliculus. *J Neurophysiol* 39:1081–1089, 1976.

Clopton BM, Silverman MS: Plasticity of Binaural Interactions; II. Critical periods and changes in midline response. *J Neurophysiol* 40(6):1275–1280, 1977.

Cohen D, Sade J: Hearing on secretory otitis media. *Can J Otol* 1:27, 1972.

Cohen ME: Neurological abnormalities in achondroplastic children. *J Pediatr* 71:367, 1967.

Cohen PE: The "D" syndrome. *Am J Dis Child* 111:235, 1966.

Cohen S, Glass DC, Singer JE: Apartment noise, auditory discrimination, and reading ability in children. *J Exp Soc Psychol* 9:407–422, 1973.

Cohen SA: Cause vs. treatment in reading achievement. *J Learning Disabil* 33:163–166, 1970.

Cokely DR, Gawlik R: A position paper on the relationship between manual English and Sign. *The Deaf American* May, 7–9, 1973.

Cole W: Hearing aid gain: a functional approach. *Hear Instruments* 26:22–24, 1975.

Coleman M: An overview of Down's syndrome. *Semin Speech Lang Hear* 1:1, 1980.

Condon WS, Sander LW: Neonate movement is synchronized with adult speech: interactional participation and language structure. *Science* 183:99–101, 1974.

Conference on Hearing Screening Services for Preschool Children, Columbus, Ohio: Maternal & Child Health Bureau, Dept. HEW, Washington, D.C., 1977.

Conway A: Mainstreaming from a school for the deaf. *Volta Rev* 81:237, 1979.

Cooper J, Langley L, Meyerhoff W, et al: The significance of negative middle ear pressure. *Laryngoscope* 87:92–97, 1977.

Cooper JC: More problems in instant medicine. *Saturday Rev* 56–61, 1967.

Cooper JC, Gates GA, Owen JH, et al: An abbreviated impedance bridge technique for school screening. *J Speech Hear Disord* 40:260–269, 1975.

Cooper L: Rubella: clinical manifestations and management. *Am J Dis Child* 118:18, 1969.

Cooper LZ, Ziring PR, Ockerse AB, et al: Rubella; clinical manifestations and management. *Am J Dis Child* 118:18–29, 1969.

Corliss E: Facts about Hearing and Hearing Aids. A consumer's guide from the National Bureau of Standards, U.S. Dept. of Commerce. Washington, D.C., U.S. Govt. Printing Office, 1971.

Cornett RO: Oralism vs manualism: cued speech may be the answer. *Hear Speech News* 35:6–9, 1967.

Cornett RO: Cued speech and oralism: an analysis. *Audiol Hear Educ* 1:26–30, 1975.

Costello A: Are mothers stimulating? In Levin R: *Child Alive*. Garden City, N.Y., Anchor Press/Doubleday, 1975.

Courtois M, Berland M: Ipsilateral no-mold fitting of hearing aids. Oti Congress II, Copenhagen, 1972, pp 3–23.

Craig W, Craig H: Verbotonal instruction for young deaf children; questions and replies. Pamphlet from Western Pennsylvania School for the Deaf, 1972.

Craig W, Dodge HW, Ross PJ: Acoustic neuromas in children. Report of two cases. *J Neurosurg* 11:505–508, 1954.

Craig WN, Craig HB, DiJohnson A: Preschool verbotonal instruction for deaf children. *Volta Rev* 74:236–246, 1972.

Craig WN, Salem JM, Craig HB: Mainstreaming and partial integration of deaf with hearing students. *Am Ann Deaf* 121:63–68, 1976.

Crarioto J: Pre-School Malnutrition. National Academy of Science, National Research Council, Publ. No. 1282, 1966.

Crispens CG Jr: *Essentials of Medical Genetics*, New York: Harper & Row, 1971.

Cross HE, Pfaffenbach DD; Duane's retraction syndrome and associated congenital malformations. *Am J Ophthalmol* 73:442–449, 1972.

Cullen JK, Thompson CL: Release from masking in subjects with temporal lobe resections. Unpublished paper, Kresge Hearing Research Laboratory of the South, New Orleans, 1973.

Cullen JK, Ellis MS, Berlin CI, et al: Human acoustic nerve action potential recordings from the tympanic membrane without anesthesia. *Acta Otolaryngol (Stockh)* 74:15–22, 1972.

Cunningham GC: Biochemical screening programs and problems. In Gold EM: *Earlier Recognition of Handicapping Conditions in Childhood: Proceedings of a Bi-Regional Institute*. University of California, Berkeley: School of Public Health, 1970, pp 37–41.

Curran J: *Four Basic Factors for Successful Hearing Aid Fittings*. Minneapolis, Minn.: Maico Hearing Instruments, Inc., 1982.

Dahl HA: Progressive hearing impairment in children with congenital CMV. *J Speech Hear Disord* 44:220, 1979.

Dahle AJ, McCollister FP: Considerations for evaluating hearing in multiply handicapped children. In *The Multiply Handicapped Child*, (Proceedings of a Symposium in Edmonton, Alta). New York: Grune & Stratton, 1983.

Dallos P: *The Auditory Periphery: Biophysics and Physiology*. New York: Academic Press, 1973.

Danaher EM, Pickett JM: Relationship between the acoustic reflex and syllable discrimination. Presented at Convention of the American Speech and Hearing Association, San Francisco, 1972.

Danaher EM, Pickett JM: Some masking effects produced by low frequency vowel formants in persons with sensorineural hearing loss. *J Speech Hear Res* 18:261–271, 1975.

Darbyshire JV: A study of the use of high power hearing aids by children with marked degrees of deafness and the possibility of deteriorations in acuity. *Br J Audiol* 10:74–78, 1976.

Darley FI: Identification audiometry for school-age children: Basic procedures, *J Speech Hear Disord* (mongr suppl) 9:26–34, 1961.

Darlington RB: Duration of pre-school effects on later school competence. *Science* 213:1145–1146, 1981.

Davey P: Hearing loss in children of low birthweight. *J Laryngol Otol* 76:274–277, 1962.

Davila RR, Brill RG: Guest editorial—P.L. 94–142. *Am Ann Deaf* 121:361, 1976.

Davis GL: CMV and hearing loss: Clinical and experimental observations. *Laryngoscope* 89:1681–1688, 1979.

Davis H: Peripheral coding of auditory information. In Rosenblith WA: *Sensory Communication*. Cambridge, Mass.: MIT Press, 1961.

Davis H: Brainstem and other responses in electric response audiometry. *Ann Otol* 85:3–13, 1976.

Davis H, Hudgins CV, Marquis RJ, et al: The selection of hearing aids. *Laryngoscope* 56:85–115, 1946.

Davis J: Utilization of audition in the education of the hearing-impaired child. In Bess F, Freeman B, Sinclair J: *Amplification in Education*, Washington, D.C.: A. G. Bell, 1981, ch 6.

Davis JM, Shepard NT, Stelmachowicz PG, et al: Characteristics of hearing-impaired children in the public schools; Part II. Psychoeducational data. *J Speech Hear Disord* 46;130–137, 1981.

Davis PA: Effects of acoustic stimuli on the waking human brain. *J Neurophysiol* 2:494–499, 1939.

Deatherage BH, Hirsh IJ: Auditory localization of clicks. *J Acoust Soc Am* 31:486–492, 1959.

DeCasper AJ, Fifer WP: Of human bonding: newborns prefer their mothers' voices. *Science* 208:1174–1176, 1980.

Dee A, Rapin I, Ruben RJ: Speech and language development in a parent-infant total communication program. Report to combined Otolaryngological Spring meetings, Palm Beach, April 30–May 2, 1982.

DeHirsch K, Jansky JJ, Langford WS: *Predicting Reading Failure*. New York: Harper & Row, 1966.

Demany I, McKenzie B, Vurpillot E: Rhythm perception in early infancy. *Nature* 266:718–719, 1977.

Denenberg VH, Morton JRC: Infantile stimulation, perpetual sexual-social interaction and emotionality. *Anim Behav* 12:11–13, 1964.

Dennis W: *Children of the Creche. Century Psychology Series*. New York: Prentice-Hall, 1973.

Denton DM, Brill RB, Kent MS, et al: Schools for

deaf children. In Fine PJ: *Deafness in Infancy and Early Childhood.* New York: Medicom Press, 1974.

Derbyshire AJ, Davis H: The action potential of the auditory nerve. *Am J Physiol* 113:476–504, 1935.

Deutsch CP: Auditory discrimination and learning: social factors. *Merrill-Palmer J Behav Dev* 10:277–296, 1964.

Dirks D: Perception of dichotic and monaural verbal material and cerebral dominance for speech. *Acta Otolaryngol* 58:73–80, 1964.

Dirks D, Carhart R: A survey of reactions from users of binaural and monaural hearing aids. *J Speech Hear Disord* 27:311–321, 1962.

Dobie RA, Berlin CI: Influence of otitis media on hearing and development. *Ann Otol Rhinol Laryngol* 88(Suppl 60):48–53, 1979.

Dodds E, Harford E: Modified earpieces and CROS for high frequency hearing loss. *J Speech Hear Res* 11:204–218, 1968.

Dodds E, Harford E: Follow-up report on modified earpieces and CROS for high frequency hearing losses. *J Speech Hear Res* 13:41–43, 1970.

Dodge HW Jr, Wood MW, Kennedy RIJ: Craniofacial dysostosis: Crouzon's disease. *Pediatrics* 23:98, 1959.

Doster M: Personal communication. Denver Public Schools Health Department, 1972.

Douek E, Dodson H, Banister L, et al: Effects of incubator noise on the cochlea of the newborn. *Lancet* 2:1110–1113, 1976.

Downs DW: Auditory brainstem response testing in the neonatal intensive care unit: a cautious response. *Asha* 24:1009–1015, 1982.

Downs M: The familiar sounds test and other tests for hearing screening in children. *J Sch Health* 26:77–87, 1956.

Downs M: Guest editorial: implanting electrodes? *Asha* 23:567–568, 1981.

Downs M, Blager FB: The otitis prone child. *Dev Behav Pediatr* 3:106–113, 1982.

Downs MP: The establishment of hearing aid use: a program for parents. *Maico Audiological Library Series* 4: V, 1966.

Downs MP: The identification of congenital deafness. *Trans Am Acad Ophthalmol Otolaryngol* 74:1208–1214, 1970.

Downs MP: Maintaining children's hearing aids. The role of parents. *Maico Audiological Library Series* 10:1, 1971.

Downs MP: The deafness management quotient. *Hear Speech News*, Jan.–Feb., 1974.

Downs MP (ed): Communication disorders in Down's syndrome. *Semin Speech Lang Hear* 1:1, 1980a.

Downs MP: The hearing of Down's individuals. *Semin Speech Lang Hear* 1:25, 1980b.

Downs MP: The team approach to congenital deafness. In Mencher G, Gerber S: *Early Management of Hearing Loss.* New York: Grune & Stratton, 1981.

Downs MP: The audiologist and the non-benign conductive hearing loss of otitis media. *Semin Speech Lang Hear* 3:295, 1982a.

Downs MP: Early identification of hearing loss. In Lass NJ, McReynolds LV, Northern JL, et al: *Speech, Language and Hearing.* Philadelphia: W. B. Saunders, 1982b, ch 41.

Downs MP, Akin J: Unpublished research on a comparison between deaf and normal hearing infant vocalizations. Denver, 1973.

Downs MP, Hemenway WG: Report on the hearing screening of 17,000 neonates. *Int Audiol* 8:72–76, 1969.

Downs MP, Sterritt GM: Identification audiometry for neonates: A preliminary report. *J Aud Res* 4:69–80, 1964.

Downs MP, Doster ME, Weaver M: Dilemmas in identification audiometry. *J Speech Hear Disord* 30:360–364, 1965.

Downs MP, Jafek B, Wood RP: Comprehensive treatment of children with recurrent serous otitis media. *Otolaryngol Head Neck Surg* 89:658–665, 1981.

Drillen CM: *The Growth and Development of the Prematurely Born Infant.* London: E & S Livingstone, 1964.

D'Souza S, McCartney E, Nolan M, et al: Hearing, speech and language in survivors of severe perinatal asphyxia. *Arch Dis Child* 56:245–252, 1981.

Dudich TM, Keiser M, Keith RW: Some relationships between loudness and the acoustic reflex. *Impedance Newsletter* (American Electromedics Corp., Acton, Mass. 4:12–15, 1975.

Dupertius SM, Musgrave RH: Experiences with the reconstruction of the congenitally deformed ear. *Plast Reconstr Surg* 23:361–373, 1959.

Dykstra R: Auditory discrimination abilities and beginning reading achievement. *Reading Res Q* 1:5–34, 1966.

Eagles EL, Wishik SM, Doerfler LG: Hearing sensitivity and ear disease in children: A prospective study. *Laryngoscope* (Monograph) 1–274, 1967.

Edwards EP: Kindergarten is too late. *Saturday Rev* 60–79, 1968.

Efron R: Temporal perception, aphasia, and déjà vu. *Brain* 86:403–424, 1963.

Eichenwald HF, Fry PC: Nutrition and learning. *Science* 163:644–648, 1969.

Eilers RE, Wilson WR, Moore JM: Developmental changes in speech discrimination in infants. *J Speech Hear Res* 20:4, 766–779, 1977.

Eimas PD: In Cohen LB, Salapatek: *Infant Perception: From Sensation to Cognition.* New York: Academic Press, 1975, vol 2.

Eimas PD, Tartter VC: On the development of speech perception: Mechanisms and analogies. *Adv Child Dev Behav* 13: 1979.

Eimas PD, Siqueland ER, Juscyzk P, et al: Speech perception in infants. *Science* 171:303, 1972.

Eisele W, Berry R, Shriner T: Infant sucking response patterns as a conjugate function of change in the sound pressure level of auditory stimuli. *J Speech Hear Res* 18:296–307, 1975.

Eisen NH: Some effects of early sensory deprivation on later behavior: The quondom hard-of-hearing child. *J Abnorm Soc Psychol* 65:338, 1962.

Eisenberg RB: Auditory behavior in the human neonate: Functional properties of sound and their ontogenetic implications. *Int Audiol* 8:34–45, 1969.

Eisenberg RB: The development of hearing in man: An assessment of current status. *Asha* 12:119–123, 1970.

Eisenberg RB: In Stark RE: *Sensory Capabilities of Hearing-Impaired Children.* Baltimore: University Park Press, 1974, pp 23–30.

Eisenberg RB: Cardiotachometry. In Bradford L: *Physiological Measures of the Audio-Vestibular System.* New York: Academic Press, 1975.

Eisenberg RB: *Auditory Competence in Early Life.* Baltimore: University Park Press, 1976.

Eisenberg RB, Coursin DB, Rupp NR: Habituation to an acoustic pattern as an index of differences among human neonates. *J Aud Res* 6:239–248, 1966.

Eldridge R, Berlin CI, Money JW, et al: Cochlear deafness, myopia, and intellectual impairment in an Amish family. *Arch Otolaryngol* 88:49–54, 1968.

Eliachar I, Northern J: Studies in tympanometry: Validation of the present technique for determining intra-tympanic pressures through the intact eardrum. *Laryngoscope* 84:247–255, 1974.

Eliachar I, Sando I, Northern J: Measurement of middle ear pressure in guinea pigs. *Arch Otolaryngol* 99:172–176, 1974.

Elliot GB, Elliot KA: Some pathological, radiological and clinical implications of the precocious development of the human ear. *Laryngoscope* 74:1160–1171, 1964.

Elliott L: Effects of noise on perception of speech of children and certain handicapped individuals. *Sound Vibration* 16:12, 1982.

Elliott L, Katz D: *Development of a New Children's Test of Speech Discrimination.* St. Louis: Auditec, 1980.

Elliott LL, Katz DR: Childrens' pure-tone detection. *J Acoust Soc Am* 67:343–344, 1980.

Ely W: Electroacoustic modifications in hearing aids. In Bess F, Freeman B, Sinclair J: *Amplication in Education.* Washington, D.C.: A. G. Bell, 1981, ch 20.

English GM: *Otolaryngology: A Textbook.* New York: Harper & Row, 1976.

English GM, Northern JL, Fria TJ: Chronic otitis media as a cause of sensorineural hearing loss. *Arch Otolaryngol* 98:17–22, 1973.

Erber NP: Use of the auditory numbers test to evaluate speech perception abilities of hearing-impaired children. *J Speech Hear Dis* 45:527, 1980.

Evans JR: Auditory and auditory-visual integration skills as they relate to reading. *The Reading Teacher* 22:625–629, 1969.

Everberg G: Further studies on hereditary unilateral deafness. *Acta Otolaryngol (Stockh)* 51:615–635, 1960.

Eviatar L, Eviatar A: Methods of vestibular testing in infants and children exposed to ototoxic drugs. In Lerner SA, Matz GJ, Hawkins JE (eds): *Aminoglycoside Ototoxicity.* Boston: Little, Brown, 1981, ch 20.

Ewing IR, Ewing AWG: The ascertainment of deafness in infancy and early childhood. *J Laryngol Otol* 59:309–338, 1944.

Falk S, Farmer J: Incubator noise and possible deafness. *Arch Otolaryngol* 97:385, 1973.

Falk SA: Combined effects of noise and ototoxic drugs. *Environ Health Perspect* 5–22, 1972.

Falk SA, Woods NF: Hospital noise-levels and potential health hazards. *N Engl J Med* 289:774, 1973.

Fant LJ Jr: An appraisal of the oral and combined methods of communication in the education of deaf children. Mimeographed manuscript prepared by Department of Education. Gallaudet College. Washington, D.C., 1963.

Fant LJ Jr: *Say It with Hands.* Washington, D.C.: Gallaudet College, 1964.

Fantz RL: The origin of form perception. *Sci Am* 204:66–72, 1961.

Fay TH: Audiologic and otologic screening of disadvantaged children. In Glorig A, Gerwin K: *Otitis Media.* Springfield, Ill.: Charles C Thomas, 1972, pp 163–170.

Fedio P, Van Buren JM: Memory deficits during electrical stimulation of the speech cortex in conscious man. *Brain Lang* 1:29–42, 1974.

Feigin RD, Dodge PR: Bacterial meningitis: newer concepts of pathophysiology and neurologic sequellae. *Pediatric Clin North Am* 23:3, 1976.'

Feldman AS, Grimes CT, Grimes LL: Hearing screening in the educational setting. *Semin Speech Lang Hear* 2:101, 1981.

Ferguson DG, Hicks DE, Pfau G: Education of hearing impaired learners. In Lass NJ, McReynolds LV, Northern JL, et al: *Speech, Language and Hearing.* Philadelphia: W. B. Saunders, 1982, ch 45.

Fernandez AO, Ronis ML: The Treacher Collins syndrome. *Arch Otolaryngol* 80:505, 1964.

Field TM, Woodson R, Greenberg R, et al: Discrimination and imitation of facial expressions by neonates. *Science* 218:179–181, 1982.

Fifield D, Earnshaw R, Smither M: A new ear impression technique to prevent acoustic feedback with high powered hearing aids. *Volta Rev* 82:33, 1980.

Finitzo-Hieber T: Classroom acoustics. In Roeser RJ, Downs MP: *Auditory Disorders in School Children.* New York: Thieme-Stratton, 1981, ch 14.

Finitzo-Hieber T: Auditory brainstem response in assessment of infants treated with aminoglycoside antibiotics. In Lerner SA, Matz GJ, Hawkins JE (eds): *Aminoglycoside Ototoxicity.* Boston: Little, Brown, 1981, ch 18.

Finitzo-Hieber T: Auditory brainstem response: its place in infant audiological evaluations. *Semin Speech Lang Hear* 3:76–87, 1982.

Finitzo-Hieber T, McCracken G, Roeser R, et al: Ototoxicity in neonates treated with gentamicin and kanamycin: results of a four-year controlled follow-up study. *Pediatrics* 63:443, 1979.

Finitzo-Hieber T, Gerling IJ, Matkin ND, et al: A sound effects recognition test for the pediatric audiologic evaluation. *Ear Hear* 1:271, 1980.

Finitzo-Hieber T, Simhadri R, Hieber JP: Auditory brainstem response assessment of postmeningitic infants and children. *Int J Pediatr Otorhinolaryngol* 3:275, 1981.

Fior R: Physiological maturation of auditory function between 3–13 years of age. *Audiology* 11:317–321, 1972.

Fisher B: An investigation of binaural hearing aids. *J Laryngol Otol* 73:658–668, 1964.

Fisher HG, Freedman SJ: The role of the pinna in auditory localization. *J Aud Res* 8:15–26, 1968.

Fitch JL, Williams TF, Etienne JE: A community based high risk register for hearing loss. *J Speech Hear Dis* 47:373–375, 1982.

Fletcher H: *Speech and Hearing.* New York: Van Nostrand, 1929.

Folsom RC, Widen JE, Wilson WR: Auditory brainstem response in Down's syndrome infants. Paper presented to the American Speech-Language-Hearing Association 1981 Annual Convention, Los Angeles.

Ford FR: *Diseases of the Nervous System in Infancy, Childhood, and Adolescence,* ed 5. Springfield, Ill.: Charles C Thomas, 1966.

Forgus RH: The effect of early perceptual learning on the behavioral organization of adult rats. *J Comp Physiol Psychol* 47:331–336, 1954.

Fosmoe RJ, Holm RS, Hildreth RC: Van Buchem's disease (hyperstosis corticalis generalisata familiaris). *Radiology* 90:771–774, 1968.

Fowler ER: Deafness from mumps. *Arch Pediatr* 77:243–246, 1960.

Fowler FP, Fletcher H: Three million deafened school children: their detection and treatment *JAMA* 87:1877–1882, 1926.

Frank R, Karlovich R: Ear canal frequency response and speech discrimination performance as a function of hearing aid mold type. *J Aud Res* 13:124–129, 1973.

Frankenburg W: Evaluation of screening procedures. In Gold EM: *Earlier Recognition of Handicapping Conditions in Childhood: Proceedings of a Biregional Institute*, University of California, Berkeley: School of Public Health, 1970, pp 42–51.

Frankenburg WK, Dodds JB: The Denver developmental screening test. *J Pediatr* 71:181–191, 1967.

Franklin B: The effect of combining low and high frequency passbands on consonant recognition in the hearing impaired. *J Speech Hear Res* 18:719–727, 1975.

Frazen LE, Elmore J, Nadler HL: Mandibulofacial dysostosis. *Am J Dis Child* 113:405, 1967.

Fraser GR: Our genetical load. *Ann Hum Genet* 25:387–415, 1962.

Fraser GR: Association of congenital deafness with goiter (Pendred's syndrome). A study of 207 families. *Ann Hum Genet* 28:201–249, 1965.

Fraser GR: The genetics of congenital deafness. *Otolaryngol. Clin North Am* 4:227–247, 1971.

Fraser GR: *The Causes of Profound Deafness in Childhood*. Baltimore: The Johns Hopkins University Press, 1976.

Fraser GR, Froggatt P, James T: Congenital deafness associated with EKG abnormalities, fainting, attacks and sudden death: a recessive syndrome. *Q J Med* 33:361, 1964.

Freedman AM, Kaplan HJ: *Comprehensive Textbook of Psychiatry*. Baltimore: Williams & Wilkins, 1967, pp 1434–1438

Freeman B, Sinclair J, Riggs D: Electroacoustic performance characteristics of FM auditory trainers. *J Speech Hear Disord* 45:16–26, 1980.

Freeman BA, Parkins C: The prevalence of middle ear disease among learning impaired children. *Clin Pediatr* 18:205–212, 1979.

French NR, Steinberg JC: Factors governing the intelligibility of speech sounds. *J Acoust Soc Am* 19:90–119, 1947.

Freud S: *Beyond the Pleasure Principle*. London: Hogarth Press, 1948.

Freyss G, Narcy P, Manac'h Y, et al: Acoustic reflex as a predictor of middle ear effusion. *Ann Otol Rhinol Laryngol* 89 (Suppl 68): 196–199, 1980.

Fria T: The auditory brain stem response: background and clinical applications. *Monogr Contemp Audiol* 2(2): 1980.

Fria T, LeBlanc J, Kristensen R, et al: Ipsilateral acoustic reflex stimulation in normal and sensorineural impaired ears; a preliminary report. *Can J Otol* 4:695–703, 1975.

Friedlander BZ: Receptive language development in infancy. *Merrill-Palmer Q Behav Dev* 16:7–51, 1970.

Friedman A, Schulman R, Weiss S: Hearing and diabetic neuropathy. *Arch Intern Med* 135:573–576, 1975.

Friedmann I, Fraser GR, Froggatt P: Pathology of the ear in the cardioauditory syndrome of Jervell and Lange-Nielsen. *J Laryngol Otol* 80:451–470, 1966.

Friel-Patti S, Finitzo-Hieber T, Conti G, et al: Language delay in infants associated with middle ear disease and mild, fluctuating hearing impairment. *Pediatric Infectious Diseases* 1:104–109, 1982.

Froeschels E, Beebe H: Testing hearing of newborn infants. *Arch Otolaryngol* 44:710–714, 1946.

Fromkin V, Krashen S, Curtiss S, et al: The development of language in Genie: a case of language acquisition beyond the "critical period." *Brain Lang* 1:81–107, 1974.

Fryer DG, Winckleman AC, Ways PO, et al: Refsum's disease. *Neurology (Minneap.)* 21:162–167, 1971.

Fulton R, Lloyd I: Hearing impairment in a population of children with Down's syndrome. *Am J Ment Defic* 73:298–302, 1968.

Fulton RT, Lamb LE: Acoustic impedance and tympanometry with the retarded: a normative study. *Audiology* 11:199–208, 1972.

Fulton RT, Lloyd LL (eds): *Audiometry for the Retarded with Implications for the Difficult-to-Test*. Baltimore: Williams & Wilkins, 1969.

Furusho T: A genetic study on the congenital deafness. *Jpn J Hum Genet* 2:35–58, 1957.

Gabbard SA: References for communication disorders related to otitis media. *Semin Speech Lang Hear* 3:351, 1982.

Gaeth JH, Lounsbury E: Hearing aids and children in elementary schools. *J Speech Hear Disord* 31:283–289, 1966.

Galambos R, Hecox KE: Clinical applications of the auditory brainstem response. *Otolaryngol Clinics North Am* 11:709–721, 1978.

Galambos R, Hicks G, Wilson MJ: Hearing loss in graduates of a tertiary intensive care nursery. *Ear Hear* 3:87–90, 1982.

Galambos R, Hicks GE, Wilson MJ: Identification audiometry in neonates: a reply to Simmons. *Ear Hear* 3:189–190, 1982.

Gallagher JC: *Histology of the Temporal Bone*. Washington, D.C.: Armed Forces Institute of Pathology, 1967.

Gallaudet College Public Service Programs, "What Every Person Should Know About Heredity and Deafness," Washington, D.C., 1975.

Gans D, Flexer C: Observer bias in the hearing testing of profoundly involved multiply handicapped children. *Ear Hear* 3:309–313, 1982.

Gardner H: The forgotten lesson of Monsieur C. *Psychology Today*, August 1973.

Gardner RA, Gardner BT: Teaching sign language to a chimpanzee. *Science* 165:664–672, 1969.

Garretson MD: The need for multiple communication skills in the education process of the deaf. *Rocky Mt Leader* 62:1–8, 1963.

Gauger JS, Clymer EW, Young M, et al: *Hearing Aid Orientation*. Rochester, N.Y.: National Technical Institute for the Deaf, 1980.

Gebhart DE: Tympanostomy tubes in the otitis media prone child. *Laryngoscope* 111:849–865, 1981.

Gerber SE, Mencher GT: Arousal responses of neonates to wide band and narrow-band noise. Paper presented to the American Speech-Language-Hearing Association, Atlanta, November 1979.

Gerber SE, Mulac A, Swain BJ: Idiosyncratic cardiovascular response of human neonates to acoustic stimuli. *J Am Audiol Soc* 1:185–192, 1976.

Gerber SE, Mulac A, Lamb ME: The cardiovascular response to acoustic stimuli. *Audiology* 16:1–10, 1977.

Gerkin KP: Infant hearing screening. *Audiol J Cont Educ* 9:3, 1984.

Gerkin KP: The high risk register for deafness: a tutorial. *Asha* 25:4, 1984.

Gerkin KP, Downs MP: The high risk register for newborn screening programs. *Semin Hear* 5:1, 1984.

Geschwind N: The anatomy of acquired disorders of reading. In Money J: *Reading Disability: Progress and Research Needs in Dyslexia*. Baltimore: Johns Hopkins, 1962.

Geschwind N, Levitsky W: Human brain: Left-right asymmetries in temporal speech region. *Science* 161:186–187, 1968.

Gershon A: Infections of fetus and newborn infants. *J Perinat Med* 9:204–206, 1981.

Gesell A: The psychological development of normal and deaf children in their preschool years. *Volta Rev* 58:117–120, 1956.

Gicomelli F, Mozzo W: An experimental and clinical study of the brainstem reticular formation on the stapedial reflex. *Int Audiol* 4:42–44, 1965.

Gilbert JHV: Babbling and the deaf child: a commentary on Lenneberg et al. (1965) and Lenneberg (1967). *J Child Lang* 9:511–515, 1981.

Giolas T, Epstein A: Comparative intelligibility of word lists and continuous disease. *J Speech Hear Res* 6:349–358, 1963.

Gladney JH, Monteleone PI: Metaphysical dysplasia. Genetic and otolaryngologic aspects. *Arch. Otolaryngol.* 92:147–153, 1970.

Glorig A, Roberts J: Hearing levels of adults by age and sex. Vital and Health Statistics, Series 11, Dept. of HEW, 1965.

Glovsky L: Audiological assessment of a mongoloid population. *Train Sch Bull* 33:27–33, 1966.

Goetzinger CP, Embrey JE, Brooks R: Auditory assessment of cleft palate adults. *Acta Otolaryngol (Stockh)* 52:551–557, 1960.

Goetzinger DP, Harrison C, Baer CJ: Small perceptive hearing loss: its effect in school-age children. *Volta Rev* 66:124–132, 1964.

Goldman R, Sanders JW: Cultural factors and hearing. *Except Child* 35:489–490, 1969.

Goldstein MA: *Problems of the Deaf*. St. Louis: The Laryngoscope Press, 1933.

Goldstein MN: Auditory agnosia for speech ("pure word-deafness"). *Brain Lang* 1:195–204, 1974.

Goldstein R: Auditory dysfunction associated with brain impairment. *Postgrad Med* 48:83–85, 1970.

Goldstein R: Electroencephalic audiometry. In Jerger J: *Modern Developments in Audiology*, ed 2. New York: Academic Press, 1973, pp 407–435.

Goldstein R: Neurophysiology of hearing. In Lass NJ, McReynolds LV, Northern JL, et al (eds): *Speech, Language and Hearing*. Philadelphia: W. B. Saunders, 1982, ch 6.

Goldstein R, Rodman LB: Early components of averaged evoked responses to rapidly repeated auditory stimuli. *J Speech Hear Res* 10:697–705, 1967.

Goldstein R, Tait C: Critique of neonatal hearing evaluation. *J Speech Hear Disord* 36:3–18, 1971.

Goldstein R, McRandle CC, Rodman LB: Site of lesion in cases of hearing loss associated with Rh incompatibility: an argument for peripheral impairment. *J Speech Hear Disord* 37:447–450, 1972.

Goodhill V: Auditory pathway lesions resulting from Rh incompatibility. In McConnell F, Ward PH: *Deafness in Childhood*. Nashville, Tenn.: Vanderbilt University Press, 1967, ch 14.

Goodhill V: *Ear Diseases, Deafness and Dizziness*. Hagerstown, Md.: Harper & Row, 1979.

Goodman RM, Lackareff S, Gwinup G: Hereditary congenital deafness with onychodystrophy. *Arch Otolaryngol* 90:474–477, 1969.

Gorlin RJ, Anderson RC, Blaw M: Multiple lentigines syndrome. *Am J Dis child* 117:652–662, 1969.

Graham MD: A longitudinal study of ear disease and hearing loss in patients with cleft lips and palates. *Trans Am Acad Opthalmol Otolaryngol* 67:213–222, 1963.

Green DS: Non-occluding earmolds with CROS and IROS hearing aids. *Arch Otolaryngol* 89:512–522, 1969.

Greenberg D, Wilson W, Moore J, et al: Visual reinforcement audiometry (VRA) with young Down's syndrome children. *J Speech Hear Dis* 43:448–458, 1978.

Greenberg MT: Hearing families with deaf children: stress and functioning as related to communication method. *Am Ann Deaf* 125:1063, 1980.

Greenough WT: Experiential modification of the developing brain. *Am Sci* 63:37–46, 1975.

Greenstein JM, Greenstein BB, McConville K, et al: Mother-Infant Communication, and Language Acquisition in Deaf Infants. New York, Lexington School for the Deaf, 1976.

Greenway EB: The communication needs of the deaf child. In Report of the Proceedings of the International Congress on the Education of the Deaf, pp. 433–439. Washington, D.C., Gallaudet College, 1964.

Gregg JB, Steele JP, Clifford S, Werthman HE: A multidisciplinary study of ear disease in South Dakota. *S. Dak. J. Med.* 23:11–20, 1970.

Grier JB, Counter SA, Shearer WM: Prenatal auditory imprinting in chickens. *Science* 155:1692–1693, 1980.

Griffing TS, Simonton KM, Hedgecock LD: Verbal auditory screening for pre-school children. *Trans Am Acad Ophthalmol Otolaryngol* 71:105–111, 1967.

Groht MA: *Natural Language for Deaf Children*. Washington, D.C.: Gallaudet College Press, 1958.

Groothuis JR, Altemeier WA, Wright PF et al: The evolution and resolution of otitis media in infants: tympanometric findings. In Harford ER, Bess FH, Bluestone CD, et al: *Impedance Screening for Middle Ear Disease in Children*. New York: Grune & Stratton, 1978, pp 105–109.

Groothuis JR, Sell SHW, Wright PF, et al: Otitis media in infancy: tympanometric findings. *Pediatrics* 63:435–442, 1979.

Grundy BL, Heros RC, Tung AS, et al: Intraoperative hypoxia detected by evoked potential monitoring. *Anesth Analg* 60:437–439, 1981.

Grusberg CM, Rudoy R, Nelson JD: Acute mastoiditis in infants and children. *Clin Pediatr* 19:8, 549–553, 1980.

Guberina P, Asp C: The verbo-tonal method for rehabilitating people with communication problems. Int. Exchange of Info. in Rehab., World Rehab. Fund, Inc., Monograph No. 13, New York, 1981.

Halfond MM, Ballenger JJ: An audiologic and otorhinologic study of cleft lip and cleft palate cases. *Arch Otolaryngol* 64:58–62, 1956.

Hall J: Predicting hearing loss from the acoustic reflex. In Jerger J, Northern JL: *Clinical Impedance Audiometry*, ed 2. Acta, Mass.: American Electromedics Corp., 1980, ch 8.

Hall J, Bleakney M: Hearing loss prediction by the acoustic reflex: comparison of seven methods. *Ear Hear* 2:156, 1981.

Hall J, Weaver T: Impedance audiometry in a young population: the effect of age, sex and tympanogram abnormalities. *J Otolaryngol* 8:211, 1979.

Hall JG, Rohrt T: The stapes in osteogenesis imperfecta. *Acta Otolaryngol (Stockh)* 65:345–348, 1968.

Hall JL II: Binaural interaction in the accessory superior olivary nucleus of the cat. *J Acoust Soc* 37:814–823, 1965.

Hall PK, Tomblin JB: A follow-up study of children with articulation and language disorders. *J Speech Hear Dis* 43:227–241, 1978.

Hallgren V: Retinitis pigmentosa combined with congenital deafness; with vestibulo-cerebellar ataxia and mental abnormality in a portion of cases. *Acta Psychiatr Scand Suppl* 138:1–101, 1959.

Hanners B, Sitton A: Ears to hear: a daily hearing aid monitoring program. *Volta Rev* 76:530–536, 1974.

Hanshaw J, Scheiner A, Moxley A, et al: School failure and deafness after "silent" congenital cytomegalovirus infection. *N Engl J Med* 295:468, 1976.

Harboyan G, Mamo J, der Kalonstian V, et al: Congenital corneal dystrophy. Progressive sensorineural deafness in a family. *Arch Ophthalmol* 85:27–32, 1971.

Harford E, Barry J: A rehabilitative approach to the problems of unilateral hearing impairment: the contralateral routing of signals (CROS). *J Speech Hear Disord* 30:121–128, 1965.

Harford E, Dodds E: The clinical application of CROS. *Arch Otolaryngol* 83:455–464, 1966.

Harford ER: Tympanometry. In Jerger J, Northern JL: *Clinical Impedance Audiometry*. Acton, Mass.: American Electromedics Corp., 1980, ch. 3.

Harford ER, Markle DM: The atypical effect of hearing aid on one patient with congenital deafness. *Laryngoscope* 65:970–972, 1955.

Harford ER, Bess FH, Bluestone CD, et al (eds): *Impedance Screening for Middle Ear Disease in Children*. New York: Grune & Stratton, 1978.

Harker LA, Van Wagoner R: Application of impedance audiometry as a screening instrument. *Acta Otolaryngol* 77:198–201, 1974.

Harker LA, Van Wagoner RS: Eustachian tube malfunction in southeast Alaska. *Alaska Med* 18:13–15, 1976.

Harris D: Action potential suppression, tuning curves and thresholds: Comparison with single fiber data. *Hear Res* 1:133, 1979.

Harris JD: Combinations of distortion in speech. The 25% safety factor by multiple-cueing. *Arch Otolaryngol* 72:227–232, 1960.

Harris JD: Pure-tone acuity and the intelligibility of everyday speech. *J Acoust Soc Am* 37:821–830, 1965.

Harris JD: Monaural and binaural speech intelligibil-

ity and the stereophonic effect based on temporal cues. *Laryngoscope* 75:428–446, 1965.

Hart BO: A child centered language program. In *Report of the Proceedings of the International Congress of the Education of the Deaf and the 41st Meeting of the Convention of American Instructors of the Deaf. Gallaudet College*. Washington, D.C.: U.S. Govt. Printing Office, 1964, pp 505–514.

Harter DH, Gordon SR: Slow virus infections of the nervous system; I. Diseases due to conventional viruses. *Medical Times* 106:28–34, April 1978.

Haskins H: A phonetically balanced test of speech discrimination for children, unpublished Master's thesis, 1949. (Cited by J O'Neill and H Oyer, in *Applied Audiometry*, New York: Dodd, Mead, 1966.)

Haskins HI, Hardy WG: Clinical studies in stereophonic listening. *Laryngoscope* 70:1427–1433, 1960.

Haug O, Baccaro P, Guilford F: A pure-tone audiogram on the infant: the PIWI technique. *Arch Otolaryngol* 86:101–106, 1967.

Hawkins JE Jr: Iatrogenic toxic deafness in children. In McConnell, Ward PH: *Deafness in Childhood*. Nashville, Tenn.: Vanderbilt University Press, 1976, pp 156–168.

Hayes E, Babin R, Platz C: The otologic manifestations of mucopolysaccharidoses. *Am J Otol* 2:65, 1980.

Hayman C, Kester F: Eye, ear, nose and throat infection in natives of Alaska. *Northwest Med* 56:423–430, 1957.

Hearing Levels of Children by Demographic and Socioeconomic Characteristics: U.S. Dept. of HEW, Nat'l. Center for Health Statistics, Pub. No. (HSM) 72–1025, 1972.

Hebb DO: The effects of early experience on problem-solving at maturity. *Am Psychol* 2:306–307, 1947.

Heber R, Garber H: An experiment in the prevention of cultural-familial mental retardation. U.S. Dept. of HEW, Office of Education, Ed. Resources Inf. Center, Washington, D.C., ED 059762, PS 005367, 1970.

Hecox K, Galambos R: Brainstem auditory evoked responses in human infants and adults. *Arch Otolaryngol* 99:30–33, 1974.

Hecox K, Squires N, Galambos R: Brainstem auditory evoked responses in man. I. Effect of stimulus rise-fall time and duration. *J Acoust Soc Am* 60:1187–1192, 1976.

Hefferman HP, Simons MR: Temporary increase in sensorineural hearing loss with hearing aid use. *Ann Otol Rhinol Laryngol* 88:86–91, 1979.

Hemenway WG, Berstrom I: Dysplasias of the inner ear. In Bergsma D: *Birth Defects, Atlas and Compendium*. Baltimore: Williams & Wilkins, published for the National Foundation—March of Dimes, 1972.

Herbets G: Otological observations on the Treacher Collins syndrome. *Acta Otolaryngol* 54:457, 1962.

Herrmann C Jr, Aguilar MJ, Sacks OW: Hereditary photomyoclonus associated with diabetes mellitus, deafness, nephropathy and cerebral dysfunction. *Neurology* 14:212–221, 1964.

Hersch B, Amon C: An approach to reporting the diagnosis of hearing loss in parents of a hearing impaired child, unpublished manuscript, University of Denver, 1973.

Hersher L: Minimal brain dysfunction and otitis media. *Percept Mot Skills* 47:723–726, 1978.

Hicks WM, Hicks DE: The Usher's syndrome adolescent: programming implications for school administrators, teachers, and resident advisors. *Am Ann Deaf* 126:422–431, 1981.

Himalstein MR: Phylogeny of the temporal bone and temporomandibular joint. *Ear Nose Throat J* 57:42, 1978.

Hinchcliffe R: Epidemiological aspects of otitis media. In Glorig A, Gerwin K: *Otitis Media.* Springfield, Ill.: Charles C Thomas, 1972, pp 36–43.

Hirsh I: Comment reported. In Levitt H, Nye P: *Proceedings of a Conference on Sensory Training Aids for the Hearing Impaired.* Washington, D.C.: National Academy of Engineering, Subcommittee on Sensory Aids, 1971.

Hirsh JE: Effect of interaural time delay on amplitude of cortical responses evoked by tones. *J Neurophysiol* 31:916–927, 1969.

Hitselberger WE, Hughes RL: Bilateral acoustic tumors and neurofibromatosis. *Arch Otolaryngol* 88:700–711, 1968.

Hodge DC, McCommons BM: Acoustical hazards of children's toys. *J Acoust Soc Am* 40:911, 1966.

Hodgson W: Audiological report of a patient with left hemispherectomy. *J Speech Hear Disord* 32:39–45, 1967.

Hodgson W, Murdock C: Effects of the earmold on speech intelligibility in hearing aid use. *J Speech Hear Res* 13:290–297, 1970.

Hodgson WR: Speech discrimination of children with suspected central nervous system impairments. Paper presented at the annual Hearing and Speech Seminar, Kansas City Medical Center, 1966.

Hodgson WR: Testing infants and young children. In Katz J: *Handbook of Clinical Audiology*, ed 2. Baltimore: Williams & Wilkins, 1978, Ch 33.

Hodgson WR, Skinner PH: *Hearing Aid Assessment and Use in Audiological Habilitation*, ed 2. Baltimore: Williams & Wilkins, 1981.

Holborow CA: Deafness associated with cleft palate. *Laryngoscope* 76:762–773, 1962.

Holcomb RK, Corbett EE: Mainstream—The Delaware Approach. Newark School District (Sterk School), Newark, Del., 1975.

Holm VA, Kunze LH: Effect of chronic otitis media on language and speech development. *Pediatrics* 43:833–839, 1969.

Holmes EM: The microtia ear. *Arch Otolaryngol* 49:243–265, 1949.

Holmes LB: Norrie's disease; an X-linked syndrome of retinal malformation, mental retardation, and deafness. *J Pediatr* 70:89–92, 1971.

Holmgren L: Can the hearing be damaged by a hearing aid? *Acta Otolaryngol (Stockh)* 28:440, 1940.

Holt R, Young W: Acute coalescent mastoiditis. *Otolaryngol Head Neck Surg* 89:317–321, 1981.

Hood DC: Evoked cortical response audiometry. In Bradford L: *Physiological Measures of the Audio-Vestibular System.* New York: Academic Press, 1975, ch 10.

Hood J, Poole J: Tolerable limit of loudness: its clinical and physiological significance. *J Acoust Soc Am* 40:47–53, 1966.

Hook PE: Learning disabilities in the hearing impaired. *Ear Nose Throat J* 58:40–52, 1979.

Horn JM: Duration of preschool effects on later school competence. *Science* 213:1145, 1981.

Horton KB: Early intervention through parent training. *Otolaryngol Clin North Am* 8:143–157, 1975.

House H, Crabtree J: Mastoiditis. In English FM: *Otolaryngology*, rev ed. Hagerstown, Md.: Harper & Row, 1978, vol 2, pp 1–9.

House WF: Subarachnoid shunt for drainage of hydrops: a report of 63 cases. *Arch Otolaryngol* 79:338–354, 1964.

Hoversten G: A public school audiology program: Amplification, maintenance, auditory management, and in-service education. In Bess F, Freeman B, Sinclair J: *Amplification in Education.* Washington, D.C.: A. G. Bell, 1981, ch 15.

Hoversten GH, Fornby D: Mainstreaming—the controversy. In Roeser R, Downs M: *Auditory Disorders in School Children*, New York: Thieme-Stratton, 1981, ch 4.

Hoverston G, Moncur J: Stimuli and intensity factors in testing infants. *J Speech Hear Res* 12:687–702, 1969.

Howie VM: Natural history of otitis media. *Ann Otol Rhinol Laryngol Suppl* 19:67–72, 1975.

Howie VM, Ploussard JH: Treatment of serous otitis media with ventilatory tubes. *Clin Pediatr* 13:919, 1974.

Howie VM, Ploussard JH, Sloyer J: The "otitis-prone" condition. *Am J Dis Child* 129:676–678, 1975.

Howie VM, Grabowski ML, Ploussard JH: Comparison between impedance audiometry and pneumatic otoscopy in the diagnosis of middle ear effusion in the young infant. Presented at the fourth annual meeting of the Society for Ear, Nose and Throat Advances in Children, New Orleans, November 1976.

Hull FM, Mielke PW, Timmons RJ, et al.: The National Speech and Hearing Survey: preliminary results. *Asha* 13:501–509, 1971.

Human Communication and its Disorders—an Overview: R Carhart (ed): Nat'l. Instit. of Neurol. Diseases and Stroke, U.S. Dept. of HEW, Bethesda, Md., 1969.

Humes L, Bess F: Tutorial on the potential deterioration in hearing due to hearing aid usage. *J Speech Hear Res* 46:3–15, 1981.

Hunt J McV: *Intelligence and Experience.* New York: Ronald Press, 1961.

Hyman CB: CNS abnormalities after neonatal hemolyte disease or hyperbilirubinemia. *Am J Dis Child* 117:395–405, 1969.

Ide CH, Wollschlaeger PP: Multiple congenital abnormalities associated with cryptophthalmia. *Arch. Ophthalmol* 81:640–644, 1969.

Illum P: The Mondini type of cochlear malformation. *Acta Otolaryngol* 96:305–311, 1972.

Illum P, Kaier HW, Hvidberg-Hansen J, et al: Fifteen cases of Pendred's syndrome. *Arch Otolaryngol* 96:297–304, 1972.

Irwin OC: Infant speech: Consonantal sounds according to manner of articulation. *J Speech Hear Disord* 12:402–404, 1947.

Irwin OC: Infant speech, the effect of family occupational status and of age on use of sound frequency. *J Speech Hear Disord* 13:320–323, 1952.

Irwin OC: Identification audiometry for school-age children: basic procedures. *J Speech Hear Disord* (monogr) 9:26–34, 1961.

Iwashita H, Inoue N, Araki S, et al: Optic atrophy, neural deafness, and distal neurogenic amyotrophy. *Arch Neurol* 22:357–364, 1970.

Jacobs JN, et al: A follow-up evaluation of the Frostig Visual Perception Training Program. *Educational Leadership Research Suppl.* 169–175, November 1968.

Jacobson JT, Morehouse CR, Johnson MJ: Strategies for infant auditory brain stem response assessment. *Ear Hear* 3:263–270, 1982.

Jaffe BF: Congenital shoulder-neck-auditory anomalies. *Laryngoscope* 58:2119–2139, 1968.

Jaffe BF: The incidence of ear diseases in the Navajo Indians. *Laryngoscope* 58:2126–2133, 1968.

Jaffe BF (ed): *Hearing Loss in Children.* Baltimore: University Park Press, 1977.

Jaffe B, Hurtado F, Hurtado E: Tympanic membrane mobility in the newborn: With seven months' follow-up. *Laryngoscope* 80:36–48, 1970.

Jarvis JF: Audiological status of children with cleft palate: A review of 350 cases. *Audiology* 15:242–248, 1976.

Jepsen O: Middle ear muscle reflexes in man. In Jerger J: *Modern Developments in Audiology.* New York: Academic Press, 1963, pp 193–239.

Jerger J: Clinical experience with impedance audiometry. *Arch Otolaryngol* 92:311–324, 1970.

Jerger J, Dirks D: Binaural hearing aids: an enigma. *J Acoust Soc* 33:537–538, 1961.

Jerger J, Hayes D: The cross-check principle in pediatric audiometry. *Arch Otolaryngol* 102:614–620, 1976.

Jerger J, Hayes D: Diagnostic applications of impedance audiometry: middle ear disorder; sensorineural disorder. In Jerger J, Northern JL: *Clinical Impedance Audiometry*, ed 2. Acton, Mass.: American Electromedics Corp., 1980, ch 6, pp 109–127.

Jerger J, Jerger S: Temporary threshold shift in rock-and-roll muscians. *J Speech Hear Res* 13:218–224, 1970.

Jerger J, Jerger S: Auditory findings in brainstem disorders. *Arch Otolaryngol* 99:342–350, 1974.

Jerger J, Lewis N: Binaural hearing aids: Are they dangerous for children? *Arch Otolaryngol* 101:480–483, 1975.

Jerger J, Northern JL (eds): *Clinical Impedance Audiometry*, ed 2. Acton, Mass.: American Electromedics Corp., 1980.

Jerger J, Thelin J: Effects of electroacoustic characteristics of hearing aids on speech understanding. *Bull Prosthet Res* 110:159–197, 1968.

Jerger J, Jerger S, Mauldin L: Studies in impedance audiometry: I. Normal and sensorineural ears. *Arch Otolaryngol* 96:513–523, 1972.

Jerger J, Anthony L, Jerger S, et al: Studies in impedance audiometry; III. Middle ear disorders. *Arch Otolaryngol* 99:165–171, 1974a.

Jerger J, Burney P, Mauldin L, et al: Predicting hearing loss from the acoustic reflex. *J Speech Hear Disord* 39:11–22, 1974b.

Jerger J, Hayes D, Anthony L, et al: Factors influencing prediction of hearing level from the acoustic reflex. *Contemp Monogr Audiol* 1:1, 1978.

Jerger J, Hayes D, Jordon C: Clinical experience with auditory brainstem response audiometry in pediatric assessment. *Ear Hear* 1:19–25, 1980.

Jerger J, Hayes D, Smith S, et al: Auditory Brainstem Response in Clinical Practice—Course Syllabus. Department of Otorhinolaryngology and Communicative Sciences, Baylor College of Medicine, 1981.

Jerger S: Speech audiometry. In Jerger J (ed): *Pediatric Audiology.* San Diego: College Hill Press, 1984.

Jerger S, Jerger J: Pediatric speech intelligibility test: performance—intensity characteristics. *Ear Hear* 4:138–145, 1983.

Jerger S, Jerger J, Mauldin L, et al: Studies in impedance audiometry; II. Children less than 6 years old. *Arch Otolaryngol* 99:1–9, 1974.

Jerger S, Lewis S, Hawkins J, et al: Pediatric speech intelligibility test: I. Generation of test materials. *Int J Pediatr Otorhinolaryngol* 2:217–230, 1980.

Jerger S, Jerger J, Lewis S: Pediatric speech intelligibility test; II. Effect of receptive language age and chronological age. *Int J Pediat Otorhinolaryngol* 3:101–118, 1981.

Jervell A, Lange-Nielsen F: Congenital deaf-mutism, functional heart disease with prolongation of the QT interval, and sudden death. *Am Heart J* 54:59–68, 1957.

Jewett D: Volume conducted potentials in response to auditory stimuli as detected by averaging in the cat. *Electroencephalogr Clin Neurophysiol* 28:609–618, 1970.

Jewett D, Williston JS: Auditory evoked far fields averaged from the scalp of humans. *Brain* 94:681–696, 1971.

Jirsa R, Norris TW: Relationship of acoustic gain to aided threshold improvement in children. *J Speech Hear Dis* 43:3, 348–351, 1978.

Johansson B: A new coding amplifier system for the severely hard of hearing. In *Proceedings of the Third International Conference on Acoustics,* Stuttgart, 1959, 2, published 1961, pp 655–657.

Johansson B: The use of the transposer for the management of the deaf child. *Int Audiol* 5:362–372, 1966.

Johansson B, Wedenberg E, Westin B: Measurement of tone response by the human fetus. *Acta Otolaryngol (Stockh)* 57:188–192, 1964.

Johnson D, Caccamise F: Hearing-impaired populations: optimizing the use of vision for academic, career and communications program planning. *Am Ann Deaf* 126:317, 1981.

Johnson J: Binaural hearing instrument system—the biphasic. *Hear Instruments* 26:20–22, 1975.

Johnson JS, Watrous BS: An acoustic impedance screening program with an American Indian population. In Harford ER, Bess FH, Bluestone CD, et al: *Impedance Screening for Middle Ear Disease in Children.* New York: Grune & Stratton, 1978.

Johnson RL: Chronic otitis media in school age Navajo Indians. *Laryngoscope* 77:1990–1995, 1967.

Johnsson LG, Arenburg K: Cochlear abnormalities in Alport's syndrome. *Arch Otolaryngol* 107:340–349, 1981.

Johnston CC, Lawy N, Lord T, et al: Osteopetrosis. A clinical, genetic, metabolic, and morphologic study of the dominantly inherited benign form. *Medicine* 47:149–167, 1968.

Joint Committee on Infant Hearing 1982 Statement. *Asha* 24:1017–1018, 1982

Jones FR, Simmons FB: Early identification of significant hearing loss; the Crib-o-gram. *Hear Instruments* 28:8–10, 1977.

Jones MD, Mulcahy ND: Osteopathia striata, osteopetrosis, and impaired hearing. *Arch Otolaryngol* 87:20–22, 1968.

Jordan IK, Gustason G, Rosen R: Current communication trends at programs for the deaf. *Am Ann Deaf* 121:527–532, 1976.

Jordan O: Mental retardation and hearing defects. *Scand Audiol* 1:29–32, 1972.

Jordan O, Greisen O, Bentzen O: Treatment with binaural hearing aids. *Arch Otolaryngol* 85:319–326, 1967.

Jordan RE, Eagles EL: The relation of air conduction audiometry to otologic abnormalities. *Ann Otol Rhinol Laryngol* 70:819–827, 1961.

Jusczyk PW, Thompson E: Perception of a phonetic contrast in multisyllabic utterances by 2-month-old infants. *Percept Psychophysics* 23:105–109, 1978.

Kaga K, Tanaka Y: Auditory brainstem response and behavioral audiometry. *Arch Otolaryngol* 106:564–566, 1980.

Kagan J: Do infants think? *Sci Am* 226:74–82, 1972.

Kahane JC: Pathophysiologic effects of Mobius syndrome on speech and hearing. *Arch Otolaryngol* 105:29–34, 1979.

Kannapell BM, Hamilton IB, Bornstein H: *Signs for Instructional Purposes.* Washington, D.C.: Gallaudet College Press, 1969.

Kaplan GK, Fleshman JK, Bender TR, et al: Long-term effects of otitis media; a 10-year cohort study of Alaska Eskimo children. *Pediatrics* 52:577–585, 1973.

Kaplan S, Goddard J, Van Kleeck M, et al: Ataxia and deafness in children due to bacterial meningitis. *Pediatrics* 68:8–12, 1981.

Karmody CS, Schuknecht HF: Deafness in congenital syphilis. *Arch Otolaryngol* 83:18–26, 1966.

Karchmer M, Trybus R: Who are the deaf children in "mainstream" programs? *Annual Survey of Hearing Impaired Children and Youth, Series R, No. 4.* Washington, D.C.: Office of Demographic Studies, Gallaudet College, 1977.

Kasten R, Braunlin R: Traumatic hearing aid usage: a case study. Presented at the American Speech and Hearing Association Convention, 1970.

Keane WM, Potsic WP, Rowe LD, et al: Meningitis and hearing loss in children. *Arch Otolaryngol* 105:39–44, 1979.

Kearsley R, Snider M, Richie R, et al: Study of relations between psychologic environment and child behavior. *Am J Dis Child* 104:12–20, 1962.

Keen RC, Chase W, Graham FK: Twenty-four hour retention by neonates of an habituated heart rate response. *Psychon Sci* 2:265–266, 1965.

Keith R: Impedance audiometry with neonates. *Arch Otolaryngol* 97:465–467, 1973.

Keith RW: Middle ear function in neonates. *Arch Otolaryngol* 101:376–379, 1975.

Keith RW (ed): *Central Auditory Dysfunction.* New York: Grune & Stratton, 1977a.

Keith RW: An evaluation of predicting hearing loss from the acoustic reflex. *Arch Otolaryngol* 103:419, 1977b.

Keith RW: Commentary. Letter to the editor. *Audiol Hear Educ* 4:28, 1978.

Keith RW (ed): Auditory perceptual problems in children. *Semin Speech Lang Hear* 1:2, 1980a.

Keith RW (ed): *Audiology for the Physician.* Baltimore: Williams & Wilkins, 1980b.

Keith RW (ed): *Central Auditory and Language Disorders in Children.* Houston: College Hill Press, 1981.

Keith RW: Central auditory tests. In Lass NJ, McReynolds LV, Northern JL, et al (eds): *Speech, Language and Hearing.* Philadelphia: W. B. Saunders, 1982, vol 3.

Keith RW, Bench RJ: Stapedial reflex in neonates. *Scand Audiol* 7:187–191, 1978.

Keith RW, Murphy KP, Martin F: Acoustic impedance measurement in the otological assessment of multiply handicapped children. *Clin Otolaryngol* 1:221–224, 1976.

Keleman G: Toxoplasmosis and congenital deafness. *Arch Otolaryngol* 68:547–561, 1958.

Keleman G: Hurler's syndrome and the hearing organ. *J Laryngol* 80:791–803, 1966.

Keleman G, Hooft C, Kluyskens P: The inner ear in autosomal trisomy. *Pract Otorhinolaryngol (Basel)* 30:251–258, 1968.

Kellman N: Noise in the intensive care nursery. *Neonatal Network,* pp 8–17, August 1982.

Kenny V: A better way to teach deaf children. *Harper's Magazine,* pp 61–65, March 1962.

Kerr G, Smyth GD, Cinnamond M: Congenital syphilitic deafness. *J Laryngol Otol* 87:1–12, 1973.

Kessler ME, Randolph K: The effects of early middle ear disease on the auditory abilities of third grade children. *J Acad Rehabil Aud* 12:6–20, 1979.

Kessner DM, Kalk CE: A strategy for evaluating health services. In *Contrasts in Health Status.* Washington, D.C.: Instit. of Med., Nat'l. Acad. of Sciences, 1973, vol 2.

Kessner DM, Snow CK, Singer J: Assessment of medical care in children. In *Contrasts in Health Status.* Washington, D.C.: Institute of Medicine, Nat'l. Acad. of Sciences, 1974, vol 3.

Killion M: Experimental wideband hearing aid (abstract). *J Acoust Soc Am* 59:562, 1976.

Killion M: Transducers, earmolds and sound quality considerations. In Studebaker G, Bess F (eds): *The Vanderbilt Hearing Aid Report: State of the Art—Research Needs. Monogr Contemp Audiol,* 1982, pp 104–111.

Kimura D: Cerebral dominance and the perception of verbal stimuli. *Can J Psychol* 15:166–171, 1961.

Kimura D: Left-right differences in the perception of melodies. *Q J Exp Psychol* 16:355–358, 1964.

Kinney CE: Pathology of hereditary deafness. *Ann Otol Rhinol Laryngol* 59:1117–1122, 1950.

Kinney CE: The further destruction of partially deafened children's hearing by the use of powerful hearing aids. *Ann Otol Rhinol Laryngol* 70:828–835, 1961.

Kirk SA, McCarthy JP, Kirk WD: *The Illinois Test of Psycholinguistic Abilities,* rev ed. Urbana: University of Illinois Press, 1968.

Kirkham TH: Duane's syndrome and familial perceptive deafness. *Br J Ophthalmol* 53:335–339, 1969.

Kittel G, Schmoll-Eskuche G: Statistische Erhebungen zur Atiologie Ererbter und fruh Erworbener Hochgradiger Perzeptionsstorungen. *Arch Ohren Nasen Kehlkopfheilkd Z Hals Nasen Ohrenheilkd* 181:310–328, 1963.

Kleffner FR: Hearing losses, hearing aids, and children with language disorders. *J Speech Hear Disord* 38:232–239, 1973.

Klein JO: Epidemiology of otitis media. In Wiet RJ, Coulthard SW: *Otitis Media: Proceedings of the Second National Conference on Otitis Media.* Columbus, Ohio: Ross Laboratories, 1979, pp 18–20.

Klein JO: Article in *Washington Post,* May 27, 1981.

Klein JO: Epidemiology and natural history of otitis media. *Pediatrics* 71:639–640, 1983.

Klockhoff I: Middle ear muscle reflexes in man: A clinical and experimental study with special reference to diagnostic problems in hearing impairment. *Acta Otolaryngol (Suppl) (Stockh)* 164:1–91, 1961.

Kloepfer HW, Laguaite JK, McLaurin JW: The hereditary syndrome of deafness in retinitis pigmentosa. *Laryngoscope* 76:850–862, 1966.

Knight CH: Auditory screening of the mentally retarded. Presented at the ASHA convention, 1973.

Kodman F: Education status of the hard-of-hearing children in the classroom. *J Speech Hear Res* 28:297–299, 1963.

Kodman P: Successful binaural hearing aid users. *Arch Otolaryngol* 74:302–314, 1961.

Koenig W: Subjective effects in binaural hearing. *J Acoust Soc* 22:61–62, 1950.

Koenigsberger MR, Chutorian AM, Gold AP, et al: Benign paroxysmal vertigo of childhood. *Neurology* 20:1108–1113, 1970.

Kohl HR: *Language and Education of the Deaf.* New York: Publication of the Center for Urban Education, Policy Study 1, 1966.

Konigsmark BW: Hereditary deafness in man. *N Engl J Med* 281:713–720, 774–778, 827–832, 1969.

Konigsmark BW: Genetic hearing loss with no associated abnormalities: a review. *J Speech Hear Disord* 37:89–99, 1972.

Konigsmark BW, Gorlin RJ: *Genetic and Metabolic Deafness.* Philadelphia: W. B. Saunders, 1976.

Konigsmark BW, Hollander MB, Berlin CI: Familial neural hearing loss and atopic dermatitis. *JAMA* 204:953–957, 1968.

Konigsmark BW, Mengel MC, Haskins H: Familial congenital moderate neural hearing loss. *J Laryngol* 84:495–506, 1970.

Kos AO, Schuknecht HF, Singer JD: Temporal bone studies in 13–15 and 18 trisomy syndrome. *Arch Otolaryngol* 83:439–445, 1966.

Kossowska E, Goralowna M: Prenatal and neonatal prophylaxis in otorhinolaryngology. *Int J Pediatr Otorhinolaryngol* 2:85–98, 1980.

Kothman W: Classroom auditory trainers: meeting students needs. *Hearing Aid J* 34:8–9, 1981.

Krause CJ, McCabe BF: Acoustic neuroma in a seven-year-old girl. *Arch Otolaryngol* 94:359–363, 1971.

Kryter K: *The Effects of Noise on Man.* New York: Academic Press, 1970.

Kryter KD: Impairment to hearing from exposure to noise. *J. Acoust Soc Am* 53:1211–1234, 1973.

Kryter KD, Ades HW: Studies on the function of the higher acoustic nervous centers in the cat. *Am J Psychol* 56:501–536, 1943.

Kryter KD, Williams C, Green DM: Auditory acuity and the perception of speech. *J Acoust Soc Am* 34:1217–1223, 1962.

Kuhl P: Speech perception in early infancy: perceptual constancy for spectrally dissimilar vowel categories. *J Acoust Soc Am* 66:1668–1679, 1979.

Kuhl P, Miller J: Discrimination of auditory target dimensions in the presence or absence of variation in a second dimension by infants. *Percept Psychophysics* 31:279–292, 1982.

Kuhl PK, Hillenbrand J: Speech perception by young infants: perceptual constancy for categories based on pitch contour. Paper presented at the meeting of the Society for Research in Child Development, San Francisco, March 1979.

Kuzniarz J: Hearing Loss and speech intelligibility in noise. In *Proceedings of the International Congress on Noise as a Public Health Problem.* Washington, D.C.: U.S. EPA, Office of Noise Abatement Control, 1973, pp 57–71.

Lamb I, Norris T: Relative acoustic impedance measurements with mentally retarded children. *Am J Ment Defic* 75:51–56, 1970.

Lamb LE, Norris T: Acoustic impedance measurement. In Fulton RT, Lloyd LI: *Audiometry for the Retarded.* Baltimore: Williams & Wilkins, 1969, pp 164–209.

Lane H: *The Wild Boy of Aveyron.* Cambridge: Harvard University Press, 1977.

Langer LO Jr: Diastrophic dwarfism in early infancy. *AJR* 93:399, 1965.

Langer LO Jr: Achondroplasia; clinical radiologic features with comment on genetic implications. *Clin Pediatr* 7:474–478, 1968.

Langer LO Jr, Baumann PA, Gorlin RJ: *Am J Roentgenol Radium Ther Nucl Med* 100:12–15, 1967.

Langford C, Bench J, Wilson I: Some effects of prestimulus activity and length of prestimulus observations of judgments of newborns' responses to sounds. *Audiology* 14:44–52, 1975.

League R, Parker J, Robertson M, et al: Acoustical environments in incubators and infant oxygen tents. *Prev Med* 1:231, 1972.

Lee L: *The Northwestern Syntax Screening Test.* Evanston, Ill.: Northwestern University Press, 1971.

Lehmann MD, et al: The effects of chronic middle ear effusion on speech and language development—a descriptive study. *Int J Pediatr Otorhinolaryngol* 1:137–144, 1979.

Lempert J, Wever EG, Lawrence M: the cochleogram and its clinical application. *Arch Otolaryngol* 45:61–67, 1947.

Lenneberg EH: *Biological Foundations of Language.* New York: John Wiley & Sons, 1967.

Leridan Audiscreen: Leridan Associates (USA), 520 Barker Pass Road, Santa Barbara, Calif. 93108.

Lerner SA, Matz G, Hawkins J: *Aminoglycoside Ototoxicity.* Boston: Little, Brown, 1981.

Leroy JG, Crocker AC: Clinical definition of Hunter-Hurler phenotypes. A review of 50 patients. *Am J Dis Child* 112:518–530, 1966.

Leshin GJ: Childhood non-organic hearing loss. *J Speech Hear Disord* 25:290–292 1960.

Leske MC: Prevalence estimates of communicative disorders in the U.S. language, hearing and vestibular disorders. *Asha* 23:229–236, 1981.

Levine RL: Bilirubin: worked out years ago? *Pediatrics* 64:380–385, 1979.

Levitt H, Nye PW: Sensory Training Aids for the Hearing Impaired. In *Proceedings of a Conference, Easton, MD., 1970.* Washington, D.C.: National Academy of Engineering, Subcommittee on Sensory Aids, 1971.

Lewin R: Starved brains. *Psychology Today*, pp 29–33, September 1975.

Lewis C: The Montana otitis media project. *Hear Instruments* 26:21–22, 1975.

Lewis JL: Semantic processing of unattended messages using dichotic listening. *J Exp Psychol* 85:225–228, 1970.

Lewis M, Goldberg S: Perceptual-cognitive development in infancy: a generalized expectancy model as a function of the mother-infant interaction. *Merrill-Palmer Q Behav Dev* 15:81–100, 1969.

Lewis N: Otitis media and linguistic incompetence. *Arch Otolaryngol* 102:387–390, 1976.

Libby ER (ed): *Binaural Hearing Aid Amplification.* Chicago: Zenetron, Inc., 1980, vols 1 and 2.

Libby ER: Achieving a transparent, smooth, wideband hearing aid response. *Hear Instruments* 32:9–12, 1981.

Libby ER: In search of transparent insertion gain hearing aid responses. In Studebaker G, Bess F (eds): *The Vanderbilt Hearing Aid Report: State of the Art—Research Needs. Monogr Contemp Audiol*, 1982, 112–123.

Liberman A M, Cooper FS, Shankweiler DP, et al: Perception of the speech code. *Psychol Rev* 74:431–461, 1967.

Liden G, Kankkonen A: Visual reinforcement audiometry. *Acta Otolaryngol (Stockh)* 67:281–292, 1961.

Liden G, Peterson JL, Bjorkman G: Tympanometry: a method for analysis of middle-ear function. *Acta Otolaryngol (Stockh)* 263:218–224, 1970.

Lieberman P: *On the Origins of Language.* New York: Macmillan, 1975.

Lieberman P, Harris KS, Wolff P, et al: Newborn infant cry and non-human primate vocalization. *J Speech Hear Res* 14:718–727, 1971.

Liebman J Graham JT: Changes in the parameters of the averaged auditory evoked potentials related to the number of data samples analyzed. *J Speech Hear Res* 10:782–785, 1967.

Lim DH: Three dimensional observation of the inner ear with the scanning electron microscope. *Acta Otolaryngol Suppl* 255, 1969.

Lindsay JR: Labyrinthitis of viral origin. In Graham B: *Sensorineural Hearing Process and Disorders.* Boston: Little, Brown, 1967a.

Lindsay JR: Congenital deafness of inflammatory origin. In McConnell F, Ward PH: *Deafness in Childhood.* Nashville, Tenn.: Vanderbilt University Press, 1967b, pp 142–155.

Lindsay JR: Inner ear histopathology in genetically determined congenital deafness. In *Birth Defects, Part IX, Ear.* Baltimore: Williams & Wilkins, published for National Foundation—March of Dimes, 1971a.

Lindsay JR: Inner ear pathology in congenital deafness. *Otolaryngol. Clin. North Am* (Symposium) 4:2, 1971b.

Lindsay JR, Black FO, Donnelly WN: Acrocephalosyndactyly (Apert's syndrome). Temporal bone findings. *Ann Otol Rhinol Laryngol* 84:174–178, 1975.

Lindsay P, Norman D: *Human Information Processing: An Introduction to Psychology.* New York: Academic Press, 1972, Fig. 7.2, p 95.

Ling D: Implications of hearing aid amplification below 300 cps. *Volta Rev* 66:723–729, 1964.

Ling D: Three experiments on frequency transposition. *Am Ann Deaf* 113:283–294, 1968.

Ling D: Rehabilitation of cases with deafness secondary to otitis media. In Glorig A, Geroin KS: *Otitis Media.* Springfield, Ill.: Charles C Thomas, 1972, pp 249–253.

Ling D: Recent developments affecting the education of hearing-impaired children. *Public Health Rev* 4:117–152, 1975.

Ling D, Maretic H: Frequency transposition in the teaching of speech to deaf children. *J Speech Hear Res* 14:37–46, 1971.

Ling D, McCoy RH, Levinson ED: The incidence of middle ear disease and its educational implications among Baffin Island Eskimo children. *Car J Public Health* 60:385–390, 1969.

Ling D, Ling AH, Doehring DG: Stimulus response and observer variables in the auditory screening of newborn infants. *J Speech Hear Res* 13:9–18, 1970.

Linthicum FH: Surgery of congenital deafness. *Otolaryngol Clin North Am* (Symposium) 4:2, 1971.

Lipscomb DM: Noise exposure and its effects. Otocongress II, Copenhagen, 1972.

Lipscomb DM: Mechanisms of the middle ear. In Northern JL: *Hearing Disorders*, ed 2. Boston: Little, Brown, 1984, ch 21.

Litke RE: Elevated high-frequency hearing in school children. *Arch Otolaryngol* 94:255–257, 1971.

Lloyd LI: Audiological aspects of mental retardation. In Ellis NR: *International Review of Research in Mental Retardation.* New York: Academic Press, 1970, pp 311–374.

Lloyd LI, Spradlin JE, Reid MJ: An operant audiometric procedure for difficult-to-test patients. *J Speech Hear Disord* 33:236–245, 1968.

Long J, Lucey J, Philip A: Noise and hypoxemia in the intensive care nursery. *Pediatrics* 65:143, 1980.

Lous J, Fiellau-Nikolajsen M: Epidemiology of middle ear effusion and tubal dysfunction. *Int J Pediatr Otorhinolaryngol* 3:303–317, 1981.

Lowe SS, Cullen JK, Thompson CL, et al: Dichotic and monotic simultaneous and time-staggered speech. *J Acoust Soc Am* 47:76, 1970.

Lowenstein B, Preger D Jr: *Diabetes, A New Look at an Old Problem.* New York: Harper & Row, 1976.

Lucker JR: Application of pass-fail criteria to middle ear screening results. *Asha* 22:839, 1980.

Luterman D: *Counseling Parents of Hearing-Impaired Children.* Boston: Little, Brown, 1979.

Luterman D, Chasin J: The deafness management quotient as an indicator of oral success. *Volta Rev* 83:405, 1981.

Luria AR: *The Mentally Retarded Child.* Oxford: Pergamon Press, 1963.

Luterman DM: A comparison of language skills of hearing impaired children trained in a visual/oral method and an auditory/oral method. *Am Ann Deaf* 121:389–393, 1976.

Lybarger S: Some comments on CROS. *Natl Hear Aid J* 21:8–33, 1968.

Lybarger S: Earmolds. In Katz J: *Handbook of Clinical Audiology*, ed 2. Baltimore: Williams & Wilkins, 1978.

Lynn GE, Gilroy J: Detection and localization of central auditory disorders. In Northern JL: *Hearing Disorders*, ed 2. Boston: Little, Brown, 1984, ch 16.

Lyon R: Auditory perceptual training: the state of the art. *J Learn Disabil* 10:564–572, 1977.

MacDonald HM: Neonatal asphyxia; I. Relationship of obstetric and neonatal complications to neonatal mortality in consecutive deliveries. *J Pediatr* 96:898–902, 1980.

MacDonald WB, Fitch KD, Lewis IC: Cockayne's syndrome. An heredo-familial disorder of growth and development. *Pediatrics* 25:997–1007, 1960.

Mackintosh HK (ed): Children and Oral Language. Joint publication of the Association for Childhood Education International, Association for Supervision and Curriculum Development, International Reading Association, and the National Council of Teachers of English, 1964.

Macklin F: Mainstreaming: the cost issue. *Am Ann Deaf* 121:364–365, 1976.

Macrae JH: TTS and recovery from TTS after use of powerful hearing aids. *J Acoust Soc Am* 43:1445–1446, 1968a.

Macrae JH: Recovery from TTS in children with sensorineural deafness. *J Acoust Soc Am* 44:1451, 1968b.

Macrae JH, Farrant RH: The effect of hearing aid use on the residual hearing of children with sensorineural deafness. *Ann Otol Rhinol Laryngol* 74:407–419, 1965.

Madell JR: Hearing aid evaluation procedures with children. In Rubin M: *Hearing Aids: Current Developments and Concepts.* Baltimore: University Park Press, 1976, pp 95–102.

Magnuson B: On the origin of the high negative pressure in the middle ear space. *Am J Otolaryngol* 2:1–12, 1981.

Malkin SF, Freeman RD, Hasting JO: Psychosocial problems of deaf children and their families: A comparative study. *Audiol Hear Educ* Part I—2:3, 21–26, Part II—2:4, 31–38, 1976.

Mandell AJ, Smith CK: Hereditary sensory radicular neuropathy. *Neurology* 10:627–630, 1960.

Mangabeira-Albernaz PL, Fukaka J, Chammas F, et al: The Mondini dysplasia—a clinical study. *ORL* 43:131–152, 1981.

Maniglia JM, Wolff D, Herques AS: Congenital deafness in 13–15 syndrome. *Arch Otolaryngol.* 92:181–188, 1970.

Marcellino GR: Neonatal hearing screening utilizing microprocessor technology. *Hear Instruments* 30:12, 1979.

Marcus RE, Valvassori G: Cochleo-vestibular apparatus; radiologic studies in hereditary and familial hearing loss. *Int Audiol* 9:95–102, 1970.

Mardel M, Hosick E, Windman T, et al: Audiometric comparison of the middle and late components of the adult auditory evoked potential awake and sleep. *Electroencephalogr Clin Neurophysiol* 38:27–33, 1975.

Margolis RH: Tympanometry in infants: State-of-the-art. In Harford ER, Bess FH, Bluestone CD et al: *Impedance Screening for Middle Ear Disease in Children.* New York: Grune & Stratton, 1978, pp 41–56.

Margolis RM: Tympanometry for prediction of middle ear effusion. Letter to the editor. *Arch Otolaryngol* 105:225, 1979.

Markides A: The effect of hearing aid use on the user's residual hearing. *Scand Audiol* 5:205, 1976.

Markle D, Zaner A: The determination of gain requirements of hearing aids; a new method. *J Aud Res* 6:371–377, 1966.

Marquardt TP, Saxman JH: Language comprehension and auditory discrimination in articulation deficient kindergarten children. *J Speech Hear Res* 15:382–389, 1972.

Marshall L, Brandt JF: Temporary threshold shift from a toy cap gun. *J Speech Hear Disord* 39:163–168, 1974.

Marshall R, Reichert T, Kerley SM, et al: Auditory function in newborn intensive care unit patients revealed by auditory brain-stem potentials. *J Pediatr* 96:731–735, 1980.

Martensson B: Dominant hereditary nerve deafness. *Arch Otolaryngol* 52:270–274, 1960.

Martin E, Pickett JM: Sensorineural hearing loss and upward spread of masking. *J Speech Hear Res* 13:426–437, 1980.

Martin FN, Clark JG: Audiologic detection of auditory processing disorders in children. *J Am Audiol Soc* 3:140–146, 1977.

Maskarinec AS, Cairns GF, Butterfield EC, et al: Longitudinal observations of individual infant's vocalizations. *J Speech Hear Disord* 46:267–273, 1981.

Masterton RB, Diamond IT: Effects of auditory cortex ablation on discrimination of small binaural time differences. *J Neurophysiol* 27:15–36, 1964.

Matkin N: Amplification for children: current status and future priorities. In Bess F, Freeman B, Sinclair J: *Amplification in Education.* Washington, D.C.: A.G. Bell, 1981, ch 12.

Matkin ND: Some essential features of a pediatric audiological evaluation. Talk presented to the Eighth Danavox Symposium, Copenhagen, June 1973.

Matkin ND, Carhart R: Auditory profiles associated with Rh incompatibility. *Arch Otolaryngol* 84:502–513, 1966.

Matkin ND, Carhart R: Hearing acuity and Rh incompatibility: electrodermal thresholds. *Arch Otolaryngol* 87:383–388, 1968.

Matkin N, Thomas J: The utilization of CROS hearing aids to children. *Maico Audiological Library Series* 10:8, 1972.

Matzker J: Two new methods for the assessment of central auditory functions in cases of brain disease. *Ann Otol Rhinol Laryngol* 68:1185–1197, 1959.

Maumenee AE: Congenital hereditary corneal dystrophy. *Am J Ophthalmol* 50:1114–1123, 1960.

Mavilya MP: Unpublished doctoral dissertation, Columbia University (University Microfilms No. 70-12879), 1969.

Mavilya MP: Spontaneous vocalization and babbling in hearing impaired infants. In Fant G: *International Symposium on Speech Communication, Ability and Profound Deafness*, Washington, D.C.: Alexander Graham Bell Association for the Deaf, 1972.

May DL, White HH: Familial myoclonus, cerebellar ataxia, and deafness. *Arch Neurol* 19:331–338, 1968.

Maynard JE: Otitis media in Alaskan Eskimo children; an epidemiologic review with observations on control. *Alaska Med* 11:93–98, 1969.

Maynard JE, Fleshman JK, Tschopp CF: Otitis media

in Alaskan Eskimo children: a prospective evaluation of chemoprophylaxis. *JAMA* 219:597–599, 1972.

McCaffrey A: Speech perception in infancy, personal communication cited in Friedlander (1970).

McCandless G: Special considerations on evaluating children and the aging for hearing aids. In Rubin M: *Hearing Aids—Current Development and Concepts*. Baltimore: University Park Press, 1976.

McCandless G, Keith R: Use of impedance measurements in hearing aid fitting. In Jerger J, Northern JL: *Clinical Impedance Audiometry*, ed 2. Acton, Mass.: American Electromedics Corp., 1980, ch 11.

McCandless G, Miller D: Loudness discomfort and hearing aids. *Natl Hear Aid J* 25:7–32, 1972.

McCandless GA: Screening for middle ear disease on the Wind River Indian Reservation. *Hear Instruments* 26:19–20, 1975.

McCandless GA, Allred PL: Tympanometry and emergence of the acoustic reflex in infants. In Harford ER, Bess FH, Bluestone CD, et al: *Impedance Screening for Middle Ear Disease in Children*. New York: Grune & Stratton, 1978, pp 56–67.

McClure WJ: The ostrich syndrome and educators of the deaf. The Kentucky Standard 100: 5 (Kentucky School for the Deaf, Danville), 1973.

McConnell F, Liff S: The rationale for early identification and intervention. *Otolaryngol Clin North Am* 8:77–87, 1975.

McConnell F, Ward PH (eds): *Deafness in Childhood*. Nashville, Tenn.: Vanderbilt University Press, 1967.

McCracken J: Rubella in the newborn. *Br Med J* 2:420–422, 1963.

McDonald A: *Children of Very Low Birthweight. MEIV Research Monograph No. 1*. London: Heinemann, 1967.

McDonald F, Studebaker G: Earmold alteration effects as measured in human auditory meatus. *J Acoust Soc Am* 48:1366–1372, 1970.

McDonough ER: Fanconi anemia syndrome. *Arch Otolaryngol* 92:284–285, 1970.

McFarlan D: The voice test of hearing. *Arch Otolaryngol* 5:1–5, 1927.

McFarland WH, Simmons FB, Jones FR: An automated hearing screening technique for newborns. *J Speech Hear Disord* 45:495, 1980.

McIntire MS, Menolascina FJ, Wiley JH: Mongolism—some clinical aspects. *Am J Ment Defic* 69:794, 1965.

McKay H, Sinisterra L, McKay A, et al: Improving cognitive ability in chronically deprived children. *Science* 200:270–278, 1978.

McLaurin JW, Kloepfer HW, Lagnaite JK, et al: Hereditary branchial anomalies and associated hearing impairment. *Laryngoscope* 76:1277–1288, 1966.

McLay K, Maran AGD: Deafness and the Klippel-Feil syndrome. *J Laryngol Otol* 83:175–184, 1969.

McLeod AC, McConnell F, Sweeney A, et al: Clinical variation in Usher's syndrome. *Arch Otolaryngol* 94:321–334, 1971.

McNeill D: Developmental psycholinguistics. In Smith F, Muller GA: *The Genesis of Language: A Psycholinguistic Approach*, Cambridge, Mass.: MIT Press, 1966.

Meadow KP: Parental response to the medical ambiguities of congenital deafness. *J Health Soc Behav* 9:299–309, 1968a.

Meadow KP: The effect of early manual communication and family climate, doctoral dissertation, University of California, Berkeley, 1968b.

Meadow KP, Trybus RJ: Behavioral and emotional problems of deaf children: an overview. In Bradford LJ, Hardy WG (eds): *Hearing and Hearing Impairment*. New York: Grune & Stratton, 1979.

Medical World News: Beyond "V.D." 21:56–63, 1980.

Mehler J, Bertonicini J, Barriere M, et al: Infant recognition of mother's voice. *Perception* 7:491–497, 1978.

Melloni BJ: *Some Pathological Conditions of Eye, Ear, Throat: An Atlas*. Chicago: Abbott Laboratories, 1957.

Melnick M, Bixler D, Nance WE, et al: Familial branchio-oto-renal dysplasia. A new addition to the branchial arch syndrome. *Clin Genet* 9:25–34, 1976.

Melnick W, Eagles EL, Levine HS: Evaluation of a recommended program of identification audiometry with school-age children. *J Hear Disord* 29:3–13, 1964.

Meltzoff AN, Moore MK: Imitation of facial and manual gestures by human neonates. *Science* 198:75–78, 1977.

Mencher G, Gerber S: *Early management of Hearing Loss*. New York: Grune & Stratton, 1981.

Mencher G, McCulloch B, Derbyshire A, et al: Observer bias as a factor in neonatal hearing screening. *J Speech Hear Res* 20:27–34, 1977.

Mencher GT: Screening infants for auditory deficits: University of Nebraska Neonatal Hearing Project. *Audiology (Suppl)* 11:69, 1972.

Mencher GT: Infant hearing screening: The state of the art. *Maico Audiological Library Series*. 12: (No. 7), 1974.

Mencher GT (ED): *Early Identification of Hearing Loss*. Basal: S. Karger, 1976.

Mencher GT, McCulloch BF: Auditory screening of kindergarten children using the VASC. *J Speech Hear Disord* 35:241–247, 1970.

Mendel M: Clinical use of primary cortical responses. *Audiology* 19:1–15, 1980.

Mendel M, Goldstein R: The effect of test conditions on the early components of the averaged electroencephalic response. *J Speech Hear Res* 12:344, 1969.

Mendel M, Goldstein R: Stability of the early components of the averaged electroencephalographic response. *J Speech Hear Res* 14:829–840, 1971

Mendel M, Hosick E, Windman T, et al: Audiometric comparison of the middle and late components of the adult auditory evoked potentials awake and asleep. *Electroencephalogr Clin Neurophysiol* 38:27–33, 1975.

Mendelson T, Salamy A, Lenoir M, et al: Brain stem evoked potential findings in children with otitis media. *Arch Otolaryngol* 105:17–20, 1979.

Mengel MC, Konigsmark BW, Berlin CI, et al. Conductive hearing loss and malformed low-set ears as a possible recessive syndrome. *J Med Genet* 6:14–21, 1969.

Menyuk P: *The Development of Speech*. New York: Bobbs-Merrill, 1972.

Menyuk P: Effects of hearing loss on babbling in the language-acquisition stage. In Jaffe B: *Hearing Loss in Children.* Baltimore: University Park Press, 1977, ch 42.

Messer SB, Lewis M: Social class and sex differences in the attachment and play behavior of the year-old infant. Paper presented at the meeting of the Eastern Psych. Assn., Atlantic City, 1970.

Metz O: The acoustic impedance measured on normal and pathological ears. *Acta Otolaryngol (Suppl) (Stockh)* 63, 1946.

Metz O: Threshold of reflex contractions of muscles of middle ear and recruitment of loudness. *Arch Otolaryngol* 55:536–543, 1952.

Miles AC: Cued speech. *American Education,* November 1967.

Miller AL, Lehman RH, Geretti R: Unusual audiological findings in cranial-metaphysical dysplasia. *Arch Orolaryngol.* 89:861–864, 1969.

Miller GA, Nicely PE: Analysis of perceptual confusions among some English consonants. *J Am Speech Assoc* 27:338–352, 1955.

Miller JD, Rothenberg SJ, Eldredge DH: Preliminary observations on the effects of exposure to noise for seven days on the hearing and inner ear of the chinchilla. *J Acoust Soc Am* 50:1199–1203, 1971.

Miller L: Creative language development. *J Colo Speech Hear Assoc* Spring, 1975.

Mills JH: Noise and children: a review of literature. *J Acoust Soc Am* 58:768–779, 1975.

Mills JH, Gengel RW, Watson CS, et al: Temporary changes for the auditory system due to exposure to noise for one or two days. *J Acoust Soc Am* 48:524–530, 1970.

Milner B, Taylor I, Sperry RW: Lateralized suppression of dichotically presented digits after commissural section in man. *Science* 161:184–186, 1968.

Mindel ED, Vernon M: *They Grow in Silence: The Deaf Child and His Family.* Silver Spring, Md.: National Association of the Deaf, 1971, p 23.

Mitchell C: Counseling for the parent. In Roeser R, Downs M: *Auditory Disorders in School Children.* New York: Thieme-Stratton, 1981, ch 19.

Mitchell O, Richards G: Effects of various anesthetic agents on normal and pathological middle ears. *Ear Nose Throat J* 55:36, 1976.

Mizrahi EM, Dorfman LJ: Sensory evoked potentials: clinical applications in pediatrics. *J Pediatr* 97:1–10, 1980.

Moffat S: Helping the Child Who Cannot Hear. The Public Affairs Committee, Public Affairs Pamphlet 479, 381 Park Ave., South New York, 1972.

Moffitt AB: Speech perception in infants, Doctoral dissertation, University of Minnesota, 1968.

Moffitt AB: Speech perception by 20 to 24 weeks old infants. Paper presented at March Meeting of Society for Research in Child Development, Santa Monica, Calif., 1969.

Molfese DL: Cerebral asymmetry in infants, children and adults: auditory evoked responses to speech and noise stimuli. *Dissertation Abstracts* 34:3, 1973.

Molfese DL: Left and right hemisphere involvement in speech perception: electrophysiological correlates. *Percept Psychophysics* 23:237–243, 1978.

Molfese DL: Hemispheric specialization for temporal information: Implications for the perception of voicing cues during speech perception. *Brain Lang* 11:285–299, 1980.

Molfese DL, Hess TM: Hemispheric specialization for VOT perception in the pre-school child. *J Exp Child Psychol* 26:71–84, 1978.

Molfese DL, Molfese VJ: Hemisphere and stimulus differences are reflected in the cortical responses of newborn infants to speech stimuli. *Dev Psychol* 15:505–511, 1979.

Molfese DL, Freeman RB, Palermo DS: The ontogeny of brain lateralization for speech and nonspeech stimuli. *Brain Lang* 2:356–368, 1975.

Moller A: The sensitivity of the contraction of the tympanic muscles in man. *Ann Otol Rhinol Laryngol* 71:86–95, 1962.

Moller P: Hearing, middle ear pressure and otopathology in a cleft palate population. *Acta Otolaryngol* 92:521–528, 1981.

Moncur J: Judge reliability in infant testing. *J Speech Hear Res* 11:348–357, 1968.

Mondini C: Anatomica surdi nati sectio; in De-Bononiensi Scientarium et Artium Instituto atque Academia Comentarii, Vol VII, pp 419–431 (Bonoia, 1791).

Montandon PP: Auditory nerve potentials from ear canals of patients with otologic problems. *Ann Otol Rhinol Laryngol* 184:1, 165–168, 1975.

Moore JM, Thompson G, Thompson M: Auditory localization of infants as a function of reinforcement conditions. *J Speech Hear Disord* 40:29–34, 1975.

Moore JM, Wilson WR, Lillis KE, et al: Earphone auditory threshold of infants utilizing visual reinforcement auditory (VR). poster session, American Speech and Hearing Assn. meeting, Houston, 1976.

Moore JM, Wilson WR, Thompson G: Visual reinforcement of head-turn responses in infants under twelve months of age. *J Speech Hear Disord* 42:328–334, 1977.

Morse PA: The discrimination of speech and nonspeech stimuli in early infancy. *J Exp Child Psychol* 14:477–492, 1972.

Mulac A, Gerber SE: Cardiovascular measures. In Gerber S: *Audiometry and Infancy.* New York: Grune & Stratton, 1977.

Murai JI: Speech developments of infants. *Psychologica* 3:27–35, 1960.

Murai JI: The sounds of infants. *Studia Phonologica* 3:21–24, 1964.

Murakami Y, Schuknecht HF: Unusual congenital anomalies in the inner ear. *Arch Otolaryngol* 87:335–349, 1968.

Murphy AT: The families of hearing-impaired children. *Volta Rev* 81:265, 1979.

Murphy KP: Development of hearing in babies. *Child Family* 1, 1962.

Murphy KP: A developmental approach to pediatric audiometry. *Hearing Aid J* 6–32, September 1979.

Mussen EF: Hearing, listening, and attending: Techniques and concepts in auditory training. In Roeser R, Downs M: *Auditory Disorders in School Children.* New York: Thieme-Stratton, 1981, ch 17.

Mussen PH, Conger JJ, Kagan J: *Child Development and Personality.* New York: Harper & Row, 1969.

Myers FN, Stool S: The temporal bone in osteoporosis. *Arch Otolaryngol* 89:44–53, 1969.

Myklebust H: *Auditory Disorders in Children.* New York: Grune & Stratton, 1954.

Nagafuchi M: Development of dichotic and monaural hearing abilities in young children. *Acta Otolaryngol (Stockh)* 69:409–414, 1970.

Nager GT: Association of bilateral VIIIth nerve tumors with meningiomas in von Recklinghausen's disease. *Laryngoscope* 74:1220–1265, 1964.

Nager GT: Congenital aural atresia: Anatomy and surgical management. In *Birth Defects, Part IX, Ear*. Baltimore: Williams & Wilkins, published for National Foundation—March of Dimes, 1971.

Nahmias AJ: The TORCH complex. *Hosp Pract* 9:65–72, 1974.

Nahmias AJ, Norrild B: Herpes simplex virus 1 and 2, basic and clinical aspects. *DM* 25:10, 1979.

Nakazima S: A comparative study of the speech development of Japanese and American English in childhood. *Studia Phonologica* 3:27–39, 1962.

Nance WE: Symposium on Usher's Syndrome, Public Service Programs. Gallaudet College, Washington, D.C., 1973.

Nassif R, Harboyan G: Madelung's deformity with conductive hearing loss. *Arch Otolaryngol* 91:175–178, 1970.

National Center for Health Statistics: Hearing Sensitivity and Related Findings Among Children, United States DHEW Pub. No. (HRA) 76-1046, 1972.

National Center for Health Statistics: Hearing Sensitivity and Related Mental Findings Among Youths 12–17 Years, United States DHEW Pub. No. (HRS) 76-1636, 1975.

Naunton RF: The effect of hearing aid use upon the user's residual hearing. *Laryngoscope* 67:569–576, 1957.

Needleman H: Effects of hearing loss from early recurrent otitis media on speech and language development. In Jaffe B: *Hearing Loss in Children*. Baltimore: University Park Press, 1977, ch 44.

Neff WD: The effects of partial section of the auditory nerve. *J Comp Physiol* 40:203–216, 1947.

Neff WD: Neural mechanisms of auditory discrimination. In Rosenblith WA: *Sensory Communications*. Cambridge, Mass.: MIT Press, 1961, pp 259–278.

Neisser A: *Cognitive Psychology*. New York: Appleton-Century-Crofts, 1967.

Nelson JM: *Agnosia, Apraxia, Aphasia: Their Value in Cerebral Localization*, ed 2. New York: Hafner Publishing, 1948.

Nelson KB, Ellenberg J: Apgar scores of predictors of chronic neurologic disability. *Pediatrics* 68:36, 1981.

Nelson M, Scott CI: Engelmann's disease (a form of craniodiaphyseal dysplasia). *Birth Defects* 5(4):301, 1969.

Neuman A, Molinelli P, Hochberg I: Post-meningitic hearing loss: report on three cases. *J Commun Disord* 14:105–111, 1981.

Newby H: *Audiology*, ed 2. New York: Appleton-Century-Crofts, 1964.

Niemeyer W, Sesterhenn G: Calculating the hearing threshold from the stapedius reflex threshold for different sound stimuli. *J Aud Commun* 11:84, 1972.

Niswander P, Ruth R: Prediction of hearing sensitivity from acoustic reflexes in mentally retarded person. *Am J Ment Defic* 81:474, 1977.

Nolte J: *The Human Brain: An Introduction to its Functional Anatomy*. St. Louis: C. V. Mosby, 1981.

Nober IW: A study of classroom noise as a factor which affects the auditory discrimination performance of primary grade children. Ed.D. thesis, Univ. Mass., Amherst, Mass., *Dissertation Abstracts*, 1973.

North FA: Chapter 4 in Frankenburg WK, Camp BW: *Pediatric Screening Tests*. Springfield, Ill.: Charles C Thomas, 1975.

Northcott W: Freedom through speech: every child's right. *Volta Rev* 83:162–181, 1981.

Northcott WH (ed): The hearing impaired child in a regular classroom: preschool, elementary and secondary years. Washington, D.C.: A. G. Bell Assoc. Deaf, 1973.

Northcott WH: *Implications of Mainstreaming for the Education of Hearing Impaired Children in the 1980's*. Washington, D.C.: A. G. Bell Publications, 1979.

Northern JL: Clinical application of acoustic impedance measurements. *Otolaryngol Clin North Am* (Symposium on Congenital Deafness) 4:359–368, 1971a.

Northern JL (ed): *Audiometric Assistant Training Guide*. U.S. Dept. HEW, Office of Education, Manpower Development and Training Program. Washington, D.C., National Association of Hearing and Speech Agencies, 1971b.

Northern JL: Acoustic impedance in the pediatric population. In Bess F: *Childhood Deafness: Causation, Assessment, and Management*, New York: Grune & Stratton, 1977a.

Northern JL: Impedance audiometry for otologic diagnosis. In Shambaugh C, Shea J: *Proceedings of the Shambaugh Fifth International Workshop on Middle Ear Microsurgery and Fluctuant Hearing Loss*. Huntsville, Ala.: Strode Publishers, 1977b, p 75.

Northern JL: Hearing aids and acoustic impedance measurements. *Monogr Contemp Audiol* 1:2, 1978a.

Northern JL: Advanced techniques for measuring middle ear function. *Pediatrics* 61:761, 1978b.

Northern JL: Impedance screening in special populations: State of the art. In Harford ER, Bess FH, Bluestone CD, et al: *Impedance Screening for Middle Ear Disease in Children*, New York: Grune & Stratton, 1978c, pp 229–248.

Northern JL: Acoustic impedance measures in the Down's population. *Semin Speech Lang Hear* 1:81, 1980a.

Northern JL: Clinical measurement procedures in impedance audiometry. In Jerger J, Northern JL: *Clinical Impedance Audiometry*, ed 2. Acton, Mass.: American Electromedics Corp., 1980b, ch 2.

Northern JL: Impedance measurements with distinctive groups. In Jerger J, Northern JL: *Clinical Impedance Audiometry*, ed 2. Acton, Mass.: American Electromedics Corp., 1980c, ch 10.

Northern JL: Impedance screening: an integral part of hearing screening. *Ann Otol Rhinol Laryngol* 89 (Suppl 68):3, 1980d.

Northern JL: Impedance measurements in infants. In Mencher G, Gerber S: *Early Management of Hearing Loss*. New York: Grune & Stratton, 1981, p 131.

Northern JL: Impedance audiometry. In Northern JL: *Hearing Disorders*, ed 2. Boston: Little, Brown, 1984a.

Northern JL (ed): *Hearing Disorders*, ed 2. Boston: Little, Brown, 1984b.

Northern J, Bergstrom L: Impedance audiometry. *Eye Ear Nose Throat Mon* 52:404–406, 1973.

Northern JL, Grimes A: Introduction to acoustic impedance. In Katz J: *Handbood of Clinical Audiology*, ed 2. Baltimore: Williams & Wilkins, 1978.

Northern JL, Hattler KW: Earmold influence on aided speech identification tasks. *J Speech Hear Res* 13:162–172, 1970.

Northern JL, Teter DL, Krug RF: Characteristics of manually communicating deaf adults. *J Speech Hear Disord* 36:71–76, 1971.

Olsen WO: The effects of noise and reverberation on speech intelligibility. In Bess F, Freeman B, Sinclair J: *Amplification in Education*. Washington, D.C.: A. G. Bell, 1981.

Olsen WO, Matkin ND: Speech audiometry. In Rintelmann WF: *Hearing Assessment*, Baltimore: University Park Press, 1979, ch 5.

Olson A, Hipskind N: The relation between levels of pure tones and speech which elicit the acoustic reflex and loudness discomfort. *J Aud Res* 13:71–76, 1973.

Omerod FC: The pathology of congenital deafness. *J Laryngol Otol* 74:919, 1960.

Opheim O: Loss of hearing following the syndrome of Van Der Hoeve-De Kleyn. *Acta Otolaryngol* 65:337, 1968.

Orchik DJ, Dunn JW, McNutt L: Tympanometry as a predictor of middle ear effusion. *Arch Otolaryngol* 104:4–6, 1978a.

Orchik DJ, Morff R, Dunn JW: Impedance audiometry in serous otitis media. *Arch Otolaryngol* 104:409–412, 1978b.

Ostwald PF, Peltzman P: The cry of the human infant. *Sci Am* March 1974.

Owens E, Telleen CC: Speech perception with hearing aids and cochlear implants. *Audecibel*, Summer 1981.

Ozdamar O, Kraus N: Auditory middle-latency response in humans. *Audiology* 22:34–49, 1983.

Ozdamar O, Stein L: Auditory brainstem response (ABR) in unilateral hearing loss. *Laryngoscope* 91:565–574, 1981.

Ozdamar O, Kraus N, Stein L: Auditory brainstem responses in infants recovering from bacterial meningitis: audiological evaluation. *Arch Otolaryngol* 109:13–18, 1982.

Palfrey JS: Commentary: P.L. 94-142: The Education for all Handicapped Children Act. *J Pediatr* 97:417–419, 1980.

Palfrey JS, Hanson MA, Pleszczynska C, et al: Selective hearing screening for young children. *Clin Pediatr* 19:474–477, 1980.

Palva T, Pulkinen K: Mastoiditis. *J Laryngol Otol* 73:573–577, 1959.

Panjvani ZFK, Henshaw JB: CMV in the perinatal period. *Am J Dis Child* 135:56–60, 1981.

Pannbacker M: Hearing loss and cleft palate. *Cleft Palate J* 6:50–56, 1969.

Pantke OA, Cohen MM Jr: The Waardenburg syndrome. *Birth Defects* 7(7):147–152, 1971.

Paparella M: Middle ear effusions: definitions and terminology. *Ann Otol Rhinol Laryngol* 85 (suppl 25):8–11, 1976.

Paparella MM: Differential Diagnosis of Childhood Deafness. In Bess F: *Childhood Deafness: Causation, Assessment and Management*. New York: Grune & Stratton, 1977.

Paparella MM, Brady DR: Sensorineural hearing loss in chronic otitis media and mastoiditis. *Arch Otolaryngol* 74:108–115, 1970.

Paparella MM, Suguira S: The patholgoy of suppurative labyrinthitis. *Ann Otol Rhinol Laryngol* 75:554–586, 1967.

Paradise JL: Pediatrician's view of middle ear effusions: More questions than answers. *Ann Otol Rhinol Laryngol* 85 (suppl 25):20, 1976a.

Paradise JL: Management of middle ear effusions in infants with cleft palate. *Ann Otol Rhinol Laryngol* (suppl 25) 85:285–288, 1976b.

Paradise JL: Otitis media in infants and children. *Pediatrics* 65:917–943, 1980.

Paradise JL: Otitis media during early life: how hazardous to development? A critical review of the evidence. *Pediatrics* 68:869–873, 1981.

Paradise JL: Editorial retrospective: tympanometry. *N Engl J Med* 307:1074–1076, 1982.

Paradise JL, Bluestone CD: Diagnosis and management of ear disease in cleft palate infants. *Trans Am Acad Ophthalmol Otolaryngol* 73:709–714, 1969.

Paradise JL, Bluestone CD: Early treatment of the universal otitis media of infants with cleft palate. *Pediatrics* 53:48–54, 1974.

Paradise JL, Smith C: Impedance screening for preschool children, state of the art. In Harford E, Bess F, Bluestone C: *Impedance Screening for Middle Ear Disease in Children*. New York: Grune & Stratton, 1978.

Paradise JL, Smith C: Impedance screening for preschool children. *Ann Otol* 88:56, 1979.

Paradise JL, Smith C, Bluestone CD: Tympanometric detection of middle ear effusion in infants and young children. *Pediatrics* 58:198–206, 1976.

Pashayan H, Fraser FC, McIntyre J, et al: Bilateral aplasia of the tibia, polydactyly and absent thumbs in a father and daughter. *J Bone Joint Surg* 53B:495–499, 1971.

Pashayan HM, Pruzansky S, Solomon L: The EEC syndrome. *Birth Defects* 10(7):105–127, 1974.

Pass RF, Stasno S: Outcome of symptomatic congenital cytomegalovirus infection results of long-term longitudinal follow-up. *Pediatrics* 66:758–762, 1980.

Passchier-Vermeer W: Noise-induced hearing loss from exposure to intermittent and varying noise. In *Proceedings of the International Congress on Noise as a Public Health Problem, v.s. EPA*. Washington, D.C.: Office of Noise Abatement Control, 1973, pp 169–200.

Patten BM: *Human Embryology*, ed 3. New York: McGraw-Hill, 1968.

Patterson MF, Bartlett PC: Hearing impairment caused by intratympanic pressure changes during general anesthesia. *Laryngoscope* 86:399–404, 1976.

Pearson AA, Jacobson AD, VanCalcar R, et al: *The Development of the Ear*. Rochester: Section on Instruction, Home Study Courses, American Academy of Otolaryngology and Ophthalmology, 1970.

Pelton S, Shurin P, Klein J: Persistence of middle ear effusion after otitis media. *Pediatr Res* 11:504, 1977.

Peltzman P, Kitterman JA, Ostwald PF, et al: Effects of incubator noise on human hearing. *J Aud Res* 10:335–339, 1970.

Penfield W, Rasmussen T: *The Cerebral Cortex of Man*. New York: Hafner Publishing, 1968.

Penfield W, Roberts L: *Speech and Brain Mechanisms*. Princeton, N.J.: Princeton University Press, 1959.

Perrin JM, Charney E, MacWhinney JB, et al: Sulfioxazole as chemoprophylaxis for recurrent otitis media. *N Engl J Med* 291:664–667, 1974.

Peterson GE, Lehiste I: Revised CNC lists for auditory testing. *J Speech Hear Disord* 27:62, 1962.

Peterson RA: Ophthalmology. In Jaffe B: *Hearing Loss in Children.* Baltimore: University Park Press, 1977.

Picton RW, Hillyard SA, Krausz H, et al: Human auditory evoked potentials; I. Evaluation of components. *Electroencephalogr Clin Neurophysiol* 36:179–190, 1974.

Pollack D: *Educational Audiology for the Limited Hearing Infant.* Springfield, Ill.: Charles C Thomas, 1970.

Pollack D: The development of an auditory function. *Otolaryngol Clin North Am* (Symposium on Congenital Deafness) 4:319–335, 1971.

Pollack D: Amplification and auditory/verbal training for the limited hearing infant 0 to 30 months. *Semin Speech Lang Hear* 3:52–67, 1982.

Pollock KC: The influence of hearing impairment. In Bzoch K: *Communicative Disorders Related to Cleft Lip and Palate.* Boston: Little, Brown, 1971, pp 77–86.

Pollack M: *Amplification for the Hearing-Impaired,* ed 2. New York: Grune & Stratton, 1980.

Polvogt LM, Crowe SJ: Anomalies of the cochlea in patients with normal hearing. *Arch Otol Rhinol Laryngol* 46:579–591, 1937.

Popelka GR: *Hearing Assessment with the Acoustic Reflex.* New York: Grune & Stratton, 1981.

Popper A, Fay R (eds): *Comparative Studies of Hearing in Vertebrates* (Proceedings in Life Science Series). Berlin: Springer-Verlag, 1980.

Portmann M, Aran JM: Electro-cochleographic sur le nourrissons et le jeune infant. *Acta Otolaryngol (Stockh)* 71:253–261, 1971.

Position Statement on Language Disorders: *Asha* 24:937–944, 1982.

Potsic WP, Marsh RR, Gursky EJ: Behavior changes associated with the resolution of middle ear effusion. *Corti's Organ,* January 1979.

Potts P, Greenwood J: Hearing aid monitoring. *Lang Speech Hear Serv Sch* 14:163, 1983.

Powers T: Individual applications for FM input hearing instruments. *Hear Instruments* 31(6):18–19, 1980.

Premack AJ, Premack D: Teaching language to an ape. *Sci Am* 227:92–99, 1972.

Preus M, Fraser FC: The lobster-claw defect with ectodermal defects, cleft lip-palate, tear duct anomaly and renal anomalies. *Clin Genet* 4:369–375, 1973.

Proctor CA, Proctor B: Understanding hereditary nerve deafness. *Arch Otolaryngol* 85:23–40, 1967.

Pumper RW, Yamashiroya HM: *Essentials of Medical Virology.* Philadelphia: W. B. Saunders, 1975.

Queen S, Moses F, Wood S, et al: The use of immitance screening by the Kansas City, Mo., public school district. *Semin Speech Lang Hear* 2:119, 1981.

Querleu Q, Renard Z, Crepin G: Perception auditive et reactivité foetale aux stimulations sonores. *J Gynecol Obstet Biol Reprod* 10:307–314, 1981.

Quigley SP: Some effects of hearing impairment upon school performance. MS prepared for the Div. of Sp. Ed. Services, Office of the Supt. of Public Instruction, State of Illinois, 1970.

Quigley SP: Environment and communication in the language development of deaf children. In Bradford LJ, Hardy WG: *Hearing and Hearing Impairment.* New York: Grune & Stratton, 1979.

Quigley SP, Frisina D: Institutionalized and Psycho-educational Development in Deaf Children. Council for Exceptional Children Research Monograph, Series A, 3, 1961.

Quisling RW, Moore GR, Jahrsdoerfer RA, et al: Osteogenesis imperfecta: a study of 160 family members. *Arch Otolaryngol* 105:207–211, 1979.

Ramaiya JJ: A study of binaural hearing aid performance, unpublished Master's thesis, directed by F McConnell, Vanderbilt University, Nashville, 1971.

Rappaport B, Tait C: Acoustic reflex threshold measurement in hearing aid selection. *Arch Otolaryngol* 102:129–132, 1976.

Rawlings BW, Trybus R: Personnel, facilities and services available in schools and classes for hearing impaired children in the United States. *Am Ann Deaf* 123:99–121, 1978.

Redding J, Hargest T, Minsky S: How noisy is intensive care? *Crit Care Med* 5:275, 1977.

Reddy JK, Rao MS: Imitation of facial and manual gestures by human neonates. *Science* 198:75–79, 1977.

Reed D, Dunn W: Epidemiologic studies of otitis media among Eskimo children. *Public Health Rep* 85:699–706, 1970.

Reed D, Struve S, Maynard JE: Otitis media and hearing deficiency among Eskimo children; a cohort study. *Am J Public Health* 57:1657–1662, 1967.

Reed WB, Store VM, Boder E, et al: Pigmentary disorders in association with congenital deafness. *Arch Dermatol* 95:176–186, 1967.

Rees N: The speech pathologist and the reading process. *Asha* 16:255–258, 1974.

Rees NS: Auditory processing factors in language disorders: the view from procrustes' bed. *J Speech Hear Disord* 38:304–315, 1973.

Refetoff A, DeWind LT, DeGroot LJ: Familial syndrome combining deaf-mutism, stippled epiphyses, goiter and abnormally high PBI. *J Clin Endocrinol* 27:279–294, 1967.

Reichert TJ, Cantekin EI, Riding KH, et al: Diagnosis of middle ear effusions in young infants by otoscopy and tympanometry. In Harford ER, Bess FH, Bluestone CD, et al: *Impedance Screening for Middle Ear Disease in Children,* New York: Grune & Stratton, 1978, pp 69–79.

Reilly K, Owens E, Uken D, et al: Progressive hearing loss in children: hearing aids and other factors. *J Speech Hear Disord* 46:328–334, 1981.

Ries P: Academic Achievement Test Results of a National Testing Program for Hearing Impaired Students. Office of Demographic Studies, Gallaudet College, Washington, D.C., 1973a.

Reisen AH: The development of visual perception in man and chimpanzee. *Science* 106:107–108, 1947.

Reisen AH: Effects of stimulus deprivation on the development and atrophy of the visual sensory system. *Am J Orthopsychiatry* 30:23–36, 1960.

Reynolds D, Stagno S, Stubbs G, et al: Inapparent congenital cytomegalovirus infection with elevated cord IGM levels. *N Engl J Med* 290:292, 1974.

Richards BW, Rundle AT: A familial hormonal disorder associated with mental deficiency, deaf mutism and ataxia. *J Ment Defic Res* 3:33–55, 1959.

Richards GB, Mitchell OC, Speight IL: Effects of pentobarbital on intra-aural muscle reflexes in retarded children. *Eye Ear Nose Throat Mon* 54:69–72, 1975.

Richards IDG, Roberts CJ: The at risk infant. *Lancet* 2:711–714, 1967.

Ridgeway J: Dumb children. *Saturday Rev* August, 19–21, 1969.

Riedner ED, Levin S, Holliday MJ: Hearing patterns in dominant osteogenesis imperfecta. *Arch Otolaryngol* 106:737–740, 1980.

Riedner ED, Levin S, Holliday MJ: Hearing patterns in dominant osteogenesis imperfecta. *Arch Otolaryngol* 106:737–740, 1980.

Riggs W Jr, Seibert J: Cockayne's syndrome; roentgen findings. *AJR* 116:623–633, 1972.

Rigrodsky S, Prunty F, Glovsky L: A study of the incidence, types and associated etiologies of hearing loss in an institutionalized mentally retarded population. *Train Sch Bull* 58:30, 1961.

Rimoin DL, Edgerton MT: Genetic and clinical heterogeneity in the oral-facial-digital syndrome. *J Pediatr* 71:94–102, 1967.

Rintelmann W, Harford E, Burchfield S: A special case of auditory localization: CROS for blind persons with unilateral hearing loss. *Arch Otolaryngol* 91:284–288, 1970.

Rintelmann WF: Auditory manifestations of Alport's Disease syndrome. *Trans Am Acad Ophthalmol Otolaryngol* 82:375–387, 1976.

Rintelmann WF, Bess FH: High-level amplification and potential hearing loss in children. In Bess FH: *Childhood Deafness: Causation, Assessment and Management.* New York: Grune & Stratton, 1977, pp 267–293.

Rintelmann EF, Borus J: Noise-induced hearing loss and rock and roll music. *Arch Otolaryngol* 88:57–65, 1968.

Rittmanic PA: The mentally retarded and mentally ill. In Rose DE: *Audiological Assessment.* Englewood Cliffs, N.J.: Prentice-Hall, 1971, pp 369–401.

Roberts C: Can hearing aids damage hearing? *Acta Otolaryngol (Stockh)* 69:123–125, 1970.

Roberts DB: The etiology of bullous myringitis and the role of mycoplasmas in ear disease. a review. *Pediatrics* 65:761–766, 1980.

Roberts JL, Davis H, Phon GL, et al: Auditory brainstem responses in preterm neonates: maturation and follow-up. *J Pediatr* 101:257–263, 1982.

Robertson EO, Peterson JL, Lamb LE: Relative impedance measurements in young children. *Arch Otolaryngol* 88:162–168, 1968.

Robinette MS, Rhodes DP, Marion MW: Effects of secobarbital on impedance audiometry. *Arch Otolaryngol* 100:351–354, 1974.

Robinson A: Genetic and chromosomal disorders. In Kempe CH, Silver HK, O'Brien D: *Current Pediatric Diagnosis and Treatment.* Los Altos, Calif.: Lange Medical Publications, 1972.

Robinson DO, Sterling GR: Hearing aids and children in school: a follow-up study. *Volta Rev* 82:229, 1980.

Robinson GC, Wildervanck LS, Chiang TP: Ectrodactyly, ectodermal dysplasia and cleft lip-palate. Its association with conductive hearing loss. *J Pediatr* 82:107–109, 1973.

Roeser R, Downs M: *Auditory Disorders in School Children: The Law, Identification, Remediation.* New York: Thieme-Stratton, 1981.

Roeser RJ, Campbell JC, Daly D: Recovery of auditory function following meningitic deafness. *J Speech Hear Disord* 40:405–411, 1975.

Roeser RJ, Glorig A, Gerken GM, et al: A hearing aid malfunction detection unit. *J Speech Hear Dis* 42:351–357, 1977.

Rogers BO: Microtic, lop, cup, and protruding ears. *Plast Reconstr Surg* 41:208–231, 1968.

Rojskjaer C: Presented at the Fifth International Congress of Audiology, Bonn, 1960.

Romer AS: *The Vertebrate Body*, ed 5. Philadelphia: W. B. Saunders, 1977.

Rood SR, Stool SE: Otologic survey of schools for the deaf. *Am Ann Deaf* 126:113–117, 1981.

Rose DE, Galambos R, Hughes JR: Microelectrode studies of the cochlear nuclei of the cat. *Johns Hopkins Med J* 104:211–251, 1959.

Rosenberg AL, Bergstrom L, Troost BT, et al: Hyperuricemia and neurologic defects. *N Engl J Med* 282:992–997, 1970.

Rosenberg P, Swogger-Rosenberg J: Hearing screening. In Lass NJ, McReynolds LV, Northern JL, et al: *Speech, Language and Hearing.* Philadelphia: W. B. Saunders, 1982, ch 42.

Rosenhall U, Kankkunen A: Hearing alterations following meningitis; 1. Hearing improvement. *Ear Hear* 1:185, 1980.

Rosenthal R: Effects of low-frequency speech bands in-intelligibility. Communication Sciences Lab. Report, No. 3, New York City University of New York, 1972.

Rosenthal RD, Lang JK, Levett H: Speech reception with low-frequency speech energy. *J Acoust Soc Am* 57:949–955, 1975.

Rosenzweig MR, Rosenblith WA: Responses to auditory stimuli at the cochlea and at the auditory cortex. *Psychol Monogr* 67:1–26, 1953.

Rosner J, Simon D: The Auditory Analysis Test: an Initial Report. Pittsburgh, Learning Research & Development Center, Univ. of Pittsburgh, 1970.

Ross M: Changing concepts in hearing aid candidacy. *Eye Ear Nose and Throat Mon* 48:27–34, 1969.

Ross M: Classroom acoustics and speech intelligibility. In Katz J: *Handbook of Clinical Audiology.* Baltimore: Williams & Wilkins, 1972.

Ross M: Hearing aid selection for the preverbal hearing-impaired child. In Pollack M: *Amplification for the Hearing-Impaired.* New York: Grune & Stratton, 1975, ch. 6.

Ross M: *Hard of Hearing Children in Regular Schools.* Englewood Cliffs, N.J.: Prentice-Hall, 1982.

Ross M, Cirmo R: Reducing feedback in a post-auricular hearing aid by implanting the receiver in an earmold. *Volta Rev* 82:41, 1980.

Ross M, Lerman J: Hearing aid usage and its effect upon residual hearing: a review of the literature and an investigation. *Arch Otolaryngol* 86:57–62, 1967.

Ross M, Lerman J: A picture identification test for hearing-impaired children. *J Speech Hear Res* 13:44–53, 1970.

Ross M, Tomassetti C: Hearing aid selection for preverbal hearing-impaired children. In Pollack M: *Amplification for the Hearing-Impaired*, ed 2. New York: Grune & Stratton, 1980, ch 6.

Ross N, Giolas T (eds): *Auditory Management of Hear-*

ing-Impaired Children. Baltimore: University Park Press, 1978.

Rossi DF: Hearing deficiency in Pueblo Indian children: results of a mass screening program. *Rocky Mt Med J* Oct., 65–69, 1972.

Rossi DF, Sims DG: Acoustic reflex measurement in the severely and profoundly deaf. *Audiol Hear Educ* 3:6–8, 1977.

Roswell F, Chall J: *Auditory Blending Test.* New York: Essay Press, 1963.

Rozin P, Poritsky S, Sotsky R: American children with reading problems can easily learn to read English represented by Chinese characters. *Science* 171:1264–1267, 1971.

Ruben RJ: Anatomical diagnosis of non-conductive deafness by physiological tests. *Arch Otolaryngol* 78:47–51, 1963.

Ruben RJ, Math R: Serous otitis media associated with sensorineural hearing loss in children. *Laryngoscope* 88:1139–1154, 1978.

Ruben RJ, Rapin I: Plasticity of the developing auditory system. *Ann Otol Rhinol Laryngol* 89:303–311, 1980.

Ruben RJ, Knickerbocker GG, Sekula J, et al: Cochlear microphonics in man. *Laryngoscope* 69:665, 1959.

Ruben RJ, Bordley JE, Nager GT, et al: Human cochlear responses to sound stimuli. *Ann Otol Rhinol Laryngol* 169:459, 1960.

Ruben RJ, Lieberman AT, Bordley JE: Some observations on cochlear potentials and nerve action potentials in children. *Laryngoscope* 5:545, 1962.

Rubin M: Hearing aids for infants and toddlers. In Rubin M: *Hearing Aids: Current Developments and Concepts,* Baltimore: University Park Press, 1976, pp 95–102.

Rubin M: Serous otitis media in severely to profoundly hearing-impaired children, ages 0 to 6. *Volta Rev* 80:81–85, 1978.

Rubin M: Management of amplification for infants. *Semin Speech Lang Hear* 1:231, 1980.

Rubin M, Ventry I: Speech detection thresholds and comfortable loudness levels for speech in children with limited hearing. *Am Ann Deaf* 120:564–567, 1975.

Ruckelshaus W: Report to the President and Congress on Noise. Rep. Admin. EPA U.S. Senate Docum. 92-63, Chapter 1, 1972, pp 38–39.

Rupp RR: An approach to the communicative needs of the very young hearing impaired child. *J Acad Rehab Audiol* 4:11–22, 1971.

Ruppert ES, Buerk E, Pfordresher MF: Hereditary hearing loss with saddle nose and myopia. *Arch Otolaryngol* 92:95–98, 1970.

Ryan AF, Dallos P: Physiology of the cochlea. In Northern JL: *Hearing Disorders,* Boston: Little, Brown, 1984, ch 22.

Sachs R, Burkhard M: Insert earphone pressure response in real ears and couplers (abstract). *J Acoust Soc Am* 52 (Part 1):183, 1972.

Saito H, Kishimoto S, Furuta M: Temporal bone findings in a patient with Mobius Syndrome. *Ann Otol* 90:80–84, 1981.

Sak RJ, Ruben RJ: Effects of recurrent middle ear effusion in pre-school years on language and learning. *J Dev Behav Pediatr* 3:7–11, 1982.

Salamy A, Mendelson T, Tooley W, et al: Contrasts in brainstem function between normal and high-risk infants in early postnatal life. *Early Human Dev* 4:179–185, 1980.

Samples JM, Franklin B: Behavioral responses in 7 to 9 month old infants to speech and non-speech stimuli. *J Aud Res* 18:115–123, 1978.

Sanchez-Longo LP, Forster FM: Clinical significance of impairment of sound localization. *Neurology (Minneap)* 8:119–125, 1958.

Sanders D: Noise conditions in normal school classrooms. *Except Child* 31:344–353, 1965.

Sanders DA: *Auditory Perception of Speech. An Introduction to Principles and Problems.* Englewood Cliffs, N.J.: Prentice-Hall, 1977.

Sanderson-Leepa M, Rintelmann WF: Articulation functions and test-retest performance of normal-hearing children on three speech discrimination tests: WIPI, PBK-50, and NU Auditory Test No. 6. *J Speech Hear Disord* 41:503, 1976.

Sando I, Wood RP: Congenital middle ear anomalies. *Otolaryngol Clin North Am* (Symposium) 4:291–318, 1971.

Sando I, Bergstrom L, Wood RP, et al: Temporal bone findings in trisomy 18 syndrome. *Arch Otolaryngol* 72:913–924, 1968.

Sando I, Hemenway WG, Morgan RW: Histopathology of the temporal bones in mandibulofacial dysostosis *Trans Am Acad Ophthalmol Otolaryngol* 72:913–924, 1968.

Sando I, Baker B, Black FO, et al: Persistence of stapedial artery in trisomy 13–15 syndrome. *Arch Otolaryngol* 96:441–447, 1972.

Sarff LS: An innovative use of free field amplification in classrooms. In Roeser R, Downs M: *Auditory Disorders in School Children.* New York: Thieme-Stratton, 1981.

Sataloff J: Medical audiology. *Arch Otolaryngol* 76:283–287, 1962.

Savage-Rumbaugh ES, Rumbaugh DM: Chimpanzee problem comprehension: insufficient evidence. *Science* 206:1201–1202, 1979.

Savage-Rumbaugh ES, Rumbaugh DM, Smith ST, et al: Reference: the linguistic essential. *Science* 210:922–925, 1980.

Schafer IA, Scriver CR, Efron ML: Familial hyperprolineamia, cerebral dysfunction, and renal anomalies occurring in a family with hereditary nephropathy and deafness. *N Engl J Med* 267:51–60, 1962.

Schein JD: *The Deaf Community Study of Washington, D.C.* Washington, D.C.: Gallaudet College Press, 1965.

Schein JD, Delk MT: *The Deaf Population of the United States.* Silver Spring, Md.: Nat'l Assn of the Deaf, 1974.

Scheiner AP: Perinatal asphyxia: factors which predict developmental outcome. *Dev Med Child Neurol* 22:102–104, 1980.

Scherz RG, Fraga JR, Reichelderfer TE: A typical example of 13–15 trisomy in a Negro boy. *Clin Pediatr* 11:246–248, 1972.

Schlesinger HS: The deaf pre-schooler and his many faces. In Lloyd L: *International Seminar of the Vocational Rehabilitation of Deaf Persons.* Washington, D.C.: U. S. Department of Health, Education and Welfare, 1973.

Schlesinger HS, Meadow KP: Emotional support to parents. In Lillie DL: *Monograph on Parent Pro-*

grams in Child Development Centers. Chapel Hill, N.C.: University of North Carolina, 1972a, pp 13–25.

Schlesinger HS, Meadow KP: *Sound and Sign; Childhood Deafness and Mental Health.* Berkeley: University of California Press, 1972b.

Schneider B, Trehub SE, Bull D: High-frequency sensitivity in infants. *Science* 207:1003–1004, 1980.

Schuchman G: An ear level hearing aid for bilateral atresia. *Arch Otolaryngol* 94:87–88, 1971.

Schuknecht HF: Pathology of sensorineural deafness of genetic origin. In McConnell F, Ward PH: *Deafness in Childhood.* Nashville, Tenn.: Vanderbilt University Press, 1967, pp 69–90.

Schuknecht HF: *Pathology of the Ear.* Cambridge, Mass.: Harvard University Press, 1974.

Schulman CA: Effects of auditory stimulation on heart rate in premature infants as a function of level of arousal, probability of CNS damage, and conceptional age. *Dev Psychobiol* 2:172–183, 1970a.

Schulman CA: Heart rate response habituation in high-risk premature infants. *Psychophysiology* 6:690–694, 1970b.

Schulman CA, Wade G: The use of heart rate in the audiological evaluation of non-verbal children; II. Clinical trials on an infant population. *Neuropaediatric* 2:197–205, 1970.

Schulman-Galambos C, Galambos R: Brain stem evoked response audiometry in newborn hearing screening. *Arch Otolaryngol* 105:86–90, 1979.

Schwartz DM, Larson V: Hearing aid selection and evaluation procedures in children. In Bess F: *Childhood Deafness: Causation, Assessment and Management.* New York: Grune & Stratton, 1977, pp 217–233.

Schwartz DM, Schwartz RH: A comparison of tympanometry and acoustic reflex measurements for detecting middle ear effusion in infants below seven months of age. In Harford ER, Bess FH, Bluestone CD, et al: *Impedance Screening for Middle Ear Disease in Children.* New York: Grune & Stratton, 1978a, pp 91–96.

Schwartz DM, Schwartz RH: Acoustic and otoscopic findings in young children with Down's syndrome. *Arch Otolaryngol* 104:652, 1978b.

Schwartz DM, Schwartz RH: Typanometric findings in young infants with middle ear effusion: Some further observations. *Int J Pediatr Otolaryngol* 2:67–72, 1980.

Schwartz RH, Stool SE, Rodriquez W, et al: Acute otitis media: Toward a more precise definition. *Clin Pediatr* 20:549–554, 1981a.

Schwartz RH, Rodriquez W, Khan W: Persistent purulent otitis media. *Clin Pediatr* 20:445–447, 1981b.

Schweinhart LJ, Weikart DP: Young children grow up: the effects of the Perry Preschool program on youths through age 15. *Monographs of the High/Scope Educational Research Foundation, N. Seven.* Ypsilanti, Mich. The High/Scope Press, 1980.

Scouten EL: The place of the Rochester method in American education of the deaf. Report of the Proceedings of the International Congress on the Education of the Deaf, 1964, pp 429–433.

Senturia BH: Classification of middle ear effusions: definitions and terminology. *Ann Otol Rhinol Laryngol* 85(Suppl 25):15–17, 1976.

Senturia BH, Bluestone CD, Klein JO, et al: Report of the Ad Hoc Committee on Definition and Classification of Otitis Media and Otitis Media with Effusion. *Ann Otol Rhinol Laryngol* 89(Suppl 68):3–4, 1980.

Shah CP, Chandler D, Dale R: Delay in referral of children with impaired hearing. *Volta Rev* 80:207, 1978.

Shankweiler D, Studdert-Kennedy M: Hemispheric specialization for speech perception. *J Acoust Soc Am* 48:579–594, 1970.

Shanon E, Himelfarb M, Gold S: Auditory function in Friedreich's ataxia. *Arch Otolaryngol* 107:254–256, 1981.

Shapiro I, et al: Ossicular discontinuity with intact acoustic reflex. *Arch Otolaryngol* 107:576–578, 1981.

Shimizu H: Editorial: clinical use of auditory brain stem response; issues and answers. *Ear Hear* 2:3–4, 1981.

Shinefield HR: Cytomegalovirus in Utero. In Bergsma D: *Birth Defects: Atlas and Compendium.* Baltimore: Williams & Wilkins, 1973, p 324.

Shulman K: Hydrocephaly. In Bergsma D: *Birth Defects: Atlas and Compendium.* Baltimore: Williams & Wilkins, 1973.

Shurin PA, Pelton SI, Klein JO: Otitis media in the newborn infant. *Ann Otol Rhinol Laryngol* 85(suppl 25):216–222, 1976.

Shurin PA, Pelton SI, Donner A, et al: Persistence of middle ear effusion after acute otitis media in children. *N Engl J Med* 300:1121–1123, 1979.

Siegel J, McCracken G: Aminoglycoside ototoxicity in children. In Lerner SA, Matz GJ, Hawkins JE (eds): *Aminoglycoside Ototoxicity.* Boston: Little, Brown, 1981, ch 24.

Siegel-Sadewitz V, Shprintzen R: The relationship of communication disorders to syndrome identification. *J Speech Hear Disord* 47:338–354, 1982.

Siegenthaler B, Haspiel G: Development of two standardized measures of hearing for speech by children. Cooperative Research Program, Project 2372, United States Office of Education, 1966.

Siervogel RM, Roche AF, Johnson DL, et al: Longitudinal study of hearing in children; II. Cross-sectional studies of noise exposure as measured by dosimetry. *J Acoust Soc Am* 71:372–377, 1982.

Silverman SR, Lane HS: Deaf children. In Davis H, Silverman SR: *Hearing and Deafness,* ed 3. New York: Holt, Rhinehart, & Winston, 1970.

Simmons FB: Automated hearing screening test for newborns: the Crib-o-gram. In Mencher G: *Early Identification of Hearing Loss.* Basel: Karger, 1976, pp 171–180.

Simmons FB: ECOG diagnosis: round table discussion. In Naunton RF, Fernandez C: *Evoked Electrical Activity in the Auditory Nervous System.* New York: Academic Press, 1978, pp 285–297.

Simmons FB: Patterns of deafness in newborns. *Laryngoscope* 90:448, 1980a.

Simmons FB: Diagnosis and rehabilitation of deaf newborns, Part II. *Asha* 22:475, 1980b.

Simmons FB: Comment on hearing loss in graduates of a tertiary intensive care nursery. *Ear Hear* 3:188, 1982.

Simmons FB, Glattke TJ: Electrocochleography. In Bradford L: *Physiological Measures of the Audio-Vestibular System,* New York: Academic Press, 1975, ch 5.

Simmons FB, Russ FN: Automated newborn hearing screening, the Crib-o-gram. *Arch Otolaryngol* 100:1–7, 1974.

Simmons FB, McFarland WH, Jones FR: An automated hearing screening technique for newborns. *Acta Otolaryngol* 87:1, 1979.

Sinclair J, Freeman B: The status of classroom amplification in American education. In Bess F, Freeman B, Sinclair J: *Amplification in Education.* Washington, D.C.: A. G. Bell, 1981.

Singh S, Bresman MJ: Menkes' "kinky hair syndrome" (trichopolio dystrophy). *Am J Dis Child* 125:572–578, 1973.

Singh SP, Rock EH, Shulman A: Klippel-Feil syndrome with unexplained conductive hearing loss. *Laryngoscope* 79:113–117, 1969.

Siqueland E, Hoenigmann N: Infant responsivity to pure tone stimulation. *J Aud Res* 13:321–327, 1973.

Siqueland ER, DeLucia CA: Visual reinforcement of nonnutritive sucking in human infants. *Science* 165:1144–1146, 1969.

Sitnick V, Rushmer N, Arpan R: *Parent-Infant Communication: A Program of Clinical and Home Training for Parents and Hearing-Impaired Infants.* Portland, Ore.: Good Samaritan Hospital and Medical Center, 1978.

Skinner MW. The hearing of speech during language acquisition. *Otolaryngol Clinics North Am* 11:631–650, 1978.

Skinner P, Glattke TJ: Electrophysiologic response audiometry: state-of-the-art. *J Speech Hear Disord* 42:170–198, 1977.

Sly RM, Sambie MF, Fernandes DA, et al: Tympanometry in kindergarten children. *Ann Allergy* 44:1–7, 1980.

Smith D, Wilson A: *The Child with Down's Syndrome (Mongolism): Causes, Characteristics and Acceptance.* Philadelphia: W. B. Saunders, 1973.

Smith DW: The number 18 trisomy syndrome. *J Pediatr* 60:513, 1962.

Smith K, Hodgson W: The effects of systematic reinforcement on the speech discrimination responses of normal and hearing-impaired children. *J Aud Res* 10:110–117, 1970.

Snell RS: *Clinical Embryology for Medical Students,* ed 2. Boston: Little, Brown, 1975.

Snow T, McCandless G: The use of impedance measures in hearing aid selection. *Natl Hear Aid J* 29:7–33, 1976.

Sohmer H, Feinmesser M: Cochlear action potentials recorded from the external ear in man. *Ann Otolaryngol* 76:427–435, 1967.

Sohmer H, Feinmesser M: Routine use of electrocochleography (cochlear audiometry) on human subjects. *Audiology* 12:167–173, 1973.

Sparkes RS, Graham CB: Camurati-Englemann disease. Genetics and clinical manifestations with a review of the literature. *J Med Genet* 9:73–85, 1972.

Sperry R: Some effects of disconnecting the cerebral hemispheres. *Science* 217:1223–1226, 1982.

Spitz RA: *A Genetic Field Theory of Ego Formation: Its Implications for Pathology.* New York: International Universities Press, 1959.

Spitz RA (In collaboration with WG Cobliner): *The First Year of Life: A Psychoanalytic Study of Normal and Deviant Development of Object Relations.* New York: International Universities Press, 1965.

Spoendlin H: The innervation of the organ of Corti. *J Laryngol Otol* 81:717–738, 1967.

Spoendlin H: Innervation patterns in the organ of Corti of the cat. *Acta Otolaryngol (Stockh)* 67:239–254, 1969.

Spoendlin H: Congenital stapes ankylosis and fusion of carpal and tarsal bones as a dominant hereditary syndrome. *Acta Otol-Rhinol-Laryngol* 206:173–179, 1974.

Spoor A, Eggermont JJ: Electrocochleography as a method of objective audiogram determination. In Hirsh SK, Eldredge DH, Hirsh IJ, et al (eds): *Hearing and Davis.* St. Louis: Washington University Press, 1976, pp 411–418.

Spradlin JE, Locke WJ, Fulton RT: Conditioning and Audiological assessment. In Fulton RT, Lloyd LL: *Audiometry for the Retarded: With Implications for the Difficult-to-Test.* Baltimore: Williams & Wilkins, 1969.

Spreng M, Keidal WG: Separierung von Cerebroaudiogramm (CAG), Neuroaudiogramm (NAG), und Otoaudiogramm (OAG) in der Objecktiven Audiometrie. *Arch Klin Exp Ohren Nasen Kehlkopfheilk* 189:225, 1967.

Spring DR, Dale PA: Discrimination of linguistic stress in early infancy. *J Speech Hear Res* 20:224–232, 1977.

Sproles ET, Azerrad J, Williamson C, et al: Meningitis due to *Haemophilus influenzae*: long-term sequela. *J Pediatr* 75:782–788, 1969.

Stagno S: Auditory and visual defects resulting from symptomatic and sub-clinical congenital CMV and toxoplasma infections. *Pediatrics* 59:669–678, 1977.

Standards and Recommendations for Hospital Care for Newborn Infants, ed 6. Evanston, Ill.: American Academy of Pediatrics, Committee of Fetus and Newborn, 1977.

Stanley RJ, Puritz EM, Birggaman RA, et al: Sensory radicular neuropathy. *Arch Dermatol* 111:760–762, 1975.

Stark EW, Borton TE: Klippel-Feil syndrome and associated hearing loss. *Arch Otolaryngol* 97:415–419, 1973.

Stark RE, Tallal P: Selection of children with specific language deficits. *J Speech Hear Disord* 46:114–122, 1981.

Stark J, Wallach GP: The path to a concept of language learning disabilities. In *Topics in Language Disorders.* Rockville, Md.: Aspen Publications, 1980, pp 1–14.

Starr A, Achor LJ: Auditory brain stem responses in neurological disease. *Arch Neurol* 32:761, 1975.

Starr A, Hamilton A: Correlation between confirmed sites of neurological lesions and abnormalities of far field auditory brainstem responses. *Electroencephalogr Clin Neurophysiol* 41:595, 1976.

Starr A, Amlie RN, Martin WH, et al: Development of auditory function in newborn infants revealed by auditory brainstem potentials. *Pediatrics* 60:831–839, 1977.

Stebbins WC: The evolution of hearing in mammals. In Fay RR, Popper RN (ed): *Comparative Studies of Hearing in Vertebrates.* New York: Springer-Verlag, 1980, ch 15.

Stechler G: Newborn attention as affected by medication during labor. *Science* 144:315–317, 1964.

Stein L, Ozdamar O, Schnabel M: Auditory brainstem

responses (ABR) with suspected deaf-blind children. *Ear Hear* 1(2):30–40, 1981.

Stein L, Ozdamar O, Kraus N, et al: Follow-up of infants screened by auditory brainstem response (ABR) in the NICU. *J Pediatr* 103:447–453,1983.

Stein LK, Jabaley T: Early identification and parent counseling. In Stein L, Mendel E, Jabaley T: *Deafness and Mental Health*. New York: Grune & Stratton, 1981.

Steinschneider A, Lipton EI, Richmond JB: Auditory sensitivity in the infant: effect of intensity on cardiac and motor responsivity. *Child Dev* 37:233–252, 1966.

Stevens PR, Macfayden WAL: Familial incidence of juvenile diabetes mellitus progressive optic atrophy, and neurogenic deafness. *Br J Ophthalmol* 56:496–500, 1972.

Stevens S, House A (1972): Cited by Eimas P: Speech perceptions in early infancy. In *From Sensation to Cognition*. New York: Academic Press, 1975, vol 2.

Stevens SS: To honor Fechner and repeal his law. *Science* 133:80–86, 1961.

Stevens SS, Warshofsky F: *Sound and Hearing*. Life Science Library. New York: Time-Life Books, 1965.

Stevenson AC, Cheeseman EA: Hereditary deaf mutism, with special reference to Northern Ireland. *Ann Hum Genet* 20:177–207, 1956.

Stewart JL, Pollack D, Downs MP: A unisensory program for the limited hearing child. *Asha* 6:151–154, 1964.

Stewart JM: Genetic counseling. In Clausen J, Flook M, Ford M, et al: *Maternity Nursing Today*. New York: McGraw-Hill, 1973.

Stewart JM, Bergstrom L: Familial hand abnormality and sensori-neural deafness, a new syndrome. *J Pediatr* 78:102–110, 1971.

Stewart TC: *Counseling Parents of Exceptional Children*. Columbus, Ohio: C. E. Merrill, 1978.

Stockard JE, Westmoreland BF: Technical considerations in the recording and interpretation of the brainstem auditory evoked potential for neonatal neurologic diagnosis. *Am J EEG Technol* 21:31–54, 1981.

Stockard JE, Stockard JJ, Westmoreland B, et al: Brainstem auditory evoked responses: normal variation as a function of stimulus and subject characteristics. *Arch Neurol* 36:823–831, 1979.

Stockard JJ, Rossiter VS: Clinical and pathologic correlates of brain stem auditory response abnormalities. *Neurology* 27:316, 1977.

Stokoe WC: *Sign Language Structure: An Outline of the Visual Communication System of the American Deaf.* Buffalo, N.Y.: University of Buffalo Press, 1960.

Stokoe WC, Casterline DC, Croneberg CG: *A Dictionary of American Sign Language on Linguistic Principles.* Washington, D.C.: Gallaudet College Press, 1965.

Stool S, Anticaglia J: Electric otoscopy—a basic pediatric skill. *Clin Pediatr* 12:420, 1973.

Stool S, Randall P: Unexpected ear disease in infants with cleft palate. *Cleft Palate J* 4:99–103, 1967.

Stool SE: Diagnosis and treatment of ear disease in cleft palate children. In Bzoch K: *Communicative Disorders Related to Cleft Lip and Palate*. Boston: Little, Brown, 1971, pp 264–273.

Stool SE, Marshak G, Stanievich J, et al: Otitis Media: Current Concepts, Incidence, Pathogenesis, Diagnosis and Management. Pamphlet Companion to an Exhibit, Dept. Otolaryngology, Children's Hosp., Pittsburgh, 1982.

Storer T, et al: *General Zoology*, ed 6. New York: McGraw-Hill, 1979.

Stratton HJM: Gonadal dysgenesis and the ears. *J Laryngol Otol* 79:343–346, 1965.

Strauss M, Davis GL: Viral disease of the labyrinth: Review of the literature and discussion of the role of cytomegalovirus in congenital deafness. *Ann Otol Rhinol Laryngol* 82:577–583, 1973.

Stream RW, Stream KS: Counseling the parents of the hearing impaired child. In Martin F: *Pediatric Audiology*. Englewood Cliffs, N.J.: Prentice-Hall, ch 9, 1978.

Strominger AS, Bashir AS: A nine-year follow-up of 50 language delayed children. Paper presented at the 1977 annual convention of the American Speech and Hearing Association, Chicago.

Stubblefield HH, Young CE: Central auditory dysfunction in learning disabled children. *J Learn Disabil* 8:89–94, 1975.

Stuckless ER (ed): Deafness and rubella: infants in the 60's, adults in the 80's. *Am Ann Deaf* 125:959, 1980.

Stuckless ER, Birch JW: The influence of early manual communication on the linguistic development of deaf children. *Am Ann Deaf* 3:452–460, 499–504, 1966.

Studdert-Kennedy M, Shankweiler D: Hemispheric specialization for speech perception. *J Acoust Soc* 48:579–594, 1970.

Studebaker G, Bess F (eds): *The Vanderbilt Hearing Aid Report: State of the Art—Research Needs.* Monogr Contemp Audiol 1982.

Studebaker GA, Hochberg I (eds): *Acoustical Factors Affecting Hearing Aid Performance*. Baltimore: University Park Press, 1980.

Sugar HS: The oculoauriculo vertebral dysplasia syndrome of Goldenhar. *Am J Ophthalmol* 62:678, 1966.

Survey of Hearing Impaired Children and Youth: Gallaudet College Office of Demographic Studies. Washington, D.C., series D, 9: 1971.

Suter AH: The ability of mildly hearing-impaired individuals to discriminate speech in noise. EPA 550/9-78-100, AMRL-TR-78-4, 1978.

Suzuki T, Ogiba Y: Conditioned orientation audiometry. *Arch Otolaryngol* 74:192–198, 1961.

Sylvester PE: Some unusual findings in a family with Friedreich's ataxia. *Arch Dis Child* 33:217–221, 1958.

Sylvester PE: Spino-cerebellar degeneration, hormonal disorder, hypogonadism, deaf-mutism, and mental deficiency. *J Ment Defic Res* 16:203–214, 1972.

Tallal P: Rapid auditory processing in normal and disordered language development. *J Speech Hear Res* 19:561–571, 1976.

Taylor AI: Autosomal trisomy syndromes: a detailed study of twenty-seven cases of Edward's syndrome and twenty-seven cases of Patan's syndrome. *J Med Genet* 5:227, 1968.

Taylor D, Mencher GT: Neonatal responses, the effect

of infant state and auditory stimuli. *Arch Otolaryngol* 95:120–124, 1972.

Teele DW, Klein JO, Rosner BA: Epidemiology of otitis media in children. *Ann Otol Rhinol Laryngol* 89 (Suppl 68):5–6, 1980.

Teele DW, Klein JO, Rosner B: Epidemiology of otitis media in children. Proceedings of 2nd International Symposium: Recurrent Advances in Otitis Media with Effusion. *Ann Otol Rhinol Laryngol* (Suppl 68) 89(3)(Part 2):5–6, 1980.

Templin M: Vocabulary problems of the deaf child. *Int Audiol* 5:349, 1966.

Terrace HS, Pettito LA, Sanders RJ, et al: Can an ape create a sentence? *Science* 206:891–902, 1979.

Tervoort B: Development of languages and the critical period. The young deaf child: Identification and management. *Acta Otolaryngol (Suppl) (Stockh)* 206:247–251, 1964.

Thelin JW, et al: Effect of middle ear dysfunction and disease on hearing and language in high risk infants. *Int J Pediatr Otorhinolaryngol* 1:125–136, 1979.

Thompson CI, Stafford MR, Cullen JK, et al: Interaural intensity differences in dichotic speech perception. Paper presented at the 83rd meeting of the Acoustical Society of America, Buffalo, 1972.

Thompson G, Folsom R: Hearing assessment of at-risk infants. *Clin Pediatr* 20:257–267, 1981.

Thompson G, Wilson W, Moore J: Application of visual reinforcement audiometry (VRA) to low-functioning children. *J Speech Hear Disord* 44:80–90, 1979.

Thompson M, Thompson G: Responses of infants and young children as a function of auditory stimuli and test month. *J Speech Hear Res* 15:699–707, 1972.

Thompson M, Thompson G: Mainstreaming: a closer look. *Am Ann Deaf* 126:395–401, 1981.

Thompson P, Northern J: Audiometric monitoring of patients treated with ototoxic drugs. In Lerner SA, Matz GJ, Hawkins JE (eds): *Aminoglycoside Ototoxicity*, Boston: Little, Brown, 1981, ch 15.

Thompson RC Jr, Gaull GE, Horwitz SJ, et al: Hereditary hyperphosphatasia. Studies of three siblings. *Am J Med* 47:209–219, 1969.

Thomsen J, Tos M: Spontaneous improvement of secretory otitis—a long-term study. *Acta Otolaryngol* 92:493–499, 1981.

Thomsen KA, Terkildsen K, Arnfred J: Middle ear pressure during anesthesia. *Arch Otolaryngol* 82:609, 1965.

Thorner M, Remein OR: Principles and procedures in the evaluation of screening for disease. *Public Health Monogr* 67, May 1967.

Tibbling L: The rotatory nystagmus response in children. *Acta Otolaryngol (Stockh)* 68:459–467, 1969.

Tietz W: A syndrome of deaf-mutism associated with albinism showing dominant autosomal inheritance. *Am J Hum Genet* 15:259–264, 1963.

Titche LL, Windrem EO, Searmel WL: Hearing aids and hearing deterioration. *Ann Otol Rhino Laryngol* 86:357, 1977.

Tos M: Spontaneous improvement of secretory otitis and impedance screening. *Arch Otolaryngol* 106:345–349, 1980a.

Tos M: Pathogenesis and pathology of chronic secretory otitis media. *Ann Otol Rhinol Laryngol* 89 (Suppl 68):91–97, 1980b.

Tos M: Treatment of cholesteatoma in children. *A J Otol* 4:189, 1983.

Townsend T, Olsen C: Performance of new hearing aids using the ANSI S3.22-1976 standard. *J Speech Hear Disord* 47:376, 1982.

Townsend T, Wavrek D: Clinical use of ANSI hearing aid measurements. *Asha* 25:25–30, 1983.

Trehub SE, Schneider BA, Endman M: Developmental changes in infants' sensitivity to octave-band noises. *J Exp Child Psychol* 29:282–293, 1980.

Trehub SE, Bull D, Schneider BA: Infants detection of speech in noise. *J Speech Hear Res* 24:202–206, 1981.

Trevarthen C: Early attempts at speech. In Levin R: *Child Alive*. Garden City, N.Y.: Anchor Press/Doubleday, 1975.

Turner G: A second family with renal, vaginal and middle ear anomalies. *J Pediatr* 76:641, 1970.

Turnure C: Response to voice of mother and stranger by babies in the first year. Presented at meeting of the Society for Research in Child Development, Santa Monica, March 1969.

Ueda K, Nishida Y, Oshima K, et al: Congenital rubella syndrome: correlation of gestational age at time of maternal rubella with type of defect. *J Pediatr* 94:763, 1979.

Ueda K, Hisanaga S, Nishida Y, et al: Low birth-weight and congenital rubella syndrome. *Clin Pediatr* 20:730–733, 1981.

Uzgiris IC: Socio-cultural factors in cognitive development. In Haywood HC: *Social-Cultural Aspects of Mental Retardation*. New York: Appleton-Century, 1970.

Uzgiris IC, Hunt JMcV: An instrument for assessing infant psychological development. Mimeographed paper, Psych. Developm. Laboratory, University of Illinois, 1966.

Valvassori GE, Naunton RF, Lindsay JR: Inner ear anomalies: clinical and histopathological considerations. *Ann Oto-Laryngol* 78:929–936, 1969.

Van Wagoner RS, Chun TH: Hearing loss in Southeast Alaska. *Alaska Med* 16:61–63, 1974.

Vaughan V, McKay RJ, Behrman R: *Nelson Textbook of Pediatrics*, ed. 11. Philadelphia: W. B. Saunders, 1979.

Ventry IM, Chaiklin JB, Boyle WF: Collapse of the ear canal during audiometry. *Arch Otolaryngol* 73:727–731, 1961.

Ventry R, et al: Implication of virus in idiopathic sudden hearing loss: primary infection of reactivation of latent viruses. *Otolaryngol Head Neck Surg* 89:137–11, 1981.

Vernon M: Tuberculous meningitis and deafness. *J Speech Hear Disord* 32:177–181, 1967a.

Vernon M: Meningitis and Deafness: The problem, its physical, audiological, and educational manifestations in deaf children. *Laryngoscope* 77:1856–1874, 1967b.

Vernon M: Multiply Handicapped Deaf Children. Research Monograph, Council for Exceptional Children. 1–112, 1969.

Vernon M, Hicks D: Relationship of rubella, Herpes simplex, cytomegalovirus and certain other viral disabilities. *Am Ann Deaf* 125:529–534, 1980.

Vernon M, Klein N: Hearing impairment in the 1980's. *Hearing Aid J* 35:17, 1982.

h SD: Effects of early manual commu-
achievement of deaf children. *Am Ann*
527–536, 1970.

, Prickett H: Mainstreaming: Issues and a
plan. *Audiol Hear Educ* 2:5–11, 1976.

DA, Hatfield HH, Kalkhoff RK: Multiple len-
nes syndrome. *Am J Med* 60:447–456, 1976.

amy DG, Normandale PA: Craniofacial dysosto-
is in a Dorset family. *Arch Dis Child* 41:375, 1966.

uorenkoski V, Wasz-Hockert O, Lind J, et al: Training the auditory perception of some specific types
of abnormal pain cry in newborn and young infants.
Quart. Prog. Stat. Report; Speech Trans. Lab.,
Royal Inst. Tech., Stockholm, No. 4, 1971, pp 37–
48.

Vuori M, Lahikainen EA, Peltonen T: Perceptive
deafness in connection with mumps. *Acta Otolaryngol* 55:231–236, 1962.

Wachs TD, Uzgiris IC, Hung JMcV: Cognitive development in infants of different age levels and from
different enviromental backgrounds: an exploratory
investigation. *Merrill-Palmer Q* 17:283–317, 1971.

Wahl RA, Dick M: Congenital deafness with cardiac
arrhythmia: The Jervell and Lange-Nielsen Syndrome. *Am Ann Deaf* 125:34, 1980.

Waldon EF: Audio-reflexometry in testing hearing of
very young children. *Audiology* 12:14–20, 1973.

Walker WG: Renal tubular acidosis and deafness.
Birth Defects 7(4):126, 1971.

Wallach GP, Less AD: Language screening in schools.
Semin Speech Lang Hear 2(2):53–68, 1981.

Ward PH, Lindsay JR, Warner NE: Cytomegalic inclusion disease affecting the temporal bone. *Laryngoscope* 75:628–636, 1965.

Ward WD, Glorig A: A case of firecracker-induced
hearing loss. *Laryngoscope* 71:1590–1596, 1961.

Warren WS, Stool SE: Otitis media in low birth weight
infants. *J Pediatr* 79:740–743, 1971.

Watrous BS, McConnell F, Sitton AB, et al: Auditory
responses of infants. *J Speech Hear Disord* 40:357–
366, 1975.

Watson DO: *Talk with Your Hands.* Winneconne,
Wis., 1964.

Watson LA: Certain fundamental principles in prescribing and fitting hearing aids. *Laryngoscope*
54:531–558, 1944.

Weber B: Validation of observer judgments in behavioral observation audiometry. *J Speech Hear Disord*
34:350–355, 1969.

Weber B: Comparison of two approaches to behavioral
observation audiometry. *J Speech Hear Res* 13:823–
825, 1970.

Weber BA: Comparison of audiometry brainstem response latency norms for premature infants. *Ear
Hear* 3:257–262, 1982.

Weber HJ, Northern JL: Selection of children's hear-
ing aids: Colorado Department of Health Program.
In Libby ER: *Binaural Hearing and Amplification,*
Chicago: Zenetron, Inc., 1980, vol 2.

Weber HJ, McGovern FJ, Zink D: An evaluation of
1000 children with hearing loss. *J Speech Hear
Disord* 32:343–354, 1967.

Webster DB, Webster M: Neonatal sound deprivation
affects brainstem auditory nuclei. *Arch Otolaryngol*
103:392–396, 1977.

Webster DB, Webster M: Effects of neonatal conductive loss on brainstem auditory nuclei. *Ann Otol
Rhinol Laryngol* 88:684–688, 1979.

Webster DB, Webster M: Mouse brainstem auditory
nuclei development. *Ann Otol Rhinol Laryngol*
89(Suppl 68):254–256, 1980.

Wedenberg E: Auditory tests on newborn infants. In
Cunningham GC: *Conference on Newborn Hearing
Screening.* California State Dept. of Public Health,
1971, pp 126–130.

Weinstein RL, Kliman B, Scully RE: Familial syndrome of primary testicular insufficiency with normal virilization, blindness, deafness, and metabolic
abnormalities. *N Engl J Med* 281:969–977, 1969.

Weir RH: Some questions on the child's learning of
phonology. In Smith F, Miller G: *The Genesis of
Language.* Cambridge, Mass.: MIT Press, 1966, pp
153–169.

Weiss KL, Goodwin MW, Moores DF: Characteristics
of young deaf children and early intervention programs. Research Report 91, Dept. of H.E.W. Bureau
of Ed. for the Handicapped, 1975.

Weiss R, Hansen K, Heubelein T: Pragmatic Psycholinguistic Therapy for Language Disorders in
Early Childhood. Short course, American Speech-
Language-Hearing Association meeting, Atlanta,
1979.

Weller TH: The cytomegaloviruses; ubiquitous agents
with protean clinical manifestations (part II). *N
Engl J Med* 285:267–274, 1971.

Wepman Test of Auditory Discrimination: Language
Research Associates, 1958.

Wever EG, Bray CW: Auditory nerve impulses. *Science* 71:215, 1930.

Wever EG, Lawrence M: *Physiological Acoustics.*
Princeton, N.J.: Princeton University Press, 1954.

Wever EG, Neff WD: A further study of the effects of
partial section of the auditory nerve. *J Comp Physiol
Psychol* 40: 217–226, 1947.

Whitely RJ: The natural history of H.S.V. infection
of mother and newborn. *Pediatrics* 66:489–494,
1980.

Wiig E, Semel E: *Language Disabilities in Children
and Adolescents.* Columbus, Ohio: Merrill, 1976.

Wiig E, Semel E: *Language Assessment and Intervention for the Learning Disabled.* Columbus, Ohio:
Merrill, 1980.

Willeford JA: Central auditory function in children
with learning disabilities. *Audiol Hear Educ* 2:12–
20, 1976.

Williams A, Williams M, Walker C, et al: The Robin
anomalad (Pierre Robin syndrome)—follow-up
study. *Arch Dis Child* 56:663–668, 1981.

Wilson MD, Evans MB, Dawson RL, et al: Disturbed
children in special schools. *Spec Educ Forward
Trends* 4:8–10, June 1977.

Wilson WR, Moore JM, Thompson G: Sound-Field
Auditory Thresholds of Infants Utilizing Visual Re-
inforcement Audiometry (VRA). Paper read at the
American Speech & Hearing Association Annual
Convention, Houston, 1976.

Wilson WR, Folson RC, Widen JE: Hearing Impairment in Down's Syndrome Children. Paper presented at the Elks 1982 International Symposium:
The Multiply Handicapped Hearing Impaired Child,
Edmont, 1982.

Windle-Taylor P, Emery PJ, Phelps PD: Ear deformities associated with the Klippel-Feil syndrome. *Ann Otol* 90:210–216, 1981.

Winter JSD, Kohn G, Mellman WJ, et al: A familial syndrome of renal, genital and middle ear anomalies. *J Pediatr* 72:88–93, 1968.

Wishik SM, Kramm EG, Koch EM: Audiometric testing of school children. *Public Health Rep* 73:265–278, 1958.

Withrow MS: The federal role in services to hearing-impaired people. In Roeser R, Downs MP: In *Auditory Disorders in School Children.* New York: Thieme-Stratton Inc., 1981.

Woolf CM, Dolowitz DA, Aldous HE: Congenital deafness associated with piebaldness. *Arch Otolaryngol* 82:244–250, 1965.

Worthington DW, Peters JF: Quantifiable hearing and no ABR: paradox or error? *Ear Hear* 1:281–285, 1980.

Yarrow LJ, Rubinstein JL, Pedersen FA, et al: Dimensions of early stimulation and their differential effects on infant development. *Merrill-Palmer Q* 18:205–218, 1971.

Yoneshige Y, Elliott LL: Pure-tone sensitivity and ear canal pressure at threshold in children and adults. *J Acoust Soc Am* 70:1272–1276, 1981.

Yoshie N: Auditory nerve action potential responses to clicks in man. *Laryngoscope* 78:198–215, 1968.

Yoshie N, Ohashi T: Clinical use of cochlear nerve action potential responses in man for differential diagnosis of hearing losses. *Acta Otolaryngol (Suppl) (Stockh)* 252:71–87, 1969.

Yoshie N, Ohashi T, Suzuki T: Nonsurgical recording of auditory nerve action potentials in man. *Laryngoscope* 77:76–85, 1967.

Yost WA, Nielsen DW: *Fundamentals of Hearing.* New York: Holt, Rinehart & Winston, 1977.

Young DF, Eldridge R, Gardner WJ: Bilateral acoustic neuroma in a large kindred. *JAMA* 214:347–353, 1970.

Yules RB: Hearing in cleft patients. *Arch Otolaryngol* 91:319–323, 1970.

Zack L, Kaufman J: How adequate is the concept of perceptual deficit for education. *J Learn Disabil* 5:351–356, 1972.

Zeaman D, Wegner H: Cardiac reflex to tones of threshold intensity. I. *Speech Hear Disord* 21:71–75, 1956.

Zeaman D, Deane G, Wegner N: Amplitude and latency characteristics of the conditioned heart response. *J Physiol* 38:235–250, 1954.

Zellweger H, Smith JK, Grutzner P: The Marshall syndrome; report of a new family. *J Pediatr* 84:868–871, 1974.

Zemlin WR: *Speech and Hearing Science* ed 2. Englewood Cliffs, N.J. Prentice-Hall, 1981.

Zigmund N: Intrasensory and intersensory processes in normal and dyslexic children, unpublished doctoral dissertation, Northwestern University, Evanston, Ill, 1966.

Zigmund N: Maturation of auditory processes in children with learning disabilities. In Tampol L: *Introduction to Learning Disabilities.* Springfield, Ill.: Charles C Thomas, 1973.

Zink GD: Hearing aids children wear: A longitudinal study of performance. *Volta Rev* 74:41–51, 1972.

Zink GD, Alpiner JG: Hearing aids: One aspect of a state public school hearing conservation program. *J Speech Hear Disord* 33:329–344, 1968.

Zinkus PW: Psychoeducational sequelae of chronic otitis media. *Semin Speech Lang Hear* 3:305, 1982.

Zinkus PW, Gottlieb ML, Schapiro M: Developmental and psychoeducational sequelae of chronic otitis media. *Am J Dis Child* 132:1100–1104, 1978.

Zonis RD: Chronic otitis media in the Southwestern American Indian. *Arch Otolaryngol* 88:40–45, 1968.

Zonis RD: Chronic otitis media in the Arizona Indian. *Ariz Med* 27:1–6, 1970.

Zurif EB, Sait PE: The laterality effect in lingual-auditory tracking. *J Acoust Soc* 49:1874–1880, 1970.

Zwislocki J: An acoustic method for clinical examination of the ear. *J Speech Hear Res* 6:303–314, 1963.

Index